DICTIONARY OF SYNONYMS
INDIAN MEDICINAL PLANTS
INCORPORATING AN APPRAISAL OF INDIAN SYSTEMS OF MEDICINE

DICTIONARY OF SYNONYMS
INDIAN MEDICINAL PLANTS
INCORPORATING AN APPRAISAL OF INDIAN SYSTEMS OF MEDICINE

C.P. KHARE
Founder President
Society for New Age Herbals
New Delhi

I.K. International Publishing House Pvt. Ltd.

NEW DELHI • BANGALORE

Editor:
C.P. Khare
khare.herbalsociety@gmail.com

Published by
I.K. International Publishing House Pvt. Ltd.
S-25, Green Park Extension
Uphaar Cinema Market
New Delhi–110 016 (India)
E-mail: info@ikinternational.com
Website: www.ikbooks.com

ISBN 978-93-81141-24-3

10 9 8 7 6 5 4 3 2 1

Published by Krishan Makhijani for I.K. International Publishing House Pvt. Ltd., S-25, Green Park Extension, Uphaar Cinema Market, New Delhi–110 016 and Printed by Rekha Printers Pvt. Ltd., Okhla Industrial Area, Phase II, New Delhi–110 020.

Dedicated to

Moodeen Sheriff
A native surgeon of Triplecane Dispensary
Madras (Chennai), 1869

who gave the first Catalogue of Indian Synonyms

See facsimile of the Preface of "A Catalogue of Indian Synonyms of the medicinal plants, products, inorganic substances, & c., proposed to be included in the Pharmacopoeia of India" also facsimile of one page of text, as appendix.

Foreword

Over the last few decades alternative medicines, which are essentially plant based, have experienced a remarkable and steady increase all over the world. This has generated a multifaceted interest in the medicinal plants. It is a time to revisit plants with an objective of developing multicomponent drug therapies with the full understanding of Systems Biology in order to develop safer and efficacious drugs.

Ayurveda is holistic and integrative in its approach to health and disease, while Allopathy is deductive and segmented. There are perhaps historical reasons for this. Ayurvedic concepts evolved at a time when the cellular and molecular structure of matter was not known and so were primarily speculative and philosophical. Now the two streams are converging, Allopathic medicine is developing holistic and integrative concepts, while Ayurveda needs to become more analytical and integrate the holistic view of the healthy body with the cellular and molecular understanding of human and animal system. Plants have substantially and significantly contributed to the drug armamentarium of the modern Allopathic system of medicine and towards traditional medicines. It becomes imperative, therefore to correctly identify the plant as a starting material.

The present dictionary of synonyms will serve as a valuable guide to modern scientists who would like to correlate scientific nomenclature with the indigenous one to understand and make the best use of ground realities of herbal drug development.

C.P. Khare covers ten chapters included in the first section of the book, *viz.*, Scientific enquiry into Indian medicine; An effort to modernise the Ayurvedic concepts; Unani medicine; Siddha medicine; Drug variants of Indian medicine; Standardisation of herbal drugs in India; Improving shelf life of herbal medicine through microcosm; Pruning process of Indian polyherbal formulations; Experimental studies in India; Adverse effects and interactions of Indian herbs. The second section covers useful tables, covering plants along with their botanical names, Indian names, English names and the systems in which these are used. The tables are sorted by botanical and Indian names.

This reference work, I am sure, would be useful to all scientists in the field of medicinal plants as well as phytomedicine, to physicians and clinicians who are interested in the alternative and adjunctive therapies and to those interested in using Ayurvedic herbs with more confidence in their practice.

Dr. Neeraj Tandon
Head, Medicinal Plant Unit
Indian Council of Medical Research
Ministry of Health & Family Welfare, Govt. of India

Why this Reference Work

All the medicinal plants incorporated in "Dictionary of Synonyms: Indian Medicinal Plants" have been studied for their medicinal properties and qualify for further research in modern labs. This work should not be confused with an exhaustive compilation on agro-forestry nor with a detailed document on botany. The purpose is to provide leads to Indian scholars who are well-versed in folk and indigenous nomenclature, but are not able to reach the latest scientific literature, which is being organised by Latin or English names. This work will also serve as a guide to modern scientists who would like to correlate scientific nomenclature with the indigenous one, to understand and make the best use of ground realities for herbal drug development.

In the text, Indian common and folk names have been spelled according to their actual pronunciation.

A coordinated reading of the following treatises will give an access to the active principles and medicinal uses of the plants incorporated in this reference work:

- Indian Medicinal Plants: An Illustrated Dictionary, C.P. Khare, 2007, Springer, New York, Heidelburg.
- The Wealth of India series, original and revised volumes, 1950-2010, Council of Scientific & Industrial Research (CSIR), New Delhi.
- The Treatise on Indian Medicinal Plants, Ashima Chatterjee and Satyesh Chandra Pakrashi, Vol I to VI, 2003, NISCAIR (CSIR), New Delhi.
- Dictionary of Indian Medicinal Plants, Akhtar Hussain et al., 1992, Central Institute of Medicinal and Aromatic Plants (CIMAP), Lucknow.

In the end, a few words of gratitude. I am thankful to Rajeev Prakash Khare, my software consultant, and Jojy Philip, my data coordinator for their untiring effort during my endeavour. My motivations include Dr. V.K. Agarwal, Mr. Sanjiv Goswami, Mr. Andrew Spencer, Mr. P.N. Venkataraman, Ms. Poonam Sharma and Ms. Sarita Joshi.

I hope, this reference work will provide a vital link to the two fag ends—the son-of-the-soil-healer and the bespectacled scientist of the lab. Somehow, I do not expect a bouquet on the section "An Insight into the Legacy, Lapses and Lifeline of Indian Systems of Medicine."

C.P. Khare
Founder President
Society for New Age Herbals, New Delhi
khare.herbalsociety@gmail.com

Contents

Part Two
THE NOMENCLATURE

Part Three
APPENDICES

INDEXES

DICTIONARY OF SYNONYMS
INDIAN MEDICINAL PLANTS

Part One

AN INSIGHT INTO THE LEGACY, LAPSES AND LIFELINE OF INDIAN SYSTEMS OF MEDICINE

1

Scientific Inquiry into Indian Systems of Medicine

Col. Sir Ram Nath Chopra (MRCS, England 1907; B. Ch, Cambridge, UK, 1908; MD, 1912; Sc D, Cantab; FRCS, London; Knighted) wrote in 1933:[1]

- Attempts at the revival of Ayurvedic and Unani systems in their present form (based on classical doctrines) are bound not to succeed.
- When it is remembered that the Ayurvedic system of medicine has been practically stationary for about 1,500 years and that no attempt has been made to advance the knowledge in conjunction with the progress of the world, one would find it very difficult to reconcile to the old theories of 2,000 years ago, however, one may stretch their significance, with the recent advances in the world of science. After imparting instruction to the Ayurvedic students in modern physiology, bacteriology, pathology, etc., to ask them to apply the doctrine of *Vayu*, *Pitta* and *Kapha* etc. (4 humours in case of Unani medicine—*Khoon*, *Balgham*, *Safra* and *Sauda* i.e., blood, phlegm, yellow bile and black bile), to explain the causation of disease, might not be convincing to them and might bring nothing but chaos and discord to their minds. The students trained under such a system might neither be good at one nor the other.
- History shows that many of our important pharmacopoeial drugs were known and were also used in some form or other possibly long before they were introduced into the Western medicine and before their actions were investigated on scientific lines. On the other hand, there are sure to be others of little therapeutic value that are given merely because they were mentioned in some old manuscripts, and no one has taken the trouble to confirm the truth of these statements. Attempts must be made to separate the good ones from the useless ones, and for this a systematic investigation of these drugs must be undertaken. Medicine is a progressive science; in every department an attempt is being made to replace empiricism by rationalism, and nowhere is this more evident than in the science of pharmacology and therapeutics.

- When it is said that a drug like *Sarca indica* is useful in menorrhagia or *Cephalandra indica* in diabetes or *Boerhavia diffusa* in dropsy, the (medical) profession will not accept these assertions, as these are symptoms and not diseases; what we (scientists) want to know is their particular value in these various conditions and how they help to restore the tissue to their normal condition.
- The scientific mind is not satisfied by mere statements, no matter from which source they originate, unless corroborated by clinical and experimental evidence.
- The active principles, responsible for their therapeutic action, have to be isolated and worked out. The active and useful drugs should be separated from those which are inactive and worthless.
- The standardisation of (herbal) drugs and preparations by chemical and biological methods of assay is an important factor to secure therapeutic uniformity, so that the amount of active principle in each dose is not subjected to irregular variations.

The first Prime Minister of India, Pt. Jawaharlal Nehru observed:[2]

"There can be no doubt that these ancient systems (Ayurveda and Unani) of India have an honourable history and that they had a great reputation. Most people know that even now they have some very effective remedies. It is necessary, however, that every approach to the problem should be made on the basis of scientific method and persons who are Ayurvedic, Unani physicians should have also a full knowledge of modern methods. This means that there should be basic training in scientific methods for all, including those who wish to practise Ayurveda or Unani systems."

A similar concern for strengthening of the research base was indicated in 1984 by PV Narasimha Rao, the then Minister of Health and Family Welfare (and later the Prime Minister of India):[2]

"The point of pride is only our being ancient. There is nothing which can be definitely said of any research that takes place in these Indian systems. To the best of my knowledge this is still the case. So it is very necessary to have a well-organised research base in each of our systems."

In 1989, Dr Nitya Anand, former Director, Central Drug Research Institute, Lucknow, wrote: "Knowledge is greatly advanced since these (traditional, Ayurvedic) systems were developed. It is necessary to examine them in the light of modern developments to rationalise their basic tenets."[3]

Dr BN Dhavan (the then) Director, Central Drug Research Institute, Lucknow, also advocated scientific evaluation of herbs and observed : "The disease pattern and health care needs of the country have changed significantly in recent years; the priorities were different when the texts of traditional systems of medicine were created."[3]

Setting aside all these observations, *The Ayurvedic Pharmacopoeia of India*, published in 1989, retained the traditional theme-line: "When we insist on a pharmacognostic study of each drug, we are really extending and expanding the Ayurvedic pharmacognosy."[4] (This has been repeated in all other volumes of the *Ayurvedic Pharmacopoeia of India.*)

Dr M Taiyab (the then) Dean, Faculty of Unani Medicine, Aligarh Muslim University, Aligarh, also supported the traditional viewpoint: "Let us accept the hard fact that the physicians of bygone era, whether on the basis of accidental revelation, logical deduction or experimentation, had determined and recorded medicinal properties of crude drugs and the same are found valid even during this scientific age. The only contribution we could make, is to provide scientific data."[3]

This superimposed concept of "Ayurvedic or Unani pharmacognosy" or classical (accidental or logical) deductions failed to attract contemporary scientists.

In 1994, VV Sivarajan and Indira Balachandran wrote:[5]

"Reflecting on the decline of Ayurveda after Brahmanic period (800 BC-1000 AD), one would find that there are three broad, all-pervading reasons for it:

- A complacent attitude among men of Ayurveda that everything is written in the ancient texts and there is little scope for further studies. The faith has, over the centuries, brought in a certain amount of lethargy among them and has taken away the spirit of questioning and experimentation.
- A self-righteous feeling that their practice reflects ancient wisdom.
- Reluctance on their part to seek and get collaboration from people working in other allied fields."

According to these authors, pharmacognosy is the most neglected area of medicinal plant research in Ayurveda. The state of affairs is extremely chaotic. A number of studies are available on prepared drugs, forgetting the fact that without standards in the herbal sources of raw drugs there cannot be any standard in prepared drugs. One has to go by materials and not by literature. The plant taxonomy can provide unambiguous, universally accepted identification of plants, yet there is a subtle but firm resistance from men of Ayurveda against this unsolicited offer of assistance. "*They are paranoid about ancient Ayurvedic texts and myopic in their approach to collaborate with other allied scientific disciplines.*"[6] (VV Sivarajan is a Professor of Botany at University of Calicut, Kerala; Indira Balachandran is a Research Officer at Herbal Garden, Arya Vaidya Sala, Kottakkal, Kerala.)

Thus, we find that the attitude of protagonists of the Indian systems of medicine did not change with time.

Col. RN Chopra initiated the process of modernisation of Indian medicine when he delivered a series of lectures on Medical Plants at Patna University, Patna, during 1920-30. He played a pivotal role when he was appointed Chairman of the Drugs Enquiry Committee appointed by the then British Government to consider the question of quality of medicinal drugs in the Indian market. The Committee's recommendation led to All India legislation for Drug Act, 1940 and Pharmacy Act, 1948.

In Unani medicine, the concept of research was originally perceived by Hakim Ajmal Khan in the 1920s. A declaration was signed by six eminent Unani physicians (Hakim Ajmal Khan, Hakim Fazul Rehman, Hakim Mohammad Ilyas Khan, Hakim Abdul Fazal Khan, Hakim Mohammad Kabiruddin and Hakim Dr Sayed Nasir Abbas) for "starting a basic and fundamental work in the Unani system of medicine for its modernisation."

Dr Salim-uz-Zaman Siddiqui, a chemist, was the first to undertake chemical studies on important medicinal plants used in the Unani system of medicine. His research on Asrol *(Rauvolfia serpentina)* was an important breakthrough in Indian medicine.

In 1969, the Government of India established a Central Council for Research in Indian Medicine and Homoeopathy (CCRIMH) to develop scientific research in different branches of Indian systems of medicine. The research activities continued under the aegis of the CCRIMH until 1978, when it was split up into four separate research councils, one each for Ayurveda and Siddha (CCRAS), Unani (CCRUM), Yoga and Naturopathy, and Homoeopathy.

All the four research councils ventured into a number of field studies and research programmes "*to further develop Indian systems in consonance with basic philosophies of the respective systems*."[7]

This "perception"/approach to "basic philosophies" resulted in a number of anomalies:

- Herbal research, in many cases, was aimed at reconfirming the validity of classical polyherbal formulations.
- An "empirical bias" reflected in many "field" trials. Over-reliance on non-clinical data and exaggerated folk claims overshadowed the scientific application of herbs.
- Anecdotal information, rather than scientific evidence, predominated. It is asserted that Indian herbs are to be screened for their toxicity, not for therapeutic activities. WHO's relaxations provided a shield to the Indian medicine.
- In academic field, an effort was made to recast more than 2000-year-old tenets of Indian medicine in the mould of modern scientific terminology.
- In spite of the best efforts of promoters of scientific herbalism, the Golden Triangle Partnership (GTP) between Council of Scientific and Industrial Research (CSIR), Indian Council of Medical Research (ICMR) and Department of Ayurveda, Yoga, Unani, Siddha and Homoeopathy (AYUSH) is still a moot point. Ministry of Health and Family Welfare, Government of India, (in a pessimistic note) admitted in its Annual Report 2004-2005: "AYUSH practitioners usually remain unaware of scientific developments and recent trends and advances in clinical practice. As a result, clinical competence of practitioners declines over the years, which may affect their clinical skill. (And herbal research.)
- Practitioners of modern medicine do not give credence to classical polyherbal formulations and bizzare concoctions; with the result, herbal research endeavours have practically been isolated from the mainstream.

Dr Sajid Husain, Chairman, Unani Pharmacopoeia Committee, gave the following suggestions in 2005:[8]

- Those who are practicing Indian Systems of Medicine should also have complete knowledge of modern trends.
- Syllabus of all Indian systems of medicine may be revised, wherein the existing relevant segments may be retained, while obsolete contents may be deleted; modern science, which is deemed vital, be introduced.
- If the old practice of diagnosis is found obsolete, the same should be dispensed and replaced with new methods.
- Attempts should be made to demonstrate the mechanism of action of ISM preparations; at least toxicity data should be provided.

Prof. (Hakim) Syed Khaleefathullah, Vice President, Central Council for Research in Unani Medicine (CCRUM), New Delhi, has put the record straight for those who are still not prepared to reconcile to the changed circumstances:[8]

- The traditional medicine in some developing countries has tended to stagnate, not exploiting the rapid discoveries of science and technology for its own development. It has kept a low pace of change in comparison with medicine as practised in industrialised countries, which keep abreast of scientific and technological innovations to the extent that it is often exclusively referred to as a modern (herbal) medicine.
- Many health professionals had tended to regard traditional medicine as a practice on a decline and of no importance. This is a serious fallacy.
- The day has come when a collective approach has to be evolved in view of the progress of the medicine under the impetus of scientific methods. Facts have led to newer facts, observations and experiments to more experimentation. Now the pace is so fast and furious that it is impossible for a single person to be abreast of the advances and innovations in various sub-branches.
- The new education policy of Indian Systems of Medicine (ISM) has made it necessary that all aspects have to be reviewed by the application of modern tools to prove its efficacy and usefulness.
- The National Policy on Indian Systems of Medicine and Homoeopathy (ISM & H) 2002 advocated the need to spend both time and energy in undertaking high quality research and clinical trials in a collaborative manner, to develop evidence-based support to ISM & H drugs and to generate data on safety factors.

At last, the importance of research on modern parameters is being formalised.

REFERENCES

1. Chopra, RN (Col.) et al., *Indigenous Drugs of India*, second edn, Academic Publishers, Kolkata.
2. Cited in *An Overview of Ayurveda, Yoga, Naturopathy, Unani, Siddha and Homoeopathy in India*, AYUSH, 2004.
3. *Research and Development of Indigenous Drugs*, 1989, Institute of History of Medicine and Medical Research, Hamdard Nagar, New Delhi-110 062.
4. *The Ayurvedic Pharmacopoeia of India*, Part I, Vol I, Preface by Prof. AN Namjoshi, Chairman, Ayurvedic Pharmacopoeia Committee, 1986.
5. Sivarajan, VV and Indira Balachandran, (1994). *Ayurvedic Drugs and their Plant Sources* (ADPS), Oxford and IBH Publishing Co. Pvt Ltd., New Delhi.
6. Sivarajan, VV, (1988). cited in ADPS.
7. *CCRUM Research Endeavours*, Ministry of Health and Family Welfare, New Delhi, 2002.
8. *Unani Medicine—Then, Now and Hereafter*, International Conference on Unani Medicine, 8-11 February 2005, New Delhi.

2

An Effort to Modernise the Ayurvedic Classical Concepts

The Ayurvedic Pharmacopoeia of India assesses the "properties and actions" of a herb on the basis of *Rasa* (taste), *Guna* (physical property), *Veerya* (potency), *Vipaaka* (again, taste indicating herb's action after ingestion) and *Karma* (therapeutic effect of the herb).

Sweet *(Madhura)*, sour *(Amla)*, salty *(Lavana)*, pungent *(Katu)*, bitter *(Tikta)* and astringent *(Kasaaya)* are 6 tastes *(Rasas)*.

Physical properties *(Guna)* of herbs have been divided into 20 categories: light, heavy, cold, hot, unctuous, dry, dull, immobile, mobile, soft, hard, clear, slim, smooth, rough, minute, bulk, solid and fluid.

Potency of herbs *(Veerya)* has been divided into cold and hot segments.

The herb is selected for medicinal use after assessing the imbalance or disharmony due to *Doshas* (morbidities)—*Vaata (Vaayu), Pitta* and *Kapha*, known as *Tridoshas* when grouped together. The entire infrastructure of Ayurvedic medicine revolves around the theory of *Tridosha*.

Once the *Dosha* (morbidity) has been identified, the first component of the herb, *Rasa* (taste), is selected. *Rasa* is considered an important marker, which indicates, initially, the right choice of the herb.

Sweet taste pacifies *Vaata* and *Pitta,* but aggravates *Kapha*.

Sour taste pacifies *Vaata*, but aggravates *Pitta* and *Kapha.*

Salty taste pacifies *Vaata,* but aggravates *Pitta* and *Kapha.*

Pungent taste pacifies *Kapha,* but aggravates *Vaata* and *Pitta.*

Bitter taste pacifies *Pitta* and *Kapha*, but aggravates *Vaata.*

Astringent taste pacifies *Pitta* and *Kapha,* but aggravates *Vaata.*[1]

In *The Ayurvedic Pharmacopoeia of India*, *Dosha* is the first component of *Karma* in the monograph, followed by important therapeutic applications. Herbs, which correct all the three *Doshas*, have also been identified and documented. Following explanation was given in 1989: "Since the effort is to compile pharmacopoeial monographs of Ayurvedic drugs, the accent on classical attributes of respective drugs according to the doctrine of *Rasa*, *Guna*, *Veerya*, *Vipaaka* and *Karma* has not been lost sight of, though some of them appear to be abstract and subjective in the absence of an established experimental method to qualify them." (Vol. I to Vol.V, 2006.) In Vol.VI, 2008, this statement was revised: "Under each monograph, classical attributes of each drug according to the doctrine *Rasa*, *Guna*, *Veerya*, *Vipaaka* and *Karma* have been kept intact. These are considered a reasonable basis and convenient reference point for a clinical classification."

Internationally, *Vaata* is equated with breath, *Pitta* with fire and *Kapha* with mucus.[2] To counteract this type of mistranslation, recently, an effort has been made to "reinterpret" the theory of *Rasas* and *Tridosha* by scholars of Ayurvedic medicine.

Arvind Chopra and Vijai V Doiphode opined that, to a certain degree, modern analytical chemistry has been used to assign properties of each of the tastes *(Rasas)*. The sour, sweet, pungent and astringent tastes are determined by acids, starches and sugars, aromatics and tannins. Bitter taste is due to chemicals such as berberine. Salty taste, uncommon in plants, is found in minerals. All the three *Doshas (Vaata, Pitta and Kapha)* should be treated as primary dynamic physiologic forces.[3]

The Ayurvedic philosophy describes a unifying hypothesis linking the universe with all living and non-living matter. Human and plant in the hierarchy of cosmic evolution consist of the same basic matter—*Panchbhootas* (earth, water, air, fire and ether). *Vaata* (material = air + ether), the most powerful force, governs motion and controls cell division, arrangement and differentiation, impulse transmission (including cardiorespiratory and all the higher functions in the brain); movement of body fluids and excreta, parturition, and, above all, the mind; it is most relevant to the nervous and musculoskeletal system. *Pitta* (material = fire) governs the metabolism and formation of tissues and waste products; it is most relevant to the digestive and endrocrine system. *Kapha* (material = earth + water) increases cell mass, promotes bonding of tissues, prevents destruction of tissues, maintains strength and immunity, and determines body growth. The six tastes *(Rasas)* transmit the properties of *Panchbhootas;* each taste has a *Dosha* related attribute, and drugs in Ayurveda have been classified according to their effect on *Dosha*. *Doshic Prakriti* (functional constitution) of the patient is diagnosed and treated by an Ayurvedic physician.

Each *Dosha* has its own characteristic, physiologic and psychologic expressions. *Vaata* is dry, cold, light and clear. *Pitta* is hot, light, fluid and clear. *Kapha* is cold, wet, heavy, cloudy and static. Although *Vaata*, *Pitta* and *Kapha* often colonise in the intestines, stomach and chest, they are ubiquitous.[3]

Bhagwan Dash, Mahadihassan, Udupa, Asima Chatterjee and Satyesh Chandra Pakrashi also tried to validate *Tridosha* hypothesis.

According to Bhagwan Dash, *Vaayu* is responsible for all movements and sensations, including motor actions inside the body. *Pitta* is responsible for all physio-chemical activities of the body in the form of metabolism, production of heat and energy, and *Kapha* is the substance which maintains compactness or cohesiveness in the body by providing the fluid matrix to it.[4]

According to Mahadihassan S and Udupa KN, the three morbidities can be easily estimated by biochemical studies. These authors have equated *Vaata* with acetylcholine liberated by cerebral cortex and peripheral and parasympathetic nerve endings, *Pitta* with catecholamines liberated by the hypothalamus, sympathetic nerve endings and adrenal medulla and *Kapha* with histamine secreted by the brain stem. The drugs, when administered, act by promoting or destroying the respective neurohumours or their precursors.[5]

According to Asima Chatterjee and Satyesh Chandra Pakrashi, the entire biological living organism is governed by *Tridosha. Vaayu (Vaata)* indicates all the biological phenomena which are controlled by the functions of the central autonomic system. The malfunction of *Vaayu,* either by itself or coupled with other functional disorders due to *Pitta* and *Kapha*, is the major factor in developing diseases. *Pitta* is the manifestation of energy in the living organism. It helps digestion, assimilation, tissue building, heat production, blood pigmentation, activities of the endrocrine glands, and so on. Many of these processes are thermogenic and metabolic. *Kapha* implies the functions of thermotaxis or heat regulation and also the formation of various preservative fluids, mucus, synovia, etc. The main function of *Kapha* is to provide nutrition to the body tissues, and to bring about coordination of the body system and regulation of all biological processes.[1]

These "modified interpretations" indicate that a concerted effort is being made to reestablish the significance of the theory of *Tridosha* and *Rasa, Guna, Veerya* and *Vipaaka*.This is a futile exercise, as a drug is to be produced for millions of people whose *Doshic Prakati* (functional constitution) is impossible to identify.

In these circumstances, survival of the theory of *Tridosha* depends upon its acceptance by the younger generation of Ayurvedic physicians who are trained in modern physiology, bacteriology, pathology and radiology, but still prefer to treat patients through individually tailored treatment.

REFERENCES

1. Chatterjee, Asima and Satyesh Chandra Pakrashi, (1999). "Basic Concepts of Ayurveda", in *Treatise on Indian Medicinal Plants*, Vol 1.
2. Balch, Phyllis A, (2002). *Prescription for Herbal Healing*.
3. Chopra, Arvind and Vijay V Doiphode, (2002). "Ayurvedic Medicine, core concept, therapeutic principles and current relevance", *Medical Clinics of North America*, Vol 86, Number 1.
4. Dash, Bhagwan and Lilitesh Kashyap, (1980). *Materia Medica of Ayurveda*, Concept Publishing Company, New Delhi-110 015.
5. Mahadihassan, S, "A Comparative Study of Early System of Indian Cosmology and Tridosha Doctrine", 1980, *Ind. J. Hist Sci*; "A Scientific Interpretation of Tridosha Doctrine of humorology", 1986, *Anc Sci Life* 6(1); "The Tridosha Doctrine Traced to Breath as Soul", 1989, *Anc Sci Life* 9(1). Udupa KN, "Ayurveda for the Service of Common Man", 1983, *Anc Sci Life*, 2(3). Cited in *Ayurvedic Drugs and their Plant Sources*, Sivarajan and Balachandran.

3

Unani Medicine: Research within Fundamental Framework

The Unani system of medicine owes its origin to Greece. The theoretical basic work of Unani medicine is based on the teachings of Hippocrates, the Greek philosopher-physician (460-377 BC).

He was the first person to establish that disease was a natural process, that its symptoms were the reactions of the body to the disease, and that the chief function of the physician was to aid the natural forces of the body. His chief contribution to the medical realm is the humoral theory. After Hippocrates, Galen (131-210 AD) and Arab physicians Rhages (850-925 AD) and Avicenna (980-1037 AD) enriched the Unani system considerably. Contemporary systems of traditional medicine in Egypt, Syria, Iraq, Persia, India, China and Middle East and Far East countries left a deep impact on the Unani medicine.

In India, the Unani system of medicine was introduced by the Arabs. The Delhi Sultans, the Khiljis, the Tughlaqs and the Mughal emperors provided state patronage to the scholars of Unani medicine. The golden period of the Unani medicine in India was during the 13th and 17th century. Abu Bakr bin Usman Kashani, Saruddin Damashqui, Bahwa bin Khwas Khan, Ali Geelani, Akbar Arzani and Mohammad Hashim Alvi Khan were the leading scholars of that period. During the British rule, Unani medicine suffered a setback due to withdrawal of governmental patronage.

Hakim Ajmal Khan (1868-1927) revived the Unani system in India with an integrated approach to Unani medicine and Ayurveda. The initiative later on emerged as the indigenous systems of medicine of India.

The humoral theory of the Unani system of medicine presupposes the presence of four *Akhlaats* (humours)—*Khoon* (blood), *Balgham* (phlegm), *Safraa* (yellow bile) and *Saudaa* (black bile) — in the body. The temperaments of persons are expressed by the words sanguine, phlegmatic, choleric and melancholic according to the preponderance of humours in them—blood, phlegm, yellow bile and black bile, respectively.

The humours themselves are assigned temperaments—blood is hot and moist, phlegm cold and moist, yellow bile hot and dry, and black bile cold and dry. Every person is supposed to have a unique humoral constitution which represents his healthy state.

Humours refer to body fluids produced after digestion and metabolism of food. They serve the functions of nutrition, growth-repair and produce the energy necessary for the maintenance of all physiological activities of an individual.[1] The importance of black bile in Unani medicine is due to its influence on pychological disorders.[2]

To maintain the correct humoral balance, there is a power of self-preservation or adjustment called *Quwwat-e-Mudabbira* (*medicatrix naturae*) in the body. If this power weakens, imbalance in the humoral composition is bound to occur which causes diseases.

In Unani medicine, great reliance is placed on this power. The medicines are used for helping the body to regain this power to an optimum level, thereby restoring humoral balance.

Another distinctive feature of the Unani system of medicine is its emphasis on diagnosing a disease through pulse *(nabz)*, a rhythmic expansion of arteries which is felt by fingers.

Research on fundamental aspects of Unani medicine has been undertaken at Central Research Institute of Unani Medicine, Hyderabad, Andhra Pradesh, with a view to correlate the fundamental principles of Unani with (modern) medicine with the help of modern laboratory investigations.[3] Side by side, pharmacological studies on Unani drugs under clinical evaluation programme are also being conducted at different centres of the Central Council for Research in Unani Medicine (CCRUM). Twenty-five Unani medicines, prepared from commonly available plants, have been validated on scientific lines (humoral considerations were not employed).

Clinical trials on infective hepatitis, hyperlipidemia, rheumatoid arthritis, proriasis and vitiligo at different centres of CCRUM provided important leads to scientist for further research. The Council has passed on quite a few coded Unani drugs to Council of Scientific and Industrial Research (CSIR), New Delhi, for extensive laboratory studies.[4]

A number of Unani herbs are of non-Indian origin and are being studied in the West. (See Table 1). This is an added advantage to the Unani medicine.

But there is a word of caution from Central Council for Research in Unani medicine: "The purpose of clinical research in Unani system of medicine is not to prove afresh its basic principles, for the efficacy of the system is time-tested. But in modern conditions, usefulness of these principles should be demonstrated. The modern criteria and parameters of research methology cannot be applied in their entirety in clinical and trials to Unani medicine."[5]

Table 1: Important Unani Herbs of non-Indian Origin[6]

Botanical Name	Common Name	English Name	Habitat	Main Source
Achillea millefolium	Biranjasif	Yarrow, Milfoil	Eurasia, North America, temperate zones	Pakistan
Agaricus albus	Ghaariqoon	White Agaric	Fungus grown on old pine trees in South and Central Europe.	Europe
Alhagi pseudalhagi syn. *Alhagi camelorum*	Turanjbeen (Alhagi Manna)	Camel Thorn Persian Manna Plant	Mediterranean and Sahara to Central Asia and the Himalayas	Pakistan
Althaea officinalis	Khatmi	Marsh Mallow	Europe, from Denmark southwards	Iran
Anacyclus pyrethrum	Akarkaraa	Spanish Pellitory	Spain and other Mediterranean countries	Morocco
Aquilaria agallocha	Dhoop-lakkar, Agar	Aloe-wood Eagle-wood	Malayan Peninsula, Assam, Manipur, Silhat, Bhutan	Malacca
Aristolochia longa	Zaraavand Taweel	Birthwort	Southern Europe	Kabul
Aristolochia rotunda	Zaraavand Madahraj	Birthwort	*A. Clematis* (Europe) *A. Longa* (North America) *A. Indica* (India)	Iran
Artemisia absinthium	Afsanteen	Worm wood	Europe, South America, North Africa, Siberia, Mangolia	Nepal
Artemisia maritima	Dirmaanaa Turki Kirmaalaa	Santonica Worm seed	North America, Brazil, Iran, Baluchistan, Pakistan, Kashmir, Nepal, Tibet	Iran
Asarun europaeum	Asaaroon Asarabacca	Wild Nard Hazelwort	Temperate Europe, North Asia (Birthwort family)	China
Asparagus officinalis	Halyun	Sperage, Sparrow Grass	Europe, Greece, Western Asia, Southern parts of Russia, Poland	Iran

Table 1: Contd.

Botanical Name	Common Name	English Name	Habitat	Main Source
Asparagus racemosus	Satawari	Asparagus var.	Upper Gangetic plains, Dehradun, Bihar plateau, Tropical and subtropical parts of India including the Himalayas and Andamans. *A. adscendens*: Western Himalayas, Himachal Pradesh, Kumaon, Chamba.	Nepal
Astragalus sarcocola	Anzaroot (gum)	Sarcocola	Iran	Iran
Bambusa arundinacea	Banslochan (Manna) Tabaasheer	Thorny bamboo manna	South-East Asia	Indonesia
Berberis vulgaris	Zarishk	Barberry	Europe and the British Isles, naturalised in parts of North America.	Afghanistan
Blepharis edulis	Uttangan seeds		Sindh, Baluchistan	Pakistan
Borago officinalis	Gaozabaan	Borage	England, Europe, North Africa North America.	Iran, Baluchistan
Cardiospermum halicacabum	Habb-e-Qilqil	Balloon Vine	Tropical America extending to Africa and Asia	Iran
Carum carvi	Kaalaa Jeeraa	Caraway	Europe, North Africa, Asia	Iran
Centaurea behen	Behman Safed	White behen	Persia	Afghanistan
Colchicum autumnale	Suranjaan Talkh	Bitter colchicum Meadow saffron	Europe, part of British Isles, North Africa, Kashmir	Afghanistan
Cinnamomum zeylanicum	Daalchini	Cinnamon Ceylon Cinnamon	South-East Asia, China	China, Indonesia
Commiphora mukul	Guggulu (exudate)	Indian Bdellium tree	Arid rocky tracts of Rajasthan, Khandesh, Berar, Mysore, Sindh, Baluchistan	Pakistan

Table 1: Contd.

Botanical Name	Common Name	English Name	Habitat	Main Source
Commiphora myrrha	Bol, Hiraabol (exudate)	Myrrh	Arabia, Somaliland, North-East Africa	Dubai
Commiphora opobalsamum	Balsaan	Balsam Tree, Gilead	In countries on both sides of Red Sea	Yemen
Convolvulus scammonia	Saqmonia	Scammony	Mediterranean region	England
Corylus avellana	Funduq	Hazel nut European Hazel	Turkey, Italy, Spain, USA	England, Turkey
Cuscuta epithymum (Lesser Dodder) *C. europaea* (Greater or Common Dodder)	Aftimoon (Dried whole plant of *Cassytha filiformis*, also of *Cuscuta reflexa* are sold as Aftimoon)	Dodder or Cuscuta	A parasite in most parts of the world	Pakistan
Dorema ammoniacum	Ushaq	Gum Ammoniac	Iran, extending into southern Siberia	Iran
Doronicum pardalianches/ Doronicum hookeri	Darunaj-akrabi	Leopard's Bane (Also equated with *Arnica montana*)	Europe	Iran, Europe
Dracaena cinnabari	Damm-ul-Akhwain	Dragon's Blood	Saudi Arabia, East Africa	Yemen
Ephedra gerardiana/ Ephedra vulgaris	Somlataa	Ephedra	West-Central China, Southern Siberia, Japan. Also Spain, Baluchistan	Pakistan
Euphorbia resinifera	Farfiyun	Euphorbium	Morocco	Morocco
Ferula assafoetida	Hing	Assafoetida	Eastern Persia, Western Afghanistan	Afghanistan, Khzakhistan, Iran

Table 1: Contd.

Botanical Name	Common Name	English Name	Habitat	Main Source
Ferula galbaniflua	Jaosheer (gum-resin)	Opopanax Tree Galbanum	Iran, Cape of Good Hope	Iran
Ferula persica	Sakbeenaj	Sagapenum	Iran	Iran
Fraxinus ornus/ F. routindifolia	Sheerkhisht (exudate)	Manna	Southern Europe, parts of Asia	Spain
Garcinia hanburyi	Usaar-e-Revand	Gamboge, Gutta (extract)	Siam, Southern Cochin-China, Cambodia, Sri Lanka	Thailand
Gentiana olivieri	Ghaafis Gul-e-Ghaafis	Persian Gentian	Iran	Afghanistan
Glycyrrhiza glabra	Asl-us-Soos	Liquorice	Spain, Germany, France, Italy, Russia	Iran, Afghanistan
Helicteres isora	Marorphali	East Indian Screw Tree	Nepal, Bihar, Bengal, central, western and southern India, Andaman Islands	Nepal
Helleborus niger	Kharbaq Siyah	Black Hellebore	Central and southern Europe, Germany, Greece, Asia Minor	Germany
Hyoscyamus niger	Bazr-ul-Banj Khoraasaani Ajwaayin	Henbane seeds Siberia	Central and southern Europe, Western Asia,	Baluchistan, Afghanistan
Hyssopus officinalis	Zufaa	Hyssop	Southern Europe	Afghanistan
Illicium verum	Star Anise	Star Anise of China	China, South-East Asia	China
Ipomoea purga/ Convolvulus jalapa	Jalaabaa, Jalaapaa	Jalap	Mexico	Mexico
Juniperus communis	Hauber, Abhal	Common Juniper	Europe, North Africa, North Asia, North America	Pakistan

Table 1: Contd.

Botanical Name	Common Name	English Name	Habitat	Main Source
Lallemantia royleana	Baalangu		Western Asia, Iran	Pakistan, Baluchistan
Laurus nobilis	Habb-ul-Ghaar	Sweet Bay, True laurel	Shores of Mediterranean Southern Europe	Saudi Arabia
Lavandula stoechas	Ustukhuddus	French Lavender	Mediterranean region	Morocco
Lepidium sativum	Habb-ul-Rashaad, Haalim	Garden Cress	Iran	Iran
Lupinus albus	Turmus	White Lupin	North and South America, Southern Europe, Egypt	Iran
Marrubium vulgare	Faraasiyun	White Horehound	England, Europe, Baluchistan, Iran	Iran
Matthiola incana	Turdi Zard (Tudri Surkh is equated with *Cheiranthus cheiri*)	Gilli Flower Wall Flower Common Stock	Mediterranean region, Western Europe	Iran
Melia azedarach	Bakaayin	Persian Lilac	China, Baluchistan, Kashmir, Western Himalayas, South India	Afghanistan
Melissa officinalis	Baadranjboyaa, Billilotan	Catmint, Catnip Mountain Balm	Europe, North America, Iran	Iran
Merendera persica	Suranjaan Shireen	Sweet Hermodactyl	Iran	Iran
Myristica fragrans	Jaiphal	Nutmeg	Native to Malacca Islands and New Guinea, Sri Lanka, West Indies	Sri Lanka
Myrtus communis	Habb-ul-Aas, Muurad	Common Myrtle	Southern Europe	Afghanistan
Myrrhis odovata	Anjudaan Roomi	Sweet Cherirel	England	Iran

Table 1: Contd.

Botanical Name	Common Name	English Name	Habitat	Main Source
Ocimum basilicum	Tukhmsharbati (Seeds)	Sweet Basil	France, Central Asia	Europe
Ocimum pilosum	Tukhm-e-Rehaan Seeds	Wild Basil	Tropical and warm temperate regions	Pakistan, Iran
Olea europea	Zaitoon	Olive	Mediterranean region	Europe
Oligochaeta ramosa syn. *Volutarella ramosa, V. divaricata* in part, *Tricholepis procumbens, Amberboa divaricata*	Baadaaward (Imported herb is actually *Fagonia arabica*)		Mediterranean region, Central Asia, India	Iran, Pakistan
Orchis latifolia/ *Orchis* spp.	Saalab Misri (root) Saalab panjaa (root) Saalab gattaa (root)	Salep	Central and southern Europe	Iran, Pakistan
Origanum vulgare	Marzanjosh	Wild Morjoram	England, Europe, North Africa, Asia	Tibet, China
Paeonia officinalis	Ood saleeb	Peony root	Southern Europe, West Asia	Pakistan
Pastinaca secacul	Shaqaq-ul-Misri		Iran, Afghanistan, Egypt	Afghanistan
Peganum harmala	Harmal	Harmal, Syrian Rue, Wild Rue, Foreign Henna	Mediterranean region, Mexico, Asia, Ladakh, Kashmir, Punjab	Pakistan, Iran
Peucedanum grande	Duku patti (seed)		Iran	Iran
Phoenix dactylifera	Gond Chhuhaaraa		North Africa, Egypt, Syria, Saudi Arabia	Iran, Pakistan
Pimpinella anisum	Anisoon	Anise	Originally from Egypt Minor. Now cultivated in warmer climates and Asia	China, Hong Kong, Taiwan, Malaysia, Vietnam

Table 1: Contd.

Botanical Name	Common Name	English Name	Habitat	Main Source
Pinus succinifera (now extinct)	Kahrubaa (fossil resin)	Amber	Baltic Amber or Malay Archipelago found in Scandinavia	Germany
Piper cubeba	Kababchini, Kankola	Cubebs	Java, Sumatra	Indonesia
Piper longum	Peeppali	Long pepper	North-eastern, Southern India, Sri Lanka, East Bengal	Indonesia
Pistacia integerrima *Rhus succedanea*	Kaakraasingi (galls)	Crab's Claw	Mediterranean region to East Asia, Himalayan ranges on the North-west	Pakistan
Pistacia lentiscus	Mastagi, Roomi Mastagi	Mastich (resin)	Mediterranean region, Iran, Afghanistan, Kabul	Kabul, Greece
Pistacia vera	Gul-e-Pistaa (flower)	Pistachio	Syria, Iran, Afghanistan	Iran, Afghanistan
Polygonum bistorta	Anjabaar	Bistort, Odewort, Snake Weed	Southern Scotland, Western Asia, Japan	
Polypodium vulgare	Bisfaayej (root)		Europe, Turkey	Turkey, Nepal
Punica granatum	Gulnaar Faarsi	Pomegranate	Iran, Saudi Arabia, Afghanistan, Baluchistan, India	Pakistan, Afghanistan
Quercus infectoria	Maazu (gall)	Gall Oak, Dyers' Oak, Aleppo or Turkey Galls (collected in Asiatic Turkey in the province of Aleppo) Mecca galls	Greece, Asia Minor, Iran, Syria. Mecca galls are from Bassorah	Iran, Turkey

Table 1: Contd.

Botanical Name	Common Name	English Name	Habitat	Main Source
Rheum emodi	Revandchini	Himalayan Rhubarb	Kashmir to Sikkim, Assam. Chinese: *R. palmatum* and *R. officinale*. English: *R. rhaponticum* (Rhapontic). Indian: *R. emodi* and *R. Webbianum.*	Nepal
Rhus coriaria	Sumaaq	Sumach, Japan Wax Tree	Mediterranean region, Spain, Italy, Sicily, Iran, Afghanistan, Saudi Arabia	
Rubia tinctorum	Majeeth	European madder	Southern Europe and parts of Asia	Iran
Salvia haemotodes	Behman Surkh	Red behen (sage)	Persia	Afghanistan
Salvia plebeia	Samundar-sokh (seeds)	Sage Seeds	Temperate and tropical regions	Pakistan
Sisymbrium irio	Khoobkalaan, Khaaksi (seeds)	London Rocket	Northern India, Iran, Europe	Iran
Smilax aristolochiaefolia	Ushbaa Maghrabi	Mexican Sarsaparilla	Central America	Mexico
Smilax china	Chobchini	China Root	Eastern Asia, China, Japan	China
Strychnos ignatii	Pipita Vilaayati	Ignatius Beans	Philippine Islands, Cochin-China	Philippines
Styrax benzoin	Lobaan	Gum benjamine	Java, Sumatra, Malay, Malacca	Penang, Indonesia
Syzygium aromaticum	Qaranful, Laung	Clove Tree	Cultivated in Tamil Nadu, Kerala, Sri Lanka, Indonesia, Malacca Islands, Tanzania, Madagascar, Penang, Brazil, other Tropical parts	Zanzibar

Table 1: Contd.

Botanical Name	Common Name	English Name	Habitat	Main Source
Tanacetum umbelliferum	Buzidaan Vilaayati	Sweet Pellitory	Iran	Iran
Teucrium chamaedrys	Usqurdiyun Kamaazarius	Wall-Germander	England, Europe	Europe
Thymus serphyllum	Haashaa	Wild Thyme	England, France, Europe	
Trifolium alexandrinum	Ispast	Trefoil berseem Egyptian Clover	England, Europe, Mediterranean region, Central and Northern Asia	Seeds of *Amaranthus retroflexus* are imported from Iran.
Trigonella uncata/ Melilotus officinalis	Naakhuunaa Ikil-ul-Malik	Meliot (bean) Tonkin bean	Iran, Afghanistan	Iran
Urginea scilla	Isqeel	Squill	Mediterranean region, Spain, Protugal, Morocco, Corsica, Southern France, Malta, Algeria, Italy, Dalmatia, Greece, Syria, Asia Minor.	Italy, Spain, Pakistan
Urtica pilulifera	Anjuraa	Roman Nettle	Europe	Europe
Valeriana hardwickii/ V. jatamansi	Sugandha-baalaa Taggar, Mushkbaalaa	Indian Valerian	Temperate Himalayas from Kashmir to Bhutan; Khasi and Jantia Hills. Valerian (*Valeriana officinalis*): Europe and Northern Asia	Nepal
Viola odorata	Banafshaa Gul-e-Banafshaa	Sweet Violet	Europe, Britain, Asia	Pakistan
Viscum album	Koli daakh, Mavizaj-e-Asli, Kishmish Kaabali	European Mistletoe	Afghanistan, Europe.	Afghanistan

Table 1: Contd.

Botanical Name	Common Name	English Name	Habitat	Main Source
Withania coagulans	Paneer, Paneer Dodaa (fruit, seed)	Vegetable Rennet	Afghanistan, Baluchistan, Sindh, Punjab	Iran, Pakistan
Withania somnifera	Asgandh	Winter Cherry	Israel, East of Mediterranean region, South Asia	Afghanistan
Zataria multiflora	Saatar faarsi	Savory	Saudi Arabia, Iran, Afghanistan, Baluchistan	Pakistan, Afghanistan
Ziziphus jujuba Mill. *Z. sativa* Gaertin	Unnaab	Jujube	China, Far East, Middle East, Africa	Kabul

REFERENCES

1. Manawar, Sultana et al., Central Research Institute of Unani Medicine, Hyderabad.
2. MSIA Aziz et al., (2005). *Role of Sauda (black bile) in Psychological Disorders*, AK Tibbia College, AMU, Aligarh.
3. Gaud, PV et al., (2000). *Research on Fundamental Principles of Unani Medicine: An Appraisal and Scope*, Central Research Institute of Unani Medicine, Hyderabad.
4. Ministry of Health & Family Welfare, Govt. of India, Annual Report 2004-2005.
5. Adhami, SM, KM Siddiqui and MK Siddiqui, (2000). *Application of Modern Research Methology in Unani Clinical Research: Some Limitations and Guidelines*, Central Council for Research in Unani Medicine, New Delhi. National Seminar on Research and Development in Unani Medicine.
6. Khare, CP, (2007). *Indian Medicinal Plants: An Illustrated Dictionary*, Springer.

4

Siddha Medicine: Slowly Moving towards Scientific Validation

Siddha medicine is confined to South India. 16035 physicians are practising Siddha medicine in Tamil Nadu and 1356 in Kerala. The system is being taught in 6 undergraduate colleges (admission capacity 320) and 2 postgraduate colleges (admission capacity 90). There are 437 licensed pharmacies of Siddha medicine, against 450 of Unani medicine and 7,778 of Ayurvedic medicine.[1]

Siddha medicine originated in South India and dates back to around 2000 BC.

According to Siddha system, the human body is composed of 96 *Tatwas*, 72000 blood vessels and 1300 nerves. Besides these, there are 10 *Nadi* (main arteries), 10 *Vayu* (vital *Pranas*) and 14 *Vegangal* (natural functions), all of which play important roles in different functions of the body.

The Siddha medicine (like Ayurvedic medicine) also recognises the role of three humours called *Mukkuthram* (*Vatham, Pittam* and *Kapam*). These humours remain in a balanced state in a normal healthy person, and disturbance in their equilibrium leads to ill health.

The diagonsis is done by the Siddha physician on the basis of *Mukkuthram* and *Ennvagal Theru* (eight entities), i.e., *Nadi* (pulse), *Na* (tongue), *Nirma* (colour), *Moozhi* (voice), *Kan* (eyes), *Sparsham* (touch), *Malam* (faeces) and *Muthiram* (urine).

The treatment is mainly directed towards restoration of equilibrium of the three humours (*Vatham, Pittam* and *Kapam*).

Siddha texts like 'Varma Kannadi' and 'Varma Suthiram' have described 108 vital points, which are located on vital junctions of arteries and veins, nerves, joints, etc., and are called *Varmanilaigal*. For the purpose of treatment, Siddha physicians give pressure by specialised technique on these points to cure ailments.

Siddha medicines are being used for the treatment of Vali Gunman (peptic ulcer); Manjal Kamalal (infective hepatitis); Kazhichal (dysenteric disorders); Veluppunoi (anaemia); Karappan (skin disorders); Putrunoi (cancer); Neerazhivu (diabetes mellitus); Kakkai Valippu (epilepsy) and Sandhi Vata Soolai (rheumatoid arthritis).[2]

For treating psoriasis, Central Council for Research in Ayurveda and Siddha has developed "777 Oil" after conducting extensive pharmacological, toxicological studies and clinical trials. The clinical trials have been conducted on 2823 patients over a period of 20 years. More than 80% patients have shown improvement. The oil contains the extract of *Wrightia tinctoria* R. Br. leaves as a main ingredient in coconut oil.[3]

A number of Siddha polyherbal formulations contain mercury, silver, arsenic, lead and sulphur, and are used for treating chronic diseases.[4]

REFERENCES

1. Ministry of Health & Family Welfare, Govt. of India, Annual Report, 2004-2005.
2. Input from Central Council for Research in Ayurveda and Siddha (CCRAS), New Delhi-110 055.
3. *CCRAS Research—An Overview*, December 2002, Dept. of AYUSH, Ministry of Health & Family Welfare, Govt. of India, New Delhi-110 001.
4. Ministry of Health & Family Planning, Govt. of India, Annual Report, 2004-2005.

5

Drug Variants of Indian Medicine: Predominantly Classical

When you enter a typical Indian drug store, you enter the 17th century or "prehistoric age" of contemporary medicine. Many segments need a detailed explanation. Our scholars should understand clearly that without contemporary nomenclature and consumer-friendly format, this legacy may not remain that popular.

Now enter a chemist's shop. A number of classical products are conspicuous because of their modified versions. Pre-mixed *Sitopaladi churna* and honey is available as *Madhuvani* (Dabur). Chyavanprasha has been converted into granular form, regular as well as for diabetics (Dabur, Baidyanath). Chyavanprasha biscuits have been launched by Yogi Pharmacy, Haridwar. Zandu *Pancharishta* is a combination of five digestive and restorative *Aasavas* and *Arishtas*. *M2 Tone* (Charak) is a combination of classical uterine tonics.

It seems changes are also creeping into the Ayurvedic Formulary of India due to contemporary compulsions. The drug "Rasapushpa" (Vol. I, 2003, page 211) is usually put inside a seedless *Vitis vinifera* (Draakshaa). Alternately, it has been officially suggested that it should be administered in a gelatine capsule. This opens up the way officially for introducing Churna, Gutikaa, Vati, Bhasma and Rasayoga in capsule form.

In practice, more than 30 classical Churnas and Kwaaths have already been converted into tablets by IMCOPS, Dabur, Baidyanath, Ayurveda Rasashala and other pharmaceutical companies.

Himalaya Drug Company took the lead; their coated tablets, capsules, and syrups proved more consumer-friendly and succeeded to a great extent in influencing the practitioners of modern medicine.

Ayurvedic medicinal oils will no more remain messy if converted into creams. At Ayurveda Rasashala, Pune, a number of herbal oils were converted into creams and put to clinical trials. Chandan Balaalaakshaadi, Vishagarbha and Narayana Taila creams gave encouraging results in accordance with the original oils.

Now, see the present nomenclature of classical Ayurvedic drugs.

Aasava and Arishta

These are medicinal preparations made by soaking the drug, either in powder form or in the form of decoction, in a solution of sugar or jaggery (as the case may be) for a specific period of time, during which it undergoes a process of fermentation generating alcohol, thus facilitating the extraction of active principles contained in the drugs. The alcohol, so generated, also serves as a preservative.

In Indian medicine, inoculum of yeast comes from the flowers of *Woodfordia fruiticosa* Kurz. (*Dhaataki*). These are nectariferous and highly tanniferous and serve the same purpose as hops (*Humulus lupulus* L.) in brewing. In some preparations, *Madhuca indica* (Madhuuka) flowers, honey or resins are used for initiating the process of fermentation.

The Aasavas are prepared from the juices of fresh plants or water-soaked dry herbs, whereas the Arishtas are prepared from the decoction of herbs.

At the final stage, the prepared medicine is moderately alcoholic (up to 12% by volume), and is taken mixed with an equal volume of water (10-30 ml twice or thrice daily).

The *Aasavas* and *Arishtas* can be kept for any length of time in well-closed bottles or jars.

Arka; Theeneer (Siddha medicine); Arq (Unani medicine)

The herbs are crushed coarsely and soaked in water overnight and transferred along with the water into the still for distillation. The final form of Arka is the distilled essence, which contains the volatile constituents of the herbs used in the preparation. It is equivalent to the "aquae" or "waters" of the Western Pharmacopoeia.

Arka is given internally mixed with an equal volume of water (15-30 ml once or thrice a day).

Avaleha, Leha, Paaka; Legiyam, Elagam (Siddha medicine); Majoon (Unani medicine)

Equivalent to confections, electuaries and conserves of the British Pharmacopoeia.

Generally the quantity of jaggery, sugar, sugar candy or honey is kept 2-3 times the weight of all the drugs.

Avaleha is given 5-10 g twice or thrice a day. It should be used within one year.

Itrifal of Unani medicine is prepared like Majoon but invariably contains the three Myrobalans (Triphala).

Churna; Choornam (Siddha medicine); Safoof (Unani medicine)

The herbs are cleaned and dried and finely powdered. The powder should be of at least 80 mesh sieve.

Churna is often taken with some vehicle such as honey, purified butter, milk, buttermilk, depending upon the formulation and indication (3-6 g daily).

Generally, powders should be used within 2 months (*Pharmacopoeial Standards of Ayurvedic Formulations*, CCRAS, 1987). If kept in tight containers, they retain potency for one year (AFI, Second Revised Edn, 2003).

Kwaatha Churna; Kudineer Choornam (Siddha medicine); Jushaandaa (Unani medicine)

Compounded coarse powders are used whenever a particular type of decoction is required. 60 g of the Kwaatha Churna is boiled in 800 ml water until the decoction is reduced to 120 ml. The decoction should be used within 24 hours after it has cooled (30-60 ml twice or thrice a day).

The Kwaatha Churna retains potency for one year and should be kept in airtight container.

Ghrita; Nei (Siddha medicine)

For preparing medicated Ghrita, purified butter is boiled with prescribed decoction and fine paste of herbs. Generally, if the paste of herbs is one part by weight, the purified butter should be four parts and decoction/liquids should be 16 parts. The mixture is boiled on mild fire till the evaporation of liquids. The Ghrita is taken after warming, generally with warm milk or water (5-10 g twice daily). It retains its potency for about 16 months.

Guggulu

Preparations having the purified (detoxified) exudate of *Commiphora mukul* are known as Guggula. Kaishore Guggulu is prescribed for gout; Kanchnaar Guggulu for tumours and enlargement of cervical glands; Triphalaa Guggulu for piles, fistula and other inflammatory conditions, and Yogaraaj Guggulu (the largest selling over-the-counter Guggulu) for rheumatic afflictions. Twelve polyherbal formulations containing Guggulu have been included in *The Ayurvedic Formulary of India*, Part I.

Gutikaa, Vati; Kulligai, Maththirai (Siddha medicine); Habb, Qurs (Unani medicine)

These are pills or tablets of contemporary medicine. Pills made of plant drugs, when kept in airtight containers, can be used for two years; if minerals are also used, then for a much longer period.

Taila; Thailam (Siddha medicine); Raughan (Unani medicine)

62 massage oils (a few for internal administration) have been included in *The Ayurvedic Formulary of India*, Part I. In an average drug store, more than 20 medicated oils are available. The oil is boiled on mild fire with prescribed

Table 2: Contd.

Botanical name/Part used	Common use/Activity	Form, Chemical marker(s)
Abutilon indicum seed	Diuretic, Nervine tonic	Powder : Mucilage 10%.
Acacia arabica bark	Astringent	Powder : Tannins 40%
Acacia catechu gum	Astringent	Powder : Tannins 60% Catechins 20%
Acacia concinna pods	Detergent	Powder/Paste: Saponins 10%-20%
Achillea millefolium seeds	Stimulant, Antispasmodic	Powder : Bitters 3%
Achyranthes aspera plant	Alterative, Diuretic	Powder/Paste : Saponins 3%
Aconitum heterophyllum plant	Antiperiodic, Antiemetic	Powder/Paste : Alkaloids 1%-1.5%
Aconitum spp. root	Antipyretic	Powder/Paste : Alkaloids 2%
Acorus calamus rhizome	Antispasmodic	Powder/Paste : Vol. Oil 1%
Adhatoda vasica leaf	Expectorant, Bronchodilatory	Powder/Paste : Alkaloids 0.5%-2.5%
Aegle marmelos leaf	Antidiabetic	Powder : Tannins 7.5%
Aegle marmelos unripe fruit	Haemostatic, Antidysenteric	Powder/Paste : Tannins 5% Mucilage 10%-15%
Albizia lebbeck bark	Anti-inflammatory	Powder/Paste : Tannins 15%
Allium cepa bulbs	Hypolipidemic, Hypocholesterolemic	Powder/Paste : Quercetin 5%
Allium sativum bulbs	Hypocholesterolemic, Antirheumatic	Powder/Paste : Alliin 1.5%-2.5% by HPLC
Aloe vera leaf	Purgative	Powder/Paste/Gel/Gum : Aloin 1.5% (3:1) Polysaccharides 50% (200:1)
Alpinia galanga rhizome	Anticatarrhal	Powder/Paste : Shagaol > 4% by HPLC
Alstonia scholaris bark	Alterative, Astringent	Powder : Alkaloids 0.3%
Anacyclus pyrethrum flowers	Stimulant, Sialogogue	Powder : Alkaloids 0.5%
Andrographis paniculata plant	Hepatoprotectant, Antiviral	Powder/Paste : Andrographolides > 10%
Anethum sowa seed	Carminative	Powder/Paste : Vol. Oil 3%
Aphanamixis rohituka bark	Astringent	Powder : Tannins 10%

Table 2: Contd.

Botanical name/Part used	Common use/Activity	Form, Chemical marker(s)
Apium graveolens seed	Carminative	Powder/Paste : Vol. Oil 5%
Argyreia speciosa root	Alterative, Nervine tonic	Powder : Resin 4.5%
Asparagus adscendens root	Nervine tonic, Galactogogue	Powder : Saponins > 10%
Asparagus racemosus root	Galactogogue	Powder/Paste : Saponins > 15%
Asteracantha longifolia herb	Diuretic	Powder/Paste : Alkaloids 0.35%
Atropa belladonna leaf	Antispasmodic, Sedative	Powder/Paste : Alkaloids 0.95%-1.6%
Atropa belladonna root	Antispasmodic, Sedative	Powder/Paste : Alkaloids 3%
Azadirachta indica bark	Astringent	Powder : Bitters 1%
Azadirachta indica leaf	Blood purifier	Powder/Paste : Bitters 2.5%
Bacopa monnieri herb	Brain tonic	Powder/Paste : Bacosides 15%- 50% Alkaloids 5%
Barleria prionitis herb	Lymphadenitis, Toothache	Powder : Tannins 5%, Alkaloids 0.5%
Bauhinia variegata bark	Alterative, antileprotic	Powder, Tannins 25%
Berberis aristata root	Emmenagogue, Cholagogue	Powder/Paste : Berberine > 8%
Bergenia ligulata root	Antiurolithiatic	Powder/Paste : Tannins 10%
Boerhavia diffusa root	Diuretic, Hepatoprotective	Powder/Paste : Alkaloids 0.01%-0.08%
Boswellia serrata gum	Anti-arthritic	Powder/Paste : Boswellic acids > 50%
Butea frondosa flowers	Astringent	Powder/Paste : Glycosides > 8%
Caesalpinia bonducella nut	Antipyretic	Powder/Paste : Bonducin 2.5%
Calotropis gigantea root	Emetic, Antiperiodic	Powder/Paste : Alkaloids 0.3%
Camellia sinensis	Antioxidant	Powder/Paste : Polyphenols > 45% by HPLC
Capparis spinosa root	Analgesic, Antirheumatic	Powder : Glycosides 15%
Capsicum spp. fruit	Antirheumatic	Powder/Paste : Capsaicin > 3%

Table 2: Contd.

Botanical name/Part used	Common use/Activity	Form, Chemical marker(s)
Cassia angustifolia leaf	Laxative	Powder : Sennosides 15%
Cassia angustifolia pods	Laxative	Paste : Sennosides 2.5%
Cassia fistula fruit	Laxative	Powder/Paste : Oxymethyl-anthraquinones > 1%
Cassia occidentalis fruit	Purgative	Powder/Paste : Oxymethyl-anthraquinones 1.2%
Cedrus deodara wood	Antirheumatic	Powder/Paste : Vol. Oil 1%
Celastrus paniculatus seed	Antirheumatic, Tranquilizer	Powder/Paste : Alkaloids 0.1%
Centella asiatica	Leprostatic, Memory tonic, Sedative	Powder/Paste : Asiaticosides > 10% Asiatic acid 2%
Cephaelis ipecacuanha root	Emetic	Powder/Paste : Alkaloids 1%
Cephalandra indica leaf	Antidiabetic	Powder : Resin 2.5%
Cicer arietinum seeds	Nutritive	Powder : Protein 15%
Cichorium intybus seeds	Liver and spleen tonic	Powder/Paste : Bitters > 1%
Cinchona ledgeriana bark	Antimalarial	Powder/Paste : Alkaloids 4%
Cissus quadrangularis stem	Bone healing	Powder : Ketosterones > 5%
Citrullus colocynthis fruit	Purgative	Powder : Bitters 4.5%
Citrullus colocynthis root	Purgative, Antirheumatic	Powder : Bitters 5%
Citrus aurantium peel	Antioxidant	Powder/Paste : Flavones > 4% Vol. Oil 1%
Citrus medica peel	Antiscurvy	Powder : Acidity as citric acid 2%, Flavones 5%
Colchicum luteum corms	In uric acid diathesis	Powder : Alkaloids > 0.5%
Coleus forskohlii root	cAMP stimulator, Hypotensive	Powder : Forskolin > 2.5%, 10% & 20% by HPLC
Commiphora mukul gum	Antarthritic, Antilipemic, Anticholesterolemic	Powder/paste : Guggul sterones 2.5% to 10% by HPLC
Commiphora myrrha gum	Astringent	Powder: Vol. Oil 5%
Coriandrum sativum seeds	Carminative	Powder/Paste : Vol. Oil 1%
Crataeva nurvala bark	Lithotriptic	Powder : Saponin > 2.5%

Table 2: Contd.

Botanical name/Part used	Common use/Activity	Form, Chemical marker(s)
Cucumis sativus seeds	Diuretic	Powder : Mucilage 24%
Cuminum cyminum fruit	Carminative	Powder/Paste : Vol. Oil 1%
Curculigo orchioides root	Uresis, Skin diseases	Powder : Saponins 20% Mucilage 30%
Curcuma amada rhizome	Carminative, Hypolipidaemic	Powder/Paste : Vol. Oil 10%
Curcuma longa rhizome	Anti-inflammatory, Stomachic	Powder/Paste : Voil. Oil > 10%, Curcumin > 10%
Cynodon dactylon herb	Astringent	Powder : Tannins 5% Alkaloids +ive
Cyperus scariosus root	Intestinal antiseptic, Anti-inflammatory	Powder/Paste : Alkaloids 0.15%-0.5%
DGL (Deglycyrrhizinated Liquorice)	Anti-ulcer, Antacid	Powder : Flavones 1% Glycyrrhizin < 3%
Dashmool (The Ten Roots)	Antirheumatic	Powder/Paste : Tannis 2%
Datura stramonium leaf	Antispasmodic, Expectorant	Powder/Paste : Alkaloids 0.5%-0.7%
Daucus carota seed	Abortifacient	Powder/Paste : Alkaloids 0.4%, Flavones 5%
Dolichos biflorus seeds	Diuretic	Powder : Saponins 20%
Eclipta alba plant	Anti-hepatotoxic	Powder/Paste : Nor-wedelolactone > 3%
Embelia ribes seed	Anthelmintic	Powder/Paste : Tannins 1%, Embelin 1%
Emblica officinalis fruit	Antioxidant, Source of Vitamin C, Antacid, Astringent	Powder/Paste : Tannins > 20%, Ellagic acid > 5%
Enicostemma littorale herb	Bitter tonic, Laxative	Powder/Paste : Bitters 4%
Ephedra vulgaris herb	Stimulant	Powder/Paste : Alkaloids 0.2%-0.5%
Eugenia jambolana seed	Antidiabetic	Powder : Saponins 4%, Alkaloids 0.4%
Euphorbia hirta herb	Antispasmodic	Powder/Paste : Flavones > 6%
Evolvulus alsinoides plant	Memory tonic	Powder/Paste : Bitters > 2.5%
Ferula foetida resin	Carminative, Stimulant	Powder : Vol. Oil 1.5%
Ficus racemosa leaf	Astringent	Powder: Tannins 5%

Table 2: Contd.

Botanical name/Part used	Common use/Activity	Form, Chemical marker(s)
Ficus racemosa bark	Astringent	Powder : Tannins 10%
Foeniculum vulgare fruit	Carminative, Spasmolytic	Powder/Paste : Vol. Oil > 1%
Fumaria officinalis herb	Diaphoretic	Powder/Paste : Bitters > 1%
Garcinia cambogia rind	Fatty acid inhibitor	Powder/ Liquid : HCA 50% by HPLC
Glycyrrhiza glabra root	Expectorant, Anti-inflammatory	Powder/Paste : Glycyrrhizin by Garratt method > 15%/24%
Gossypium herbaceum root	Emmenagogue, Galactagogue	Powder : Alkaloids 0.4% Falvones 1.5%
Gymnema sylvestre leaf	Antidiabetic	Powder : Gymnemic acids 25%-75%
Hemidesmus indicus root	Alterative, antiseptic	Powder/Paste : Saponins 7.5%
Holarrhena antidysenterica seed	Antidysenteric	Powder : Alkaloids 3% seed
Holarrhena antidysenterica bark	Antidysenteric, Anthelmintic	Powder/Paste : Alkaloids > 4%
Hydrastis Indian root	Emmenagogue	Powder/Paste : Hydrastin 1%
Hyoscyamus niger herb	Antispasmodic, Sedative	Powder/Paste : Alkaloids 0.28%-0.3%
Hypericum perforatum herb	Antidepressant	Powder : Hypericin 0.3%
Indigofera tinctoria plant	Antiseptic, Astringent	Powder : Saponins 10%
Inula racemosa root	Antirheumatic, In chronic bronchitis	Powder/Paste : Alantolactone 2.5% by HPLC
Juglans regia bark	Astringent, Antiseptic	Powder : Tannins 12%
Lawsonia alba leaf	Antimicrobial, Anti-inflammatory	Powder/Paste : Tannins > 5%
Leptadenia reticulata herb	Spermatogenic, Galactagogue	Powder/Paste : Alkaloids 0.5%
Lobelia nicotianaefolia leaf	Antispasmodic	Powder/Paste : Alkaloids 0.5%
Mangifera indica bark	Astringent	Powder : Tannins 20%
Matricaria chamomilla flower	Antiseptic	Paste : Vol. Oil 1%
Mentha spicata	Carminative, Stimulant, Spasmolytic	Powder/Paste : Flavones > 2%
Mesua ferrea fruit and flower bud	Astringent, Styptic	Powder/Paste : Bitters > 2.5%

Table 2: Contd.

Botanical name/Part used	Common use/Activity	Form, Chemical marker(s)
Mimusops elengi bark	Astringent	Powder : Tannins 10%
Momordica charantia fruit	Blood-purifier	Powder : Bitters > 2.5%
Morinda citrifolia fruit	Stimulant	Powder/Liquid : Morindin 15% Scopoletin 0.17%
Moringa oleifera bark	Emmenagogue, Abortifacient	Powder : Glycosides > 5%
Moringa oleifera leaf	Anti-inflammatory	Powder/Paste : Alkaloids 0.1%
Mucuna pruriens seeds	Antiparkinsonian, Aphrodisiac	Powder : L-Dopa by IP method > 15%
Myrica nagi bark	Astringent, Carminative	Powder : Tannins 5%
Myristica fragrans fruit	Hypocholesterolemic, Carminative	Powder/Paste : Vol. Oil 4%
Nardostachys jatamansi root	Sedative	Powder/Paste : Vol. Oil 0.1%-0.5%
Nelumbo nucifera seed	Stimulant	Powder : Saponins 30%
Nigella sativa seed	Anthelmintic, Carminative, Antimicrobial	Powder/Paste : Bitters 3% Saponins 15%
Nyctanthes arbortristis leaf	Antirheumatic, Anthelmintic	Powder, Alkaloids 0.15%
Ocimum basilicum leaf	Carminative, Vermifuge	Powder/Paste : Tannins 5% Vol. Oil 1.5%
Ocimum sanctum herb/leaf	Immunomodulator, Expectorant	Powder/Paste : Tannins > 7% Ursolic acid > 2%
Oldenlandia corymbosa plant	Liver tonic, Febrifuge	Powder/Paste : Alkaloids 0.35%
Onosma echioides root	Anticutaneous	Powder/Paste : Alkamine 1%
Operculina turpethum root	Purgative	Powder : Resin > 10%
Opuntia dillenii herb	Antispasmodic	Powder : Tannins 10%
Orchis mascula tubers	Nervine tonic	Powder : Saponins 4% Mucilage 20%
Phyllanthus niruri herb	Antihepatotoxic, Antiviral	Powder/Paste : Bitters 1.4%-2%

Table 2: Contd.

Botanical name/Part used	Common use/Activity	Form, Chemical marker(s)
Picrorhiza kurroa root	Antihepatotoxic, Bitter tonic	Powder/Paste : Kutkin 4% - 6% Bitters > 6%
Piper cubeba fruit	Carminative, Expectorant	Paste, Vol. Oil 8% Piperine 10%
Piper longum fruit	Carminative, Bioavailability enhancer	Powder/Paste Vol. Oil 10% Piperine 5%
Piper nigrum fruit	Carminative, Antiperiodic, Bioavailability enhancer	Vol. Oil 7% Piperine > 10%
Pistacia integerrima galls	Astringent, Antispasmodic	Powder/Paste : Tannins 20%
Plumbago indica root	Anticutaneus	Powder : Alkaloids 0.08%-0.15%
Podophyllum emodi rhizome	Purgative	Powder : Resin > 20%
Polygala chinensis root	Anticatarrhal	Powder/Paste : Saponins 5%
Pongamia glabra seed	Antileprotic	Powder/Paste : Fixed Oil 10%
Prunus serotina bark	Astringent	Paste : Tannins 10%
Psoralea corylifolia seed	Antipsoriatic	Powder/Paste : Psoralen > 5%
Pterocarpus marsupium wood	Antidiabetic	Powder : Alkaloids 0.4% Pterostilbene 4%-5% Flavones 5%
Pterocarpus santalinus bark	Astringent, Antidiarrhoeal	Powder/Paste : Santalin > 3%
Pueraria tuberosa root	Demulcent, Nervine tonic	Powder/Paste : Flavones 6%
Punica granatum rind	Astringent	Powder : Ellagic acid by HPLC > 8%, Tannins 10-20%
Putranjiva roxburghii berries	Immunogenic	Powder : Alkaloids 0.5%
Pyrus malus fruit	Nutritive. Natural source of Iron	Powder/Paste : Iron 4%
Quercus infectoria galls	Astringent	Powder/Paste : Tannins 40%
Randia dumetorum fruit	Antioxidant, Liver protectant	Powder/Paste : Oleonolic acid > 5%
Rauvolfia serpentina root	Hypotensive	Powder/Paste : Alkaloids > 8%

Table 2: Contd.

Botanical name/Part used	Common use/Activity	Form, Chemical marker(s)
Rheum emodi root	Blood purifier, Liver protectant, Laxative	Powder/Paste : Oxymethyl anthraquinones > 5%
Ricinus communis leaf	Hepatoprotective, Anti-inflammatory	Powder : Alkaloids 2.5%
Ricinus communis root	Laxative	Powder : Alkaloids 0.5%
Rubia cordifolia root	Blood purifier	Powder/Paste : Tannins > 2%
Salacia reticulata root	Antivenereal, Antirheumatic	Powder : Glycosides > 15% Flavones > 5%
Santalum album wood	Coolant, Antibacterial	Powder/Paste : Vol. Oil 2%
Sapindus trifoliatus fruit cortex	Detergent	Paste : Saponins 20%
Saraca indica bark	Uterine tonic	Powder/Paste : Tannins > 2.5%
Saussurea lappa root	Antispasmodic, Carminative	Powder/Paste : Alkaloids > 0.2%
Semecarpus anacardium kernal	Antiseptic	Powder : Anacardic acid 0.4%
Sida cordifolia root	Nervine tonic	Powder/Paste : Alkaloids > 0.1%
Silybum marianum seeds	Hepatoprotectant, Diuretic, Anti-inflammatory	Powder : Flavones > 50% Silymarin 50%
Solanum nigrum berries	Expectorant, Liver tonic	Powder/Paste : Alkaloids 0.2% Bitters > 1%
Solanum xanthocarpum plant	Antiasthmatic, Expectorant	Powder/Paste : Solasodin > 1%
Spinacia oleracea leaves	Antioxidant	Paste : Vit K. by TLC
Strychnos nux-vomica seeds	CNS stimulant, Analeptic	Powder/Paste : Alkaloids 3%-6%
Swertia chirayita plant	Antidiabetic, Blood purifier	Powder : Bitters 4%
Symplocos racemosa bark	Uterine tonic	Powder/Paste : Alkaloids 0.5%
Taraxacum officinale herb	Hepatic stimulant	Powder/Paste : Bitters 2.5% Alkaloids 0.5%
Tecomella undulata bark	Astringent	Powder : Tannins 10%

Table 2: Contd.

Botanical name/Part used	Common use/Activity	Form, Chemical marker(s)
Tephrosia purpurea plant	Antioxidant, Antihepatotoxic	Powder/Paste : Rutin 2%-6% by HPLC
Terminalia arjuna bark	Cardiovascular support, Antiarrhythemic	Powder/Paste : Tannins > 25% Arjunic acid > 1%
Terminalia bellirica fruit	Detoxificant, Spasmolytic	Powder : Tannins > 10%
Terminalia chebula fruit	Detoxificant, Purgative	Powder : Tannins 20%-40%
Tinospora cordifolia root	Hepatoprotective	Powder/Paste : Bitters > 1.5%
Trachyspermum ammi fruit	Carminative	Powder/Paste : Vol. Oil 10%
Tribulus terrestris fruit	Spermatogenic, Diuretic, Nephroprotective	Powder/paste : Saponins 15%-45%
Trichosanthes dioica leaf	Antidiabetic	Powder : Saponins 10%
Trigonella foenum-graecum seed	Antilipemic, Anticholesterolemic	Powder : Saponins 15%-40%
Trikatu : Dry ginger, Long pepper and Black pepper	Bioavailability enhancer	Powder/Paste : Vol. Oil > 1% Piperine > 2%
Triphala: The Three Myrobalans	Detoxificant	Powder : Tannins > 25%
Triticum sativum bran	Nutritive	Powder : Vit B1 = 40 mcg/g B2 = 6.28 mcg/g B5 = 1130 mcg/g
Triticum sativum germ	Skin protectant	Oil, Vit. E 0.8% by HPLC
Tylophora indica leaf	Antiasthmatic, Anti-inflammatory	Powder/Paste : Alkaloids > 0.1%
Urginea indica bulbs	Cardiac stimulant, Diuretic	Paste : Glycosides 10%
Valeriana wallichii root	Sedative	Powder/Paste : Valeric acid 0.8%
Viburnum spp. bark	Emmenagogue	Powder/Paste : Tannins > 1.4%
Viola odorata flowers/leaf	Expectorant, antiseptic	Powder/Paste : Saponins 2.5%
Vitex negundo leaf	Anti-inflammatory	Powder/Paste : Alkaloids 0.15%
Vitis vinifera fruit/seed	Antioxidant	Powder/paste : Polyphenols > 20% by HPLC

Table 2: Contd.

Botanical name/Part used	Common use/Activity	Form, Chemical marker (s)
Wedelia calendulacea herb	Hepatoprotective	Powder/Paste : Tannins 5% Saponins 2%
Withania somnifera root	Immunomodulator, Antioxidant	Powder/Paste : Withanolides > 2.5%
Woodfordia floribunda flowers	Antileucorrhoeic	Powder/Paste : Tannins 7%
Zingiber officinale rhizome	Anti-inflammatory, Carminative, Antinauseant	Powder/Paste : Gingerols by HPLC > 5%

REFERENCES

1,2,3. Mowrey, Daniel, B. (1993). *Herbal Tonic Therapies*, 15-16.
Miller, Lucinda G. and Murray, Wallace J (1998). *Herbal Medicinals: A Clinician's Guide*, 2-3.
Rotblatt, Michael and Irwin Ziment, (2002). *Evidence-Based Herbal Medicine*, 18.

4. White, Linda B and Steven Foster, (2002). *The Herbal Drug Store*, 23-24.
5. Prof. BB Date, (Ed.) (1999). *Ayurved Research Papers*, 107.
6. *Vaidya Yog Ratnavali*, IMPCOPS, (2000). 291, Chennai.
7. Khare, CP (2007). *Indian Medicinal Plants: An Illustrated Dictionary*, Springer, inputs from Vikram Naharwar.

See also "*Improving Shelf Life of Herbal Medicine through Microcosm.*"

Now we go back to 2000 BC to find out how herbal medicines were processed and how they were impregnated for the preservation of their therapeutic properties.

Charaka advocated the use of *Sukshma Churna* (micro-pulverised powder), introduced the process of impregnating the herb with its own juice or decoction and *Jarjarikaran* (trituration) of the micro-pulverised powder.[3]

According to Sushruta, the *Churna*, the powder of essential parts of the plant belonging to a group, is saturated for 7 days with the equal quantity of decoction of plants belonging to a separate group, but having same properties, and the final product is to be accepted as the *Churna* with required medicinal properties.[4]

At this point, we would like to remember the seer who gave the Ayurvedic dictum: *mardanam gunavardhanam* (trituration accentuates and hidden medicinal properties of the herb). *Chatusshashti Prahari Pippali* (*Ayurveda Sarsangriha, Kasa Chikitsa Adhikar*) should be prepared by triturating *Piper longum* (in its own decoction) for 72 hours, if the triturating machine is run by an electric motor.

Thus, impregnating and triturating the herb was of utmost importance in the mind of the physician. It was important to ensure that the herb, as soon as administered, enters the body as a dynamic agent.

According to Sushruta, subtlety is the quality by virtue of which a drug can penetrate into the smallest capillary and channels of the biological system.[5] This theory has also been propounded in *Bhavaprakash* (1600 AD). Earlier, Hemadri elaborated it in his commentary on the 700 AD text of *Ashtanghridaya.*

In Ayurveda, impregnating the herb and its trituration go together. The process of impregnating the herb is called *Bhaavanaa.* Out of 100 g micro-pulverised powder, 20 g powder is boiled in 4 parts of water till 3 parts of the water evaporates. This paste is mixed well with the remaining powder, and after drying it at 50°C, trituration is done in a porcelain mortar for 6 to 8 hours. This process is repeated 6 times. After 7 *Bhaavanaa*, the herb is transformed into a *Rasaayana* (tonic or a potent medicinal agent).

In 1918, J & J DeChane of Hyderabad introduced micro-herbal medicines and incorporated the theory of Rasayana in the manufacturing process, reviving the process enunciated in *Samhitas*. DeChane produced herbal medicines by micro-pulverising and "atomising" the herbs so that the medicine gets absorbed from the mucous membrane into the system before reaching the stomach. The medicine starts working within minutes, while crude herbs take hours. The results achieved are not because of the quantity of the medicine but due to "ions" absorbed in the system.

Recently, solid extract (*Ghana-saar*) of herbs has shown promising results. It has been tried successfully in Pune by Dr Kulkarni PH and Dr Date BB in a number of clinical trials.[6]

For preparing solid extract *(Ghana-saar)* of herbs, first soak fine powders of herbs overnight (herb-water ratio 1:16 by weight) and then stir the mixture vigorously and filter it. Boil the filtrate continuously until it becomes semisolid. Convert the semi-solid mass into granular form and prepare tablets.[7] Only water-soluble constituents remain in the final product.

In case, all the constituents are to be retained, the micro-pulverised herbal powder should be triturated for 6 to 8 hours in its own decoction, following *Bhaavanaa* process, as described above, at least 7 times. According to the nature of the compound, herbs like *Piper longum* (Pippali), *Crocus sativum* (Kesar) or *Emblica officinalis* (Aamalaki) can also be used. These herbs increase the bioavailability of the herbal compound. By adopting these processes, the dose of herb can be reduced from 4-15 g to 1 to 1.5 g and the final product is ideal for preparing capsules.

While resorting to microcosm, it is advisable that the total herb, standardised to a particular marker, should be used. (See earlier chapter on Standardisation.) The total herb, besides active principles, also contains other constituents like resins, gum, sugar, vitamins, inorganic salts and a number of vegetable substances, which initiate a balancing mechanism during assimilation.[8]

For example, the ingestion of whole liquorice root does not produce "liquorice toxicity."[9]

The leaf of *Digitalis purpurea* and *D. lanata* has been shown to be less toxic and is required in smaller doses than digitoxin and digoxin.

Ephedrine, isolated from *Ephedra sinica*, may raise blood pressure, while the whole plant is safer, as it contains ingredients that help to lower blood pressure.

Spiraea ulmaria, known as meadowsweet, is the source of salicylic acid and aspirin-like painkiller. Using the whole plant, instead of the extracted active principle, is found safer, as it does not cause stomach bleeding, which is common with aspirin and related drugs.[10]

Arbutin, the most active constituent of *Arctostaphylos uva–ursi*, has marked antiseptic and diuretic action. To achieve this, arbutin must be converted into hydroquinone in the urinary tract. However, when extracted arbutin is administered, bacteria in the intestines break it down before it can be absorbed. When the whole herb is administered, bacterial breakdown of arbutin does not occur. Full antibiotic activity of arbutin depends on the alkalinity of the urine, and other constituents of the herb help increase the alkalinity of urine.

Thus the "working" parts of the plant—whether roots, buds, leaves or bark—are the repository of more than just one active compound, and act as potentiators and buffers.[11]

Daniel B Mowrey recommends that the extract of the herb should be placed back into whole herb material, so that the delicate balances of the herb are not disturbed. The standardisation process must ensure the presence of all constituents, or at least those responsible for the bidirectional action of the plant.[11]

REFERENCES

1. *The Ayurvedic Formulary of India*, (2003). Part I, Second Revised Edition.
2. Singh, Ram Sushil, (1983). *Vanoshadhi Nidarshika*, Uttar Pradesh Hindi Sansthan, Lucknow, (Hindi).
3. *Charaka Samhita*, Vimanasthan 7, 22; ibid 7, 16; Chikitsasthan 26, 244.

4. *Sushruta Samhita*, Chikitsasthan, 10,3; 12, 10.
5. *Sushruta Samhita*, Sutrasthan 46, 158.
6. Date, BB (Ed.) (1999). *Ayurveda Research Papers*, Ayurveda Rasashala, Pune.
7. *Theory & Practice of Ghanasaar* (Solid extracts of medicinal plants), 1996, Ayurveda Education Series, 36, Kothrud, Pune-411 029.
8. Taiyab, M, (1989). Dean, Faculty of Unani Medicine, Aligarh Muslim University, Aligarh.
9. Mowrey, Daniel B, (1990). *Herbal Tonic Therapies*, Wing Books, New York.
10. Polunin, Miriam and Christopher Robbins, (1992). *The Natural Pharmacy*, Macmillan, New York, 99, 100, 103.
11. Antol, Marie Nadine (1996). *Healing Teas*, Avery Publishing Group, New York, 210, 48.

Additional references for further study on microcosm:

Deerghayu International, 1990, 6(3), 5; 1995, 11 (41), 24-26.

Journal of Research in Ayurveda and Siddha, CCRAS, 1992, XIII (1-2), 35-47.

Ibid, 1993, XIV (1-2), 10-24.

8

Pruning Process of Indian Polyherbal Formulations

Col. Ram Nath Chopra raised the issue in 1933 when he suggested that attempts must be made to separate the good herbs from the useless ones and for this a systematic investigation of these drugs must be undertaken.[1]

Prof. (Dr) AJ Baxi (Gujarat Ayurved University, Jamnagar) wrote in 1986:

"Dashamuula Kwaath Churna and Dashamuulaarishta contain powders of the roots of ten different plants. These plants belong to different families and some of them contain chemical compounds, which under favourable conditions may interact or undergo enzymatic reactions causing oxidation of the hydroxyl group or reduction of keto group or breaking up of double bounds, etc., forming altogether different compounds in the final product. To study this possibility, it is necessary to plan an elaborate scheme. We may take each plant separately one by one and process it under similar experimental conditions and study the changes in chemical constituents at every stage. Then permutations and combinations will have to be carried out by mixing plant 1 and 2; 1 and 3; 1 and 4; 2 and 3; 2 and 4; 2 and 5; 1, 2 and 3; 1, 2, 3 and 4; and like that as many combinations as possible will be required to be studied. Such an elaborate study would indicate as to what were the intermediate products and what is the final constitution. An instrumental study at every stage will be more helpful and would give us the information about the genuineness and quality of each drug and final product."[2]

Dashamuulaarishta is the largest selling tonic for women in India (followed by Ashokaarishta, Drakshaasava, Arjunaarishta, Lohaasava, Kumaryaasava and Saaraswataarishta).

Ayurvedic Formulary of India (AFI), Part I, first edn, 1978, included the roots of all the ten plants (*Aegle marmelos, Oroxylum indicum, Gmelina arborea, Stereospermum suaveolens, Premna integrifolia, Desmodium gangeticum, Uraria picta, Solanum indicum, Solanum xanthocarpum* and *Tribulus terrestris)* in the compound, while in its second revised edition, 2003, an option has been provided to use either the root or stem-bark of the first five herbs and aboveground parts of the remaining herbs. (In classical Ayurvedic medicine, plant parts like root, bark, flower, seed, fruit and leaves are used for their specific therapeutic activities. Improper parts of the plant may affect the treatment and may exhibit even harmful effects.)[3]

Dashamuulaarishta was originally formulated for neurological disorders. But due to non-availability of proper plant parts, its profile changed with the passage of time. AFI recommended it for the following important therapeutic uses in 1978: emesis, malabsorption syndrome, abdominal lump, cough, asthma, tissue wasting, neurological afflictions and piles. This was expanded in its second edition, 2003: fistula-in-ano, anaemia, jaundice, diseases of the skin, excessive flow of urine, digestive impairment, diseases of the abdomen, gravel in urine, calculus, dysuria, infertility, emaciation, deficiency of semen and debility. (This expansion is obviously arbitrary.)

Dabur recommends Dashamuulaarishta as a general tonic and restorative for women; Baidyanath Ayurved Bhavan as a bitter tonic and alterative for nervous diseases, anaemia, cough, piles and as a general tonic; Zandu Pharmaceutical for cough, piles, aneroxia, alcoholism, asthma, vomiting, as a stimulant, alterative and bitter tonic; Indian Medical Practitioner's Cooperative Pharmacy (IMPCOPS), Chennai, as a restorative, digestive, cardiac and nervine tonic.

Muzaffer Alam et al. analysed Dashamuulaarishta, prepared according to textual procedure, on scientific parameters. The reduced decoction of specified herbs showed vitamin C 33 mg/100 ml. At the completion of fermentation (on 30th day), pH was 3.9, specific gravity 1.13, solid content 21.3% (w/w), reducing sugar 17.2% (w/v), non-reducing sugar nil, total sugar 17.2% (w/v), alcohol 6.9% (v/v). Microbiological analysis showed 25680 cells/ml. (*Bacillus* sp.).[4]

Dashamuula Kwaath extract produced CNS depressant effect in albino-mice. It reduced the spontaneous motor activity, potentiated the pentobarbitone hypnosis and antagonised the amphetamine-induced hyperactivity. It also exhibited a tranquilo-sedative activity like a major tranquilliser and blocked the condition avoidance response in rats.[5] Another study indicated that Dashamuula Kwaath extract effectively produced aspirin-like analgesic, antipyretic and anti-inflammatory effect in mice.[6]

Dey et al., (1968) reported that *Solanum indicum* induced drowsiness, decreased motor activity, alertness in mice and significantly potentiated barbiturate hypnosis in mice.[7] Dhawan et al., (1977) reported that the entire plant extract of *Uraria picta* exhibited CNS depressant activity.[8] Marmin, a coumarin, isolated from the root of *Aegle marmelos*, showed anti-inflammatory effect against carrageenan-induced inflammation in rats. The methanolic extract of the rootbark inhibited the beating rate of cultured mouse myocardial cells. Among the isolated constituents, aurapten is found to be the most potent inhibitor comparable with verapamil.[9] The root of *Desmodium gangeticum* gave gangetin, one of the pterocarpans isolated from hexane extract of the root. It showed significant anti-inflammatory activity in rats.[10] Alcoholic extract of the stembark of *Gmelina arborea* showed anti-inflammatory activity comparable to phenylbutazone."[11]

Thus, if we scan the published literature, on the basis of leads already available, the number of herbs can be reduced (Dashamuulaarishta contains not only the "ten roots" but 60 additional herbs) and efficacy of the drug can be improved.

Now, we give an example of a contemporary polyherbal formulation labelled as "the effective cardioprotective". As old habits diehard, we find, even pioneers of evidence-based herbal medicine in India are sometimes swayed away by the classical craving. The product contains the "ten roots" of Dashamuula along with most of the tonic herbs including *Terminalia arjuna, Nepeta hindostana, Convolvulus pluricaulis, Nardostachys jatamansi, Centella asiatica* (47 herbs, 10 mineral drugs). The tonic has been recommended in hypertension, as an adjuvant in the therapy of angina in patients with cardiac risk factors and cardiovascular and cerebrovascular conditions requiring inhibition of platelet aggregation.

This product has been validated by 105 experimental and clinical trials. But, then, can we ignore some studies with single herbs or at the most two to five herbs which exhibited equally encouraging results in the same area.

A clinical trial with 4 single drugs—*Commiphora mukul* oleoresin, *Acorus calamus*, *Inula racemosa* and *Terminalia arjuna*—(against placebo) may provide sufficient leads for pruning complicated cardioprotective formulations.[12]

All the four drug-treated groups showed mild to moderate improvement in symptoms of chest pain and dyspnoea. *Commiphora mukul* oleoresin and *Inula racemosa* groups showed significant reduction in body weight as well as correction of lipid profile. However, restoration of HDL was significant only in *Terminalia arjuna* group. Favourable ECG changes of mild to moderate degree were noted in all the four groups. Total Lipid Atherogenicity Index was significant in *Inula racemosa* group: *Commiphora mukul* oleoresin+, *Acorus calamus*–, *Inula racemosa* ++, *Terminalia arjuna* +.

In an earlier clinical trial, dried and powdered roots of *Inula racemosa* and purified oleoresin of *Commiphora mukul* in 1:1 (w/w) proportion were prescribed (6-8 g/day in divided doses) for 6 months, and gave encouraging results in hyperlipidemia.[13]

A Sri Lankan compound formulation, Karvi Panchakadasha Kashaaya, was shortened to 5 herbs: *Carum carvi*, *Inula racemosa*, *Ricinus communis*, *Bacopa monnieri* and *Boerhavia diffusa*, and was prescribed in the form of decoction (made by boiling 50 g crude drugs in 400 ml water, reducing to one-eighth) to 80 randomly selected patients of essential hypertension as an adjuvant with modern hypertensive drugs, also as an independent drug). At the end of 28 days, both the groups showed significant symptomatic improvement and reduction in systolic and diastolic blood pressure.[14]

These findings again take us back to the product containing 47 herbs and 10 minerals drugs. Dr SA Dahanukar (Seth GS Medical College and KEM Hospital, Mumbai) included it among anti-hypertensives. In normotensive rats it produced a significant lowering of blood pressure, enhancement of vaso-pressor responses to low dose of noradrenaline (with no effect on dopamine beta-hydroxylase activity) and no effect on vaso-depressor responses of acetylcholine and isopernaline. It, however, protected against ethinyl oestradiol-induced hypertension and increased dopamine beta-hydroxylase activity in these hypertensive animals, thus suggesting that it produces effects against ethinyl oestradiol-induced hypertension by its sympatholytic property.[15]

Now that a good number of single herbs are exhibiting CNS-CVS active, antihypertensive, hypolipidemic and cardioprotective potential in experimental and clinical trials, a concerted effort should be made to review and restructure complicated compound formulations of Indian medicine.

Hard core Ayurvedic scholars are creating a serious problem for drug industry. They have assigned botanical names to a host of classical herbs arbitrarily, coined Sanskritized synonyms for non-Ayurvedic herbs to give them a classical touch and did not apply scientific parameters to examine ambiguous and controversial herbs. North-South divide still continues.

Immediate steps should be taken to prune Indication Pluralism from *The Ayurvedic Pharmacopoeia of India.* Only scientifically validated and therapeutically substantiated information should be retained. It is no more possible to accept the therapeutics and guidelines of the 17th century in 21st century.

Divergent sources of important classical herbs are also creating a lot of confusion in polyherbal formulations and herbal research. These must be sorted out by Central Council for Research in Ayurveda and Siddha. (See Table 3). A good number of classical herbs need stringent scientific screening.

Table 3: Divergent Plant Sources of Important Classical Herbs[16]

Plant Drug	Accepted Source	Other Sources
Agaru	*Aquilaria agallocha* (*Thymelaeaceae*)	South India: *Dysoxylum malabaricum* (*Meliaceae*)
Bhaarangi	*Clerodendrum serratum* (*Verbanaceae*)	South India: *Premna herbacea*(*Verbanaceae*) Bengal: *Picrasma quassioides* (*Simarubaceae*)
Bhuunimba Kiraatatikta	*Swertia chirayita* (*Gentianaceae*)	South India: *Andrographis paniculata* (*Acanthaceae*)
Daaruharidraa	*Berberis aristata* (*Berberidaceae*)	South India: *Coscinium fenestratum* (*Menispermaceae*)
Duraalabha/ Dhanvayaasa	*Fagonia cretica* (*Zygophyllaceaea*)	South India: *Tragia involucrata* (*Euphorbiaceae*)
Hapushaa/ Havushaa	*Juniperus communis* (*Pinaceae*)	South India: *Sphaeranthus indicus* (*Asteraceae*)
Jivanti	*Leptadenia reticulata* (*Asclepiadaceae*)	South India: *Holostemma rheedei* (*Asclepiadaceae*)
Muurvaa	*Marsdenia tenacissima* (*Asclepiadaceae*)	South India: *Chonemorpha macrophylla* (*Apocynaceae*) *Sansevieria roxburghiana* (*Liliaceae*) (IMPCOPS, Chennai)
Naagakeshara	*Mesua ferrea* (*Clusiaceae*)	South India: *Calophyllum inophyllum* (*Clusiaceae*) Tamil Nadu: *Cinnamomum wightii* (*Lauraceae*) and *Dillenia pentagyna* (*Dilleniaceae*) fruits

(Table Contd.)

Table 3: Contd.

Plant Drug	Accepted Source	Other Sources
Paashaanabheda	*Bergenia ligulata* (*Saxifragaceae*) Substitute: *Aerva lanata* (*Amaranthaceae*)	South India: *Rotula aquatica* (*Boraginaceae*), *Homonoia riparia* (*Euphorbiaceae*) Gujarat: *Iris pseudacorus* (*Iridaceae*)
Prasaarini	*Paederia foetida* (*Rubiaceae*)	South India: *Merremia tridentata* (*Convolvulaceae*) (An altogether different plant)
Priyangu	*Callicarpa macrophylla* (*Verbenaceae*) Substitute: *Prunus mahaleb* (*Rosaceae*)	South India: *Callicarpa tomentosa* (*Verbenaceae*); *Zanthoxylum rhetsa* (*Rutaceae*); *Aglaia roxburghiana* fruits (*Meliaceae*); *Myristica malabarica* (*Myristicaceae*) dried flowers (IMPCOPS, Chennai)
Prishniparni	*Uraria picta* (*Fabaceae*)	South India: *Pseudarthria viscida* (*Fabaceae*) Kerala: *Desmodium gangeticum* (*Papilionaceae*)
Raasnaa	*Pluchea lanceolata* (*Asteraceae*) Substitute: *Alpinia galanga* (*Zingiberaceae*)	South India: *Alpinia calcarata* and *Alpinia galanga* (*Zingiberaceae*) Andhra Pradesh: *Dodonaea viscosa* (*Sapindaceae*) Eastern India: *Vanda roxburghii* (*Orchidaceae*) Bihar: *Lepidagathis trinervis* (*Acanthaceae*) Madhya Pradesh: *Blepharispermum subsessile* (*Compositae*, *Asteraceae*)
Renukaa	*Vitex agnus-castus* (*Verbenaceae*)	South India: *Vitex altissima*, *Vitex negundo* (*Verbenaceae*) South India: fruits of *Vitex* spp. sold as Arenuka. Fruits of *Piper aurantiacum* (*Piperaceae*) are used as Harenukaa/ Renukaa. (IMPCOPS, Chennai)
Sahachara	*Barleria prionitis* (*Acanthaceae*)	South India: *Niligirianthus ciliatus*, (*Acanthaceae*) Kerala: *Ecbolium viride* (Nila Sahachara), *Justica betonica* (Shveta Sahachara) (*Acanthaceae*)
Saarivaa Shveta Saarivaa	*Hemidesmus indicus* (*Asclepiadaceae*)	South India: *Decalepis hamiltonii*; *Cryptolepis buchanani* (*Asclepiadaceae*); *Ichnocarpus frutescens* used as Krishna Saarivaa (*Apocynaceae*) Kerala, Tamil Nadu, Karnataka: *Decalepis hamiltonii* (*Asclepiadaceae*)
Shati	*Hedychium spicatum* (*Zingiberaceae*)	South India: *Kaempeferia galanga* (Zingiberaceae), *Curcuma zedoaria* (*Zingiberaceae*)

(Table Contd.)

Table 3: Contd.

Plant Drug	Accepted Source	Other Sources
Shankhapushpi	*Convolvulus pluricaulis* (*Convolvulaceae*)	South India: *Evolvulus alsinoides*, *Clitoria ternatea* (*Convolvulaceae* and *Fabaceae* respectively) Bengal: *Canscora decussata* (*Gentianaceae*), *Lavandula bipinnata* (*Labiateae*; *Lamiaceae*)
Shringi Karkatashringi	*Pistacia integerrima* (galls) (*Anacardiaceae*)	South India: *Rhus semialata* galls, *Rhus succedanea* galls (*Anacardiaceae*).
Vidhaari	*Pueraria tuberosa* (*Fabaceae*)	South India: *Adenia hondala* (*Passifloraceae*); *Ipomoea paniculata* (*Convolvulaceae*); *Cycas circinalis* (*Cycadaceae*)

Accepted Source: Appendix of *Ayurvedic Formulary of India*, Second Revised Edition, 2003.

Other sources: Ayurvedic Drugs and their Plant Sources, V V Sivarajan and Indira Balachandran, 1994; *Formulary of Ayurvedic Medicines*, IMPCOPS, Chennai, 1987; K. Vasudevan Nair et al., *Ancient Sc Life*, 5(1): 49–53, 1985; *Plants of Bhava Prakash*, Rashtriya Ayurveda Vidyapeeth, 1999; *Medicinal Plants used in Ayurveda*, Rashtriya Ayurveda Vidyapeeth, 1998.

REFERENCES

1. *Indigenous Drugs of India*, (1933), first edn 1958, second reprint 1994, p. 6, Academic Publishers, Kolkata-700 009.
2. *Perspectives in Pharmaceutical Aspects of Indian Medicinal Plants*, (1986). Scientific Seminar on Medicinal Plants Research, CCRAS, Pune.
3. Shah, DC and SN Sannd, *Scope of Research and Development on Ayurvedic Medicinal Plants with Reference to their useful parts*, Regional Research Centre, CCRAS, Jammu.
4. Studies on the Fermentation of Dashmulaarishta, *Journal of Res. in Ayurveda and Siddha*, (*JRAS*) 1988, IX, 3-4, 150-55.
5. Gupta, RA et al., (1983). *Pharmacological Studies on Dashamula Kwaath*, *JRAS*, Vol IV, 73-84.
6. *Ibid.*, (1984). JRAS, Vol. V, 1-4, 38, 50.
7. Neuropharmological Properties of Several Indian Medicinal Plants, *Jour Res Ind Med*, Vol 3, No 1, 9-18.
8. Screening of Indian Plants for Biological Activity, Part IV, *Ind Jour Exp Biol*, Vol 15, 208-219.
9. Kakiuchi et al., (1991). *Planta Med*, 57, 43; Handa *et al.*, Fitoterapia, (1992), 63, 3.
10. Handa et al., (1992). *Fitoterapia*, 63, 12.
11. Agrawal et al., (1994). *Ind J Nat Prod*, 19(1), 14.
12. Singh, RH, Institute of Medical Sciences, Banaras Hindu University, Varanasi; *Ayu International*, Vol 1, No 1, Jan-March 2001, Gujarat Ayurved University, Jamnagar.
13. Ramji Singh et al., (1991). *JRAS*, Vol XIII, 1-18.
14. Ariyawansa HAS and RH Singh, (supervisor) (1999). Ph.D. Thesis, Dept. of Kayachikitsa, Banaras Hindu University, Varanasi.
15. Bhatt, JD et al., (1998). *Indian J Pharmacol*, 30, 399-403.
16. Khare, CP, (2007). *Indian Medicinal Plants: An Illustrated Dictionary*, Springer.

9

Experimental Studies in India: Scientific Edge over Classical Concepts

In India, Central Council for Research in Ayurveda and Siddha (CCRAS), since its inception in 1978, is making efforts to present pharmacodynamics of Ayurvedic drugs as available in classical treatises and proximate them with modern research investigations.[1] While presenting pharmacological investigations of Ayurvedic medicinal plants and their compounds, the then Director of CCRAS (Dr VN Pandey) wrote in 1996: "The ambitions, expectations and demands of youth for 20-40 years to come, has to be looked into by planners of the renaissance of Ayurveda. We are now precisely on the crossroads to do a technical appraisal. What we have done in the name of the renaissance during post-independent era of first two (1946-66) and later two (1966-1986) decades, and taking an account of the situations, what is to be done in the next four decades (1986-2026) is to pondered over."[2]

Dr Ranjit Roy Chaudhury advocated the continuance of dialogue and interaction between the old and new generations of medical scientists.[1]

In 2005, Central Council for Research in Unani Medicine (CCRUM) brought out "Pharmacological and Toxicological studies on Unani Single and Compound Drugs". The Director of CCRUM, Dr Mohammed Khalid Siddiqui, asserted that these studies will generate necessary information on rational therapy, particularly pharmacokinetics for determining dosing schedule and safety/toxicity.

In India, general pharmacological screening comprises evaluating the drug action on a variety of intact animals as well as tissues and organs isolated from their bodies. Guinea pigs, albino rats, rabbits, frogs and dogs are commonly used animals. The organs usually employed are rabbit and frog heart, isolated as well as intact. Among the isolated tissues (both skeletal as well as smooth muscles), the most easily available are rectus abdominis muscle of frog, guinea pig ileum and rabbit intestine. Experiments on anaesthetised animals involve carrying out a series of standard tests, as well as after injecting the test drug to animals. These include vagal stimulation, carotid artery occlusion, injecting ACh; adrenaline or noradrenaline. An effort is made to classify a herb or compound on the basis of pharmacological screening. Toxicity tests are generally carried out in inbred rats and mice (in vertebrates or non-vertebrates).[3]

A brief review of models adopted for screening biological activities of herbs will prove that India is now consolidating its position on the scientific platform:[4]

1. Activity on A.N.S.

Effect on mammalian blood pressure.
Effect on frog heart.
Effect of aconitine induced arrhythmias in dogs.
Effect of herbal drugs on isolated guinea pig ileum or the isolated ileum of rabbit.
Effect of herbal drugs on the oestrogenprimed uterus of female rats
Effect of herbal drugs on the eyes of rabbits.

2. Activity on Muscles

Effect of drugs on cat's polysynaptic lingo-mandibular reflex for central muscle relaxant activity.
Frog's rectus or rat phrenic nerve diaphragm for effects on neuromuscular junction for peripheral muscle relaxants.
Sciatic nerve gastrocnemius preparation of frog or cat.

3. Activity on C.N.S.

Anaesthetic and hypnotic activity

Rabbit or dog by giving inhalational or general inhalational anaesthetic (not used with herbal drugs).
Rabbit's cornea for assessing local anaesthetic activity.
Hypnotic activity model of rats or mice to assess various righting, pinna, sound reflexes or motor activity.

Antiepileptic activity

Supramaximal electroshock seizure pattern test in rats.
Metrazol induced seizure threshold test in rats.

Analgesic activity

Hardy Woolfe and Goodel method.
Stimulation of tooth pulp in dogs, rabbits or even in man.
Mechanical (Tail Clip method using analgesiometer), thermal (Eddy's hot plate method) or mechanical (Hollander's method), chemical stimulation by using acids, croton oil, 2 phenyl 4 benzo quinine, bradykinin or by producing aconitine-induced writhing response in mice or rats.

Tranquillising activity

(a) Effect on gross behaviour

Decrease of spontaneous locomotor activity.
Catalepsy.

Hypothermia.
Prolongation of pentobarbital/ hexobarbital sleeping time.

(b) Effect on unlearnt behaviour
Taming effect on cats and monkeys.
Abolition of fighting behavior in beta spiendens (Siamese fighting fish).
Abolition of "Shamrage" in decorticated and diencephalic cats.

(c) Effect on learnt behaviour
Impairment of performance in Maize, or skinner's box or light discrimination box. Blockade of conditioned avoidance responses.
Decrease in lever pressing rate of rats with chronically implanted electrodes in "pleasure centres".

(d) Effect on stress-induced behaviour
Conflict neurosis in rats and cats.

(e) Adaptogenic activity
Mice and rats, swimming endurance test; stress-induced gastric ulcer in rats; milk-induced leucocytosis in mice; stress-induced increase in adrenal weight; rats in cold-hypoxia-restraint (C-H-R) model, recently developed by the scientists of the Defence Institute of Physiology and Allied Sciences, New Delhi (Dr Srivastava KK and associates).

(f) Antagonism of C.N.S. stimulants
Amphetamine induced stimulation.
Methods used for assessing anti-depressant activity.
Reserpine reversal test.
Amphetamine potentiation test in rats.
Swimming despair test in mice.

(g) Anti-emetic effects
Apomorphine induced vomiting in dogs.
CT-zone ablated dogs.

4. Autacoid Activity

Anti-allergic/antihistaminic activity
Model: Mast cell degranulation produced by diazoxide or compound 48/80 in rats, antigen or histamine-induced bronchospasm in guinea pigs, antigen induced histamine release from peritoneal mast cells sensitized rats *in vitro*, isolated guinea pig lung preparations, egg-induced passive cutaneous anaphylaxis (PCA) in albino rats.

5. Anti-inflammatory and Anti-pyretic Activity

Carrageenine and cotton pellet-induced oedema in rats and mice, formaline or adjuvant induced arthritis akin to that of human rheumatoid arthritis, croton oil-induced oedema in rats, oedema induced by chemical mediators like histamine, serotonin, bradykinin, etc. Brewer's yeast-induced pyrexia in rats for anti-pyretic activity.

6. Activity on GIT

Anti-ulcerogenic activity

Prednisolone or histamine or aspirin/ phenylbutazone or stress-induced ulcers in rats and guinea pigs. Gastric pouch studies and analysis of gastric juices.
Antiemetic activity models in dogs or cats as described above.
Spasmolytic activity as described above.

7. Hepatoprotective Activity

Model: Carbon tetrachloride-induced hepatotoxicity in rats and rabbits; stimulated viral hepatitis; fatty infiltration and cirrhosis; alcohol-induced liver damage on non-hepatectomised and partially hepatectomised rats; galactosamine-induced hepatic damage in rats.

8. Metabolic Disorders

Hypoglycaemic activity

Model: Normal and alloxan-induced diabetic rats, rabbits, guinea pigs and dogs; streptozotocin-induced diabetic rats; pancreatectomised dogs; hormone-induced diabetic models in rats, guinea pigs and rabbits; insulin deficient models using insulin antibodies in guinea pigs; viral-induced diabetic model and in spontaneous diabetic mice, transgenic animals.

Hypolipidaemic activity

Model: Cholesterol fed rabbits or guinea pigs, albino rats or dogs.

9. Urinary Activity

Diuretic and anti-diuretic activity on the urinary flow in rats.

10. Antifertility Activity

Female rats for oestrogenic/anti-oestrogenic activity; male rats for inhibition of spermatogenesis.

11. Antimalarial Activity

In malarial mice and rhesus monkeys.

12. Anti-infective Activity

Plant (alcoholic, ethanolic and aqueous) extracts, essential oil and seed extracts tested *in vitro* for their antibacterial, antifungal, antiviral and anthelmintic activity.

13. Anticancer or Effects on Genomic Structure

Besides routine toxicity studies (mostly not done with herbal drugs), studies are being done by using cell lines or even human cancerous or rat's tissue using Western Blotting technique and other similar methods to find changes in genomic proteins and the cell dividing enzymes. Occasionally, Amese test is used for toxicity studies.

On the basis of pharmacological and toxicological studies (350 by CCRAS, 72 by Central Research Institute for Siddha, Chennai, 92 by CCRUM and more than 13,000 by Central Drug Research Institute, Lucknow, during the last 42 years), a new classification of Indian medicinal plants has emerged. This has facilitated further research in the right direction and paved the way for appropriate clinical trials. Adaptogenic, anti-inflammatory, cardio-protective, CNS active, CVS active, hypolipidaemic, hepatoprotective, hypoglycaemic, ulcero-protective, chemoprotective, cytoprotective activities of Indian medicinal plants are being studied experimentally, but scientific validation will depend upon the results of clinical trials.[5]

Dr CK Katiyar, Former Director, Herbal Drug Research, Ranbaxy Laboratory Ltd, Gurgaon, Haryana, presented an analysis of 68 clinical trials conducted in India (during 1980-2004):

Randomised open	:	28
Open comparative	:	13
Double-blind placebo controlled	:	7
Single-blind placebo controlled	:	5
Single-blind reference controlled	:	4
Double-blind comparative	:	3
Open comparative placebo-controlled	:	3
Open add-on, flexi-dose open, Double-blind cross-over, Open add-on comparative, Open non-comparative	:	1 each

All the clinical trials (except two) showed significant efficacy. But majority of the trails, according to Dr Katiyar, did not fulfil the criteria of well-conducted, well-planned trials in terms of designing, statistics and parameters of evaluation. Various researchers followed varying clinical trial methodologies herbal products, leading sometimes to inconsistent results. While summarising the analysis, Dr Katiyar observed: "Almost all clinical trials (with Ayurvedic medicines) prove efficacy, but surprisingly, effective Ayurvedic medicines in the market (are) literally none!"[6]

Table 4: Contd.

Botanical Name	Ayurvedic/Native Name	Adverse Effects and Interactions
Areca catechu Linn.	Puga	Interactions: High tannin of the nut may cause alkaloids to become insoluble and precipitate. The cholinergic activity of arecoline interacts with anti-cholinergic drugs.[5,14] Toxic constituents: Arecoline, arecain (pyridine alkaloids).[11] Asthmatic and chronic obstructive pulmonary disease (COPD) patients may be at risk.[14]
Argemone mexicana Linn.	Svarnakshiri	Adulteration of edible oil with sanguinarine containing argemone oil has led to widespread epidemic of dropsy and glaucoma. Sanguinarine is also carcinogenic.[4b] Traditional medicinal uses attributed to this plant are based on wrong identity.[4b] Drugs interacting with the herbs: Anticholinergic drugs, cholinergic drugs, procycline.[2]
Argyreia speciosa Sweet	Vriddhadaaruka	Seeds contain 0.5-0.9% ergoline alkaloids; a few are reported to be hallucinogenic. LD_{50}: 500 mg/kg body wt.[4b]
Aristolochia indica Linn.	Ishvari	Toxic constituents: Aristolochin, aristolochic acid.[11] Toxic to kidneys. Carcinogenic in animals and human cells.[2,11] Many cases of nephropathy associated with the use of aristolochia have been reported worldwide.[2] Any product, which contains plants known or suspected to contain aristolochic acid, is detained in the U.S.[2] A cytotoxic lignan, savinin, has been isolated from the root.[4c] Root: Oxytocic, emmenagogue, abortifacient.[4b]
Artemesia nilagirica (C.B. Clarke) Pamp.	Damanaka	Emmenagogue, uterine stimulant.[4b,10] Toxic constituent: Thujone.[11,4c] May interact with anticonvulsants, may lower seizure threshold.[12] *A. absinthium*: Plant extract decreased hepatotoxicity of acetaminophen in mice.[5] Contraindicated in pregnancy.[17(2)]
Artocarpus heterophyllus Lam.	Panasa	A lectin, jacalin, a potent polyclonal activator for human lymphocytes has been isolated from the seeds.[4c]
Artocarpus lakoocha Roxb.	Lakucha	A lectin, artocarpin, isolated from the seeds precipitates several galactomannans. Besides human and animal erythrocytes, it agglutinates rat lymphocytes and mouse ascites cells.[4c]
Asparagus adscendens Roxb.	Mushali (Safed)	*A. officinalis*: Contraindicated in inflammatory kidney diseases; in oedema due to functional heart or kidney disorders.[1,10]
Asparagus racemosus Willd.	Shataavari	The alkaloid asparagamine A (in the root) showed antioxytocic activity *in vitro*.[4d] Roots are reported to show inhibitory effects on digestive enzymes, lipase and trypsin may lead to stoppage of degradation of food material in the intestinal tract.[4c]

Table 4: Contd.

Botanical Name	Ayurvedic/Native Name	Adverse Effects and Interactions
Azadirachta indica A. Juss.	Nimba	The oil might cause morphological changes in sperm; leaf can affect sperm motility and viability. Avoid in couples with infertility.[2] Might decrease the effectiveness of immunosuppressants in organ transplant patients.[2] Cardiac arrest due to Neem leaf poisoning reported.[16(3)]
Bacopa monnieri (Linn.) Wettst.	Brahmi	Herb: Prolongs hypnotic effect of pentobarbitone; may antagonise the haloperidol-induced catalepsy, suggesting an involvement of GABA-ergic system. Potentiates phenothiazines.[5] Herb's CNS action does not include serious sedation; caution with phenothiazine co-administration is indicated.[3] Taking 300 mg extract per day for 12 weeks improved verbal learning, memory and information processing in healthy men and women. (Psychopharmacology, Berl, 2001,156: 481-84).[2]
Bambusa arundinacea Willd.	Vansha	Tender shoots and root contain a cyanogenic glucoside.[4b] Ethanolic extract of tender shoots adversely affects the sperm count and motility in rats.[4e]
Bambusa arundinacea (Retz.) Roxb.	Vansa Rochana	Manna consists of silica 90.5, potash 1.1, alumina 0.4 and iron peroxide 0.9%.[4b]
Bauhinia variegata Linn.	Kaanchanaara	Seeds exhibit hemagglutinating activity.[4c]
Berberis asiatica DC.	Daruharidraa	Toxic constituent: Berberine (isoquinoline alkaloids). Berberine containing herbs: Not recommended during pregnancy.[10] Berberine is well tolerated up to 0.5 g, equivalent to about 8 g dried root. Therapeutic dose. Powder 0.32-2.6 g.[11] Drugs interaction with berberine: Cyclosorine, Cytochrome P450 3A4 (CYP3A4) substrates.[2]
Bergenia ciliata (Haw.) Sternb.	Paashaanabheda	*Bergenia ciliata* rhizome: Acetone extract reported to be cardiotoxic in higher doses and depressant on CNS. Mildly diuretic; in higher doses anti-diuretic in experimental animals.[4b]
Boerhavia diffusa Linn.	Punarnavaa	Official as a diuretic in IP. The cholinergic activity of the root was observed *in vitro* but not *in vivo*.[4d]
Boswellia serrata Roxb.	Shallaki	For osteoarthritis (effective adult dose): 250-1200 mg of alcoholic dry extract (4.2-5.9:1, to contain approximately 65% of total organic acids) divided into 3 doses.[8b] Boswellic acids might prevent organ rejection and ischemia/reperfusion injury.[2]

Table 4: Contd.

Botanical Name	Ayurvedic/Native Name	Adverse Effects and Interactions
Brassica alba Boiss	Sarshapa Gaura	Isothiocyanates can cause endemic goitre.[2] Irritant poisoning (on ingestion of a large quantity) can occur in people with kidney disorders.[2] GRAS status in the US.
Brassica campestris Hook. f. & Thoms.	Sarshapa	The pollen grains act as allergens causing bronchial and bronchopulmonary problems. Glycoprotein containing 11.4% of carbohydrate is the main allergin.[4d]
Brassica juncea (Linn.), Czern. & Coss.	Raajikaa	Toxic constituent: Glucosinolates.[11] Vegetables containing glucosinolates are goitrogenic.[5] Drugs interacting with black mustard: Antacids, H_2 Blockers, and Proton Pump Inhibitors.[2]
Butea monosperma (Lam.) Kuntze	Palaasha	Flower and seed: Anti-oestrogenic. Seed: Nephrotoxic. Anthelmintic principle: Palasonin.[4b]
Calotropis gigantea (Linn.) Ait. f.	Arka	Root: Cardiac glycosides[2] may be additive with digoxin.[5] Drugs interacting with the herb: Digoxin, diuretic drugs, stimulant laxatives.[2]
Cannabis sativa Linn.	Bhangaa	Toxic constituents: Tetrahydrocannabinol (cannabinoids 15-20%).[11] Oxytocic, crosses human placenta, high doses damage developing embryos.[11] Dried, crushed mature leaves and flower shoots, known as Bhaang, are an ingredient in cannabis chocolates in the U.S. and New Mexico.
Carthamus tinctorius Linn.	Kusumbha	Flowers: Sedative, emmenagogue.[4b] The plant contains a propanetriol derivative, which can be used for the treatment of circulatory disorders.[4c] Inhibits platelet aggregation.[16(3)]
Carum carvi Linn.	Jeeraka Krishna	Seed: May lower blood glucose and test results.[2] Should not be used in gastro-oesophageal reflux disease or during pregnancy (uterine relaxation may occur). Side effects include renal dysfunction.[7] Drugs interacting with the herbs: Antidiabetic drugs.[2]
Cassia fistula Linn.	Aaragvadha	Pulp of pod and Senna spp: Contraindicated in abdominal pain of unknown origin, pregnancy, lactation, appendicitis, Crohn's disease, ulcerative colitis, ileus, intestinal inflammation or obstruction, children under 12 year of age;[15,8(a)] in haemorrhoids.[10] With chronic use or abuse: Electrolyte imbalance, potassium deficiency, albuminuria, hematuria.[1] May potentiate toxicity of digitalis and diuretics.[12] Toxic constituents in senna spp.—anthraquinone glycosides, dianthrones, anthrones.[11] Drugs interacting with the herbs: Digoxin, diuretic drugs.[2]
Celastrus paniculatus Willd.	Jyotishmati	Seed oil: CNS depressant, additive to pentobarbitol.[4b]

Table 4: Contd.

Botanical Name	Ayurvedic/Native Name	Adverse Effects and Interactions
Centella asiatica (Linn.) Urban	Manduukaparni	Emmenagogue.[3,6] Excessive internal use is contraindicated in early pregnancy.[6] Canadian regulations do not allow the use of herb as a non-medical ingredient for oral use products.[10] In majority of randomised and placebo controlled studies, in which daily dose of 60-180 mg of *Centella* triterpene fractions have been taken orally for periods upto 12 months, no side effects were reported.[8(b)]
Chenopodium album Linn.	Vaastuka	Toxic constituents of *C. ambrosioides*. (American wormseed): Ascaridole (unsaturated terpene peroxide of volatile oxide); nitrates. Emmenagogue, abortifacient.[11]
Cinnamomum camphora (Linn.) Nees & Eberm.	Karpura	Contraindicated externally on injured skin, burns[1], preparation not to be used in the facial region of infants and small children, especially in the nasal area.[1,10] Not for long-term use.[10] Toxic constituents: Camphor (volatile saturated ketone), 30-50% of volatile oil; safrole, cincole, (volatile oxides) in crude camphor oil.[11] Camphorated oil (20% camphor in cottonseed oil) was removed from the US market due to toxicity in 1980s. Available without a prescription in Canada.[2]
Cinnamomum zeylanicum Blume	Tvak	Contraindicated in pregnancy,[1,17(1)] stomach and duodenal ulcers.[16(1)] Large doses caused stimulation of vasomotor center.[5,10] Drugs interacting with the herb: Antidiabetic drugs.[2]
Cissampelos pareira Linn.	Paathaa	Root: Alkaloid haytine (methiodide and methochloride derivatives), reported to be potent neuromuscular-blocking agent.[4b]
Cissus quadrangularis Linn.	Asthisamhaara	Total alcoholic extract of the plant, on parenteral administration, neutralises antianabolic effect of cortisone in healing fractures.[4b]
Citrullus colocynthis (Linn.) Schrad.	Indravaaruni	Toxic constituents in dried pulp or unripe fruit: Up to 3% E-, I- and L-cucurbitacins and 0.21% alpha-elaterin (glycosides). Toxic dose: 0.6-1 g.[11] Contraindicated in infections or inflammatory gastrointestinal conditions. Death has resulted from the consumption of as little as 1½ teaspoons of powder.[2] Drugs interacting with the herb: Digoxin, diuretic drugs.[2]
Citrus limon (Linn.) Burm. f.	Jambira	The furocoumarins, bergapten and oxypeucedanin in oil are photosensitising. Topically photosensitivity can occur.[2]
Clematis gouriana Roxb.	Muurvaa (substitute)	Leaves: Protoanemonin is a direct irritant to the skin and mucous membranes, check after drying the herb.[10]

Table 4: Contd.

Botanical Name	Ayurvedic/Native Name	Adverse Effects and Interactions
Cyperus rotundus Linn.	Mustaa	Methanolic extract of plant stimulates the production of melanin in cultured melanocytes.[4c] Alcoholic and aqueous extract of tubers possess lipolytic action.[4c]
Datura metel Linn.	Dhattura	Toxic constituents: Hyoscine, hyoscyamine.[11] Adverse reactions: Agitation, blurred vision, dilated pupils, disorientation, hallucinations, mydriasis, tachycardia, seizures, xerostomia and coma.[5] Lethal dose for adults: 15-25 g seeds; 100 mg atropine.[11] Contraindicated in tachycardiac arrhythmia, glaucoma.[17(1)]
Desmodium gangeticum DC.	Shaalparni	Root extract exhibited significant antifertility activity at 50 and 100 mg/kg in rats.[4c]
Dolichos biflorus Linn.	Kulattha	A dipeptide, pyroglutamyglutamine, is diuretic, found to be 2-3 times that of acetazolamide in albino rats.[4c]
Dorema ammoniacum D. Don	Ushaka	Oleo-gum resin is the source of the drug Amoniacum.[4a]
Echinochloa frumentacea Link	Shyaamaaka	Contains glutelin.[4a]
Elettaria cardamomum Maton	Elaa	Contraindicated in case of gallstones (to be used only after consultation with physician);[1,16(4)] in gastro-oesophageal reflux disease,[7] cholagogue.[1]
Embelia ribes Burm. f.	Vidang	A potential contraceptive plant.[4c] Embelin: antispermatogenic, changes can be reversed.[4c]
Ephedra nebrodensis Tineo/ *gerardiana* Wall.	"Soma" (component)	Toxic constituents: Ephedrine, pseudoephedrine, (2-aminophenylpropane alkaloids),[11] contraindicated in coronary thrombosis, diabetes, glaucoma,[16(1)] anxiety, high blood pressure, glaucoma, impaired circulation of the cerebrum, adenoma of the prostate with residual urine accumulation, pheochromocytoma, thyrotoxicosis, may potentiate MAO inhibition.[3,10,13] Interacts with methyldopa, beta blockers, caffeine, monoamine oxidase inhibitors, theophylline sympathomimetics, St John's Wort, Guanethidine, cardiac glycosides, oxytocin.[12]
Erythrina variegata Linn.	Paaribhadra	Alkaloids: Muscle relaxants, increase the sedative effect of hexabarbitol, LD_{50} in mice 306.4 mg/kg.[4c]
Euphorbia hirta Linn.	Dugdhikaa	Contraindicated in individuals with infection or inflammatory gastrointestinal conditions.[2]
Euphorbia neriifolia auct. non Linn.	Snuhi	Canadian regulations do not allow Euphorbia in foods.[10]

Table 4: Contd.

Botanical Name	Ayurvedic/Native Name	Adverse Effects and Interactions
Ferula foetida Regel.	Hingu	Emmenagogue, uterine stimulant,[10] contraindicated in infant colic,[17(1)] in bleeding disorders, pregnancy, infection or inflammatory GI diseases,[5] peptic ulcers,[6] 50-100 mg of gum resin may cause convulsions in persons suffering from nervousness.[2,10] Drugs interacting with the herb: Anticoagulant/antiplatelet drugs, antihypertensive drugs.[2]
Ficus beng(h)alensis Linn.	Vata	Bark extracts due to leucodelphinidin and bengalenoside, not to be taken concurrently with diabetes medications.[5] These constituents decreased blood glucose in research animals.[5]
Ficus hispida Linn. f.	Kaakodumbara	Fruits, seeds, bark: Emetic.[4c]
Foeniculum vulgare Mill.	Mishreyaa/ Shatapushpaa	Fennel oil: Not to be used for infants and toddlers.[1] Estragole (5-10% of essential oil): a procarcinogen,[10] concomittant use of fennel may reduce ciprofloxacin bioavailability by nearly 50%, possibly due to calcium, iron and magnesium contained in fennel. Fennel increases tissue distribution and slows the elimination of ciprofloxacin.[2,14] Similar effects from fluroquinolones.[14] Seed oil and anethole: emmenagogue.[16(3)] Avoid during pregnancy.[17(2)]
Fumaria parviflora Lam.	Parpataka	Should not be used by persons with seizure disorders or increased intraocular pressure.[7] *Fumaria officinalis* contraindicated in biliary obstructions. In cases of gallstones, not to be used without medical advice.[8b] Raised intraocular pressure and oedema.[17(1)]
Garcinia indica Choisy	Vrikshaamla	Garcinia cambogia: Mixed evidence of the use of garcinia fruit rind extract for weight loss. An extract containing 50% hydroxycitric acid, 1000 mg three times daily and 500 mg four times daily has been used.[(2)]
Gentiana kurroo Royle	Traayamaana	Toxic constituents in *G. lutea* root are: Amarogentine, gentiopicrin, swertiamarin, sweroside, (iridoid monoterpenes).[11] Contraindicated in gastric and duodenal ulcers.[1] Emmenagogue.[16(3)]
Gloriosa superba Linn.	Laangali	Young sprouts, seeds, tubers: Source of colchicine.[4a]
Glycyrrhiza glabra Linn.	Yashtimadhu	Toxic constituent in the root: 6-14% Glycyrrhizic acid (saponin glycoside) interacts with spironolactone (antagonises diuretic effect), cardiac glycosides, thiazide diuretics (can cause hypokalemia, may potentiate digoxin toxicity, corticosteroids, cyclosporine, monoamine oxidase inhibitors (immunostimulating effect may decrease response to the drugs). Sympathomimetic

Table 4: Contd.

Botanical Name	Ayurvedic/Native Name	Adverse Effects and Interactions
		amines may increase the risk of hypertensive crisis.[12,10] Contraindicated in cholestatic liver disorders, liver cirrhosis, hypertonia, hypokalemia, severe kidney insufficiency, pregnancy[1], bleeding disorders, diabetes (on insulin), impotence, male infertility.[5] Deglycyrrhizinized licorice (DGL) is usually free of side effects.[10] French regulation limits daily consumption to 5 g or as tea 8 g.[10]
Gossypium arboreum Linn.	Kaarpaasaka	Root bark: Abortifacient, emmenagogue, uterine stimulant, contraindicated in urogenital irritation or tendency to inflammation. Chronic use may cause sterility in man.[10] Gossypol decreases sperm count, interacts with diuretics and potentiates hypokalemia, with NSAIDs, increases gastrointestinal irritations; concurrent use with thyroid replacement therapy may require an increase in dosage of the drug.[5] Canadian regulation does not allow an excess of 450 ppm of free gossypol in foods (cotton seed meal and oils).[10] Drugs interacting with gossypol: Digoxin, diuretic drugs, NSAIDs, stimulant laxatives, theophylline.[2]
Gymnema sylvestre R. Br.	Ajashringi	Gymnemic acid and gurmarin inhibit the ability to taste bitter (quinine) or sweet (sugar), without affecting the ability to taste sour, astringent or pungent flavours.[2]
Hemidesmus indicus R. Br.	Anantamuula	Known as Indian or false Sarsaparilla, in Western herbals; according to Tyler (Honest herbals), does not contain same saponins or other principal constituents found in Sarsaparilla.
Hibiscus rosa-sinensis Linn.	Japaa	Alcoholic extract of flowers showed anti-implantation activity.[4c,d]
Holarrhena antidysenterica (Linn.) Wall.	Kutaja	Latex: Irritant, high doses affect blood vascular system.[4c]
Hordeum vulgare Linn.	Yava	Seeds contain gliadin, a component of gluten.[5] May suppress the secretion of milk in women whose children have died after birth. (Chinese *Materia Medica*, GA Stuart).
Hyoscyamus niger Linn.	Khuraashaanikaa	Toxic constituents in whole plant: Scopolamine (hyoscine), hyoscyamine, butyrine (tropane alkaloids), hyospicrin (glucoside).[11] Leaf: Contraindicated in tachycardiac arrythmias,[17(1)] prostatic adenoma with urine retention, narrow angle glaucoma, acute pulmonary oedema, mechanical stenosis in any part of the gastrointestinal tract, megacolon.[1] Hyoscymine and scopolamine alkaloids are anti-cholinergic.[5] Therapeutic dose: 130-325 mg powder, Hyoscine hydrobromate 0.33-0.93 mg.[11]

Table 4: Contd.

Botanical Name	Ayurvedic/Native Name	Adverse Effects and Interactions
Imperata cylindrica Beauv.	Darbha	Leaves and stem contain cyanophoric compounds.[4c] Plant can be used as a substitute for Ephedra (as an anti-fatigue agent).[4c]
Indigofera tinctoria Linn.	Nili	The plant contains an appreciable amount of conjugated indoxyl, together with rotenoids. Can be used in endogenous depression.[4c] Indirubin isolated from the plant : An antitumour constituent.[4d]
Inula racemosa Hook. f.	Pushkarmula	The root powder has been found to possess beta blocking activity.[4c]
Juniperus communis Linn.	Hapushaa	Fruits are contraindicated in pregnancy and inflammatory kidney diseases.[1,10,17(2)] Not for use exceeding four to six weeks in succession. Canadian regulation does not allow juniper as a non-medical ingredient for oral use products.[10] The volatile monoterpenes are irritant to the urinary mucosa.[11]
Lathyrus sativus Linn.	Kalaaya	Seeds: Neurotoxic.[4c]
Lawsonia inermis Linn.	Madayanti	Leaf: History of internal use as an abortifacient is recorded in Africa.[10] Leaf juice (50 g) is an oral herbal contraceptive in both the sexes; prolonged use may cause permanent sterility.[4c]
Linum usitatissimum Linn.	Atasi	Contraindicated in intestinal obstruction of any origin,[1,8(a)] bleeding disorders, elevated prolactin, hypokalemia.[5] Use during pregnancy or lactation, only on medical advice.[5] Toxic constituents: Linatine, (glutamic acid derivatives) from seed; lotaustralin (cyanogenic glycosides) from leaves, stems and roots; 0.1-1.5 % linustatin and neolinustatin (cyanogenic glycosides) in seeds.[11] In spite of cyanogenic glycosides, single dose of upto 150-300 g of powdered linseed is not toxic.[8(a)]
Loranthus longiflorus Desr.	Vandaaka	Plant: Diuretic, antilithiatic.[4c]
Madhuca indica J. F. Gmel.	Madhuuka	Seed oil causes total but reversible sterility in male rats; shows testicular atrophy and degeneration of seminiferous tubules.[4c]
Malva rotundifolia Linn.	Suvarchalaa	Leaves: Emmenagogue.[4a]
Maranta arundinacea Linn.	Tikhura	Roots: Canadian regulations do not allow arrow roots as a non-medical ingredient for oral use products.[10] The tuber contains a protease inhibitor, which inhibits the proteolytic activity of human and bovine pancreatic secretion.[4d]
Marsdenia tenacissima W. & A.	Muurvaa	The roots are used as a substitute for Black Nishoth (*Ipomoea turpethium*) [4c]

Table 4: Contd.

Botanical Name	Ayurvedic/Native Name	Adverse Effects and Interactions
Melia azedarach Linn.	Mahaanimba	Fruits: Poisonous. Cases of severe poisoning have been reported.[4a]
Mimosa pudica Linn.	Lajjaalu	Feeding trials with horses in large doses caused toxic symptoms including loss of hairs. Leaf meal caused stunted growth in chicks.[4a]
Momordica charantia Linn.	Kaaravella	Potentiates the effects of hypoglycemic drugs.[12] Safety in pregnancy is not established. Red arils should not be consumed by children. Excessive amount can cause diarrhoea and GI distress.[5] Juice: Emmenagogue and abortifacient.[6]
Moringa oleifera Lam.	Shigru	Root and bark extract: Antifertility activity in experimental animals.[4c] Root more potent than bark.[4c] Due to levodopa, the herb might cause false urine glucose test, elevated liver function test, elevated urine uric acid levels.[2] Drugs interacting with the herb: Antidiabetic drugs, antipsychotic drugs, guanethidine, methyldopa, MAOs inhibitors, tricyclic antidepressants.[2]
Myrica nagi Hook. f./*Myrica esculenta* Buch.-Ham.	Katphala	Canadian regulations do not allow bayberry (Myrica) as a non-medical ingredient for oral use products.[10] Fruits are sedative.[4a]
Myristica fragrans Houtt.	Jaatiphala	Toxic constituents: Myristicin, elemicine, safrole. More than 5 gm of powdered nutmeg, or mace affects the central nervous system, producing hallucinations, headache, dizziness, drowsiness, nausea, stomach pain, liver pain, excessive thirst, rapid pulse, anxiety, double vision and sometimes acute panic, coma or death.[1,5,10] Upon ingestion of 9 teaspoons of nutmeg powder per day, an atropine like effect was observed.[1,5] When taken in larger amount, the herb has abortifacient effect.[1]
Nardostachys jatamansi DC.	Jataamaansi	Rhizome: Emmenagogue, uterine stimulant.[10] Oil: Potentiated phenobarbital narcosis, reduced brain serotonin content in rats.[4c] Action at variance with that of reserpine, which has direct action on cell to liberate serotonin.[4c]
Nelumbo nucifera Gaertn.	Kamala	Contraindicated in constipation and stomach distention.[10]
Nerium indicum Mill.	Karavira	Powdered extract of leaf: Contraindicated in hypercalcaemia.[5] Entire plant is toxic, has caused fatal poisonings. Contains cardiac glycosides.[5] Between 65-86% of the cardioactive glycosides are absorbed and about 50% are protein bound. The duration of effect is about 2.65 days.[11]

Table 4: Contd.

Botanical Name	Ayurvedic/Native Name	Adverse Effects and Interactions
Ocimum basilicum Linn.	Barbari Shveta	Not recommended for infants or toddlers or for extended period of time.[10] The herb contains about 0.5% of essential oil with upto 85% of estragole (a procarcinogen).[1,5]
Ocimum sanctum Linn.	Surasaa	Essential oil contains estragole (a procarcinogen).[5] In mice, leaf extract decreased serum T4. To be used with caution in thyroid diseases.[5] Conflicting reports on embryotoxicity.[16(2)]
Origanum majorana Linn.	Phanijjaka	Emmenagogue,[6] has the potential to stimulate menstruation.[2] Should be avoided in early pregnancy.[6]
Paederia foetida Linn.	Prasaarani	Root and bark: Emetic.[4a]
Papaver somniferum Linn.	Ahiphena	Toxic constituents in latex from unripe seed capsules: Morphine, codeine, papaverine (isoquinoline alkaloids).[11] Opium is a controlled substance in many countries.[10]
Picrorhiza kurroa Royle ex Benth.	Katuki	There is some concern that Picrorhiza might adversely affect patients with autoimmune disorders because of its immune stimulating effects. Avoid using in patients with multiple sclerosis, systemic lupus erythomatosus, rheumatoid arthritis and other autoimmune disorders.[2] Interacts with immunosuppressants.[2] 70% methanol extract not teratogenic.[16(4)]
Piper cubeba Linn. f.	Kankola	Contraindicated in nephritis,[2,10] also in individuals with infections or inflammatory GI conditions.[2] Drugs interacting with the herb: Antacids, H_2 Blockers, Proton Pump Inhibitors.[2]
Piper longum Linn.	Pippali	Contraindicated in pregnancy in large doses.[5,6] Piperine inhibits gastric emptying and GI transit. Also increases drug induced sleep.[5]
Piper nigrum Linn.	Maricha	Contraindicated in pregnancy in large doses.[5,6] Phenytoin was more rapidly and completely absorbed and eliminated more slowly when taken with piperine.[6] Piperine can augment the therapeutic effects of phenobarbital, phenytoin, rifampicin, theophylline and other drugs. It can also predispose the patient to an increased risk of side effects of drugs with a narrow therapeutic window that are liver metabolised (e.g., theophylline).[14] Drugs interacting with the herbs: CYP 3A4 substrates, P-glycoprotein substrates, phenytoin, propranolol, rifampicin, sparteine, theophylline.[2]
Pisum sativum Linn.	Harenu	An antifertility agent. m-xylohydroquinone, isolated from peas, produced fatal resorption in rats; in humans reduced fertility rate by 50%.[4d]

Table 4: Contd.

Botanical Name	Ayurvedic/Native Name	Adverse Effects and Interactions
Polygonatum verticillatum All.	Medaa	Plant: Diuretic, contains a digitalis glucoside.[4a] Rhizomes may be used as a source of diosgenin.[4c]
Prunus amygdalus Batsch	Vaataama	A Japanese patent claims isolation of low molecular weight peptides with analgesic and anti-inflammatory properties.[2] Drugs interacting with the herb: ACE inhibitors, antihypertensive drugs.[2]
Prunus cerasus Linn.	Elavaaluka	Leaves: Anticonvulsant. Seed kernel: Nervine tonic.[4a]
Psoralea corylifolia Linn.	Baakuchi	Toxic symptoms of seeds: Nausea, vomiting, malaise, GI disturbances. External application of oil: Irritant to skin, causes blistering.[4a] Oil even in high dilutions (upto 1 in 100,000) increases tone of the uterus and stimulates smooth muscles of experimental animals.[4a] A mixture of psoralen and isopsoralen (in 1:3 ratio) is recommended in leucoderma.[4d] A powder has been patented in China containing salt as the main ingredient with *P. corylifolia* extract for odontopathy, dental caries and peri-odontal diseases. In Japan, oral compositions are being patented containing extracts of *P. corylifolia* for controlling *Streptococcus mutans* related dental caries.[4d]
Pterocarpus santalinus Linn. f.	Chandana (Rakta)	Regulated in the US as an allowable flavouring agent in alcoholic beverages only.[10]
Punica granatum Linn.	Daadima	Dried root bark, stem bark, seeds contain: toxic constituents pelletrin, piperidine alkaloids 0.4%, punicalagin, punicacontein C, casurin (tannins 20-25%).[10,11]
Quercus infectoria Olivier	Maajuuphalaka	Oak bark: Contraindicated in cardiac insufficiency, hypertonia and externally on broken skin.[5] Tannins may interfere with absorption of drugs.[5]
Randia dumetorum Poir.	Madanaphala	Fruit pulp: Emetic and abortificient, potentiates pentobarbitone, depresses heart, relaxes ileum, antagonises effect of acetylcholine (in animal studies).[4a,c]
Randia uliginosa DC.	Pinditaka	Roasted pulp is used during pregnancy in GI distress.[4a]
Raphanus sativus Linn.	Muulaka	Contraindicated in cholelithiasis.[1] It might cause biliary colic.[2] Seeds contain glycosidically bound mustard oils.[4a] Red raddish contains anthocyanins.[4d]
Rauvolfia serpentina Benth. ex Kurz	Sarpagandhaa	Contraindicated in depression, ulcer, pheochromocytoma, pregnancy and lactation,[1] Parkinson's disease.[7] Toxic constituents: Reserpine, serpentine, raupine, ajmaline and other indole alkaloids.[11]

Table 4: Contd.

Botanical Name	Ayurvedic/Native Name	Adverse Effects and Interactions
Rheum emodi Wall. ex Meisn	Vetasaamala	Rhubarb root: Contraindicated with other stimulant laxatives,[16(1)] renal disorders,[17(1)] in intestinal obstruction, Crohn's disease, colitis ulcerosa, appendicitis, abdominal pain of unknown origin,[1] pregnancy and children under 12 years of age.[1] Toxic constituents: Emodin, anthraquinones.[11]
Ricinus communis Linn.	Eranda	Seed oil: Contraindicated in intestinal obstruction and abdominal pain of unknown origin, appendicitis, ulcerative colitis.[5,10] Must be used with caution during pregnancy and menstruation;[10] with cardiac glycosides, antiarrhythmic drugs, diuretics, cortisol, liquorice, antihistamines and fat-soluble vitamins.[16(4)] Toxic constituents (seeds, leaves): 3% ricin (toxalbumin), ricinine.[11]
Salvia plebeia R. Br.	Samudrashosha	Sage leaf: Essential oil and alcoholic extracts contraindicated during pregnancy.[1,10] Sage oil contains more thujone than absinthium oil, yet it has not been reported as toxic.[10.] Alcoholic preparations to be used with caution due to the presence of thujone.[8(a)] Essential oil not recommended during pregnancy or lactation.[8(a)]
Santalum album Linn.	Chandana (Shveta)	Contraindicated in the diseases of parenchyma of kidney.[1,10] Oil is considered to be kidney irritant.[2] Use longer than six weeks not advised.[2] Extracts of alpha and beta-santols are sedative and could be considered neuroleptic by resemblance to pharmacological activities of chloropromazine.[4d]
Sarcostemma brevistigma W. & A.	Somavalli (Soma component)	Dried stem: Emetic. Active constituents of the plant: Toxic.[4(a)]
Saussurea lappa C. B. Clarke	Kustha	The root is commonly contaminated with aristolochic acid which is nephrotoxic and carcinogenic. Any product which contains plants, known or suspected to contain aristolochic acid is detained in the US.[2]
Sesamum indicum Linn.	Tila	Anaphylaxis associated with the sesame consumption has been described, especially in persons with a known history of asthma or with other anaphylactic sensitivity.[10]
Sida cordifolia Linn.	Balaa	Ephedrine is reported to be present in the plant.[4a] Drugs interacting with the herb: Antidiabetic drugs, dexamethasone, ergot derivatives, methylxnathine, MAOs, tricyclic antidepressants.[2]
Solanum indicum Linn.	Brihati	Utilization of the fruit as an alternative source of steroidal material for the preparation of cortisone and steroid sex hormones has been suggested.[4a]

Table 4: Contd.

Botanical Name	Ayurvedic/Native Name	Adverse Effects and Interactions
Solanum nigrum Linn.	Kaakamaachi	Toxic constituents: Glycosidal alkaloids, solamargine and solasonine. Total alkaloids in fruits and leaves: 0.101 and 0.431% respectively.[4a]
Solanum xanthocarpum Schrad. and Wendl.	Kantakaari	Glycoalkaloids and fatty fractions of the herbs cause depletion of histamine from bronchial and lung tissues.[4a]
Spinacia oleracea Linn.	Paalankya	Spinach is not recommended in diets of growing children, pregnant women and patients suffering from calcium deficiency (due to high content of oxalate in leaves).[4a] (Oxalates can be eliminated by boiling the vegetable for 15 minutes and rejecting the water. Discarding the cooking water reduces nitrate content.)[4a]
Streblus asper Lour.	Shaakhota	The Central Drug Research Institute, Lucknow, India, has developed an antifilarial elephantiasis drug (glycoside asperoside- K029 and glycoside strebloside-K030) from the crude extracts of the stem.[4c]
Strychnos nux-vomica Linn.	Vishatinduka	Toxic constituents of dried ripened seeds: 1-2%, strychnine and brucine, vomicine and other indole alkaloids, glycoside loganin, caffeotannic acid.[11] Toxic dose: 5 mg strychnine.[11]
Swertia chirayita (Roxb. ex Flem.) Karst.	Kiraatikta	May exacerbate duodenal ulcers.[2] Unlike most other bitters, it does not constipate the bowels, may nauseate and oppress in overdoses.[4a] GRAS status in the U.S.
Syzygium aromaticum (Linn.) Merrill & Perry	Lavanga	Contraindicated in bleeding disorders.[5] Smoking cloves may cause haemoptysis and irritation of mucous membrane.[5] (Clove cigarettes generally contain 60-80% tobacco and 20-40% ground clove).[2] Drugs interacting with the herbs: Anticoagulant/antiplatelet drugs.[2] Eugenol and acetyl eugenol in clove oil inhibit platelet aggregation, which may be additive with anticoagulants.[5] Case reports of acute liver toxicity, intravascular coagulation, acidosis, CNS depression and coma.[5]
Syzygium cuminii (Linn.) Skeels	Jambu	Seed extract exhibited protection against the effect of exposure to gamma radiation[2] (*J Radiat Res*, Tokyo, 2005, 46:59-65). Fruit extract not to be used concurrently with aspirin or ibuprofen.[2]
Taxus baccata Linn.	Sthauneya	The cancer chemotherapeutic compounds, taxol (paclitaxel) from the bark of *T. brevifolia* and semisynthetic docetaxel from *T. baccata*, are not present in nature in effective therapeutic quantities. Taxol in taxus media cultivars "Hicksy" fresh needles is at 0.0086-0.0094 g% and in microwave and oven dried needles at 0.0052 and 0.0029 g% respectively.[11]

Table 4: Contd.

Botanical Name	Ayurvedic/Native Name	Adverse Effects and Interactions
Terminalia arjuna (Roxb.) W. & A.	Arjuna	Crude extract of the bark showed anti-implantation as well as foetus absorption activity; ethanolic extract showed only anti-implantation activity. The drug had no effect on spermatogenesis.[4d]
Terminalia chebula Retz.	Haritaki	Fruit: Contraindicated in acute cough, acute diarrhoea, and early stage dysentery. Contains tannins (25-30%).[10]
Thevetia neriifolia Juss. ex Steud.	Karavira (Fita)	The oral absorbability of peruvoside is comparable to that of digoxin. It has very low toxicity. Peruvoside containing drug, Endocordin, has been marketed in Germany for cardiac insufficiency.[4d]
Tinospora cordifolia (Willd.) Miers ex Hook. f. Thoms.	Guduchi	Root: Emetic. Alkadoidal constituents include berberine.[4(a)]
Trachyspermum ammi (Linn.) Sprague	Yavaani	Thymol, produced from *ajowan* oil, is toxic in high doses, and may lead to fatal poisoning.[4a]
Trapa natans Linn.	Shringaata	Dentrifrices, containing collagenase inhibitor extracted from the seed extract are used for periodontal disease control.[4d] The collagenase inhibitor is anti-inflammatory, and can be incorporated into the skin lotions and creams.[4d]
Trianthema portulacastrum Linn.	Vasuka	The leaves and stems, eaten as vegetables, may produce toxic effects, even paralysis. Roots: cathartic, contraindicated in pregnancy due to use in traditional medicine as an abortifacient.[4a]
Tribulus terrestris Linn.	Gokshura	Hormonal activity is attributed to protodioscin constituent of *T. terrestris*.[2] (*J Ethnopharmacol*, 2005, 96: 127-32). In Bulgaria, the plant is used for impotency. A pharmaceutical preparation developed from the plant, Tribestan, has been found to increase the libido, the number and motility of sperm in men; in women it improves ovarial functions.[4d] Plant can cause neurotoxicity when used in high doses over a long period.[4d]
Trigonella foenum-graecum Linn.	Methikaa	Contraindicated with all medications, may reduce absorption if used concurrently. Not to be used concurrently with anti-coagulants.[6] The crude steroidal extract of seeds exert both antifertility and antiandrogenic activity in male albino rats; fed orally 100 mg/day for 60 days significantly declined the sperm count.[4c] ESCOP recommends 25 g powdered seeds or equivalent preparations daily as adjuvant therapy in diabetes or for hypercholesterolemia.[8(a)]
Triticum aestivum Linn.	Godhuma	Gluten sensitivity has been reported.[4a]

Table 4: Contd.

Botanical Name	Ayurvedic/Native Name	Adverse Effects and Interactions
Urginea indica Kunth	Vajrakanda	White squill: Contraindicated with digitalis glycosides, in potassium deficiency,[1] hypercalcaemia and hyperkalaemia.[5, 17(1)] Toxic constituents: Scillarin A and B, proscillaridin A (bufadienolides) and other glycosides.[11] New York Heart Association: 100-500 mg standardised squill bulb powder per day in stage I and II heart disease.[2] Squill contains cardiac glycosides.[5]
Valeriana wallichii DC.	Tagara	Lethal dose: Valerenic acid 400 mg/kg IP in mice. Valepotriates LD_{50} 64-150 mg/kg. IP in mice, non-toxic at 4.6 g/kg orally in mice.[11] Valerian: Interacts with opiates, alcohol, CNS depressants.[12,5]
Vetiveria zizanioides (Linn.) Nash	Ushira	Root: Emmenagogue, uterine stimulant. Regulated in the US as an allowable flavouring agent in alcoholic beverages only.[10]
Vitex negundo Linn.	Nirgundi	*Vitex agnus castus* berry: Contraindicated in depression associated with reduced oestrogen level.[6] Not to be used during pregnancy and lactation.[7] Mutual attenuation effects might occur in patients under concomittant treatment with dopamine receptor antagonists.[8(a),12] *Vitex agnus castus* has dopaminergic effect, may antagonise effects of dopamine receptor antagonists (phenothiazines).[12] Possible harmful interaction: Bromocriptine and related drugs; may augment prolactin inhibitory effects.[14] Drugs interacting with *V. agnus castus*: Antipsychotic drugs, contraceptive drugs, dopamine agonists, oestrogens, metoclopramide,[2] hormones that affect the pituitary.[5]
Vitex negundo Linn. (seeds)	Renukaa	*Vitex agnus castus* fruit: May counteract the effectiveness of birth control pills.[10] An amphoteric hormone-regulating herb.[10] Not to be used during pregnancy.[1]
Vitis vinifera Linn.	Draakshaa	Red vine leaf, aqueous dry extract (4-7:1): for chronic venous insufficiency,[8b] Grape seed extracts are standardised to 85-95% procynacidins.[7]
Wendlandia exserta DC.	Prapaundarika/ Tilaka	An oral contraceptive of folk medicine. (20-25 g paste of young leaves, mixed with sugar, on empty stomach on third or fourth day of menstruation.)[4c]
Withania somnifera Dunal	Ashvagandhaa	Ashwagandhaa may increase serum T4.[2,5] Contraindicated in pregnancy.[5,6,10] May potentiate barbiturates.[10] Possible harmful interaction: Antipsychotic agents, benzodiazepines, carbamazepines, phenobarbital, phenytoin, primidone, valproic acid, tricyclic antidepressants, zolpidem.[13] Methanolic extract induced marked impairment of sexual performance in male rats. (*Asian J Androl*, 2002, 295-298.)

Table 4: Contd.

Botanical Name	Ayurvedic/Native Name	Adverse Effects and Interactions
Zanthoxylum alatum Roxb.	Tejovati	Essential oil from seeds: Strong antibacterial against *Escherichia coli*, *Vibrio cholerae*, *Mycrococcus pyogens* var *aureus*, *Shigella dysenteriae* and *Salmonella typhi*. In a dilution of 1 in 40,000, the oil killed 50% of ciliates.[4a]
Zingiber officinale Rosc.	Aardraka	Contraindicated in gallstones, (only to be used after consultation with a physician).[1] Safety of large doses in pregnancy not established[5] due to emmenagogue and abortifacient effects.[6] For nausea and vomiting in pregnancy: only under medical supervision.[8b] FDA considers ginger as GRAS.[3] Drugs interacting with the herb: Calcium channel blockers.[2]
Ziziphus jujuba (Lam.) Gaertn. non Mill.	Badara	Kernels: Reported to have sedative effects, are prescribed to stop nausea and vomiting and for relief from abdominal pain in pregnancy, also given as an antidote to aconite poisoning.[4a]

Table 5: By Ayurvedic/Native Names

Ayurvedic/Native Name	Botanical Name	Adverse Effects and Interactions
Aakaarakarabha	*Anacyclus pyrethrum* DC.	Seeds: Abortifacient.[4c]
Aaragvadha	*Cassia fistula* Linn.	Pulp of pod and Senna spp: Contraindicated in abdominal pain of unknown origin, pregnancy, lactation, appendicitis, Crohn's disease, ulcerative colitis, ileus, intestinal inflammation or obstruction, children under 12 year of age;[1,5,8(a)] in haemorrhoids.[10] With chronic use or abuse: Electrolyte imbalance, potassium deficiency, albuminuria, hematuria.[1] May potentiate toxicity of digitalis and diuretics.[12] Toxic constituents in senna spp.; anthraquinone glycosides, dianthrones, anthrones.[11] Drugs interacting with the herbs: Digoxin, diuretic drugs.[2]
Aardraka	*Zingiber officinale* Rosc.	Contraindicated in gallstones, (only to be used after consultation with a physician).[1] Safety of large doses in pregnancy not established[5] due to emmenagogue and abortifacient effects.[6] For nausea and vomiting in pregnancy: only under medical supervision.[8b] FDA considers ginger as GRAS.[3] Drugs interacting with the herb: Calcium channel blockers.[2]
Aguru	*Aquilaria agallocha* Roxb.	Benzene extract of the wood exhibited potent CNS depressant activity in mice.[4c]
Ahiphena	*Papaver somniferum* Linn.	Toxic constituents in latex from unripe seed capsules: Morphine, codeine, papaverine (isoquinoline alkaloids).[11] Opium is a controlled substance in many countries.[10]
Ajamoda	*Apium graveolens* Linn.	Contraindicated in pregnancy and kidney disorders,[17(1)] furanocoumarin constituents may cause photosensitivity.[9] Seed tablets interact with thyroxine and anticoagulants. Potential allergenicity, including anaphylactic shock reported.[1] Furanocoumarin content increases 100-fold in injured or diseased celery.[2]
Ajashringi	*Gymnema sylvestre* R. Br.	Gymnemic acid and gurmarin, inhibit the ability to taste bitter (quinine) or sweet (sugar), without affecting the ability to taste sour, astringent or pungent flavours.[2]
Anantamuula	*Hemidesmus indicus* R. Br.	Known as Indian or false Sarsaparilla, in Western herbals; according to Tyler (Honest herbals), does not contain same saponins or other principal constituents found in Sarsaparilla.
Ankola	*Alangium salviifolium* (Linn. f.) Wang.	Flowers contain deoxytubulosine, a potent antiplatelet aggregation component.[4c]

Table 5: Contd.

Ayurvedic/Native Name	Botanical Name	Adverse Effects and Interactions
Apaamaarga	*Achyranthes aspera* Linn.	The benzene extract of the plant exhibited (100%) abortifacient activity experimentally.[4c] Acetone and methanolic extract of the root exhibited anti-implantation activity in rats.[4d]
Aparaajitaa	*Clitoria terrnatea* Linn.	Seeds: Contain a nucleoprotein with its amino acid sequence similar to insulin, but for the absence of histidine, threonine, proline and cystine.[4c]
Aralu	*Ailanthus excelsa* Roxb.	An alcoholic extract of leaf and stem bark showed anti-implantation and early abortifacient activities in female rats.[4c]
Arjuna	*Terminalia arjuna* (Roxb.) W. & A.	Crude extract of the bark showed anti-implantation as well as foetus absorption activity; ethanolic extract showed only anti-implantation activity. The drug had no effect on spermatogenesis.[4d]
Arka	*Calotropis gigantea* (Linn.) Ait. f.	Root: Cardiac glycosides[2] may be additive with digoxin.[5] Drugs interacting with the herb: Digoxin, diuretic drugs, stimulant laxatives.[2]
Ashvagandhaa	*Withania somnifera* Dunal	Ashwagandhaa may increase serum T4.[2,5] Contraindicated in pregnancy.[5,6,10] May potentiate barbiturates.[10] Possible harmful interaction: Antipsychotic agents, benzodiazepines, carbamazepines, phenobarbital, phenytoin, primidone, valproic acid, tricyclic antidepressants, zolpidem.[13] Methanolic extract induced marked impairment of sexual performance in male rats. (*Asian J. Androl*, 2002, 295-298.)
Asthisamhaara	*Cissus quadrangularis* Linn.	Total alcoholic extract of the plant, on parenteral administration, neutralises the antianabolic effect of cortisone in healing fractures.[4b]
Atasi	*Linum usitatissimum* Linn.	Contraindicated in intestinal obstruction of any origin,[1,8(a)] bleeding disorders, elevated prolactin, hypokalaemia.[5] Use during pregnancy or lactation only on medical advice.[5] Toxic constituents: Linatine, (glutamic acid derivatives) from seed; lotaustralin (cyanogenic glycosides) from leaves, stems and roots; 0.1-1.5% linustatin and neolinustatin (cyanogenic glycosides) in seeds.[11] In spite of cyanogenic glycosides, single dose of upto 150-300 g of powdered linseed is not toxic.[8(a)]
Atibalaa	*Abutilon indicum* (Linn.) Sweet	Plant considered an abortifacient.[4c] Country Mallow with ephedrine content is banned in the U.S.

Table 5: Contd.

Ayurvedic/Native Name	Botanical Name	Adverse Effects and Interactions
Ativishaa	*Aconitum heterophyllum* Wall. ex Royle	Atisine: Much less toxic than aconitine, although produces hypotension.[4b]
Baakuchi	*Psoralea corylifolia* Linn.	Toxic symptoms of seeds: Nausea, vomiting, malaise, GI disturbances. External application of oil: Irritant to skin, causes blistering.[4a] Oil even in high dilutions (upto 1 in 100,000) increases tone of the uterus and stimulates smooth muscles of experimental animals.[4a] A mixture of psoralen and isopsoralen (in 1:3 ratio) is recommended in leucoderma.[4d] A powder has been patented in China containing salt as the main ingredient with *P. corylifolia* extract for odontopathy, dental caries and peri-odontal diseases. In Japan, oral compositions containing the extracts of *P. corylifolia* are being patented for controlling *Streptococcus mutans* related dental caries.[4d]
Babbula	*Acacia arabica* auct. (non Lam.) Willd.	Acacia gum: Contains peroxidase enzyme which forms coloured complexes with certain amines and phenols and enhances the destruction of many pharmaceutical products, including alkaloids.[3] Contraindicated in intestinal obstruction.[5] When exposed to alcohol, becomes unsoluble and will form a precipitate.[5,6] Drugs interacting with the herb: Amoxicillin.[2]
Badara	*Ziziphus jujuba* (Lam.) Gaertn. non Mill.	Kernels: Reported to have sedative effects, are prescribed to stop nausea and vomiting and for relief from abdominal pain in pregnancy, also given as an antidote in aconite poisoning.[4a]
Balaa	*Sida cordifolia* Linn.	Ephedrine is reported to be present in the plant.[4a] Drugs interacting with the herb: Antidiabetic drugs, dexamethasone, ergot derivatives, methylxnathine, MAOs, tricyclic antidepressants.[2]
Barbari Shveta	*Ocimum basilicum* Linn.	Not recommended for infants or toddlers or for extended period of time.[10] The herb contains about 0.5% of essential oil with upto 85% of estragole (a procarcinogen).[1,5]
Bhadraa	*Aerva lanata* (L.) Juss.	(A subsitute for Paasaanabheda. AFI.) Plant extract did not show any significant diuretic activity in healthy human volunteers (*Indian J. Physiol Pharmacol*, 1993, 37:135)
Bhangaa	*Cannabis sativa* Linn.	Toxic constituents: Tetrahydrocannabinol (cannabinoids 15-20%)[11] Oxytocic, crosses human placenta, high doses damage developing embryos.[11] Dried, crushed mature leaves and flower shoots, known as Bhaang, are an ingredient in cannabis chocolates in the U.S. and New Mexico.

Table 5: Contd.

Ayurvedic/Native Name	Botanical Name	Adverse Effects and Interactions
Bhunimba	*Andrographis paniculata* Wall. ex Nees	Contraindicated in bleeding disorders, hypotension, male sterility.[5] Adverse reactions: GI distress[5,10] anaphylaxis, infertility.[5] Patients with autoimmune diseases, including rheumatoid arthritis to use with caution.[2] Drugs interacting with the herbs: Anticoagulant drugs, immunosuppressants.[2] Extracts may have a synergistic effect with isoniazid.[16(2)]
Bhuutikaa	*Cymbopogon citratus* (DC.) Stapf	Emmenagogue, uterine stimulant.[10] Contraindicated in glaucoma, (citral raised ocular pressure in very low doses in experimental studies), benign prostatic hyperplasia (due to citral),[6] and pregnancy.[5] Adverse reactions include slight elevation of direct bilirubin and amylase.[2,5]
Bilva	*Aegle marmelos* (L.) Correa Serr.	Aqueous and alcoholic extract of leaves are reported to possess effect like digitalis on amphibian and mammalian hearts.[4b] Aurapten is found comparable with verapamil.[4c] Marmelosin, like psoralen, causes an increased deposition of pigment melanin by augmenting enzymic activity.[4d]
Bimbi	*Coccinia indica* W. & A.	Pectin extracted from the fruit enhanced glycolysis, glycogenesis and decreased glycogenolysis.[4c]
Bola	*Commiphora myrrha* (Nees) Engl.	Amounts greater than 2-4 g can cause kidney irritation and diarrhoea; large amounts can affect heart rate.[2] Emmenagogue.[16(3)]
Brahmi	*Bacopa monnieri* (Linn.) Wettst.	Herb: Prolongs hypnotic effect of pentobarbitone, may antagonise the haloperidol-induced catalepsy, suggesting an involvement of GABA-ergic system. Potentiates phenothiazine.[5] Herb's CNS action does not include serious sedation; caution with phenothiazine co-administration is indicated.[3] Taking 300 mg extract per day for 12 weeks improved verbal learning, memory and information processing in healthy men and women. (Psychopharmacology, Berl, 2001, 156: 481-84).[2]
Brihati	*Solanum indicum* Linn.	Utilization of the fruit as an alternative source of steroidal material for the preparation of cortisone and steroid sex hormones has been suggested.[4a]

Table 5: Contd.

Ayurvedic/Native Name	Botanical Name	Adverse Effects and Interactions
Chandaa/Choraka	*Angelica archangelica* Linn.	Root contains furanocoumarins; intense UV radiation should be avoided.[1,2,10] Emmenagogue, uterine stimulant,[10] and induce miscarriage,[7] and cause uterine contractions.[2] GRAS status in the U.S. Canada does not allow Archangelica species as food ingredients.[2] *A. sinensis*: Contraindicated in bleeding disorders,[16(2)] lactation, pregnancy.[5] Osthole and ferulic acid may inhibit platelet aggregation.[5] Herb interacts with anticoagulants, antiplatelet agents, oestrogen replacement therapy/ oral contraceptives.[12] Contraindicated in gastric and duodenal ulcers,[17(2)] also during pregnancy.[16(2)]
Chandana (Rakta)	*Pterocarpus santalinus* Linn. f.	Regulated in the US as an allowable flavouring agent in alcoholic beverages only.[10]
Chandana (Shveta)	*Santalum album* Linn.	Contraindicated in the diseases of parenchyma of kidney.[1,10] Oil is considered to be the kidney irritant.[2] Use longer than six weeks not advised.[2] Extracts of the alpha and beta-santols are sedative and could be considered neuroleptic by resemblance to pharmacological activities of chloropromazine.[4d]
Daadima	*Punica granatum* Linn.	Dried root bark, stem bark, seeds contain toxic constituents pelletrin, piperidine alkaloids 0.4%, punicalagin, punicacontein C, casurin (tannins 20-25%).[10,11]
Damanaka	*Artemesia nilagirica* (C.B. Clarke) Pamp.	Emmenagogue, uterine stimulant.[4b,10] Toxic constituent: Thujone.[11,4c] May interact with anticonvulsants, may lower seizure threshold.[12] *A. absinthium*: Plant extract decreased hepatotoxicity of acetaminophen in mice.[5] Contraindicated in pregnancy.[17(2)]
Darbha	*Imperata cylindrica* Beauv.	Leaves and stem contain cyanophoric compounds.[4c] Plant can be used as a substitute for Ephedra (as an anti-fatigue agent).[4c]
Daruharidraa	*Berberis asiatica* DC.	Toxic constituent: Berberine (isoquinoline alkaloids). Berberine containing herbs: Not recommended during pregnancy.[10] Berberine is well tolerated up to 0.5 g, equivalent to about 8 g dried root. Therapeutic dose. Powder 0.32-2.6 g.[11] Drugs interacting with berberine: Cyclosorine, Cytochrome P450 3A4 (CYP3A4) substrates.[2]
Dhaanyaka	*Coriandrum sativum* Linn.	Contraindications: May interact with hypoglycemic agents.[5]
Dhattura	*Datura metel* Linn.	Toxic constituents: Hyoscine, hyoscyamine.[11] Adverse reactions: Agitation, blurred vision, dilated pupils, disorientation, hallucinations, mydriasis, tachycardia, seizures, xerostomia and coma.[5] Lethal dose for adults: 15-25 g seeds; 100 mg atropine.[11] Contraindicated in tachycardiac arrhythmia, glaucoma.[17(1)]

Table 5: Contd.

Ayurvedic/Native Name	Botanical Name	Adverse Effects and Interactions
Dhava	*Anogeissus latifolia* (Roxb.) Wall. ex Bedd.	Alcoholic extract of the stem bark: CNS depressant, hypothermic, responds to amphatamine hyperactivity test.[4d]
Draakshaa	*Vitis vinifera* Linn.	Red vine leaf, aqueous dry extract (4-7:1): for chronic venous insufficiency,[8b] Grape seed extracts are standardised to 85-95% procynacidins.[7]
Dugdhikaa	*Euphorbia hirta* Linn.	Contraindicated in individuals with infection or inflammatory gastrointestinal conditions.[2]
Elaa	*Elettaria cardamomum* Maton	Contraindicated in case of gallstones (to be used only after consultation with physician);[1,16(4)] in gastro-oesophageal reflux disease,[7] cholagogue.[1]
Elavaaluka	*Prunus cerasus* Linn.	Leaves: Anticonvulsant. Seed kernel: Nervine tonic.[4a]
Eranda	*Ricinus communis* Linn.	Seed oil: Contraindicated in intestinal obstruction and abdominal pain of unknown origin, appendicitis, ulcerative colitis.[5,10] Must be used with caution during pregnancy and menstruation;[10] with cardiac glycosides, antiarrhythmic drugs, diuretics, cortisol, liquorice, antihistamines and fat-soluble vitamins.[16(4)] Toxic constituents (seeds, leaves): 3% ricin (toxalbumin), ricinine.[11]
Gavedhu	*Coix lacryma-jobi* Linn.	Seeds and leaves: May promote fertility in women; trans-ferulyl stigmastanol and trans-ferulyl campestanol (isolated from the seed) may induce ovulation.[4c]
Ghitakumaari	*Aloe barbadensis* Mill.	Dried latex: Contraindicated in intestinal obstruction, acutely inflammed intestinal diseases, e.g., Crohn's disease, ulcerative colitis, appendicitis, abdominal pain of unknown origin. Not to be prescribed during pregnancy or to children under 12 years of age.[1,10] Toxic constituents in dried latex: Anthraquinone glycosides.[11] (not in *A. vera* gel.)[11] *A. vera* latex: Interacts with cardiac glycosides and thiazide diuretics; can cause electrolyte imbalance, may potentiate drug toxicity.[12] Avoid during the first trimester of pregnancy or take under medical supervision.[8b] Drugs interacting with the herb: Antidiabetic drugs, digoxin, diuretic drugs, sevoflurane, stimulant laxatives.[2] Chronic use of anthraquinone stimulant laxatives can lead to hepatitis.[16(1)] Aloe turns the urine red.[17(1)]
Godhuma	*Triticum aestivum* Linn.	Gluten sensitivity has been reported.[4a]

Table 5: Contd.

Ayurvedic/Native Name	Botanical Name	Adverse Effects and Interactions
Gokshura	*Tribulus terrestris* Linn.	Hormonal activity is attributed to protodioscin constituent of *T. terrestris*.[2] (*J. Ethnopharmacol*, 2005, 96: 127-32). In Bulgaria, the plant is used for impotency. A pharmaceutical preparation developed from the plant, Tribestan, has been found to increase the libido, the number and motility of sperm in men; in women it improves ovarial functions.[4d] Plant can cause neurotoxicity when used in high doses over a long period.[4d]
Guduchi	*Tinospora cordifolia* (Willd.) Miers ex Hook. f. Thoms.	Root: Emetic.[4a] Alkadoidal constituents include berberine.[4(a)]
Guggulu	*Commiphora mukul* (Hook. ex Stocks) Engl.	Emmenagogue, uterine stimulant.[10] In contrast to studies of guggulu in Indian population, taking guggulu in dose of 3000 or 6000 mg per day does not seem to lower total cholesterol or triglycerides, or raise HDL cholesterol in people on western diet. It seems to increase LDL cholesterol by 9 to 10%[2] (*JAMA*, 2003, 290: 765-72). Drugs interacting with the herbs: Antiplatelet/anticoagulant drugs, contraceptive drugs, calcium channel blockers, thyroid hormones.[2]
Gunjaa (Sweta, Rakta)	*Abrus precatorius* Linn.	Toxic constituent: Alkaloid abrin; Cytotoxic potential.[4b] 5 mg of abrin is reported to be toxic in humans.[3] (0.15% in the seed. LD_{50} is 0.029 mg/kg body wt of mice.)[4b]
Hapushaa	*Juniperus communis* Linn.	Fruits are contraindicated in pregnancy and inflammatory kidney diseases.[1,10,17(2)] Not for use exceeding four to six weeks in succession. Canadian regulation does not allow juniper as a non-medical ingredient for oral use products.[10] The volatile monoterpenes are irritant to the urinary mucosa.[11]
Harenu	*Pisum sativum* Linn.	An antifertility agent. m-xylohydroquinone, isolated from peas, produced fatal resorption in rats; in humans reduced fertility rate by 50%.[4d]
Haridraa	*Curcuma longa* Linn.	Root: Contraindicated in obstruction of bile passage, in cases of gallstones use only after consulting a physician.[1,10,5] Not to be administered to patients of stomach ulcers or hyperacidity.[10,5] Emmenagogue, uterine stimulant.[10,5] Curcumin may potentiate antiplatelet activity, interacts with antiplatelet agents.[12] Not teratogenic in mice.[16(1)]
Haritaki	*Terminalia chebula* Retz.	Fruit: Contraindicated in acute cough, acute diarrhoea, early stage dysentery. Contains tannins (25-30%).[10]

Table 5: Contd.

Ayurvedic/Native Name	Botanical Name	Adverse Effects and Interactions
Hingu	*Ferula foetida* Regel.	Emmenagogue, uterine stimulant,[10] contraindicated in infant colic,[17(1)] in bleeding disorders, pregnancy, infection or inflammatory GI diseases,[5] peptic ulcers,[6] 50-100 mg of Gum resin may cause convulsions in persons suffering from nervousness.[2,10] Drugs interacting with the herb: Anticoagulant/antiplatelet drugs, antihypertensive drugs.[2]
Indravaaruni	*Citrullus colocynthis* (Linn.) Schrad.	Toxic constituents in dried pulp or unripe fruit: Up to 3% E-, I- and L- cucurbitacins and 0.21% alpha-elaterin (glycosides). Toxic dose: 0.6-1 g.[11] Contraindicated in infections or inflammatory gastrointestinal conditions. Death has resulted from the consumption of as little as 1½ teaspoons of powder.[2] Drugs interacting with the herb: Digoxin, Diuretic drugs.[2]
Irimeda	*Acacia leucophloea* Willd.	Root: Abortifacient.[4c] Roots-contain anthraquinone glycosides.[4d]
Ishvari	*Aristolochia indica* Linn.	Toxic constituents: Aristolochin, aristolochic acid.[11] Toxic to kidneys. Carcinogenic in animals and human cells.[2,11] Many cases of nephropathy associated with the use of aristolochia have been reported wordwide.[2] Any product which contains plants known or suspected to contain aristolochic acid, is detained in the U.S.[2] A cytotoxic lignan, savinin, has been isolated from the root.[4c] Root: Oxytocic, emmenagogue, abortifacient.[4b]
Jaatiphala	*Myristica fragrans* Houtt.	Toxic constituents: Myristicin, elemicine, safrole. More than 5 gm of powdered nutmeg, or mace affects the central nervous system, producing hallucinations, headache, dizziness, drowsiness, nausea, stomach pain, liver pain, excessive thirst, rapid pulse, anxiety, double vision and sometimes acute panic, coma or death.[1,5,10] With ingestion of 9 teaspoons of nutmeg powder per day, an atropine-like effect was observed.[1,5] When taken in larger amount, the herb has abortifacient effect.[1]
Jaipaala	*Croton tiglium* Linn.	Toxic constituents in oil from seeds: Phorbols (terpenoids) from nonvolatile oil. Crotin, a toxic albuminous substance, is not extracted in the oil.[11] Phorbol esters: Tumour promoting.[4c]
Jambira	*Citrus limon* (Linn.) Burm. f.	The furocoumarins, bergapten and oxypeucedanin in oil are photosensitising. Topically photosensitivity can occur.[2]
Jambu	*Syzygium cumini* (Linn.) Skeels	Seed extract exhibited protection against the effect of exposure to gamma radiation[2] (*J. Radiat Res*, Tokyo, 2005, 46: 59-65). Fruit extract not to be used concurrently with aspirin or ibuprofen.[2]

Table 5: Contd.

Ayurvedic/Native Name	Botanical Name	Adverse Effects and Interactions
Karpura	*Cinnamomum camphora* (Linn.) Nees & Eberm.	Contraindicated externally on injured skin, burns,[1] preparation not to be used in the facial region of infants and small children, especially in the nasal area.[1,10] Not for long-term use.[10] Toxic constituents: Camphor (volatile saturated ketone), 30-50% of volatile oil; safrole, cincole, (volatile oxides) in crude camphor oil.[11] Camphorated oil (20% camphor in cottonseed oil) was removed from the US market due to toxicity in 1980s. Available without a prescription in Canada.[2]
Katabhi	*Albizia procera* Benth.	Seed saponin: Spermicidal.[4c]
Katphala	*Myrica nagi* Hook. f. *Myrica esculenta* Buch.-Ham.	Canadian regulations do not allow bayberry (Myrica) as a non-medical ingredient for oral use products.[10] Fruits are sedative.[4a]
Katuki	*Picrorhiza kurroa* Royle ex Benth.	There is some concern that *Picrorhiza* might adversely affect patients with autoimmune disorders because of its immune stimulating effects. Avoid using in patients with multiple sclerosis, systemic lupus erythomatosus, rheumatoid arthritis and other autoimmune disorders.[2] Interacts with immunosuppressants.[2] 70% methanol extract not teratogenic.[16(4)]
Kebuka	*Costus speciosus* (Koenig) Sm.	Rhizomes: Abortifacient. Diosgenin, isolated from the plant, is the raw material for the synthesis of corticosteroids, sex hormones, oral contraceptives and anabolic agents.[4c]
Khadir	*Acacia catechu* Willd.	Leukoagglutinating activity of saline extract of seeds against leukaemic cells is inhibited by simple sugars.[4c] Catechin (cianidanol) is associated with fatal hemolytic anaemia. Unstandardised products may contain high amount of aflatoxin, metabolite of *Aspergillus*, which is toxic and may lead to certain cancers.[2] Drugs interacting with the herb: Antihypertensive drugs.[2]
Khuraashaanikaa	*Hyoscyamus niger* Linn.	Toxic constituents in whole plant: Scopolamine (hyoscine), hyoscyamine, butyrine (tropane alkaloids), hyospicrin (glucoside).[11] Leaf: Contraindicated in tachycardiac arrythmias,[17(1)] prostatic adenoma with urine retention, narrow angle glaucoma, acute pulmonary oedema, mechanical stenosis in any part of the gastrointestinal tract, megacolon.[1] Hyoscymine and scopolamine alkaloids are anti-cholinergic.[5] Therapeutic dose: 130-325 mg powder, Hyoscine hydrobromate 0.33-0.93 mg.[11]
Kiraatikta	*Swertia chirayita* (Roxb. ex Flem.) Karst.	May exacerbate duodenal ulcers.[2] Unlike most other bitters, it does not constipate the bowels, may nauseate and oppress in overdoses.[4a] GRAS status in the U.S.

Table 5: Contd.

Ayurvedic/Native Name	Botanical Name	Adverse Effects and Interactions
Kulattha	*Dolichos biflorus* Linn.	A dipeptide, pyroglutamyglutamine, is diuretic, found to be 2-3 times that of acetazolamide in albino rats.[4c]
Kumkuma	*Crocus sativus* Linn.	Toxic constituents in stigma and styles: Alpha-crocin (carotenoids), picrocrocin (volatile glycoside).[11] Emmenagogue, uterine stimulant, abortifacient.[10] Side effects occur on 5 g,[16(3)] lethal dose 20 g, therapeutic dose 1.5 g/day.[10] Abortifacient dose 10 g.[1] Side effects include severe purpura, a thrombocytopenia of 24,000, hypothrombinemia of 41 per cent, severe collapse with uremia, bleeding from uterus, bloody diarrhoea, bleeding from nose and eyelids, vertigo, dizziness, numbness.[1]
Kustha	*Saussurea lappa* C.B. Clarke	The root is commonly contaminated with aristolochic acid, which is nephrotoxic and carcinogenic. Any product that contains plants, known or suspected to contain aristolochic acid, is detained in the US.[2]
Kusumbha	*Carthamus tinctorius* Linn.	Flowers: Sedative, emmenagogue.[4b] The plant contains a propanetriol derivative, which can be used for the treatment of circulatory disorders.[4c] Inhibits platelet aggregation.[16(3)]
Kutaja	*Holarrhena antidysenterica* (Linn.) Wall.	Latex: Irritant, high doses affect blood vascular system.[4c]
Laangali	*Gloriosa superba* Linn.	Young sprouts, seeds, tubers: Source of colchicine.[4a]
Lajjaalu	*Mimosa pudica* Linn.	Feeding trials with horses in large doses caused toxic symptoms including loss of hairs. Leaf meal caused stunted growth in chicks.[4a]
Lakucha	*Artocarpus lakoocha* Roxb.	A lectin, artocarpin, isolated from the seeds precipitates several galactomannans. Besides human and animal erythrocytes, it agglutinates rat lymphocytes and mouse ascites cells.[4c]
Lasuna	*Allium sativum* Linn.	Contraindicated in bleeding disorders, gastric ulcer, and thyroid disease.[5] Inhibits platelet aggregation, and shows additive anticoagulant, antiplatelet effects.[12] Harmful interaction with heparin, warfarin, NSAIDs.[13] For hyperlipidemia and hypertension, extract (containing 1.3% allicin) 600-1200 mg, divided and given three times daily, has been used in clinical trials.[2] Average daily dose: 4 g fresh garlic (to be chewed) or equivalent preparations.[1] To be discontinued at least 7 days prior to surgery.[5] Enteric coated tablets, containing alliin and alliinase, enhance allicin.[9]

Table 5: Contd.

Ayurvedic/Native Name	Botanical Name	Adverse Effects and Interactions
Lavanga	*Syzygium aromaticum* (Linn.) Merrill & Perry	Contraindicated in bleeding disorders.[5] Smoking cloves may cause haemoptysis and irritation of mucous membrane.[5] (Clove cigarettes generally contain 60-80% tobacco and 20-40% ground clove.)[2] Drugs interacting with the herbs: Anticoagulant/antiplatelet drugs.[2] Eugenol and acetyl eugenol in clove oil inhibit platelet aggregation, which may be additive with anticoagulants.[5] Case reports of acute liver toxicity, intravascular coagulation, acidosis, CNS depression and coma.[5]
Maajuuphalaka	*Quercus infectoria* Olivier	Oak bark: Contraindicated in cardiac insufficiency, hypertonia and externally on broken skin.[5] Tannins may interfere with absorption of drugs.[5]
Maanakanda	*Alocasia indica* (Roxb.) Schott.	Leaves, stalks, tubers and roots contain high concentration of soluble oxalates. Prolonged use may lead to calcium deficiency and oxaluria. All parts, except rhizome, contain cyanogenic principle.[4b]
Madanaphala	*Randia dumetorum* Poir.	Fruit pulp: Emetic and abortifacient, potentiates pentobarbitone, depresses heart, relaxes ileum, antagonises effect of acetylcholine (in animal studies).[4a,c]
Madayanti	*Lawsonia inermis* Linn.	Leaf: History of internal use as an abortifacient is recorded in Africa.[10] Leaf juice (50 g) is an oral herbal contraceptive in both the sexes; prolonged use may cause permanent sterility.[4c]
Madhuuka	*Madhuca indica* J.F. Gmel.	Seed oil causes total but reversible sterility in male rats; shows testicular atrophy and degeneration of seminiferous tubules.[4c]
Mahaanimba	*Melia azedarach* Linn.	Fruits: Poisonous. Cases of severe poisoning have been reported.[4a]
Manduukaparni	*Centella asiatica* (Linn.) Urban	Emmenagogue.[3,6] Excessive internal use is contraindicated in early pregnancy.[6] Canadian regulations do not allow the herb as a non-medical ingredient for oral use products.[10] In majority of randomised and placebo controlled studies, in which daily dose of 60-180 mg of *Centella* triterpene fractions have been taken orally for periods upto 12 months, no side effects were reported.[8(b)]

Table 5: Contd.

Ayurvedic/Native Name	Botanical Name	Adverse Effects and Interactions
Maricha	*Piper nigrum* Linn.	Contraindicated in pregnancy in large doses.[5,6] Phenytoin was more rapidly and completely absorbed and eliminated more slowly when taken with piperine.[6] Piperine can augment the therapeutic effects of phenobarbital, phenytoin, rifampicin, theophylline and other drugs. It can also predispose the patient to an increased risk of side effects of drugs with a narrow therapeutic window that are liver metabolized (e.g., theophylline).[14] Drugs interacting with the herbs: CYP 3A4 substrates, P-glycoprotein substrates, phenytoin, propranolol, rifampicin, sparteine, theophylline.[2]
Matsyaakshi	*Alternanthera sessilis* (Linn.) DC.	Alkaloidal extract of the plant in moderate and high dose levels produces slight hepatotoxic and nephrotoxic effects.[4d]
Medaa	*Polygonatum verticillatum* All.	Plant: Diuretic, contains a digitalis glucoside.[4a] Rhizomes may be used as a source of diosgenin.[4c]
Methikaa	*Trigonella foenum-graecum* Linn.	Contraindicated with all medications, may reduce absorption if used concurrently. Not to be used concurrently with anti-coagulants.[6] The crude steroidal extract of seeds exert both antifertility and antiandrogenic activity in male albino rats; fed orally 100 mg/day for 60 days significantly declined the sperm count.[4c] ESCOP recommends 25 g powdered seeds or equivalent preparations daily as adjuvant therapy in diabetes or for hypercholesterolemia.[8(a)]
Mishreyaa/ Shatapushpaa	*Foeniculum vulgare* Mill.	Fennel oil: Not to be used for infants and toddlers.[1] Estragole (5-10% of essential oil): a procarcinogen,[10] concomittant use of fennel may reduce ciprofloxacin bioavailability by nearly 50% possibly due to calcium, iron and magnesium contained in fennel. Fennel increases tissue distribution and slows elimination of ciprofloxacin.[2,14] Similar effects from fluroquinolones.[14] Seed oil and anethole: emmenagogue.[16(3)] Avoid during pregnancy.[17(2)]
Mushali (Safed)	*Asparagus adscendens* Roxb.	*A. officinalis*: Contraindicated in inflammatory kidney diseases; in oedema due to functional heart or kidney disorders.[1,10]
Mustaa	*Cyperus rotundus* Linn.	Methanolic extract of plant stimulates the production of melanin in cultured melanocytes.[4c] Alcoholic and aqueous extract of tubers possess lipolytic action.[4c]
Muulaka	*Raphanus sativus* Linn.	Contraindicated in cholelithiasis.[1] It might cause biliary colic.[2] Seeds contain glycosidically bound mustard oils.[4a] Red raddish contains anthocyanins.[4d]

Table 5: Contd.

Ayurvedic/Native Name	Botanical Name	Adverse Effects and Interactions
Muurvaa	*Marsdenia tenacissima* W & A	The roots are used as a substitute for Black Nishoth (*Ipomoea turpethium*).[4c]
Muurvaa (substitute)	*Clematis gouriana* Roxb.	Leaves: Protoanemonin is a direct irritant to the skin and mucous membranes, check after drying the herb.[10]
Naarikela	*Cocos nucifera* Linn.	Coconut oil, in amounts commonly found in food, has GRAS status in the U.S. Coconut or coconut oil consumption is not associated with an increased risk of atherosclerosis and coronary heart disease, though it can increase LDL levels.[2]
Nili	*Indigofera tinctoria* Linn.	The plant contains appreciable amount of conjugated indoxyl, together with rotenoids. Can be used in endogenous depression.[4c] Indirubin isolated from the plant: An antitumour constituent.[4d]
Nimba	*Azadirachta indica* A. Juss.	The oil might cause morphological changes in sperm; leaf can affect sperm motility and viability. Avoid in couples with infertility.[2] Might decrease the effectiveness of immunosuppressants in organ transplant patients.[2] Cardiac arrest due to Neem leaf poisoning reported.[16(3)]
Nirgundi	*Vitex negundo* Linn.	*Vitex agnus castus* berry: Contraindicated in depression associated with reduced oestrogen level.[6] Not to be used during pregnancy and lactation.[7] Mutual attenuation effects might occur in patients under concomittant treatment with dopamine receptor antagonists.[8(a),12] *Vitex agnus castus* has dopaminergic effect, may antagonise effects of dopamine receptor antagonists (phenothiazines).[12] Possible harmful interaction: Bromocriptine and related drugs; may augment prolactin inhibitory effects.[14] Drugs interacting with *V. agnus castus*: Antipsychotic drugs, contraceptive drugs, dopamine agonists, oestrogens, metoclopramide.[2] Hormones that affect the pituitary.[5]
Paalankya	*Spinacia oleracea* Linn.	Spinach is not recommended in the diets of growing children, pregnant women and patients' suffering from calcium deficiency (due to high content of oxalate in leaves).[4a] (Oxalates can be eliminated by boiling the vegetable for 15 minutes and rejecting the water. Discarding the cooking water reduces nitrate content.)[4a]
Paaribhadra	*Erythrina variegata* Linn.	Alkaloids: Muscle relaxants, increase the sedative effect of hexabarbitol, LD_{50} in mice 306.4 mg/kg.[4c]

Table 5: Contd.

Ayurvedic/Native Name	Botanical Name	Adverse Effects and Interactions
Paashaanabheda	*Bergenia ciliata* (Haw.) Sternb.	*Bergenia ciliata* rhizome: Acetone extract reported to be cardiotoxic in higher doses and depressant on CNS. Mildly diuretic; in higher doses anti-diuretic in experimental animals.[4b]
Paathaa	*Cissampelos pareira* Linn.	Root: Alkaloid haytine (methiodide and methochloride derivatives), reported to be potent neuromuscular-blocking agent.[4b]
Palaandu	*Allium cepa* Linn.	Contraindicated in bleeding disorders, uncontrolled diabetes. Daily maximum amount of diphenylamine: 0.035g.[1]
Palaasha	*Butea monosperma* (Lam.) Kuntze	Flower and seed: Anti-oestrogenic. Seed: Nephrotoxic. Anthelmintic principle: Palasonin.[4b]
Panasa	*Artocarpus heterophyllus* Lam.	A lectin, jacalin, a potent polyclonal activator for human lymphocytes has been isolated from the seeds.[4c]
Parpataka	*Fumaria parviflora* Lam.	Should not be used by persons with seizure disorders or increased intraocular pressure.[7] *Fumaria officinalis* contraindicated in biliary obstructions. In cases of gallstones, not to be used without medical advice.[8b] Raised intraocular pressure and oedema.[17(1)]
Phanijjaka	*Origanum majorana* Linn.	Emmenagogue,[6] has the potential to stimulate menstruation.[2] Should be avoided in early pregnancy.[6]
Pinditaka	*Randia uliginosa* DC.	Roasted pulp is used during pregnancy in GI distress.[4a]
Pippali	*Piper longum* Linn.	Contraindicated in pregnancy in large doses.[5,6] Piperine inhibits gastric emptying and GI transit. Also increases drug induced sleep.[5]
Prapaundarika/Tilaka	*Wendlandia exserta* DC.	An oral contraceptive of folk medicine. (20-25 g paste of young leaves, mixed with sugar, on empty stomach on third or fourth day of menstruation.)[4c]
Prasaarani	*Paederia foetida* Linn.	Root and bark: Emetic.[4a]
Prativishaa	*Aconitum palmatum* D. Don	Root: Toxicity of diterpenoid alkaloids not reported. Feebly toxic.[4b]
Priyangu (variety)	*Aglaia roxburghiana* M.q.	The leaves contain bisamide alkaloids, found to inhibit the growth of vinblastin-resistant KB cells by enhancing anticancer activity of vinblastine.[4c]

Table 5: Contd.

Ayurvedic/Native Name	Botanical Name	Adverse Effects and Interactions
Puga	*Areca catechu* Linn.	Interactions: High tannin of the nut may cause alkaloids to become insoluble and precipitate. The cholinergic activity of arecoline interacts with anti-cholinergic drugs.[5,14] Toxic constituents: Arecoline, arecain (pyridine alkaloids).[11] Asthmatic and chronic obstructive pulmonary disease (COPD) patients may be at risk.[14]
Punarnavaa	*Boerhavia diffusa* Linn.	Official as a diuretic in IP. The cholinergic activity of the root was observed *in vitro* but not *in vivo*.[4d]
Pushkarmula	*Inula racemosa* Hook. f.	The root powder has been found to possess beta blocking activity.[4c]
Raajikaa	*Brassica juncea* (Linn.) Czern & Coss.	Toxic constituent: Glucosinolates.[11] Vegetables containing glucosinolates are goitrogenic.[5] Drugs interacting with black mustard: Antacids, H_2 Blockers, and Proton Pump Inhibitors.[2]
Renukaa	*Vitex negundo* Linn. (seeds)	*Vitex agnus castus* fruit: May counteract the effectiveness of birth control pills.[10] An amphoteric hormone-regulating herb.[10] Not to be used during pregnancy.[1]
Samudrashosha	*Salvia plebeia* R. Br.	Sage leaf: Essential oil and alcoholic extracts contraindicated during pregnancy.[1,10] Sage oil contains more thujone than absinthium oil, yet it has not been reported as toxic.[10] Alcoholic preparations to be used with caution due to the presence of thujone.[8(a)] Essential oil not recommended during pregnancy or lactation.[8(a)]
Sankhapushpi	*Convolvulus pluricaulis* Choisy	Multiple doses of "Shankhapushpi syrup" decreased serum level of phenytoin and half life (Dilantin);[5] Loss of seizure control was reported.[9,12,4c]
Saptalaa	*Acacia concinna* DC.	Bark saponins: Spermicidal. Pods: Used for fish poisoning.[4b]
Saptaparna	*Alstonia scholaris* R. Br.	Alkaloid echitamine (from the bark) is found to be toxic to mice in doses of 0.3-0.5 mg/20 g body wt.[4b]
Sarpagandhaa	*Rauvolfia serpentine* Benth. ex Kurz	Contraindicated in depression, ulcer, pheochromocytoma, pregnancy and lactation,[1] Parkinson's disease.[7] Toxic constituents: Reserpine, serpentine, raupine, ajmaline and other indole alkaloids.[11]
Sarshapa Gaura	*Brassica alba* Boiss	Isothiocyanates can cause endemic goitre.[2] Irritant poisoning (on ingestion of a large quantity) can occur in people with kidney disorders.[2] GRAS status in the US.

Table 5: Contd.

Ayurvedic/Native Name	Botanical Name	Adverse Effects and Interactions
Sarshapa	*Brassica campestris* Hook. f. & Thoms.	The pollen grains act as allergens causing bronchial and bronchopulmonary problems. Glycoprotein containing 11.4% of carbohydrate is the main allergen.[4d]
Shaakhota	*Streblus asper* Lour.	The Central Drug Research Institute, Lucknow, India, has developed an antifilarial elephantiasis drug (glycoside asperoside-K029 and glycoside strebloside-K030) from the crude extracts of the stem.[4c]
Shaalparni	*Desmodium gangeticum* DC.	Root extract exhibited significant antifertility activity at 50 and 100 mg/kg in rats.[4c]
Shallaki	*Boswellia seratta* Roxb.	For osteoarthritis (effective adult dose): 250-1200 mg of alcoholic dry extract (4.2-5.9:1, to contain approximately 65% of total organic acids) divided into 3 doses.[8b] Boswellic acids might prevent organ rejection and ischemia/reperfusion injury.[2]
Shana	*Crotalaria juncea* Linn.	Seeds: An ethanolic extract (90%) exhibited antiplantation activity in albino rats (200 mg/kg for 7 days after coitus), abortifacient activity when given for 3 days after coitus.[4c]
Shataavari	*Asparagus racemosus* Willd.	The alkaloid asparagamine A (in the root) showed antioxytocic activity *in vitro*.[4d] Roots are reported to show inhibitory effects on digestive enzymes, lipase and trypsin may lead to stoppage of degradation of food material in the intestinal tract.[4c]
Shigru	*Moringa oleifera* Lam.	Root and bark extract: Antifertility activity in experimental animals.[4c] Root more potent than bark.[4c] Due to levodopa, the herb might cause false urine glucose test, elevated liver function test, and elevated urine uric acid levels.[2] Drugs interacting with the herb: Antidiabetic drugs, antipsychotic drugs, guanethidine, methyldopa, MAOs inhibitors, tricyclic antidepressants.[2]
Shirisha	*Albizia lebbeck* Benth.	Seed saponin: Spermicidal.[4c]
Shringaata	*Trapa natans* Linn.	Dentrifrices, containing collagenase inhibitor extracted from the seed extract, are used for periodontal disease control.[4d] The collagenase inhibitor is anti-inflammatory, and can be incorporated into the skin lotions and creams.[4d]
Shukanaasaa	*Corallocarpus epigaeus* Benth. ex Hook.	Root: Emetic; contains cucurbitacin B.[4c]

Table 5: Contd.

Ayurvedic/Native Name	Botanical Name	Adverse Effects and Interactions
Shurana	*Amorphophallus campanulatus* Blume ex Decne	Alcoholic extract of the plant: Oxytocic.[4d]
Shyaamaaka	*Echinochloa frumentacea* Link	Contains glutelin.[4a]
Snuhi	*Euphorbia nerrifolia* auct. non Linn.	Canadian regulations do not allow Euphorbia in foods.[10]
"Soma" (component)	*Amanita muscaria* Linn.	Toxic constituents: Ibotenic acid and muscimol (isoxazole derivatives), muscazone (oxazole derivative), small amount of muscarine (alkaloid), stizolic acid, tricholomic acid. Isoxazole constituents are psychoactive.[2,11]
"Soma" (component)	*Ephedra nebrodensis* Tineo/*gerardiana* Wall.	Toxic constituents: Ephedrine, pseudoephedrine, (2-aminophenylpropane alkaloids),[11] contraindicated in coronary thrombosis, diabetes, glaucoma,[16(1)] anxiety, high blood pressure, glaucoma, impaired circulation of the cerebrum, adenoma of the prostate with residual urine accumulation, pheochromocytoma, thyrotoxicosis, may potentiate MAO inhibition.[3,10,13] Interacts with methyldopa, beta blockers, caffeine, monoamine oxidase inhibitors, theophylline sympathomimetics, St. John's Wort, Guanethidine, cardiac glycosides, oxytocin.[12]
Somavalli ("Soma" component)	*Sarcostemma brevistigma* W. & A.	Dried stem: Emetic. Active constituents of the plant: Toxic.[4a]
Sprukkaa	*Anisomeles malabarica* R. Br. ex Sims	Aqueous extract of the shoot: Spermicidal effect in albino rats (*in vitro*), also on human semen.[4b]
Sthauneya	*Taxus baccata* Linn.	The cancer chemotherapeutic compounds, taxol (paclitaxel) from the bark of *T. brevifolia* and semisynthetic docetaxel from *T. baccata*, are not present in nature in effective therapeutic quantities. Taxol in taxus media cultivars "Hicksy" fresh needles is at 0.0086-0.0094 g%, and in microwave and oven dried needles at 0.0052 and 0.0029 g% respectively.[11]
Sthula elaa	*Ammomum subulatum* Roxb.	Seeds: Promote elimination of bile; used in congestion of liver.[4b]
Surasaa	*Ocimum sanctum* Linn.	Essential oil contains estragole (a procarcinogen).[5] In mice, leaf extract decreased serum T4. To be used with caution in thyroid diseases.[5] Conflicting reports on embryotoxicity.[16(2)]

Table 5: Contd.

Ayurvedic/Native Name	Botanical Name	Adverse Effects and Interactions
Suvarchalaa	*Malva rotundifolia* Linn.	Leaves: Emmenagogue.[4a]
Svarnakshiri	*Argemone mexicana* Linn.	Adulteration of edible oil with sanguinarine containing argemone oil has led to widespread epidemic of dropsy and glaucoma. Sanguinarine is also carcinogenic.[4b] Traditional medicinal uses, attributed to this plant, are based on wrong identity.[4b] Drugs interacting with the herbs: Anticholinergic drugs, Cholinergic drugs, Procycline.[2]
Taalisa	*Abies webbiana* Lindl.	*Abies alba* (needle oil): Bronchospasm can be increased.[1] Can exacerbate asthma and whooping cough.[1,2]
Tagara	*Valeriana wallichii* DC.	Lethal dose: Valerenic acid 400 mg/kg IP in mice. Valepotriates LD_{50} 64-150 mg/kg. IP in mice, non-toxic at 4.6 g/kg orally in mice.[11] Valerian: Interacts with opiates, alcohol, CNS depressants.[12,5]
Tanduliyaka	*Amaranthus spinosus* Linn.	The plant gave negative antibiotic tests, but has a high phagocytic index.[4b]
Tarkaari	*Clerodendrum phlomidis* Linn.	Plant: Exhibited antiovulatory activity and prevented pregnancy in albino rats.[4c]
Tejovati	*Zanthoxylum alatum* Roxb.	Essential oil from seeds: Strong antibacterial against *Escherichia coli*, *Vibrio cholerae*, *Mycrococcus pyogens var aureus*, *Shigella dysenteriae* and *Salmonella typhi*. In a dilution of 1 in 40,000, the oil killed 50% of ciliates.[4a]
Tikhura	*Maranta arundinacea* Linn.	Roots: Canadian regulations do not allow arrow roots as a non-medical ingredient for oral use products.[10] The tuber contains a protease inhibitor, which inhibits the proteolytic activity of human and bovine pancreatic secretion.[4d]
Tila	*Sesamum indicum* Linn.	Anaphylaxis associated with the sesame consumption has been described, especially in persons with a known history of asthma or with other anaphylactic sensitivity.[10]
Traayamaana	*Gentiana kurroo* Royle	Toxic constituents in *G. lutea* root are: Amarogentine, gentiopicrin, swertiamarin, sweroside, (iridoid monoterpenes).[11] Contraindicated in gastric and duodenal ulcers.[1] Emmenagogue.[16(3)]
Tvak	*Cinnamomum zeylanicum* Blume	Contraindicated in pregnancy.[1,17(1)] stomach and duodenal ulcers.[16(1)] Large doses caused stimulation of vasomotor center.[5,10] Drugs interacting with the herb: Antidiabetic drugs.[2]
Ushaka	*Dorema ammoniacum* D. Don	Oleo-gum resin is the source of the drug Amoniacum.[4a]

Table 5: Contd.

Ayurvedic/Native Name	Botanical Name	Adverse Effects and Interactions
Ushira	*Vetiveria zizanioides* (Linn.) Nash	Root: Emmenagogue, uterine stimulant. Regulated in the US as an allowable flavouring agent in alcoholic beverages only.[10]
Vaasaka	*Adhatoda vasica* Nees	Vasicine and vasicinone may potentiate bronchodilatory activity of theophylline and isoprenaline.[9] Vasicine was formerly used as a starting substance for the production of mucolytics, Bromhexin and Ambroxol. Now, not available in the US.[2]
Vaastuka	*Chenopodium album* Linn.	Toxic constituents of *C. ambrosioides*. (American wormseed): Ascaridole (unsaturated terpene peroxide of volatile oxide); nitrates. Emmenagogue, abortifacient.[11]
Vaataama	*Prunus amygdalus* Batsch	A Japanese patent claims isolation of low molecular weight peptides with analgesic and anti-inflammatory properties.[2] Drugs interacting with the herb: ACE inhibitors, antihypertensive drugs.[2]
Vachaa	*Acorus calamus* Linn.	Calamus oil: Beta-isoasarone is carcinogenic.[11] North American variety: isoasarone-free. European variety: less than 10% isoasarone; type III and IV: up to 96% isoasarone (in volatile oil).[2] Tincture therapeutic dose: 1.85-3.7 ml. Tincture (1:2). LD_{50} 5 ml/kg IP in mice.[11] Drugs interacting with the herbs: Antacids, CNS depressants, H_2 Blockers, Monoamine Oxidase Inhibitors, Proton Pump Inhibitors.[2] Contraindicated during pregnancy.[17(2)]
Vahirshikhaa	*Actiniopteris dichotoma* Kuhn	Ethanolic extract (50%) of the plant showed antispermatogenic activity in male rats.[4d]
Vajrakanda	*Urginea indica* Kunth	White squill: Contraindicated in digitalis glycosides, in potassium deficiency,[1] hypercalcaemia and hyperkalaemia.[5,17(1)] Toxic constituents: Scillarin A and B, proscillaridin A (bufadienolides) and other glycosides.[11] New York Heart Association: 100-500 mg standardised squill bulb powder per day in stage I and II heart disease.[2] Squill contains cardiac glycosides.[5]
Vandaaka	*Loranthus longiflorus* Desr.	Plant: Diuretic, antilithiatic.[4c]
Vansa Rochana	*Bambusa arundinacea* (Retz.) Roxb.	Manna consists of silica 90.5, potash 1.1, alumina 0.4 and iron peroxide 0.9%.[4b]
Vansha	*Bambusa arundinacea* Willd.	Tender shoots and root contain a cyanogenic glucoside.[4b] Ethanolic extract of tender shoots adversely affects the sperm count and motility in rats.[4c]

Table 5: Contd.

Ayurvedic/Native Name	Botanical Name	Adverse Effects and Interactions
Vasuka	*Trianthema portulacastrum* Linn.	The leaves and stems, eaten as vegetables, may produce toxic effects even paralysis. Roots: cathartic, contraindicated in pregnancy due to use in traditional medicine as an abortifacient.[4a]
Vata	*Ficus beng(h)alensis* Linn.	Bark extracts due to leucodelphinidin and bengalenoside, not to be taken concurrently with diabetes medications.[5] These constituents decreased blood glucose in research animals.[5]
Vatsanaabha	*Aconitum ferox* Wall. ex Ser.	Aconitine: 2 to 5 mg may cause death. Even external application is reported to cause toxic symptoms.[3] Contraindicated with antiarrhythmics, antihypertensives, cardiac glycosides.[5] Confined to homoeopathic medicine.[2] Toxic constituents: Aconitine, mesaconitine, hypaconitine, diteropenoid-ester alkaloids.[11] Processed aconite may be devoid of toxicity.[3]
Vetasaamla	*Rheum emodi* Wall. ex Meisn	Rhubarb root: Contraindicated with other stimulant laxatives,[16(1)] renal disorders,[17(1)] in intestinal obstruction, Crohn's disease, colitis ulcerosa, appendicitis, abdominal pain of unknown origin,[1] pregnancy and children under 12 years of age.[1] Toxic constituents: Emodin, anthraquinones.[11]
Vidang	*Embelia ribes* Burm. f.	A potential contraceptive plant.[4c] Embelin: antispermatogenic, changes can be reversed.[4c]
Vishatinduka	*Strychnos nux-vomica* Linn.	Toxic constituents of dried ripened seeds: 1-2%, strychnine and brucine, vomicine and other indole alkaloids, glycoside loganin, caffeotannic acid.[11] Toxic dose: 5 mg strychnine.[11]
Vriddhadaaruka	*Argyreia speciosa* Sweet	Seeds contain 0.5-0.9% ergoline alkaloids; a few are reported to be hallucinogenic. LD_{50}: 500 mg/kg body wt.[4b]
Vrikshaamla	*Garcinia indica* Choisy	Garcinia cambogia: Mixed evidence of the use of garcinia fruit rind extract for weight loss. An extract containing 50% hydroxycitric acid, 1000 mg three times daily and 500 mg four times daily has been used.[(2)]

Table 5: Contd.

Ayurvedic/Native Name	Botanical Name	Adverse Effects and Interactions
Yashtimadhu	*Glycyrrhiza glabra* Linn.	Toxic constituent in the root: 6-14% Glycyrrhizic acid (saponin glycoside) interacts with spironolactone (antagonises diuretic effect), cardiac glycosides, thiazide diuretics (can cause hypokalaemia, may potentiate digoxin toxicity, corticosteroids, cyclosporine, monoamine oxidase inhibitors (immunostimulating effect may decrease response to the drugs). Sympathomimetic amines may increase the risk of hypertensive crisis.[12,10] Contraindicated in cholestatic liver disorders, liver cirrhosis, hypertonia, hypokalaemia, severe kidney insufficiency, pregnancy,[1] bleeding disorders, diabetes (on insulin), impotence, male infertility.[5] Deglycyrrhizinized licorice (DGL) is usually free of side effects.[10] French regulation limits daily consumption to 5 g or as tea 8 g.[10]
Yava	*Hordeum vulgare* Linn.	Seeds contain gliadin, a component of gluten.[5] May supress the secretion of milk in women whose children have died after birth. (*Chinese Materia Medica*, GA Stuart).
Yavaani	*Trachyspermum ammi* (Linn.) Sprague	Thymol, produced from *ajowan* oil, is toxic in high doses, and may lead to fatal poisoning.[4a]

Sanskrit Names: *Plants of Bhavaprakash*, National Academy of Ayurveda, New Delhi. (The last classical reference work of Ayurveda, 1550 AD.)

A number of obsolete Sanskrit names appear in the table. These will lead the researchers of classical texts to proper botanical names.

REFERENCES

1. Blumenthal et al., (1998). *The Complete German Commission E Monographs*, American Botanical Council, Austin, Texas.
2. *Natural Medicines Comprehensive Database*, (2007). Therapeutic Research Faculty, Stockton, CA.
3. *The Review of Natural Products, Facts and Comparisons*, (2005) Wolter Kluwer, St. Louis, Missouri.
4. *The Wealth of India*, CSIR, Original Series, Vol 2 to 11 (a); Revised Vol 1 to 3 (b), First Supplement Series, Vol 1 to 5 (c), Second Supplement Series Vol 1 to 3 (d), (1976-2009). NISCAIR (CSIR), New Delhi.
5. Herr, Sharon M, (2002). *Herb-Drug Interaction Handbook*, Second edition. Church Street Books, Nassau, NY.
6. Francis & Brinker, (2001). *Herb Contraindications & Drug Interactions*, Eclectic Medical Publications, Sandy, Oregon.
7. More-Roth, Linda Skid, (2004). *Handbook of Herbs and Naturals Supplements*, Mosby, St. Lois, Missourie.
8. *ESCOP (European Scientific Co-operative on Phytotherapy), Monographs*, Second edn, 2003 (a), Second edn Supplement, 2009 (b), Thieme, Stuttgart, Germany.
9. Miller, Lucinda G and Wallace I Murray, (1998). *Herbal Medicinals: A Clinician's Guide*, Haworth Press, New York.
10. Guffin, Michel Mac et al., (1997). *Botanical Safety Handbook* (American Product Association), CRC, Boca Raton.
11. Brinker, Francis, (2000). *Toxicology of Botanical Medicines*, Eclectic Medical Publications, Sandy, Oregon.
12. University of Michigan Health System: *http://www.umich/edu*, 2010.
13. Harkness, Richard and Steven Bratman, (2000). *Drug-Herb-Vitamin Interactions Bible*, Prima Publishing.
14. Harkness, Richard and Steven Bratman, (2003). *Handbook of Drug-Herb and Drug-Supplement Interactions*, Mosby, St. Lois, Missouri.
15. PAGM, De Smet et al., (Eds.) *Adverse Effects of Herbal Drugs*-1(1991), 2(1993), 3(1995), Springer-Verlag, Germany.
16. WHO monographs on selected medicinal plants, Vol. 1, 1999; Vol. 2, 2002; Vol. 3, 2007, Vol. 4, 2009, World Health Organization, Geneva.
17. British Herbal Compendium, Vol. 1, 1992; Vol. 2, 2006; Peter Bradley, British Herbal Medicine Association, Bournemouth.

Part Two

THE NOMENCLATURE

COORDINATED READING
(for Active Principles, research findings and medicinal uses):

Indian Medicinal Plants: An Illustrated Dictionary
C.P. Khare, 2007, Springer, New York, Heidelburg.
The Wealth of India series, original and Revised volumes, 1950-2009, Council of Scientific & Industrial Research (CSIR), New Delhi.
The Treatise on Indian Medicinal Plants, Ashima Chatterjee and Satyesh Chandra Pakrashi, Vol I to VI, 2003, NISCAIR (CSIR), New Delhi.
Dictionary of Indian Medicinal Plants, Akhtar Hussain *et al.* 1992, Central Institute of Medicinal an Aromatic Plants (CIMAP), Lucknow.

Table Contd.

Botanical Name	Indian Name	English Name	Medicinal System
Abies webbiana	Taalispatra	Indian Silver Fir, The West-Himalayan High-Level Fir, The East-Himalayan Fir	Folk
Abies webbiana	Dhaatriparni	Indian Silver Fir, The West-Himalayan High-Level Fir, The East-Himalayan Fir	Ayurvedic
Abies webbiana	Dhaatripatra	Indian Silver Fir, The West-Himalayan High-Level Fir, The East-Himalayan Fir	Ayurvedic
Abies webbiana	Patraadhya	Indian Silver Fir, The West-Himalayan High-Level Fir, The East-Himalayan Fir	Ayurvedic
Abies webbiana	Taalisa	Indian Silver Fir, The West-Himalayan High-Level Fir, The East-Himalayan Fir	Ayurvedic
Abies webbiana	Taalisapatra	Indian Silver Fir, The West-Himalayan High-Level Fir, The East-Himalayan Fir	Ayurvedic
Abies webbiana	Taalisha	Indian Silver Fir, The West-Himalayan High-Level Fir, The East-Himalayan Fir	Ayurvedic
Abroma augusta	Pishaacha Kaarpaasa	Perennial Indian Hemp, Devil's Cotton	Ayurvedic
Abroma augusta	Pivari	Perennial Indian Hemp, Devil's Cotton	Ayurvedic
Abroma augusta	Ulat-kambal	Perennial Indian Hemp, Devil's Cotton	Unani
Abroma augusta	Sivapputtutti	Perennial Indian Hemp, Devil's Cotton	Siddha/Tamil
Abroma augusta	Kumal	Perennial Indian Hemp, Devil's Cotton	Folk
Abroma augusta	Sanukapaasi	Perennial Indian Hemp, Devil's Cotton	Folk
Abrus precatorius	Chirihintikaa	Indian Wild Liquorice, Jequirity, Crab's Eye, Precatory Bean	Ayurvedic
Abrus precatorius	Chirmiti	Indian Wild Liquorice, Jequirity, Crab's Eye, Precatory Bean	Ayurvedic
Abrus precatorius	Gunjaa	Indian Wild Liquorice, Jequirity, Crab's Eye, Precatory Bean	Ayurvedic

Table Contd.

Botanical Name	Indian Name	English Name	Medicinal System
Abrus precatorius	Gunjaka	Indian Wild Liquorice, Jequirity, Crab's Eye, Precatory Bean	Ayurvedic
Abrus precatorius	Kakanti	Indian Wild Liquorice, Jequirity, Crab's Eye, Precatory Bean	Ayurvedic
Abrus precatorius	Kabjaka	Indian Wild Liquorice, Jequirity, Crab's Eye, Precatory Bean	Ayurvedic
Abrus precatorius	Kaakananti	Indian Wild Liquorice, Jequirity, Crab's Eye, Precatory Bean	Ayurvedic
Abrus precatorius	Kaakchinchi	Indian Wild Liquorice, Jequirity, Crab's Eye, Precatory Bean	Ayurvedic
Abrus precatorius	Raktikaa	Indian Wild Liquorice, Jequirity, Crab's Eye, Precatory Bean	Ayurvedic
Abrus precatorius	Tiktikaa	Indian Wild Liquorice, Jequirity, Crab's Eye, Precatory Bean	Ayurvedic
Abrus precatorius	Ghunghchi	Indian Wild Liquorice, Jequirity, Crab's Eye, Precatory Bean	Unani
Abrus precatorius	Ghamchi	Indian Wild Liquorice, Jequirity, Crab's Eye, Precatory Bean	Unani
Abrus precatorius	Kunri	Indian Wild Liquorice, Jequirity, Crab's Eye, Precatory Bean	Siddha/Tamil
Abrus precatorius	Chirmiti	Indian Wild Liquorice, Jequirity, Crab's Eye, Precatory Bean	Folk
Abrus precatorius	Ratti	Indian Wild Liquorice, Jequirity, Crab's Eye, Precatory Bean	Folk
Abutilon indicum	Atibalaa	Country Mallow, Flowering Maples, Chinese Bell-flowers	Ayurvedic
Abutilon indicum	Kankatikaa	Country Mallow, Flowering Maples, Chinese Bell-flowers	Ayurvedic
Abutilon indicum	Rishyaproktaa	Country Mallow, Flowering Maples, Chinese Bell-flowers	Ayurvedic

Table Contd.

Botanical Name	Indian Name	English Name	Medicinal System
Abutilon indicum	Kanghi	Country Mallow, Flowering Maples, Chinese Bell-flowers	Unani
Abutilon indicum	Musht-ul-Ghaul	Country Mallow, Flowering Maples, Chinese Bell-flowers	Unani
Abutilon indicum	Darkht-e-Shaan	Country Mallow, Flowering Maples, Chinese Bell-flowers	Unani
Abutilon indicum	Thutthi	Country Mallow, Flowering Maples, Chinese Bell-flowers	Siddha/Tamil
Abutilon indicum	Kanghi	Country Mallow, Flowering Maples, Chinese Bell-flowers	Folk
Abutilon indicum	Kakahi	Country Mallow, Flowering Maples, Chinese Bell-flowers	Folk
Abutilon indicum	Kakahiyaa	Country Mallow, Flowering Maples, Chinese Bell-flowers	Folk
Acacia arabica	Aabhaa	Babul, Black Babul, Indian Gum Arabic Tree	Ayurvedic
Acacia arabica	Baavari	Babul, Black Babul, Indian Gum Arabic Tree	Ayurvedic
Acacia arabica	Babbuula	Babul, Black Babul, Indian Gum Arabic Tree	Ayurvedic
Acacia arabica	Babbuuri	Babul, Black Babul, Indian Gum Arabic Tree	Ayurvedic
Acacia arabica	Shuulikaa	Babul, Black Babul, Indian Gum Arabic Tree	Ayurvedic
Acacia arabica	Shitaka	Babul, Black Babul, Indian Gum Arabic Tree	Ayurvedic
Acacia arabica	Kinkiraata	Babul, Black Babul, Indian Gum Arabic Tree	Ayurvedic
Acacia arabica	Yugmakantaka	Babul, Black Babul, Indian Gum Arabic Tree	Ayurvedic
Acacia arabica	Sukshmapatra	Babul, Black Babul, Indian Gum Arabic Tree	Ayurvedic
Acacia arabica	Pitapushpaka	Babul, Black Babul, Indian Gum Arabic Tree	Ayurvedic
Acacia arabica	Aqaaqia	Babul, Black Babul, Indian Gum Arabic Tree	Unani
Acacia arabica	Babuul	Babul, Black Babul, Indian Gum Arabic Tree	Unani
Acacia arabica	Kikar	Babul, Black Babul, Indian Gum Arabic Tree	Unani

Table Contd.

Botanical Name	Indian Name	English Name	Medicinal System
Acacia arabica	Mughilaan	Babul, Black Babul, Indian Gum Arabic Tree	Unani
Acacia arabica	Samur	Babul, Black Babul, Indian Gum Arabic Tree	Unani
Acacia arabica	Karu-velamaram	Babul, Black Babul, Indian Gum Arabic Tree	Siddha/Tamil
Acacia arabica	Karuvelei	Babul, Black Babul, Indian Gum Arabic Tree	Siddha/Tamil
Acacis arabica	Velampisin (gum)	Babul, Black Babul, Indian Gum Arabic Tree	Siddha/Tamil
Acacia canescens	Aadaari	Climbing Acacia	Ayurvedic
Acacia canescens	Araara	Climbing Acacia	Folk
Acacia canescens	Ari	Climbing Acacia	Folk
Acacia catechu	Khadira	Cutch tree, Catechu	Ayurvedic
Acacia catechu	Kadara	Cutch tree, Catechu	Ayurvedic
Acacia catechu	Somavalka	Cutch tree, Catechu	Ayurvedic
Acacia catechu	Gaayatri	Cutch tree, Catechu	Ayurvedic
Acacia catechu	Dantdhaavan	Cutch tree, Catechu	Ayurvedic
Acacia catechu	Kantaki	Cutch tree, Catechu	Ayurvedic
Acacia catechu	Raktasaara (Heartwood extract)	Cutch tree, Catechu	Ayurvedic
Acacia catechu	Kaat	Cutch tree, Catechu	Unani
Acacia catechu	Katthaa (Heartwood extract)	Cutch tree, Catechu	Unani
Acacia catechu	Khair	Cutch tree, Catechu	Unani
Acacia catechu	Karunkaali (Bark)	Cutch tree, Catechu	Siddha/Tamil
Acacia catechu	Karangalli	Cutch tree, Catechu	Siddha/Tamil
Acacia catechu	Kadiram	Cutch tree, Catechu	Siddha/Tamil
Acacia catechu	Kaasukkatti (Heartwood extract)	Cutch tree, Catechu	Siddha/Tamil
Acacia chundra	Khadira	Red Cutch	Ayurvedic
Acacia chundra	Katthakkaambu (Heartwood extract)	Red Cutch	Siddha/Tamil

Table Contd.

Botanical Name	Indian Name	English Name	Medicinal System
Acacia chundra	Laal Khair	Red Cutch	Folk
Acacia concinna	Saptalaa	Soap-nut Acacia	Ayurvedic
Acacia concinna	Shitalaa	Soap-nut Acacia	Ayurvedic
Acacia concinna	Saatalaa	Soap-nut Acacia	Ayurvedic
Acacia concinna	Shrivalli	Soap-nut Acacia	Ayurvedic
Acacia concinna	Kantvalli	Soap-nut Acacia	Ayurvedic
Acacia concinna	Shikaakaai	Soap-nut Acacia	Unani
Acacia concinna	Kharunb Nabti	Soap-nut Acacia	Unani
Acacia concinna	Seekai	Soap-nut Acacia	Siddha/Tamil
Acacia concinna	Sigakai	Soap-nut Acacia	Siddha/Tamil
Acacia concinna	Ban-Reethaa	Soap-nut Acacia	Folk
Acacia farnesiana	Arimeda	Cassie Flower, Cassie Absolute, Sweet Acacia	Ayurvedic
Acacia farnesiana	Vitakhadira	Cassie Flower, Sweet Acacia	Ayurvedic
Acacia farnesiana	Vilaayati Kikar	Cassie Flower, Sweet Acacia	Unani
Acacia farnesiana	Durgandh Khair	Cassie Flower, Sweet Acacia	Unani
Acacia farnesiana	Gandbabuul	Cassie Flower, Sweet Acacia	Unani
Acacia farnesiana	Guyaa Babuul	Cassie Flower, Sweet Acacia	Unani
Acacia farnesiana	Kastuurivelam	Cassie Flower, Sweet Acacia	Siddha/Tamil
Acacia farnesiana	Veddayala	Cassie Flower, Sweet Acacia	Siddha/Tamil
Acacia leucophloea	Arimanja	White Babul	Ayurvedic
Acacia leucophloea	Arimeda	White Babul	Ayurvedic
Acacia leucophloea	Arimedaka	White Babul	Ayurvedic
Acacia leucophloea	Godhaa-skandha	White Babul	Ayurvedic
Acacia leucophloea	Irimeda	White Babul	Ayurvedic
Acacia leucophloea	Vitakhadir	White Babul	Ayurvedic
Acacia leucophloea	Raamaka	White Babul	Ayurvedic
Acacia leucophloea	Guyaa Babuul	White Babul	Unani
Acacia leucophloea	Kath Safed	White Babul	Unani
Acacia leucophloea	Vilaayati Babuul	White Babul	Unani
Acacia leucophloea	Valval	White Babul	Siddha/Tamil
Acacia leucophloea	Velvayalam	White Babul	Siddha/Tamil
Acacia leucophloea	Safed Babul	White Babul	Folk

Table Contd.

Botanical Name	Indian Name	English Name	Medicinal System
Acacia leucophloea	Safed Kikar	White Babul	Folk
Acacia leucophloea	Renvaa	White Babul	Folk
Acacia pennata	Aadaari	Feathery-shoot Acacia	Ayurvedic
Acacia pennata	Ari	Feathery-shoot Acacia	Ayurvedic
Acacia pennata	Lataakhadira	Feathery-shoot Acacia	Ayurvedic
Acacia pennata	Aila	Feathery-shoot Acacia	Folk
Acacia pennata	Indan	Feathery-shoot Acacia	Siddha/Tamil
Acacia pennata	Indu, Iyak Koluntu (Tender leaves)	Feathery-shoot Acacia	Siddha/Tamil
Acacia senegal	Shveta Babbuula	Gum Arabic Tree	Ayurvedic
Acacia suma	Shveta Khadira	White Babul	Ayurvedic
Acacia suma	Kadara	White Babul	Ayurvedic
Acacia suma	Somavalkala	White Babul	Ayurvedic
Acacia suma	Khor	White Babul	Unani
Acacia suma	Safed Khair	White Babul	Unani
Acacia torta	Aadaari	Twisted Acacia	Ayurvedic
Acacia torta	Lataa Khadira	Twisted Acacia	Ayurvedic
Acacia torta	Araar	Twisted Acacia	Folk
Acacia torta	Chilar	Twisted Acacia	Folk
Acacia torta	Aila	Twisted Acacia	Folk
Acacia torta	Kariyundu	Twisted Acacia	Siddha/Tamil
Acacia torta	Ingu	Twisted Acacia	Siddha/Tamil
Acalypha ciliata	Daadari	Smaller var. Acalypha	Folk
Acalypha ciliata	Kuppi (Smaller variety)	Smaller var. Acalypha	Ayurvedic
Acalypha fruticosa	Kuppaimeni	Birch-leaved Acalypha	Siddha/Tamil
Acalypha fruticosa	Chinnivara	Birch-leaved Acalypha	Folk
Acalypha indica	Aamaabhaaji	Copperleaf Acalypha	Folk
Acalypha indica	Khokli	Copperleaf Acalypha	Folk
Acalypha indica	Kuppi	Copperleaf Acalypha	Folk
Acalypha indica	Kuppi	Copperleaf Acalypha	Ayurvedic
Acalypha indica	Muktavarchaa	Copperleaf Acalypha	Ayurvedic

Table Contd.

Botanical Name	Indian Name	English Name	Medicinal System
Acalypha indica	Haritamanjari	Copperleaf Acalypha	Ayurvedic
Acalypha indica	Kuppaimeni	Copperleaf Acalypha	Siddha/Tamil
Acanthospermum hispidum	Trikantaka	Bristly Starbur	Ayurvedic
Acanthus ilicifolius	Krishna Saraiyaka	Sea Holly	Ayurvedic
Acanthus ilicifolius	Kollimulli	Sea Holly	Siddha/Tamil
Acanthus ilicifolius	Hargozaa	Sea Holly	Folk
Achillea millefolium	Biranjaasif	Milfoil, Yarrow, Thousand Leaf	Unani
Achillea millefolium	Gandana	Milfoil, Yarrow, Thousand Leaf	Folk
Achillea millefolium	Rojmari	Milfoil, Yarrow, Thousand Leaf	Folk
Achras zapota	Cheeku	Sapota, Sapodilla Plum, Chicle	Unani
Achras zapota	Sapotaa	Sapota, Sapodilla Plum, Chicle	Unani
Achras zapota	Shimai eluppai	Sapota, Sapodilla Plum, Chicle	Siddha/Tamil
Achyranthes aspera	Aaghaat	Prickly Chaff Flower	Ayurvedic
Achyranthes aspera	Adahshalya	Prickly Chaff Flower	Ayurvedic
Achyranthes aspera	Apaamaarga	Prickly Chaff Flower	Ayurvedic
Achyranthes aspera	Chirchitaa	Prickly Chaff Flower	Ayurvedic
Achyranthes aspera	Shikhari	Prickly Chaff Flower	Ayurvedic
Achyranthes aspera	Shaikharika	Prickly Chaff Flower	Ayurvedic
Achyranthes aspera	Mayura	Prickly Chaff Flower	Ayurvedic
Achyranthes aspera	Mayuraka	Prickly Chaff Flower	Ayurvedic
Achyranthes aspera	Kharamanjari	Prickly Chaff Flower	Ayurvedic
Achyranthes aspera	Kharapushpaa	Prickly Chaff Flower	Ayurvedic
Achyranthes aspera	Pratyakpushpaa	Prickly Chaff Flower	Ayurvedic
Achyranthes aspera	Vashira	Prickly Chaff Flower	Ayurvedic
Achyranthes aspera	Kanihi	Prickly Chaff Flower	Ayurvedic
Achyranthes aspera	Chirchitaa	Prickly Chaff Flower	Unani
Achyranthes aspera	Naayuruvi	Prickly Chaff Flower	Siddha/Tamil
Achyranthes aspera	Chirchitta	Prickly Chaff Flower	Folk
Achyranthes aspera	Chichidaa	Prickly Chaff Flower	Folk
Achyranthes aspera	Latjeeraa	Prickly Chaff Flower	Folk
Achyranthes bidentata	Shveta Apaamaarga	White Chaff Flower	Ayurvedic
Achyranthes bidentata	Naayurivi	White Chaff Flower	Siddha/Tamil

Table Contd.

Botanical Name	Indian Name	English Name	Medicinal System
Aconitum atrox	Banwaa	Himalayan Napellus	Folk
Aconitum atrox	Vatsanaabha	Himalayan Napellus	Ayurvedic
Aconitum chasmanthum	Visha	Indian Napellus	Ayurvedic
Aconitum chasmanthum	Shringika-Visha	Indian Napellus	Ayurvedic
Aconitum chasmanthum	Vatsanaabha	Indian Napellus	Ayurvedic
Aconitum chasmanthum	Mohri	Indian Napellus	Folk
Aconitum chasmanthum	Meethaa Zahar	Indian Napellus	Folk
Aconitum deinorrhizum	Bashahr-Mohra	Indian Aconite	Folk
Aconitum deinorrhizum	Dudhiyaa Bish	Indian Aconite	Folk
Aconitum deinorrhizum	Safed Bikh	Indian Aconite	Folk
Aconitum deinorrhizum	Vatsanaabha	Indian Aconite	Ayurvedic
Aconitum falconeri	Bikh	Indian Aconite	Folk
Aconitum falconeri	Bish	Indian Aconite	Folk
Aconitum falconeri	Meethaa Telia	Indian Aconite	Folk
Aconitum falconeri	Vatsanaabha	Indian Aconite	Ayurvedic
Aconitum ferox	Amrita	Indian Aconite, Wolfsbane, Monkshood	Ayurvedic
Aconitum ferox	Garala	Indian Aconite, Wolfsbane, Monkshood	Ayurvedic
Aconitum ferox	Shrangikavisha	Indian Aconite, Wolfsbane, Monkshood	Ayurvedic
Aconitum ferox	Sthaavaravisha	Indian Aconite, Wolfsbane, Monkshood	Ayurvedic
Aconitum ferox	Vajraanga	Indian Aconite, Wolfsbane, Monkshood	Ayurvedic
Aconitum ferox	Vatsanaabha	Indian Aconite, Wolfsbane, Monkshood	Ayurvedic
Aconitum ferox	Vatsanaagaka	Indian Aconite, Wolfsbane, Monkshood	Ayurvedic
Aconitum ferox	Visha	Indian Aconite, Wolfsbane, Monkshood	Ayurvedic
Aconitum ferox	Bish	Indian Aconite, Wolfsbane, Monkshood	Unani
Aconitum ferox	Bishnaag	Indian Aconite, Wolfsbane, Monkshood	Unani
Aconitum ferox	Vasanaavi	Indian Aconite, Wolfsbane, Monkshood	Siddha/Tamil

Table Contd.

Botanical Name	Indian Name	English Name	Medicinal System
Aconitum ferox	Karunaabhi	Indian Aconite, Wolfsbane, Monkshood	Siddha/Tamil
Aconitum ferox	Bacchanaag	Indian Aconite, Wolfsbane, Monkshood	Folk
Aconitum ferox	Bish	Indian Aconite, Wolfsbane, Monkshood	Folk
Aconitum ferox	Mitha Zahar	Indian Aconite, Wolfsbane, Monkshood	Folk
Aconitum ferox	Telia Vish	Indian Aconite, Wolfsbane, Monkshood	Folk
Aconitum heterophyllum	Ativisha	Atis Root, Aconite	Ayurvedic
Aconitum heterophyllum	Arunaa	Atis Root, Aconite	Ayurvedic
Aconitum heterophyllum	Vishaa	Atis Root, Aconite	Ayurvedic
Aconitum heterophyllum	Shuklakandaa	Atis Root, Aconite	Ayurvedic
Aconitum heterophyllum	Bhanguraa	Atis Root, Aconite	Ayurvedic
Aconitum heterophyllum	Ghunapriyaa	Atis Root, Aconite	Ayurvedic
Aconitum heterophyllum	Ghunavallabhaa	Atis Root, Aconite	Ayurvedic
Aconitum heterophyllum	Kaashmiraa	Atis Root, Aconite	Ayurvedic
Aconitum heterophyllum	Shishubhaishajyaa	Atis Root, Aconite	Ayurvedic
Aconitum heterophyllum	Vishwaa	Atis Root, Aconite	Ayurvedic
Aconitum heterophyllum	Atis	Atis Root, Aconite	Unani
Aconitum heterophyllum	Athividayam	Atis Root, Aconite	Siddha/Tamil
Aconitum heterophyllum	Patis	Atis Root, Aconite	Folk
Aconitum laciniatum	Vatsanaabha	Himalayan Aconite	Ayurvedic
Aconitum laciniatum	Kalo Bikhmo	Himalayan Aconite	Folk
Aconitum luridum	Vatsanaabha	Himalayan Aconite	Ayurvedic
Aconitum palmatum	Bikhamaa	Himalayan Aconite	Folk
Aconitum palmatum	Prativishaa	Himalayan Aconite	Ayurvedic
Aconitum palmatum	Shyaamkandaa	Himalayan Aconite	Ayurvedic
Aconitum palmatum	Patis	Himalayan Aconite	Ayurvedic
Aconitum spicatum	Vatsanaabha	Nepal Aconite	Ayurvedic
Aconitum violaceum	Vatsanaabha	Himalayan Aconite	Ayurvedic
Aconitum violaceum	Tilia Kachnaag	Himalayan Aconite	Folk
Aconitum violaceum	Dudhia	Himalayan Aconite	Folk
Acorus calamus	Vachaa	Sweet Flag, Calamus	Ayurvedic

Table Contd.

Botanical Name	Indian Name	English Name	Medicinal System
Acorus calamus	Ugragandhaa	Sweet Flag, Calamus	Ayurvedic
Acorus calamus	Ugraa	Sweet Flag, Calamus	Ayurvedic
Acorus calamus	Golomi	Sweet Flag, Calamus	Ayurvedic
Acorus calamus	Shadgranthaa	Sweet Flag, Calamus	Ayurvedic
Acorus calamus	Shataparvaa	Sweet Flag, Calamus	Ayurvedic
Acorus calamus	Tikshnagandhaa	Sweet Flag, Calamus	Ayurvedic
Acorus calamus	Kshudra-patra	Sweet Flag, Calamus	Ayurvedic
Acorus calamus	Maangalyaa	Sweet Flag, Calamus	Ayurvedic
Acorus calamus	Ghorbach	Sweet Flag, Calamus	Ayurvedic
Acorus calamus	Waj-e-Turki	Sweet Flag, Calamus	Unani
Acorus calamus	Waj	Sweet Flag, Calamus	Unani
Acorus calamus	Vasambu	Sweet Flag, Calamus	Siddha/Tamil
Acorus gramineus	Haimavati	Calamus, White var.	Ayurvedic
Actaea spicata	Visha-phala	Baneberry Grapewort	Folk
Actiniopteris dichotoma	Mayurshikhaa	Peacock's Tail	Ayurvedic
Actiniopteris dichotoma	Madhuchhadaa	Peacock's Tail	Ayurvedic
Actiniopteris dichotoma	Sahastrahi	Peacock's Tail	Ayurvedic
Actiniopteris dichotoma	Vahrishikhaa	Peacock's Tail	Ayurvedic
Actinodaphne hookeri	Thali	Pisa	Siddha/Tamil
Actinodaphne hookeri	Paratathali	Pisa	Siddha/Tamil
Actinodaphne hookeri	Pisaa	Pisa	Folk
Adansonia digitata	Sheet-phala	Baobab, Monkey Bread Tree, African Calabash	Ayurvedic
Adansonia digitata	Ravanaamlikaa	Baobab, Monkey Bread Tree, African Calabash	Ayurvedic
Adansonia digitata	Gorakshi	Baobab, Monkey Bread Tree, African Calabash	Ayurvedic
Adansonia digitata	Panchparni	Baobab, Monkey Bread Tree, African Calabash	Ayurvedic
Adansonia digitata	Gorakh amli	Baobab, Monkey Bread Tree, African Calabash	Unani
Adansonia digitata	Papparapuli	Baobab, Monkey Bread Tree, African Calabash	Siddha/Tamil
Adansonia digitata	Gorakh Imli	Baobab, Monkey Bread Tree, African Calabash	Folk

Table Contd.

Botanical Name	Indian Name	English Name	Medicinal System
Adansonia digitata	Gorakh Chinchaa	Baobab, Monkey Bread Tree, African Calabash	Folk
Adenanthera pavonina	Rakta Kanchana	Coral Wood, Red Wood	Ayurvedic
Adenanthera pavonina	Rakta Kambal	Coral Wood, Red Wood	Ayurvedic
Adenanthera pavonina	Anai-gundumani	Coral Wood, Red Wood	Siddha/Tamil
Adenanthera pavonina	Ghumchi	Coral Wood, Red Wood	Folk
Adhatoda vasica	Vaasaa	Malabar Nut, Vasaca	Ayurvedic
Adhatoda vasica	Vaasaka	Malabar Nut, Vasaca	Ayurvedic
Adhatoda vasica	Vaasikaa	Malabar Nut, Vasaca	Ayurvedic
Adhatoda vasica	Simhaasya	Malabar Nut, Vasaca	Ayurvedic
Adhatoda vasica	Simhaparni	Malabar Nut, Vasaca	Ayurvedic
Adhatoda vasica	Simhavadanaa	Malabar Nut, Vasaca	Ayurvedic
Adhatoda vasica	Vaajidanta	Malabar Nut, Vasaca	Ayurvedic
Adhatoda vasica	Vrisha	Malabar Nut, Vasaca	Ayurvedic
Adhatoda vasica	Aataruushaka	Malabar Nut, Vasaca	Ayurvedic
Adhatoda vasica	Arusaa	Malabar Nut, Vasaca	Unani
Adhatoda vasica	Aadaathodai	Malabar Nut, Vasaca	Siddha/Tamil
Adhatoda vasica	Vasaakaa	Malabar Nut, Vasaca	Folk
Adiantum aethiopicum	Hansapadi	Nilgiri Fern	Ayurvedic
Adiantum capillus-veneris	Hansaraaja	American Maidenhair Fern, Venus Hair, Rock Fern	Ayurvedic
Adiantum capillus-veneris	Hansapadi	American Maidenhair Fern, Venus Hair, Rock Fern	Ayurvedic
Adiantum capillus-veneris	Parsiaavashaan	American Maidenhair Fern, Venus Hair, Rock Fern	Unani
Adiantum capillus-veneris	Seruppadai	American Maidenhair Fern, Venus Hair, Rock Fern	Siddha/Tamil
Adiantum capillus-veneris	Mubaaraka	American Maidenhair Fern, Venus Hair, Rock Fern	Folk
Adiantum incisum	Nilakantha-shikhaa	Peacock's Tail	Ayurvedic
Adiantum incisum	Mayurshikhaa	Peacock's Tail	Ayurvedic
Adiantum incisum	Vahrishikhaa	Peacock's Tail	Ayurvedic
Adiantum lunulatum	Hansaraaja	Walking Maidenhair Fern, Black Maidenhair	Ayurvedic

Table Contd.

Botanical Name	Indian Name	English Name	Medicinal System
Adiantum lunulatum	Hansapadi	Walking Maidenhair Fern, Black Maidenhair	Ayurvedic
Adiantum lunulatum	Hansapaadi	Walking Maidenhair Fern, Black Maidenhair	Ayurvedic
Adiantum lunulatum	Raktapaadi	Walking Maidenhair Fern, Black Maidenhair	Ayurvedic
Adiantum lunulatum	Kitamaataa	Walking Maidenhair Fern, Black Maidenhair	Ayurvedic
Adiantum lunulatum	Tripaadikaa	Walking Maidenhair Fern, Black Maidenhair	Ayurvedic
Adiantum lunulatum	Seruppadai	Walking Maidenhair Fern, Black Maidenhair	Siddha/Tamil
Adiantum lunulatum	Raajhans	Walking Maidenhair Fern, Black Maidenhair	Folk
Adiantum lunulatum	Mubaaraka	Walking Maidenhair Fern, Black Maidenhair	Folk
Adina cordifolia	Haridru	Yellow Teak, Saffron Teak	Ayurvedic
Adina cordifolia	Haraduaa-kadamba	Yellow Teak, Saffron Teak	Ayurvedic
Adina cordifolia	Gaur-kadamba	Yellow Teak, Saffron Teak	Ayurvedic
Adina cordifolia	Girikadamba	Yellow Teak, Saffron Teak	Ayurvedic
Adina cordifolia	Dhaaraa-kadamba	Yellow Teak, Saffron Teak	Ayurvedic
Adina cordifolia	Pitadaaru	Yellow Teak, Saffron Teak	Ayurvedic
Adina cordifolia	Kadambaka	Yellow Teak, Saffron Teak	Ayurvedic
Adina cordifolia	Manjakadambu	Yellow Teak, Saffron Teak	Siddha/Tamil
Adina cordifolia	Haladu	Yellow Teak, Saffron Teak	Folk
Adina cordifolia	Kheta Kadam	Yellow Teak, Saffron Teak	Folk
Aegle marmelos	Bilva	Bael Tree, Bengal Quince	Ayurvedic
Aegle marmelos	Shriphala	Bael Tree, Bengal Quince	Ayurvedic
Aegle marmelos	Shaandilya	Bael Tree, Bengal Quince	Ayurvedic
Aegle marmelos	Shailuusha	Bael Tree, Bengal Quince	Ayurvedic
Aegle marmelos	Shalya	Bael Tree, Bengal Quince	Ayurvedic
Aegle marmelos	Sadaaphala	Bael Tree, Bengal Quince	Ayurvedic
Aegle marmelos	Mahaakapittha	Bael Tree, Bengal Quince	Ayurvedic
Aegle marmelos	Maaluura	Bael Tree, Bengal Quince	Ayurvedic
Aegle marmelos	Rudrajataa	Bael Tree, Bengal Quince	Ayurvedic

Table Contd.

Botanical Name	Indian Name	English Name	Medicinal System
Albizia amara	Vaagei	Siris Tree, East Indian Walnut	Siddha/Tamil
Albizia lebbeck	Shirisha	Siris Tree, East Indian Walnut	Ayurvedic
Albizia lebbeck	Bhandi	Siris Tree, East Indian Walnut	Ayurvedic
Albizia lebbeck	Bhandila	Siris Tree, East Indian Walnut	Ayurvedic
Albizia lebbeck	Shitapushpa	Siris Tree, East Indian Walnut	Ayurvedic
Albizia lebbeck	Mridupushpa	Siris Tree, East Indian Walnut	Ayurvedic
Albizia lebbeck	Kapitana	Siris Tree, East Indian Walnut	Ayurvedic
Albizia lebbeck	Siras	Siris Tree, East Indian Walnut	Unani
Albizia lebbeck	Vaagei	Siris Tree, East Indian Walnut	Siddha/Tamil
Albizia procera	Shirisha Shveta	White Siris	Ayurvedic
Aleurites moluccana	Akshota	Candlenut Tree	Ayurvedic
Aleurites moluccana	Jangali Akharot	Candlenut Tree	Ayurvedic
Aleurites moluccana	Naatuakrottu	Candlenut Tree	Siddha/Tamil
Alhagi pseudalhagi	Yavaasaka	Camel Thorn, Persian Manna Plant	Ayurvedic
Alhagi pseudalhagi	Yavaasa	Camel Thorn, Persian Manna Plant	Ayurvedic
Alhagi pseudalhagi	Yaasa	Camel Thorn, Persian Manna Plant	Ayurvedic
Alhagi pseudalhagi	Duhsparshaa	Camel Thorn, Persian Manna Plant	Ayurvedic
Alhagi pseudalhagi	Duraalabhaa	Camel Thorn, Persian Manna Plant	Ayurvedic
Alhagi pseudalhagi	Kunaashak	Camel Thorn, Persian Manna Plant	Ayurvedic
Alhagi pseudalhagi	Yaasa-sharkaraa (Manna)	Camel Thorn, Persian Manna Plant	Ayurvedic
Alhagi pseudalhagi	Jawaasaa	Camel Thorn, Persian Manna Plant	Unani
Alhagi pseudalhagi	Turanjabeen (Manna)	Camel Thorn, Persian Manna Plant	Unani
Alhagi pseudalhagi	Poonaik-kanchori	Camel Thorn, Persian Manna Plant	Siddha/Tamil
Alhagi pseudalhagi	Khaar-e-shutur	Camel Thorn, Persian Manna Plant	Unani
Alkanna tinctoria	Ratanjot	Alkanet, Dyers' or Spanish Bugloss	Unani

Table Contd.

Botanical Name	Indian Name	English Name	Medicinal System
Alkanna tinctoria	Ratthapaalai	Alkanet, Dyers' or Spanish Bugloss	Siddha/Tamil
Alkanna tinctoria	Surulpattai	Alkanet, Dyers' or Spanish Bugloss	Siddha/Tamil
Alkanna tinctoria	Dineshavalli	Alkanet, Dyers' or Spanish Bugloss	Siddha/Tamil
Allemanda cathartica	Zahari Sontakkaa	Golden Trumpet	Folk
Allium ascalonicum	Grnjana	Shellot	Ayurvedic
Allium ascalonicum	Gandanaa	Shellot	Unani
Allium ascalonicum	Ek-daanaa Lehsun	Shellot	Unani
Allium ascalonicum	Ek-potia Lehsum	Shellot	Unani
Allium cepa	Palaandu	Onion	Ayurvedic
Allium cepa	Durgandh	Onion	Ayurvedic
Allium cepa	Piyaaz	Onion	Unani
Allium cepa	Venkaayam	Onion	Siddha/Tamil
Allium macleanii	Baadshaahi Saalab	Oriental Royal Salep	Unani
Allium porrum	Vilaayati Piyaaz	Leek	Folk
Allium porrum	Praan	Leek	Folk/Kashmir
Allium porrum	Seemevangayam	Leek	Folk/Tamil
Allium sativum	Arishta	Garlic	Ayurvedic
Allium sativum	Lashuna	Garlic	Ayurvedic
Allium sativum	Mahaushadh	Garlic	Ayurvedic
Allium sativum	Rasona	Garlic	Ayurvedic
Allium sativum	Ugragandha	Garlic	Ayurvedic
Allium sativum	Yavaneshta	Garlic	Ayurvedic
Allium sativum	Seer	Garlic	Unani
Allium sativum	Lahsun	Garlic	Unani
Allium sativum	Ullippoondu	Garlic	Siddha/Tamil
Allium sativum	Rasonaka	Garlic	Ayurvedic
Alocasia indica	Maanaka	Giant Taro	Ayurvedic
Alocasia indica	Maana	Giant Taro	Ayurvedic
Alocasia indica	Maankanda	Giant Taro	Ayurvedic

Table Contd.

Botanical Name	Indian Name	English Name	Medicinal System
Alocasia indica	Kasaalu	Giant Taro	Ayurvedic
Alocasia indica	Hastikarni	Giant Taro	Ayurvedic
Alocasia indica	Merukan kizhangu	Giant Taro	Siddha/Tamil
Aloe barbadensis	Kanyaasaara (Dried leaf juice)	Curacao Aloe, Barbados Aloe, Indian Aloe, Jaffarabad Aloe	Ayurvedic
Aloe barbadensis	Eleyaka (Dried leaf juice)	Curacao Aloe, Barbados Aloe, Indian Aloe, Jaffarabad Aloe	Ayurvedic
Aloe barbadensis	Kumaari	Curacao Aloe, Barbados Aloe, Indian Aloe, Jaffarabad Aloe	Ayurvedic
Aloe barbadensis	Kumaarikaa	Curacao Aloe, Barbados Aloe, Indian Aloe, Jaffarabad Aloe	Ayurvedic
Aloe barbadensis	Kanyaa	Curacao Aloe, Barbados Aloe, Indian Aloe, Jaffarabad Aloe	Ayurvedic
Aloe barbadensis	Grihkanyaa	Curacao Aloe, Barbados Aloe, Indian Aloe, Jaffarabad Aloe	Ayurvedic
Aloe barbadensis	Ghritkumaarika	Curacao Aloe, Barbados Aloe, Indian Aloe, Jaffarabad Aloe	Ayurvedic
Aloe barbadensis	Gheekuwaar	Curacao Aloe, Barbados Aloe, Indian Aloe, Jaffarabad Aloe	Unani
Aloe barbadensis	Sibr (Dried leaf juice)	Curacao Aloe, Barbados Aloe, Indian Aloe, Jaffarabad Aloe	Unani
Aloe barbadensis	Kattraazhai	Curacao Aloe, Barbados Aloe, Indian Aloe, Jaffarabad Aloe	Siddha/Tamil
Aloe barbadensis	Kumaari	Curacao Aloe, Barbados Aloe, Indian Aloe, Jaffarabad Aloe	Siddha/Tamil
Aloe barbadensis	Moosaambaram (Dried leaf juice)	Curacao Aloe, Barbados Aloe, Indian Aloe, Jaffarabad Aloe	Siddha/Tamil

Table Contd.

Botanical Name	Indian Name	English Name	Medicinal System
Aloe barbadensis	Elwaa (Dried leaf juice)	Curacao Aloe, Barbados Aloe, Indian Aloe, Jaffarabad Aloe	Folk
Aloe barbadensis	Musabbar (Dried leaf juice)	Curacao Aloe, Barbados Aloe, Indian Aloe, Jaffarabad Aloe	Folk
Alpinia galanga	Kulanjana	Greater Galangal	Ayurvedic
Alpinia galanga	Sthuulagranthi	Greater Galangal	Ayurvedic
Alpinia galanga	Sugandhaa	Greater Galangal	Ayurvedic
Alpinia galanga	Ugragandhaa	Greater Galangal	Ayurvedic
Alpinia galanga	Malaya Vachaa	Greater Galangal	Ayurvedic
Alpinia galanga	Mahaabhari-Vachaa	Greater Galangal	Ayurvedic
Alpinia galanga	Khulanjaan	Greater Galangal	Unani
Alpinia galanga	Perarattai	Greater Galangal	Siddha/Tamil
Alpinia malaccensis	Saliyeridumpa	Malacca Galangal	Folk/Tamil
Alpinia officinarum	Kulanjan	Lesser Galangal, Alpinia, Catarrh Root, Chinese Ginger	Ayurvedic
Alpinia officinarum	Khulanjaan	Lesser Galangal, Alpinia, Catarrh Root, Chinese Ginger	Unani
Alpinia officinarum	Chitraraththai	Lesser Galangal, Alpinia, Catarrh Root, Chinese Ginger	Siddha/Tamil
Alpinia speciosa	Chitraraththai	Light Galangal	Siddha/Tamil
Alstonia scholaris	Chhaatim	Devil's Tree, Dita Bark Tree	Unani
Alstonia scholaris	Kaasim	Devil's Tree, Dita Bark Tree	Unani
Alstonia scholaris	Saptaparna	Devil's Tree, Dita Bark Tree	Ayurvedic
Alstonia scholaris	Saptachhada	Devil's Tree, Dita Bark Tree	Ayurvedic
Alstonia scholaris	Saptaparni	Devil's Tree, Dita Bark Tree	Ayurvedic
Alstonia scholaris	Saptaahvaa	Devil's Tree, Dita Bark Tree	Ayurvedic
Alstonia scholaris	Vishaaltvak	Devil's Tree, Dita Bark Tree	Ayurvedic
Alstonia scholaris	Shaarada	Devil's Tree, Dita Bark Tree	Ayurvedic
Alstonia scholaris	Vishamchhada	Devil's Tree, Dita Bark Tree	Ayurvedic
Alstonia scholaris	Ezhilamippalai	Devil's Tree, Dita Bark Tree	Siddha/Tamil
Alstonia scholaris	Mukkampalai	Devil's Tree, Dita Bark Tree	Siddha/Tamil
Alstonia scholaris	Chhitavan	Devil's Tree, Dita Bark Tree	Folk
Alstonia scholaris	Sataunaa	Devil's Tree, Dita Bark Tree	Folk

Table Contd.

Botanical Name	Indian Name	English Name	Medicinal System
Alstonia venenata	Pazh-munipala	Devil's Tree, Dita Bark Tree	Folk/Tamil
Alstonia venenata	Addasarpa	Devil's Tree, Dita Bark Tree	Folk/Kannada
Alstonia venenata	Palamunpala	Devil's Tree, Dita Bark Tree	Folk/Malayalam
Alternanthera sessilis	Matsyaakshi	Sessile Joyweed	Ayurvedic
Alternanthera sessilis	Matsyaakshika	Sessile Joyweed	Ayurvedic
Alternanthera sessilis	Matsyagandhaa	Sessile Joyweed	Ayurvedic
Alternanthera sessilis	Matsyaadani	Sessile Joyweed	Ayurvedic
Alternanthera sessilis	Minaakshi	Sessile Joyweed	Ayurvedic
Alternanthera sessilis	Matsya-gandhi	Sessile Joyweed	Ayurvedic
Alternanthera sessilis	Toya-pippali	Sessile Joyweed	Ayurvedic
Alternanthera sessilis	Gartkalambukaa	Sessile Joyweed	Ayurvedic
Alternanthera sessilis	Vahlikaa	Sessile Joyweed	Ayurvedic
Alternanthera sessilis	Machhechhi	Sessile Joyweed	Unani
Alternanthera sessilis	Ponnankanni Keerai	Sessile Joyweed	Siddha/Tamil
Alternanthera sessilis	Gudari Saag	Sessile Joyweed	Folk
Althaea officinalis	Khatmi	Marshmallow, Hollyhock	Unani
Althaea officinalis	Gul-Khairu	Marshmallow, Hollyhock	Unani
Althaea officinalis	Shemai-tutti	Marshmallow, Hollyhock	Siddha/Tamil
Altingia excelsa	Shilaarasa	Storax, Oriental Sweet Gum	Ayurvedic
Altingia excelsa	Turushka	Storax, Oriental Sweet Gum	Ayurvedic
Altingia excelsa	Silhaka	Storax, Oriental Sweet Gum	Ayurvedic
Altingia excelsa	Neriyurishippal	Storax, Oriental Sweet Gum	Siddha/Tamil
Amanita muscaria	Visha-chhatraka	Fly Agaric, Aga, Soma (Constituent)	Ayurvedic
Amaranthus blitum	Alpamaarisha	Trailing Amaranth, Wild Blite	Ayurvedic
Amaranthus blitum	Aarumatha-thandu	Trailing Amaranth, Wild Blite	Folk/Tamil
Amaranthus blitum	Kiraitandu	Trailing Amaranth, Wild Blite	Folk/Tamil
Amaranthus blitum	Marasaa	Trailing Amaranth, Wild Blite	Folk
Amaranthus caudatus	Chuko	Love-Lies-Bleeding, Tassel Flower	Folk
Amaranthus caudatus	Raam-daanaa (Grain)	Love-Lies-Bleeding, Tassel Flower	Ayurvedic

Table Contd.

Botanical Name	Indian Name	English Name	Medicinal System
Amaranthus caudatus	Pungikeerai	Love-Lies-Bleeding, Tassel Flower	Siddha/Tamil
Amaranthus caudatus	Sirukeerai	Love-Lies-Bleeding, Tassel Flower	Siddha/Tamil
Amaranthus spinosus	Alpamaarish	Spiny Amaranth, Thorny Amaranth, Spiny Pigweed	Ayurvedic
Amaranthus spinosus	Meghnaad	Spiny Amaranth, Thorny Amaranth, Spiny Pigweed	Ayurvedic
Amaranthus spinosus	Megharava	Spiny Amaranth, Thorny Amaranth, Spiny Pigweed	Ayurvedic
Amaranthus spinosus	Tanduliya	Spiny Amaranth, Thorny Amaranth, Spiny Pigweed	Ayurvedic
Amaranthus spinosus	Tandulaka	Spiny Amaranth, Thorny Amaranth, Spiny Pigweed	Ayurvedic
Amaranthus spinosus	Vishaghn	Spiny Amaranth, Thorny Amaranth, Spiny Pigweed	Ayurvedic
Amaranthus spinosus	Mullukkeerai	Spiny Amaranth, Thorny Amaranth, Spiny Pigweed	Siddha/Tamil
Amaranthus spinosus	Katili-chaulai	Spiny Amaranth, Thorny Amaranth, Spiny Pigweed	Folk
Amaranthus tricolor	Maarisha-rakta	Chinese Spinach, Garden Amaranth, Fountain Plant	Ayurvedic
Amaranthus tricolor	Arai-keerai	Chinese Spinach, Garden Amaranth, Fountain Plant	Folk/Tamil
Amaranthus tricolor	Siru-keerai	Chinese Spinach, Garden Amaranth, Fountain Plant	Folk/Tamil
Amaranthus tricolor	Thandu-keerai	Chinese Spinach, Garden Amaranth, Fountain Plant	Folk/Tamil
Amaranthus tricolor	Mulakkeerai	Chinese Spinach, Garden Amaranth, Fountain Plant	Folk/Tamil
Amaranthus tricolor	Laal Shaak	Chinese Spinach, Garden Amaranth, Fountain Plant	Folk
Amaranthus tricolor	Laal Marashaa	Chinese Spinach, Garden Amaranth, Fountain Plant	Folk
Amberboa divaricata	Baadaavard	Volutarella	Unani
Amberboa divaricata	Brahmadandi	Volutarella	Ayurvedic
Ammannia baccifera	Agnipatri	Blistering Ammannia	Ayurvedic
Ammannia baccifera	Daadmaari	Blistering Ammannia	Folk

Table Contd.

Botanical Name	Indian Name	English Name	Medicinal System
Ammi majus	Itarilaal	Bishop's Weed-Amee, Greater Ammi	Unani
Ammi majus	Khalah	Bishop's Weed-Amee, Greater Ammi	Unani
Ammi visnaga	Paashaanabhedi	Khella	Folk
Amomum aromaticum	Sthula-elaa	Bengal Cardamom, Cardamom	Ayurvedic
Amomum aromaticum	Perelam	Bengal Cardamom, Cardamom	Folk/Tamil
Amomum aromaticum	Morang-elaichi	Bengal Cardamom, Cardamom	Folk
Amomum subulatum	Bahulaa	Greater or Nepal Cardamom	Ayurvedic
Amomum subulatum	Bhadraa	Greater or Nepal Cardamom	Ayurvedic
Amomum subulatum	Bhadrailaa	Greater or Nepal Cardamom	Ayurvedic
Amomum subulatum	Prithivikaa	Greater or Nepal Cardamom	Ayurvedic
Amomum subulatum	Sthula-elaa	Greater or Nepal Cardamom	Ayurvedic
Amomum subulatum	Triputaa	Greater or Nepal Cardamom	Ayurvedic
Amomum subulatum	Truti	Greater or Nepal Cardamom	Ayurvedic
Amomum subulatum	Heel Kalaan	Greater or Nepal Cardamom	Unani
Amomum subulatum	Qaaqule Kubaar	Greater or Nepal Cardamom	Unani
Amomum subulatum	Peria elam	Greater or Nepal Cardamom	Folk/Tamil
Amomum subulatum	Kattu elam	Greater or Nepal Cardamom	Folk/Tamil
Amomum subulatum	Kakolaa	Greater or Nepal Cardamom	Folk
Amoora cucullata	Amur	Rohitak	Folk
Amoora cucullata	Latmi	Rohitak	Folk
Amoora cucullata	Natmi	Rohitak	Folk (Bengal)
Amphicome emodi	Kaur	False Chirayita	Folk (Kashmir)
Amorphophallus campanulatus	Suurana	Elephant's Foot Yam	Ayurvedic
Amorphophallus campanulatus	Kanduula	Elephant's Foot Yam	Ayurvedic
Amorphophallus campanulatus	Arshoghna	Elephant's Foot Yam	Ayurvedic
Amorphophallus campanulatus	Kand-naayaka	Elephant's Foot Yam	Ayurvedic
Amorphophallus campanulatus	Kandala	Elephant's Foot Yam	Ayurvedic
Amorphophallus campanulatus	Vajra-kanda	Elephant's Foot Yam	Ayurvedic

Table Contd.

Botanical Name	Indian Name	English Name	Medicinal System
Amorphophallus campanulatus	Zamikand	Elephant's Foot Yam	Unani
Amorphophallus campanulatus	Chenai-kkizhangu	Elephant's Foot Yam	Siddha/Tamil
Amorphophallus campanulatus	Kaathukarunai	Elephant's Foot Yam	Siddha/Tamil
Amygdalus communis	Vaataama	Almond	Ayurvedic
Amygdalus communis	Vaataada	Almond	Ayurvedic
Amygdalus communis	Badaam	Almond	Unani
Amygdalus communis	Loz	Almond	Unani
Amygdalus communis	Vaadumai	Almond	Siddha/Tamil
Amygdalus persica	Aaruka	Peach Tree	Ayurvedic
Amygdalus persica	Aaduu	Peach Tree	Unani
Amygdalus persica	Khokh	Peach Tree	Unani
Anacardium occidentale	Kaaju	Cashew Nut Tree	Unani
Anacardium occidentale	Mindiri	Cashew Nut Tree	Siddha/Tamil
Anacyclus pyrethrum	Aakaarakarabha	Spanish, Pellitory, Pyrethrum Root	Ayurvedic
Anacyclus pyrethrum	Aakallaka	Spanish, Pellitory, Pyrethrum Root	Ayurvedic
Anacyclus pyrethrum	Aakulakrit	Spanish, Pellitory, Pyrethrum Root	Ayurvedic
Anacyclus pyrethrum	Agragraahi	Spanish, Pellitory, Pyrethrum Root	Ayurvedic
Anacyclus pyrethrum	Aaqarqarhaa	Spanish, Pellitory, Pyrethrum Root	Unani
Anacyclus pyrethrum	Akkiraakaaram	Spanish, Pellitory, Pyrethrum Root	Siddha/Tamil
Anagallis arvensis	Anaaghaalis	Bird's Eye, Bird's Tongue, Blue Pimpernel, Scarlet Pimpernel	Unani
Anagallis arvensis	Jonkmaari	Bird's Eye, Bird's Tongue, Blue Pimpernel, Scarlet Pimpernel	Folk
Anagallis arvensis	Dhabbar	Bird's Eye, Bird's Tongue, Blue Pimpernel, Scarlet Pimpernel	Folk (Punjab)

Table Contd.

Botanical Name	Indian Name	English Name	Medicinal System
Anagallis arvensis	Jighanaa	Bird's Eye, Bird's Tongue, Blue Pimpernel, Scarlet Pimpernel	Folk
Anagallis arvensis	Jenghani	Bird's Eye, Bird's Tongue, Blue Pimpernel, Scarlet Pimpernel	Folk
Anamirta cocculus	Kaakaadani	Levant Berry, Fish Berry, Poison Berry, Crow Killer	Ayurvedic
Anamirta cocculus	Kaakamaari	Levant Berry, Fish Berry, Poison Berry, Crow Killer	Ayurvedic
Anamirta cocculus	Kaakkaik-kollividai	Levant Berry, Fish Berry, Poison Berry, Crow Killer	Siddha/Tamil
Ananas comosus	Anaanaasa	Pineapple	Ayurvedic
Ananas comosus	Bahunetra	Pineapple	Ayurvedic
Ananas comosus	Anannaas	Pineapple	Unani
Ananas comosus	Annanshippa-zham	Pineapple	Siddha/Tamil
Ananas comosus	Annasi	Pineapple	Siddha/Tamil
Anaphalis neelgerriana	Raktaskandana	Katplaster	Ayurvedic
Anaphalis neelgerriana	Katplaaster	Katplaster	Folk
Anastatica hierochuntica	Garbha-phool	Jericho Rose	Folk
Anastatica hierochuntica	Kafemariyam	Jericho Rose	Unani
Anastatica hierochuntica	Kafe-aaishaa	Jericho Rose	Unani
Anchusa italica	Gojihvikaa	Cow's Tongue Plant	Ayurvedic
Anchusa italica	Gaozabaan	Cow's Tongue Plant	Unani
Andrographis echioides	Ranchimani	Creat	Folk
Andrographis paniculata	Kaalmegha	Creat	Ayurvedic
Andrographis paniculata	Bhuunimba	Creat	Ayurvedic
Andrographis paniculata	Bhuuminimbaka	Creat	Ayurvedic
Andrographis paniculata	Vishwambharaa	Creat	Ayurvedic
Andrographis paniculata	Yavtikta	Creat	Ayurvedic
Andrographis paniculata	Kalpanaatha	Creat	Ayurvedic
Andrographis paniculata	Kiraata-tikta	Creat	Ayurvedic
Andrographis paniculata	Kiryaat	Creat	Unani
Andrographis paniculata	Nilavembu	Creat	Siddha/Tamil
Andropogon muricatus	Ushira	Vetiver, Cuscus	Ayurvedic

Table Contd.

Botanical Name	Indian Name	English Name	Medicinal System
Andropogon muricatus	Khas	Vetiver, Cuscus	Unani
Andropogon muricatus	Vettiveru	Vetiver, Cuscus	Siddha/Tamil
Anemone obtusiloba	Gul-laalaa	Wind-Flower, Wood Anemone, Pasque Flower, Pulsatilla	Unani
Anemone obtusiloba	Shaqaaq-un-Nomaan	Wind-Flower, Wood Anemone, Pasque Flower, Pulsatilla	Unani
Anethum sowa	Shataahvaa	Indian Dill, Sowa	Ayurvedic
Anethum sowa	Shatapushpaa	Indian Dill, Sowa	Ayurvedic
Anethum sowa	Shibt	Indian Dill, Sowa	Unani
Anethum sowa	Soyaa	Indian Dill, Sowa	Unani
Anethum sowa	Sadakuppai	Indian Dill, Sowa	Siddha/Tamil
Angelica archangelica	Chandaa	Angelica	Ayurvedic
Angelica archangelica	Chandaam-shuka	Angelica	Ayurvedic
Angelica archangelica	Kathachoraa	Angelica	Ayurvedic
Angelica glauca	Choraka	Angelica	Ayurvedic
Angelica glauca	Chorakaa	Angelica	Ayurvedic
Angelica glauca	Kopanaa	Angelica	Ayurvedic
Angelica glauca	Chorakaakhya	Angelica	Ayurvedic
Angelica glauca	Nishaachara	Angelica	Ayurvedic
Angelica glauca	Dhanhar	Angelica	Ayurvedic
Angelica glauca	Taskara	Angelica	Ayurvedic
Angelica glauca	Kshemaka	Angelica	Ayurvedic
Anisochilus carnosus	Karpuravalli	Wild Violet	Folk (South)
Anisomeles malabarica	Sprikkaa	Malabar Catmint	Ayurvedic
Anisomeles malabarica	Irattaipeya-meraii	Malabar Catmint	Siddha/Tamil
Annona reticulata	Raamaphala	Bull's Heart, Common Custard Apple	Ayurvedic
Annona reticulata	Aninuna	Bull's Heart, Common Custard Apple	Siddha/Tamil
Annona reticulata	Luvuni	Bull's Heart, Common Custard Apple	Folk
Annona squamosa	Gandagaatra	Custard Apple, Sugar Apple, Sweet-sop	Ayurvedic

Table Contd.

Botanical Name	Indian Name	English Name	Medicinal System
Annona squamosa	Sitaaphala	Custard Apple, Sugar Apple, Sweet-sop	Ayurvedic
Annona squamosa	Sharifaa	Custard Apple, Sugar Apple, Sweet-sop	Unani
Annona squamosa	Sitaaphalam	Custard Apple, Sugar Apple, Sweet-sop	Siddha/Tamil
Annona squamosa	Atta	Custard Apple, Sugar Apple, Sweet-sop	Siddha/Tamil
Anogeissus latifolia	Dhava	Axle-wood, Button Tree, Ghatti Tree	Ayurvedic
Anogeissus latifolia	Dhurandhara	Axle-wood, Button Tree, Ghatti Tree	Ayurvedic
Anogeissus latifolia	Shakataahya	Axle-wood, Button Tree, Ghatti Tree	Ayurvedic
Anogeissus latifolia	Indravrksha	Axle-wood, Button Tree, Ghatti Tree	Ayurvedic
Anogeissus latifolia	Dhaavaa	Axle-wood, Button Tree, Ghatti Tree	Unani
Anogeissus latifolia	Vellaynaga	Axle-wood, Button Tree, Ghatti Tree	Siddha/Tamil
Anogeissus latifolia	Ghatti (Gum)	Axle-wood, Button Tree, Ghatti Tree	Folk
Anthemis nobilis	Shimai chamantipu	Roman Chamomile, Double Chamomile	Folk/Tamil
Anthemis nobilis	Gul-e-Baabuuna	Roman Chamomile, Double Chamomile	Unani
Anthocephalus cadamba	Kadamba	Wild Cinchona	Ayurvedic
Anthocephalus cadamba	Priyaka	Wild Cinchona	Ayurvedic
Anthocephalus cadamba	Vrtta-pushpa	Wild Cinchona	Ayurvedic
Anthocephalus cadamba	Nipa	Wild Cinchona	Ayurvedic
Anthocephalus cadamba	Halipriya	Wild Cinchona	Ayurvedic
Anthocephalus cadamba	Kolaoyila	Wild Cinchona	Folk/Tamil
Anthocephalus cadamba	Vellai Kadambam	Wild Cinchona	Siddha/Tamil
Antiaris toxicaria	Valkala vrksha	Sacking Tree, Upas Tree	Ayurvedic
Antiaris toxicaria	Aranthellia	Sacking Tree, Upas Tree	Folk/Tamil
Antiaris toxicaria	Mara-uri	Sacking Tree, Upas Tree	Folk/Tamil
Antiaris toxicaria	Nettavil	Sacking Tree, Upas Tree	Folk/Tamil

Table Contd.

Botanical Name	Indian Name	English Name	Medicinal System
Aphanamixis polystachya	Rohitaka	Amoora	Ayurvedic
Aphanamixis polystachya	Daadimachhada	Amoora	Ayurvedic
Aphanamixis polystachya	Daadima-pushpaka	Amoora	Ayurvedic
Aphanamixis polystachya	Plihaghna	Amoora	Ayurvedic
Aphanamixis polystachya	Malampuluvan	Amoora	Siddha/Tamil
Apium graveolens	Ajmoda	Celery	Ayurvedic
Apium graveolens	Ajmodaa	Celery	Ayurvedic
Apium graveolens	Ajmodikaa	Celery	Ayurvedic
Apium graveolens	Dipyaka	Celery	Ayurvedic
Apium graveolens	Karafs	Celery	Unani
Apium graveolens	Celery-keerai	Celery	Siddha/Tamil
Apium graveolens	Randhuni	Celery	Folk
Apium leptophyllum	Ajmodaa	Celery	Ayurvedic
Apium leptophyllum	Dipyaka	Celery	Ayurvedic
Apium leptophyllum	Ajmod	Celery	Unani
Apium leptophyllum	Karafs-e-Hindi	Celery	Unani
Apium leptophyllum	Omam	Celery	Siddha/Tamil
Aquilaria agallocha	Aguru	Aloewood, Eaglewood, Agarwood	Ayurvedic
Aquilaria agallocha	Krimij	Aloewood, Eaglewood, Agarwood	Ayurvedic
Aquilaria agallocha	Krishnaaguru	Aloewood, Eaglewood, Agarwood	Ayurvedic
Aquilaria agallocha	Jongaka	Aloewood, Eaglewood, Agarwood	Ayurvedic
Aquilaria agallocha	Maaliyaka	Aloewood, Eaglewood, Agarwood	Ayurvedic
Aquilaria agallocha	Loha	Aloewood, Eaglewood, Agarwood	Ayurvedic
Aquilaria agallocha	Kaalaloha	Aloewood, Eaglewood, Agarwood	Ayurvedic
Aquilaria agallocha	Asitaka	Aloewood, Eaglewood, Agarwood	Ayurvedic
Aquilaria agallocha	Ood-ul Hindi	Aloewood, Eaglewood, Agarwood	Unani
Aquilaria agallocha	Ood Gharqi	Aloewood, Eaglewood, Agarwood	Unani
Aquilaria agallocha	Akil kattai	Aloewood, Eaglewood, Agarwood	Siddha/Tamil
Aquilaria agallocha	Aggali-chandanam	Aloewood, Eaglewood, Agarwood	Folk/Tamil
Arachis hypogaea	Mandapi	Groundnut, Peanut, Monkeynut	Ayurvedic
Arachis hypogaea	Tailamudga	Groundnut, Peanut, Monkeynut	Ayurvedic
Arachis hypogaea	Bhuumimudga	Groundnut, Peanut, Monkeynut	Ayurvedic

Table Contd.

Botanical Name	Indian Name	English Name	Medicinal System
Arachis hypogaea	Moongphali	Groundnut, Peanut, Monkeynut	Unani
Arachis hypogaea	Nelakadalai	Groundnut, Peanut, Monkeynut	Siddha/Tamil
Arachis hypogaea	Verkadalai	Groundnut, Peanut, Monkeynut	Siddha/Tamil
Aralia bipinnatifida	Taapamaari	Himalayan pseudo-ginseng	Folk
Arctium lappa	Phaggarmuul	Common/Great Burdock	Folk (Kashmir)
Arctostaphylos uva-ursi	Angur-e-khiras	Bearberry	Unani
Arctostaphylos uva-ursi	Inbud-dub	Bearberry	Unani
Arctostaphylos uva-ursi	Reechh Daakh	Bearberry	Unani
Areca catechu	Puuga	Areca Nut, Betel Nut	Ayurvedic
Areca catechu	Puugi	Areca Nut, Betel Nut	Ayurvedic
Areca catechu	Kramuka	Areca Nut, Betel Nut	Ayurvedic
Areca catechu	Ghontaa	Areca Nut, Betel Nut	Ayurvedic
Areca catechu	Guwaak	Areca Nut, Betel Nut	Ayurvedic
Areca catechu	Ghorant	Areca Nut, Betel Nut	Ayurvedic
Areca catechu	Fufal	Areca Nut, Betel Nut	Unani
Areca catechu	Chhaalia	Areca Nut, Betel Nut	Unani
Areca catechu	Supaari	Areca Nut, Betel Nut	Unani
Areca catechu	Kottai Paakku	Areca Nut, Betel Nut	Siddha/Tamil
Areca catechu	Kamugu	Areca Nut, Betel Nut	Folk/Tamil
Argemone mexicana	Katuparni	Prickly Poppy, Mexican Poppy	Ayurvedic
Argemone mexicana	Svarnkshiri	Prickly Poppy, Mexican Poppy	Ayurvedic
Argemone mexicana	Kaanchan-kshiri	Prickly Poppy, Mexican Poppy	Ayurvedic
Argemone mexicana	Pitadugdhaa	Prickly Poppy, Mexican Poppy	Ayurvedic
Argemone mexicana	Hemaahvaa	Prickly Poppy, Mexican Poppy	Ayurvedic
Argemone mexicana	Himaavati	Prickly Poppy, Mexican Poppy	Ayurvedic
Argemone mexicana	Hemavati	Prickly Poppy, Mexican Poppy	Ayurvedic
Argemone mexicana	Satyaanaashi	Prickly Poppy, Mexican Poppy	Unani
Argemone mexicana	Piramathandu	Prickly Poppy, Mexican Poppy	Siddha/Tamil
Argemone mexicana	Kudiyotti	Prickly Poppy, Mexican Poppy	Siddha/Tamil
Argyreia speciosa	Vriddhadaaruka	Elephant Creeper	Ayurvedic
Argyreia speciosa	Vriddhadaaru	Elephant Creeper	Ayurvedic
Argyreia speciosa	Vriddhadaaraka	Elephant Creeper	Ayurvedic

Table Contd.

Botanical Name	Indian Name	English Name	Medicinal System
Argyreia speciosa	Bastaantri	Elephant Creeper	Ayurvedic
Argyreia speciosa	Sthavira	Elephant Creeper	Ayurvedic
Argyreia speciosa	Sthaviradaaru	Elephant Creeper	Ayurvedic
Argyreia speciosa	Atarunadaaru	Elephant Creeper	Ayurvedic
Argyreia speciosa	Samudrashosha	Elephant Creeper	Ayurvedic
Argyreia speciosa	Samundersokh	Elephant Creeper	Unani
Argyreia speciosa	Ambgar	Elephant Creeper	Siddha/Tamil
Argyreia speciosa	Samuddira-pacchai	Elephant Creeper	Siddha/Tamil
Argyreia speciosa	Bidhaaraa	Elephant Creeper	Folk
Aristolochia bracteolata	Kitamaari	Bracteated Birthwort	Ayurvedic
Aristolochia bracteolata	Dhumrapatra	Bracteated Birthwort	Ayurvedic
Aristolochia bracteolata	Naakuli	Bracteated Birthwort	Ayurvedic
Aristolochia bracteolata	Kiraamaar	Bracteated Birthwort	Unani
Aristolochia bracteolata	Aadutheenda-appaalai	Bracteated Birthwort	Siddha/Tamil
Aristolochia bracteolata	Kattusuragam	Bracteated Birthwort	Siddha/Tamil
Aristolochia indica	Ishvari	Indian Birthwort	Ayurvedic
Aristolochia indica	Gandhnaakuli	Indian Birthwort	Ayurvedic
Aristolochia indica	Naagadamani	Indian Birthwort	Ayurvedic
Aristolochia indica	Arkamuula	Indian Birthwort	Ayurvedic
Aristolochia indica	Zaraavand-Hindi	Indian Birthwort	Unani
Aristolochia indica	Adagam	Indian Birthwort	Siddha/Tamil
Aristolochia indica	Isarmuula	Indian Birthwort	Folk
Aristolochia indica	Isrola	Indian Birthwort	Folk
Aristolochia longa	Zaraawand Taweel	European Birthwort	Unani
Armoracia lapathifolia	Horse-radish	Red Cole, Pepperrot, Great Raifort	Folk
Arnebia benthamii	Kashmiri Gaozabaan	Himalayan Arnebia	Folk
Arnebia benthamii	Kashmiri Kahzabaan	Himalayan Arnebia	Folk
Artabotrys hexapetalus	Panasagandhi	Yling-Yling Vine	Ayurvedic

Table Contd.

Botanical Name	Indian Name	English Name	Medicinal System
Bacopa monnieri	Braahmi	Thyme-leaved Gratiola	Ayurvedic
Bacopa monnieri	Aindri	Thyme-leaved Gratiola	Ayurvedic
Bacopa monnieri	Neerabraahmi	Thyme-leaved Gratiola	Ayurvedic
Bacopa monnieri	Kapotavankaa	Thyme-leaved Gratiola	Ayurvedic
Bacopa monnieri	Bhaarati	Thyme-leaved Gratiola	Ayurvedic
Bacopa monnieri	Darduradalaa	Thyme-leaved Gratiola	Ayurvedic
Bacopa monnieri	Matsyaakshaka	Thyme-leaved Gratiola	Ayurvedic
Bacopa monnieri	Shaaluraparni	Thyme-leaved Gratiola	Ayurvedic
Bacopa monnieri	Brahmi	Thyme-leaved Gratiola	Unani
Bacopa monnieri	Piramivazhukkai	Thyme-leaved Gratiola	Siddha/Tamil
Bacopa monnieri	Brahmi-vazhukkai	Thyme-leaved Gratiola	Siddha/Tamil
Bacopa monnieri	Jalaneem	Thyme-leaved Gratiola	Folk
Bacopa monnieri	Safed-Chammi	Thyme-leaved Gratiola	Folk
Balanites aegyptiaca	Ingudi	Desert Date	Ayurvedic
Balanites aegyptiaca	Angaar Vrksha	Desert Date	Ayurvedic
Balanites aegyptiaca	Taapasadrum	Desert Date	Ayurvedic
Balanites aegyptiaca	Taapasa vrksha	Desert Date	Ayurvedic
Balanites aegyptiaca	Dirghkantaka	Desert Date	Ayurvedic
Balanites aegyptiaca	Hingan	Desert Date	Unani
Balanites aegyptiaca	Hanguul	Desert Date	Unani
Balanites aegyptiaca	Nanjundan	Desert Date	Siddha/Tamil
Balanites aegyptiaca	Hingol	Desert Date	Folk
Balanites aegyptiaca	Hingota	Desert Date	Folk
Balanites aegyptiaca	Hingothaa	Desert Date	Folk
Balanophora involucrata	Chavya	Knotted-Cup Vine	Ayurvedic
Baliospermum montanum	Danti	False Croton	Ayurvedic
Baliospermum montanum	Nikumbha	False Croton	Ayurvedic
Baliospermum montanum	Udumbarparni	False Croton	Ayurvedic
Baliospermum montanum	Erandphalaa	False Croton	Ayurvedic
Baliospermum montanum	Shighraa	False Croton	Ayurvedic
Baliospermum montanum	Pratyak-shreni	False Croton	Ayurvedic
Baliospermum montanum	Vishaalya	False Croton	Ayurvedic

Table Contd.

Botanical Name	Indian Name	English Name	Medicinal System
Baliospermum montanum	Neeradimuthu	False Croton	Siddha/Tamil
Baliospermum montanum	Nervaalam	False Croton	Siddha/Tamil
Baliospermum montanum	Jangli Jamaalgotaa	False Croton	Folk
Balsamodendron mukul	Guggul	Indian Bdellium, Gum Guggul	Ayurvedic
Balsamodendron mukul	Devadhoop	Indian Bdellium, Gum Guggul	Ayurvedic
Balsamodendron mukul	Kaushika	Indian Bdellium, Gum Guggul	Ayurvedic
Balsamodendron mukul	Pur	Indian Bdellium, Gum Guggul	Ayurvedic
Balsamodendron mukul	Mahishaaksha	Indian Bdellium, Gum Guggul	Ayurvedic
Balsamodendron mukul	Palankash	Indian Bdellium, Gum Guggul	Ayurvedic
Balsamodendron mukul	Kumbha	Indian Bdellium, Gum Guggul	Ayurvedic
Balsamodendron mukul	Uluukhala	Indian Bdellium, Gum Guggul	Ayurvedic
Balsamodendron mukul	Aflaatuun	Indian Bdellium, Gum Guggul	Unani
Balsamodendron mukul	Muql	Indian Bdellium, Gum Guggul	Unani
Balsamodendron mukul	Bu-e-Jahudaan	Indian Bdellium, Gum Guggul	Unani
Balsamodendron mukul	Erumaikan Kungiliyam	Indian Bdellium, Gum Guggul	Siddha/Tamil
Balsamodendron myrrha	Bola	Myrrh, Herabol	Ayurvedic
Balsamodendron myrrha	Hiraabola	Myrrh, Herabol	Ayurvedic
Balsamodendron myrrha	Surasa	Myrrh, Herabol	Ayurvedic
Balsamodendron myrrha	Barbara	Myrrh, Herabol	Ayurvedic
Balsamodendron myrrha	Gandharasa	Myrrh, Herabol	Ayurvedic
Balsamodendron myrrha	Murmakki	Myrrh, Herabol	Unani
Balsamodendron myrrha	Al-murr	Myrrh, Herabol	Unani
Balsamodendron myrrha	Vellaibolam	Myrrh, Herabol	Siddha/Tamil
Balsamodendron opobalsamum	Balsaan	Balsam Tree, Balsam of Mecca, Balsam of Gilead	Unani
Balsamodendron opobalsamum	Roghan-e-Balsaan (Oil)	Balsam Tree, Balsam of Mecca, Balsam of Gilead	Unani
Balsamodendron opobalsamum	Habb-e-Balsaan (Fruit)	Balsam Tree, Balsam of Mecca, Balsam of Gilead	Unani
Balsamodendron opobalsamum	Ood-e-Balsaan (Wood)	Balsam Tree, Balsam of Mecca, Balsam of Gilead	Unani
Bambusa bambos	Vansha	Spiny or Thorny Bamboo	Ayurvedic

Table Contd.

Botanical Name	Indian Name	English Name	Medicinal System
Bambusa bambos	Venu	Spiny or Thorny Bamboo	Ayurvedic
Bambusa bambos	Kichaka	Spiny or Thorny Bamboo	Ayurvedic
Bambusa bambos	Trinadhwaj	Spiny or Thorny Bamboo	Ayurvedic
Bambusa bambos	Shatparvaa	Spiny or Thorny Bamboo	Ayurvedic
Bambusa bambos	Yavphala	Spiny or Thorny Bamboo	Ayurvedic
Bambusa bambos	Vanshalochana (Manna)	Spiny or Thorny Bamboo	Ayurvedic
Bambusa bambos	Vansharochanaa (Manna)	Spiny or Thorny Bamboo	Ayurvedic
Bambusa bambos	Shubhaa	Spiny or Thorny Bamboo	Ayurvedic
Bambusa bambos	Tugaa	Spiny or Thorny Bamboo	Ayurvedic
Bambusa bambos	Tugaakshiri (Manna)	Spiny or Thorny Bamboo	Ayurvedic
Bambusa bambos	Tvakkshiri (Manna)	Spiny or Thorny Bamboo	Ayurvedic
Bambusa bambos	Qasab	Spiny or Thorny Bamboo	Unani
Bambusa bambos	Tabaashir (Manna)	Spiny or Thorny Bamboo	Unani
Bambusa bambos	Moongil	Spiny or Thorny Bamboo	Siddha/Tamil
Bambusa bambos	Mongiluppu (Manna)	Spiny or Thorny Bamboo	Siddha/Tamil
Barbarea vulgaris	Cress, Indian Posey	Bitter Cress, Hedge Mustard, Yellow Rocket, Winter Cress	Folk
Barleria buxifolia	Sahachara	Box-leaved Barleria	Ayurvedic
Barleria buxifolia	Jhinti	Box-leaved Barleria	Folk
Barleria cristata	Saireyaka Shveta-Rakta-pushpa	Crested Philippine Violet	Ayurvedic
Barleria cristata	Ottamulli	Crested Philippine Violet	Siddha/Tamil
Barleria cristata	Katsaraiyaa	Crested Philippine Violet	Folk
Barleria cristata	Raktajhinti	Crested Philippine Violet	Folk
Barleria prionitis	Sahachara	Common Yellow Nail Dye Plant	Ayurvedic
Barleria prionitis	Baana	Common Yellow Nail Dye Plant	Ayurvedic
Barleria prionitis	Kurantaka	Common Yellow Nail Dye Plant	Ayurvedic
Barleria prionitis	Kuranta	Common Yellow Nail Dye Plant	Ayurvedic
Barleria prionitis	Koranda	Common Yellow Nail Dye Plant	Ayurvedic

Table Contd.

Botanical Name	Indian Name	English Name	Medicinal System
Barleria prionitis	Korandaka	Common Yellow Nail Dye Plant	Ayurvedic
Barleria prionitis	Saireyaka	Common Yellow Nail Dye Plant	Ayurvedic
Barleria prionitis	Saireyaka (Pita)	Common Yellow Nail Dye Plant	Ayurvedic
Barleria prionitis	Piyaabaansaa	Common Yellow Nail Dye Plant	Unani
Barleria prionitis	Chemmulli	Common Yellow Nail Dye Plant	Siddha/Tamil
Barleria prionitis	Jhinti	Common Yellow Nail Dye Plant	Folk
Barleria prionitis	Katsaraiyaa	Common Yellow Nail Dye Plant	Folk
Barleria strigosa	Sahachara	Blue-flowered Barleria	Ayurvedic
Barleria strigosa	Nili	Blue-flowered Barleria	Siddha/Tamil
Barleria strigosa	Koilekhaa	Blue-flowered Barleria	Folk
Barringtonia acutangula	Nichula	Indian Oak	Ayurvedic
Barringtonia acutangula	Hijjala	Indian Oak	Ayurvedic
Barringtonia acutangula	Ijjala	Indian Oak	Ayurvedic
Barringtonia acutangula	Vidula	Indian Oak	Ayurvedic
Barringtonia acutangula	Ambuj	Indian Oak	Ayurvedic
Barringtonia acutangula	Samandarphal	Indian Oak	Unani
Barringtonia acutangula	Kadappai	Indian Oak	Siddha/Tamil
Barringtonia acutangula	Samudra-phullarni	Indian Oak	Siddha/Tamil
Basella alba	Amritvallari	Indian Spinach	Ayurvedic
Basella alba	Maalvaa	Indian Spinach	Ayurvedic
Basella alba	Potaki	Indian Spinach	Ayurvedic
Basella alba	Upodikaa	Indian Spinach	Ayurvedic
Basella alba	Vaslakkirai	Indian Spinach	Siddha/Tamil
Basella alba	Poi	Indian Spinach	Folk
Bassia longifolia	Madhuuka (Bheda)	Mowra Butter Tree, South Indian Mahua	Ayurvedic
Bassia longifolia	Elupa	Mowra Butter Tree, South Indian Mahua	Folk/Tamil
Bassia longifolia	Naatu	Mowra Butter Tree, South Indian Mahua	Folk/Tamil
Bassia longifolia	Iluppei	Mowra Butter Tree, South Indian Mahua	Folk/Tamil
Bassia longifolia	Iruppei	Mowra Butter Tree, South Indian Mahua	Siddha/Tamil

Table Contd.

Botanical Name	Indian Name	English Name	Medicinal System
Bauhinia acuminata	Kaanchnaara	Dwarf White Bauhinia	Ayurvedic
Bauhinia acuminata	Kovidaara	Dwarf White Bauhinia	Ayurvedic
Bauhinia acuminata	Kachnaal	Dwarf White Bauhinia	Unani
Bauhinia acuminata	Vellaimandarai	Dwarf White Bauhinia	Siddha/Tamil
Bauhinia malabarica	Ashmantaka	Malabar Mountain Ebony	Ayurvedic
Bauhinia malabarica	Kaanchanaara	Malabar Mountain Ebony	Ayurvedic
Bauhinia malabarica	Malaiyatti	Malabar Mountain Ebony	Siddha/Tamil
Bauhinia malabarica	Aapataa	Malabar Mountain Ebony	Folk
Bauhinia malabarica	Amli	Malabar Mountain Ebony	Folk
Bauhinia malabarica	Amlosaa	Malabar Mountain Ebony	Folk
Bauhinia purpurea	Kovidaara	Camel's Foot Tree, Pink Bauhinia, Butterfly Tree, Geramium Tree, Orchid Tree	Ayurvedic
Bauhinia purpurea	Kaanchanaara (Rakta)	Camel's Foot Tree, Pink Bauhinia, Butterfly Tree, Geramium Tree, Orchid Tree	Ayurvedic
Bauhinia purpurea	Sivappu Mandaarai	Camel's Foot Tree, Pink Bauhinia, Butterfly Tree, Geramium Tree, Orchid Tree	Siddha/Tamil
Bauhinia purpurea	Koilaara	Camel's Foot Tree, Pink Bauhinia, Butterfly Tree, Geramium Tree, Orchid Tree	Folk
Bauhinia purpurea	Khairwaal	Camel's Foot Tree, Pink Bauhinia, Butterfly Tree, Geramium Tree, Orchid Tree	Folk
Bauhinia purpurea	Kaliaar	Camel's Foot Tree, Pink Bauhinia, Butterfly Tree, Geramium Tree, Orchid Tree	Folk
Bauhinia purpurea	Rakta Kanchan	Camel's Foot Tree, Pink Bauhinia, Butterfly Tree, Geramium Tree, Orchid Tree	Folk
Bauhinia racemosa	Ashmantaka	Kachnar Tree	Ayurvedic
Bauhinia racemosa	Kanchini	Kachnar Tree	Ayurvedic
Bauhinia racemosa	Kachnaar	Kachnar Tree	Unani
Bauhinia racemosa	Aapataa	Kachnar Tree	Folk
Bauhinia racemosa	Kachnaala	Kachnar Tree	Folk
Bauhinia racemosa	Kokku-mandarai	Kachnar Tree	Siddha/Tamil

Table Contd.

Botanical Name	Indian Name	English Name	Medicinal System
Bauhinia retusa	Nirpa	Semla Gum Tree	Siddha/Tamil
Bauhinia retusa	Semalaa	Semla Gum Tree	Folk
Bauhinia retusa	Kathmahuli	Semla Gum Tree	Folk
Bauhinia retusa	Gum–Thaur	Semla Gum Tree	Folk
Bauhinia tomentosa	Pita Kovidaara	Yellow Bauhinia, St. Thomas Tree, Bell Bauhinia	Ayurvedic
Bauhinia tomentosa	Pita Kanchana	Yellow Bauhinia, St. Thomas Tree, Bell Bauhinia	Ayurvedic
Bauhinia tomentosa	Kokkumandarai	Yellow Bauhinia, St. Thomas Tree, Bell Bauhinia	Siddha/Tamil
Bauhinia tomentosa	Tiruvaatti	Yellow Bauhinia, St. Thomas Tree, Bell Bauhinia	Siddha/Tamil
Bauhinia tomentosa	Kanchini	Yellow Bauhinia, St. Thomas Tree, Bell Bauhinia	Siddha/Tamil
Bauhinia tomentosa	Kachnaar	Yellow Bauhinia, St. Thomas Tree, Bell Bauhinia	Folk
Bauhinia variegata	Kaanchanaara	Mountain Ebony, Buddhist Bauhinia	Ayurvedic
Bauhinia variegata	Kaanchanaaraka	Mountain Ebony, Buddhist Bauhinia	Ayurvedic
Bauhinia variegata	Kanchanak	Mountain Ebony, Buddhist Bauhinia	Ayurvedic
Bauhinia variegata	Kaanchana	Mountain Ebony, Buddhist Bauhinia	Ayurvedic
Bauhinia variegata	Gandhaari	Mountain Ebony, Buddhist Bauhinia	Ayurvedic
Bauhinia variegata	Sonapushpaka	Mountain Ebony, Buddhist Bauhinia	Ayurvedic
Bauhinia variegata	Ashmantaka	Mountain Ebony, Buddhist Bauhinia	Ayurvedic
Bauhinia variegata	Sivappuman-chori	Mountain Ebony, Buddhist Bauhinia	Siddha/Tamil
Begonia laciniata	Hooirjo	Beefsteak Geraniums, Elephant's Ear	Folk/Bengal
Belamcanda chinensis	Surajkaanti	Leopard Lily	Folk/Assam
Belamcanda chinensis	Dasbaha	Leopard Lily	Folk/Bengal
Belamcanda chinensis	Dasbichandi	Leopard Lily	Folk/Bengal

Table Contd.

Botanical Name	Indian Name	English Name	Medicinal System
Benincasa hispida	Kuushmaanda	Ash Gourd, White Gourd, Wax Gourd, White Pumpkin	Ayurvedic
Benincasa hispida	Kuushmaandaka	Ash Gourd, White Gourd, Wax Gourd, White Pumpkin	Ayurvedic
Benincasa hispida	Kuushmaandi	Ash Gourd, White Gourd, Wax Gourd, White Pumpkin	Ayurvedic
Benincasa hispida	Pethaa	Ash Gourd, White Gourd, Wax Gourd, White Pumpkin	Unani
Benincasa hispida	Mahdabah	Ash Gourd, White Gourd, Wax Gourd, White Pumpkin	Unani
Benincasa hispida	Kaddu-e-Roomi	Ash Gourd, White Gourd, Wax Gourd, White Pumpkin	Unani
Benincasa hispida	Ven-poosani	Ash Gourd, White Gourd, Wax Gourd, White Pumpkin	Siddha/Tamil
Benincasa hispida	Saambalpushani	Ash Gourd, White Gourd, Wax Gourd, White Pumpkin	Siddha/Tamil
Berberis aristata	Daaruharidraa	Indian Barberry	Ayurvedic
Berberis aristata	Daaru	Indian Barberry	Ayurvedic
Berberis aristata	Daarvi	Indian Barberry	Ayurvedic
Berberis aristata	Daarunishaa	Indian Barberry	Ayurvedic
Berberis aristata	Daarurajani	Indian Barberry	Ayurvedic
Berberis aristata	Vrahitaphala	Indian Barberry	Ayurvedic
Berberis aristata	Valliphala	Indian Barberry	Ayurvedic
Berberis aristata	Sthirphala	Indian Barberry	Ayurvedic
Berberis aristata	Pushpaphala	Indian Barberry	Ayurvedic
Berberis aristata	Somakaa	Indian Barberry	Ayurvedic
Berberis aristata	Parjanyaa	Indian Barberry	Ayurvedic
Berberis aristata	Parjani	Indian Barberry	Ayurvedic
Berberis aristata	Kantkateri	Indian Barberry	Ayurvedic
Berberis aristata	Taarthya	Indian Barberry	Ayurvedic
Berberis aristata	Pachampachaa	Indian Barberry	Ayurvedic
Berberis aristata	Daarhald	Indian Barberry	Unani
Berberis aristata	Rasaut (Extract)	Indian Barberry	Unani
Berberis aristata	Zarishk (Fruit)	Indian Barberry	Unani

Table Contd.

Botanical Name	Indian Name	English Name	Medicinal System
Berberis aristata	Marmanjal	Indian Barberry	Siddha/Tamil
Berberis chitria	Daaruharidraa	Barberry	Ayurvedic
Berberis chitria	Totaro	Barberry	Folk
Berberis chitria	Kintodaa	Barberry	Folk
Berberis vulgaris	Daruharidraa	Common Barberry, True Barberry	Ayurvedic
Berberis vulgaris	Chatrod	Common Barberry, True Barberry	Folk
Berberis vulgaris	Kashmal	Common Barberry, True Barberry	Folk
Bergenia ligulata	Paashaanabheda	Elephant-Ear, Siberian Saxifrage	Ayurvedic
Bergenia ligulata	Ashmaribhadikaa	Elephant-Ear, Siberian Saxifrage	Ayurvedic
Bergenia ligulata	Ashmaribhit	Elephant-Ear, Siberian Saxifrage	Ayurvedic
Bergenia ligulata	Ashmghna	Elephant-Ear, Siberian Saxifrage	Ayurvedic
Bergenia ligulata	Shilaabhit	Elephant-Ear, Siberian Saxifrage	Ayurvedic
Bergenia ligulata	Shilaabheda	Elephant-Ear, Siberian Saxifrage	Ayurvedic
Bergenia ligulata	Padanbethi	Elephant-Ear, Siberian Saxifrage	Siddha/Tamil
Beta vulgaris	Rakta-Granjana	Beet Root, Garden Beet, Chard	Ayurvedic
Beta vulgaris	Chukandar	Beet Root, Garden Beet, Chard	Folk
Betula alnoides	Bhojapatra	Indian Birch, Naga Birch	Ayurvedic
Betula utilis	Bhuurja	Himalayan Silver Birch, Indian Paper Tree	Ayurvedic
Betula utilis	Bahulvalkala	Himalayan Silver Birch, Indian Paper Tree	Ayurvedic
Betula utilis	Bahuputa	Himalayan Silver Birch, Indian Paper Tree	Ayurvedic
Betula utilis	Lekhyapatraka	Himalayan Silver Birch, Indian Paper Tree	Ayurvedic
Betula utilis	Charmi	Himalayan Silver Birch, Indian Paper Tree	Ayurvedic
Betula utilis	Chitrapatra	Himalayan Silver Birch, Indian Paper Tree	Ayurvedic
Betula utilis	Mardu tvak	Himalayan Silver Birch, Indian Paper Tree	Ayurvedic
Betula utilis	Sukshm patraka	Himalayan Silver Birch, Indian Paper Tree	Ayurvedic

Table Contd.

Botanical Name	Indian Name	English Name	Medicinal System
Betula utilis	Boorjapattirum (Leaves)	Himalayan Silver Birch, Indian Paper Tree	Siddha/Tamil
Bidens pilosa	Phutium	Beggar's Tick, Devil's Needle	Folk
Bidens pilosa	Kuri	Beggar's Tick, Devil's Needle	Folk
Biophytum sensitivum	Lajjaalu	Life Plant	Ayurvedic
Biophytum sensitivum	Vipareet Lajjaalu	Life Plant	Ayurvedic
Biophytum sensitivum	Alambushaa	Life Plant	Ayurvedic
Biophytum sensitivum	Lajoni	Life Plant	Folk
Biophytum sensitivum	Jhalai	Life Plant	Folk
Biophytum sensitivum	Lakajana	Life Plant	Folk
Bixa orellana	Sinduri	Annatto	Ayurvedic
Bixa orellana	Sinduriyaa	Annatto	Ayurvedic
Bixa orellana	Jabara	Annatto	Siddha/Tamil
Bixa orellana	Manjitti	Annatto	Siddha/Tamil
Blepharis edulis	Utangana	Acanthus	Ayurvedic
Blepharis edulis	Kaamavridhi	Acanthus	Ayurvedic
Blepharis edulis	Chatushpatri	Acanthus	Ayurvedic
Blepharis edulis	Shikhi	Acanthus	Ayurvedic
Blepharis edulis	Uchchattaa	Acanthus	Folk
Blepharis edulis	Anjrah	Acanthus	Unani
Blepharis linariaefolia	Ushtrakaandi	Acanthus	Ayurvedic
Blepharis linariaefolia	Utangan (Sindh)	Acanthus	Ayurvedic
Blepharis linariaefolia	Bhangari	Acanthus	Folk/Rajasthan
Blepharis linariaefolia	Asad	Acanthus	Unani
Blumea balsamifera	Kukundara	Nagai Camphor	Ayurvedic
Blumea balsamifera	Gangaapatri	Nagai Camphor	Ayurvedic
Blumea balsamifera	Kakarondaa	Nagai Camphor	Unani
Blumea densiflora	Kukundara	Nagai Camphor	Ayurvedic
Blumea eriantha	Kukundara	Nagai Camphor	Ayurvedic
Blumea eriantha	Kakaronda	Nagai Camphor	Unani
Blumea eriantha	Nirmudi	Nagai Camphor	Folk
Blumea fastulosa	Kukundara	Nagai Camphor	Ayurvedic
Blumea fastulosa	Kakarondaa	Nagai Camphor	Unani

Table Contd.

Botanical Name	Indian Name	English Name	Medicinal System
Blumea lacera	Kukundara	Nagai Camphor	Ayurvedic
Blumea lacera	Kukuradru	Nagai Camphor	Ayurvedic
Blumea lacera	Taamrachuuda	Nagai Camphor	Ayurvedic
Blumea lacera	Kakarondaa	Nagai Camphor	Unani
Blumea lacera	Narakkarandai	Nagai Camphor	Siddha/Tamil
Blumea lacera	Kaatu Mullangi	Nagai Camphor	Siddha/Tamil
Blumea lacera	Kakranda	Nagai Camphor	Folk
Boerhavia diffusa	Rakta-punarnavaa	Red- flowered Hogweed	Ayurvedic
Boerhavia diffusa	Punarnavaa	Red-flowered Hogweed	Ayurvedic
Boerhavia diffusa	Katthilla	Red-flowered Hogweed	Ayurvedic
Boerhavia diffusa	Shothahrit	Red-flowered Hogweed	Ayurvedic
Boerhavia diffusa	Shothaghni	Red-flowered Hogweed	Ayurvedic
Boerhavia diffusa	Varshaabhu	Red-flowered Hogweed	Ayurvedic
Boerhavia diffusa	Itsit	Red-flowered Hogweed	Unani
Boerhavia diffusa	Bishkhaparaa	Red-flowered Hogweed	Unani
Boerhavia diffusa	Mookkirattai	Red-flowered Hogweed	Siddha/Tamil
Boerhavia diffusa	Gadaha-purnaa	Red-flowered Hogweed	Folk
Boerhavia verticillata	Shveta Punarnavaa	White-flowered Hogweed	Ayurvedic
Boerhavia verticillata	Vrshchira	White-flowered Hogweed	Ayurvedic
Boerhavia verticillata	Vrshchiraka	White- flowered Hogweed	Ayurvedic
Borago officinalis	Gaozabaan	Borage, Cow's Tongue Plant	Unani
Borassus flabellifer	Taala	Palmyra Palm, Brab Tree	Ayurvedic
Borassus flabellifer	Taada	Palmyra Palm, Brab Tree	Ayurvedic
Borassus flabellifer	Trinraj	Palmyra Palm, Brab Tree	Ayurvedic
Borassus flabellifer	Mahonnata	Palmyra Palm, Brab Tree	Ayurvedic
Borassus flabellifer	Lekhyapatra	Palmyra Palm, Brab Tree	Ayurvedic
Borassus flabellifer	Panai	Palmyra Palm, Brab Tree	Siddha/Tamil
Borassus flabellifer	Panaimaram	Palmyra Palm, Brab Tree	Siddha/Tamil
Borreria articularis	Madana-ghanti	Shaggy Button Weed	Ayurvedic
Borreria articularis	Nathaichoori	Shaggy Button Weed	Siddha/Tamil
Borreria articularis	Ghanti-chi-bhaaji	Shaggy Button Weed	Folk

Table Contd.

Botanical Name	Indian Name	English Name	Medicinal System
Borreria articularis	Gatbhanjan	Shaggy Button Weed	Folk
Borreria articularis	Satgathiyaa	Shaggy Button Weed	Folk
Boswellia serrata	Shallaki	Indian Frankincense, Indian Olibanum	Ayurvedic
Boswellia serrata	Susravaa	Indian Frankincense, Indian Olibanum	Ayurvedic
Boswellia serrata	Gajabhakshyaa	Indian Frankincense, Indian Olibanum	Ayurvedic
Boswellia serrata	Salai	Indian Frankincense, Indian Olibanum	Ayurvedic
Boswellia serrata	Kunduru (Gum)	Indian Frankincense, Indian Olibanum	Ayurvedic
Boswellia serrata	Kundur (Gum)	Indian Frankincense, Indian Olibanum	Unani
Boswellia serrata	Parangisaam-birani	Indian Frankincense, Indian Olibanum	Siddha/Tamil
Boswellia serrata	Kungli	Indian Frankincense, Indian Olibanum	Siddha/Tamil
Boswellia serrata	Salai Guggul	Indian Frankincense, Indian Olibanum	Folk
Brassica alba	Siddhaartha	White Mustard	Ayurvedic
Brassica alba	Shveta Sarshapa	White Mustard	Ayurvedic
Brassica alba	Sarshapa-Gaura	White Mustard	Ayurvedic
Brassica alba	Khardal Safed	White Mustard	Unani
Brassica alba	Venkadugu	White Mustard	Siddha/Tamil
Brassica alba	Safed Raai	White Mustard	Folk
Brassica campestris	Sarshapa	Field Mustard, Turnip Rape	Ayurvedic
Brassica campestris	Siddhaartha	Field Mustard, Turnip Rape	Ayurvedic
Brassica campestris	Sarson	Field Mustard, Turnip Rape	Unani
Brassica campestris	Kadugu	Field Mustard, Turnip Rape	Siddha/Tamil
Brassica juncea	Raajikaa	Chinese Mustard, Brown Mustard	Ayurvedic
Brassica juncea	Aasuri Raai	Chinese Mustard, Brown Mustard	Ayurvedic
Brassica juncea	Tikshnagandhaa	Chinese Mustard, Brown Mustard	Ayurvedic
Brassica juncea	Kadugu	Chinese Mustard, Brown Mustard	Siddha/Tamil
Brassica juncea	Raai	Chinese Mustard, Brown Mustard	Folk

Table Contd.

Botanical Name	Indian Name	English Name	Medicinal System
Brassica napus	Krishna-Sarshapa	Mustard, Indian Rape	Ayurvedic
Brassica napus	Raajakshavaka	Mustard, Indian Rape	Ayurvedic
Brassica napus	Kattaka	Mustard, Indian Rape	Ayurvedic
Brassica napus	Katusneha	Mustard, Indian Rape	Ayurvedic
Brassica napus	Tantubha	Mustard, Indian Rape	Ayurvedic
Brassica napus	Siddhaartha	Mustard, Indian Rape	Ayurvedic
Brassica napus	Siddhaarthaka	Mustard, Indian Rape	Ayurvedic
Brassica napus	Siddhaartha-sita	Mustard, Indian Rape	Ayurvedic
Brassica napus	Rakshogna	Mustard, Indian Rape	Ayurvedic
Brassica napus	Kaali Sarson	Mustard, Indian Rape	Unani
Brassica nigra	Banarasi Raai	Black Mustard	Ayurvedic
Brassica nigra	Raajika	Black Mustard	Ayurvedic
Brassica nigra	Khardal Siyah	Black Mustard	Unani
Brassica nigra	Kadugu	Black Mustard	Siddha/Tamil
Brassica nigra	Raai	Black Mustard	Folk
Brayera anthelmintica	Kousso	Cusso, Brayera	Folk
Breynia retusa	Bahuprajaa	Cup Saucer Plant	Ayurvedic
Breynia retusa	Kaamboji	Cup Saucer Plant	Ayurvedic
Breynia retusa	Kaali Kamboi	Cup Saucer Plant	Folk
Bridelia montana	Ekaviraa	Spinous Kino Tree	Ayurvedic
Bridelia montana	Venge maram	Spinous Kino Tree	Siddha/Tamil
Bridelia montana	Gondni	Spinous Kino Tree	Folk
Bridelia montana	Asaanaa	Spinous Kino Tree	Folk
Bridelia retusa	Mahaaviraa	Spinous Kino Tree	Ayurvedic
Bridelia retusa	Asana	Spinous Kino Tree	Ayurvedic
Bridelia retusa	Mulluvengai	Spinous Kino Tree	Siddha/Tamil
Bridelia retusa	Gondani	Spinous Kino Tree	Folk
Bridelia retusa	Gondui	Spinous Kino Tree	Folk
Bridelia retusa	Khaajaa	Spinous Kino Tree	Folk
Brugmansia suaveolens	Datura (American)	Angel's Trumpet, Angel's Tears	Folk
Brunella vulgaris	Ustukhudduus	Self-heal	Unani

Table Contd.

Botanical Name	Indian Name	English Name	Medicinal System
Brunella vulgaris	Dhaaru	Self-heal	Folk
Bryonopsis laciniosa	Lingini	Bryony	Ayurvedic
Bryonopsis laciniosa	Shivalingi	Bryony	Ayurvedic
Bryonopsis laciniosa	Chitraphalaa	Bryony	Ayurvedic
Bryonopsis laciniosa	Lingikaa	Bryony	Ayurvedic
Bryonopsis laciniosa	Ishalingi	Bryony	Ayurvedic
Bryonopsis laciniosa	Lingadonda	Bryony	Folk/Telugu
Bryophyllum pinnatum	Parnabija	Air Plant, Mexican Love Plant	Ayurvedic
Bryophyllum pinnatum	Airaavati	Air Plant, Mexican Love Plant	Ayurvedic
Bryophyllum pinnatum	Zakhm-e-Hayaat	Air Plant, Mexican Love Plant	Unani
Buchanania axillaris	Priyaal	Buchanan's Mango, Cuddapah Almond	Ayurvedic
Buchanania axillaris	Habb-us-Simanaa	Buchanan's Mango, Cuddapah Almond	Unani
Buchanania axillaris	Mudaima	Buchanan's Mango, Cuddapah Almond	Siddha/Tamil
Buchanania axillaris	Saraparuppu (Seeds)	Buchanan's Mango, Cuddapah Almond	Siddha/Tamil
Buchanania lanzan	Priyaala	Almondette Tree, Cheronjee, Buchanan's Mango	Ayurvedic
Buchanania lanzan	Piyaar	Almondette Tree, Cheronjee, Buchanan's Mango	Ayurvedic
Buchanania lanzan	Kharskandha	Almondette Tree, Cheronjee, Buchanan's Mango	Ayurvedic
Buchanania lanzan	Bahulvalkala	Almondette Tree, Cheronjee, Buchanan's Mango	Ayurvedic
Buchanania lanzan	Taapaseshtha	Almondette Tree, Cheronjee, Buchanan's Mango	Ayurvedic
Buchanania lanzan	Habb-us-Simanaa	Almondette Tree, Cheronjee, Buchanan's Mango	Unani
Buchanania lanzan	Chironjee	Almondette Tree, Cheronjee, Buchanan's Mango	Ayurvedic
Buchanania lanzan	Nuql-e-khwazaa (Seeds)	Almondette Tree, Cheronjee, Buchanan's Mango	Unani
Buchanania lanzan	Mudaima	Almondette Tree, Cheronjee, Buchanan's Mango	Siddha/Tamil

Table Contd.

Botanical Name	Indian Name	English Name	Medicinal System
Buchanania lanzan	Moriamaram	Almondette Tree, Cheronjee, Buchanan's Mango	Siddha/Tamil
Bupleurum flacutum	Shingu	Hare's Ear	Folk
Bupleurum flacutum	Sipil	Hare's Ear	Folk
Bupleurum flacutum	Thaanyo	Hare's Ear	Folk
Butea monosperma	Paalasha	Flame of the Forest, Butea Gum, Bengal Kino	Ayurvedic
Butea monosperma	Kimshuka	Flame of the Forest, Butea Gum, Bengal Kino	Ayurvedic
Butea monosperma	Raktapushpaka	Flame of the Forest, Butea Gum, Bengal Kino	Ayurvedic
Butea monosperma	Kshaarshreshtha	Flame of the Forest, Butea Gum, Bengal Kino	Ayurvedic
Butea monosperma	Brahmavriksha	Flame of the Forest, Butea Gum, Bengal Kino	Ayurvedic
Butea monosperma	Samidvar	Flame of the Forest, Butea Gum, Bengal Kino	Ayurvedic
Butea monosperma	Dhaak	Flame of the Forest, Butea Gum, Bengal Kino	Unani
Butea monosperma	Samagh Dhaak (Gum)	Flame of the Forest, Butea Gum, Bengal Kino	Unani
Butea monosperma	Kamar-kas (Gum)	Flame of the Forest, Butea Gum, Bengal Kino	Unani
Butea monosperma	Palasam	Flame of the Forest, Butea Gum, Bengal Kino	Siddha/Tamil
Butea monosperma	Murukkan	Flame of the Forest, Butea Gum, Bengal Kino	Siddha/Tamil
Butea monosperma	Tesu	Flame of the Forest, Butea Gum, Bengal Kino	Folk
Butea superba	Lataa-Palaash	Flame of the Forest	Ayurvedic
Buxus wallichiana	Chikri	Himalayan Boxwood Tree	Folk
Buxus wallichiana	Shamshaad	Himalayan Boxwood Tree	Folk
Buxus wallichiana	Paapari	Himalayan Boxwood Tree	Folk
Caccinia crassifolia	Gaozabaan	False Gaozaban	Unani
Cadaba fruticosa	Kattagatti	Indian Cadaba	Siddha/Tamil
Cadaba fruticosa	Vilivi	Indian Cadaba	Siddha/Tamil
Cadaba fruticosa	Dabi	Indian Cadaba	Folk

Table Contd.

Botanical Name	Indian Name	English Name	Medicinal System
Callicarpa macrophylla	Habb-ul-Mihlb	Perfumed Cherry	Unani
Callicarpa macrophylla	Gnazhal	Perfumed Cherry	Siddha/Tamil
Callicarpa macrophylla	Chokkala	Perfumed Cherry	Siddha/Tamil
Calophyllum apetalum	Shirupinnai	Poonspar of Travancore	Siddha/Tamil
Calophyllum inophyllum	Punnaaga	Indian Laurel, Alexandrian Laurel	Ayurvedic
Calophyllum inophyllum	Tunga	Indian Laurel, Alexandrian Laurel	Ayurvedic
Calophyllum inophyllum	Sultaan Champaa	Indian Laurel, Alexandrian Laurel	Ayurvedic
Calophyllum inophyllum	Naagchampaa	Indian Laurel, Alexandrian Laurel	Ayurvedic
Calophyllum inophyllum	Raajchampaa	Indian Laurel, Alexandrian Laurel	Ayurvedic
Calophyllum inophyllum	Punnai	Indian Laurel, Alexandrian Laurel	Siddha/Tamil
Calophyllum inophyllum	Punnagam	Indian Laurel, Alexandrian Laurel	Siddha/Tamil
Calotropis gigantea	Alarka	Swallow Wort	Ayurvedic
Calotropis gigantea	Raajaarka	Swallow Wort	Ayurvedic
Calotropis gigantea	Shvetaarka	Swallow Wort	Ayurvedic
Calotropis gigantea	Vasuka	Swallow Wort	Ayurvedic
Calotropis gigantea	Mandaar	Swallow Wort	Ayurvedic
Calotropis gigantea	Bhaasvanmuula	Swallow Wort	Ayurvedic
Calotropis gigantea	Dinesh	Swallow Wort	Ayurvedic
Calotropis gigantea	Prabhaakara	Swallow Wort	Ayurvedic
Calotropis gigantea	Ravi	Swallow Wort	Ayurvedic
Calotropis gigantea	Bhaanu	Swallow Wort	Ayurvedic
Calotropis gigantea	Tapana	Swallow Wort	Ayurvedic
Calotropis gigantea	Madaar	Swallow Wort	Unani
Calotropis gigantea	Aak	Swallow Wort	Unani
Calotropis gigantea	Erukku	Swallow Wort	Siddha/Tamil
Calotropis procera	Alarka	Swallow-wort, Milk Weed, King's Crown	Ayurvedic
Calotropis procera	Surya	Swallow-wort, Milk Weed, King's Crown	Ayurvedic
Calotropis procera	Suuryaahvya	Swallow-wort, Milk Weed, King's Crown	Ayurvedic
Calotropis procera	Vikirna	Swallow-wort, Milk Weed, King's Crown	Ayurvedic

Table Contd.

Botanical Name	Indian Name	English Name	Medicinal System
Calotropis procera	Vasuka	Swallow-wort, Milk Weed, King's Crown	Ayurvedic
Calotropis procera	Tapana	Swallow-wort, Milk Weed, King's Crown	Ayurvedic
Calotropis procera	Tuulaphala	Swallow-wort, Milk Weed, King's Crown	Ayurvedic
Calotropis procera	Kshirparna	Swallow-wort, Milk Weed, King's Crown	Ayurvedic
Calotropis procera	Arkaparna	Swallow-wort, Milk Weed, King's Crown	Ayurvedic
Calotropis procera	Aasphota	Swallow-wort, Milk Weed, King's Crown	Ayurvedic
Calotropis procera	Aakh	Swallow-wort, Milk Weed, King's Crown	Unani
Calotropis procera	Madaar	Swallow-wort, Milk Weed, King's Crown	Unani
Calotropis procera	Ashar	Swallow-wort, Milk Weed, King's Crown	Unani
Calotropis procera	Vellerukku	Swallow-wort, Milk Weed, King's Crown	Siddha/Tamil
Calotropis procera	Arkkam	Swallow-wort, Milk Weed, King's Crown	Siddha/Tamil
Caltha palustris	Mamiri	American Cowslip, Marsh Marigold, Water Buttercup	Folk
Calycopteris floribunda	Sushavi	White Daisy	Ayurvedic
Calycopteris floribunda	Paaniyavalli	White Daisy	Ayurvedic
Calycopteris floribunda	Minnargodi	White Daisy	Siddha/Tamil
Camellia sinensis	Chaai	Tea Plant	Unani
Camellia sinensis	Chaah	Tea Plant	Unani
Camellia sinensis	Shaay	Tea Plant	Unani
Camellia sinensis	Thacyilai	Tea Plant	Siddha/Tamil
Canarium commune	Jangali Baadaam	Jave Almond, Kenari Nut	Folk
Canarium strictum	Raal Dhuup	Black Dammar	Ayurvedic
Canarium strictum	Mand Dhuup	Black Dammar	Ayurvedic
Canarium strictum	Karunkungiliyam	Black Dammar	Siddha/Tamil
Cannabis sativa	Vijayaa	Hemp, Indian Hemp	Ayurvedic

Table Contd.

Botanical Name	Indian Name	English Name	Medicinal System
Cassia fistula	Aarevata	Indian Laburnum, Purging Cassia, Golden Shower	Ayurvedic
Cassia fistula	Suvarnaka	Indian Laburnum, Purging Cassia, Golden Shower	Ayurvedic
Cassia fistula	Khyaarshambar	Indian Laburnum, Purging Cassia, Golden Shower	Unani
Cassia fistula	Sarakkonrai	Indian Laburnum, Purging Cassia, Golden Shower	Siddha/Tamil
Cassia fistula	Amaltaasa	Indian Laburnum, Purging Cassia, Golden Shower	Unani
Cassia obovata	Maarkandikaa	Spanish, Sudan Senna	Ayurvedic
Cassia obovata	Svarnapattri	Spanish, Sudan Senna	Ayurvedic
Cassia obovata	Sonaamukhi	Spanish, Sudan Senna	Folk
Cassia obovata	Sanaai	Spanish, Sudan Senna	Folk
Cassia obtusifolia	Chakramarda	Arsenic Weed, Sicklepod	Ayurvedic
Cassia obtusifolia	Prapunnaada	Arsenic Weed, Sicklepod	Ayurvedic
Cassia obtusifolia	Chakondaa	Arsenic Weed, Sicklepod	Folk
Cassia obtusifolia	Chakwar	Arsenic Weed, Sicklepod	Folk
Cassia obtusifolia	Pumariaa	Arsenic Weed, Sicklepod	Folk
Cassia occidentalis	Kaasamarda	Coffee Senna, Foetid Cassia, Negro Coffee	Ayurvedic
Cassia occidentalis	Kaasaari	Coffee Senna, Foetid Cassia, Negro Coffee	Ayurvedic
Cassia occidentalis	Kasondi	Coffee Senna, Foetid Cassia, Negro Coffee	Unani
Cassia occidentalis	Paeyaavarai	Coffee Senna, Foetid Cassia, Negro Coffee	Siddha/Tamil
Cassia occidentalis	Ponnaavaarai	Coffee Senna, Foetid Cassia, Negro Coffee	Siddha/Tamil
Cassia occidentalis	Kalkashunda	Coffee Senna, Foetid Cassia, Negro Coffee	Folk/Bengal
Cassia sophera	Kaasamarda	Sophera Senna	Ayurvedic
Cassia sophera	Kasondi	Sophera Senna	Unani
Cassia sophera	Ponnaavaarai	Sophera Senna	Folk
Cassia tora	Chakramarda	Sickle Senna, Ringworm Plant	Ayurvedic
Cassia tora	Chakri	Sickle Senna, Ringworm Plant	Ayurvedic
Cassia tora	Prapunnaada	Sickle Senna, Ringworm Plant	Ayurvedic

Table Contd.

Botanical Name	Indian Name	English Name	Medicinal System
Cassia tora	Dadrughna	Sickle Senna, Ringworm Plant	Ayurvedic
Cassia tora	Meshalochana	Sickle Senna, Ringworm Plant	Ayurvedic
Cassia tora	Padmaata	Sickle Senna, Ringworm Plant	Ayurvedic
Cassia tora	Aedagaja	Sickle Senna, Ringworm Plant	Ayurvedic
Cassia tora	Penwaad Taarutaa	Sickle Senna, Ringworm Plant	Unani
Cassia tora	Ushittgarai	Sickle Senna, Ringworm Plant	Siddha/Tamil
Cassia tora	Chakavad	Sickle Senna, Ringworm Plant	Folk
Cassia tora	Daadamaari	Sickle Senna, Ringworm Plant	Folk
Cassytha filiformis	Amarvalli	Doddar-Laurel, Love-Vine	Ayurvedic
Cassytha filiformis	Aakaashbel	Doddar-Laurel, Love-Vine	Ayurvedic
Cassytha filiformis	Erumaikkottan	Doddar-Laurel, Love-Vine	Siddha/Tamil
Castanea sativa	Singhaaraa	Spanish Chestnut, Sweet Chestnut	Folk
Casuarina equisetifolia	Jhaau	Casuarina, She-Oak, Australian or Whistling Pine, Beefwood	Ayurvedic
Casuarina equisetifolia	Vilaayati Saru	Casuarina, She-Oak, Australian or Whistling Pine, Beefwood	Folk (Gujarat)
Casuarina equisetifolia	Savukkumaram	Casuarina, She-Oak, Australian or Whistling Pine, Beefwood	Siddha/Tamil
Catharanthus roseus	Sadaabahaar	Madagascar Periwinkle	Folk
Catharanthus roseus	Nayantaaraa	Madagascar Periwinkle	Folk
Catharanthus roseus	Nityakalyaani	Madagascar Periwinkle	Folk
Cayratia carnosa	Gandira	Cayratia	Ayurvedic
Cayratia carnosa	Tumans	Cayratia	Siddha/Tamil
Cayratia pedata	Godhaapadi	Cayratia	Ayurvedic
Cayratia pedata	Kattuppirandai	Cayratia	Siddha/Tamil
Cedrela toona	Tuunikaa	Red Cedar, Toon, Indian Mahogany Tree	Ayurvedic
Cedrela toona	Nandi Vrksha	Red Cedar, Toon, Indian Mahogany Tree	Ayurvedic
Cedrela toona	Tunumaram	Red Cedar, Toon, Indian Mahogany Tree	Siddha/Tamil
Cedrela toona	Santhanavembu	Red Cedar, Toon, Indian Mahogany Tree	Siddha/Tamil

Table Contd.

Botanical Name	Indian Name	English Name	Medicinal System
Centratherum anthelminticum	Kamoon Barri	Purple Flea-bane, Achenes	Unani
Centratherum anthelminticum	Kaatu Seerakam	Purple Flea-bane, Achenes	Siddha/Tamil
Cephaelis ipecacuanha	Ipecac	Ipecac, Ipecacuanha	Unani
Ceratonia siliqua	Kharnuub Shaami	Locust Bean, St. John's Bread, Carob Tree	Unani
Ceratophyllum demersum	Shaivaala	Coontail, Hornwort	Ayurvedic
Ceratophyllum demersum	Jalnili	Coontail, Hornwort	Ayurvedic
Ceratophyllum demersum	Jalaja	Coontail, Hornwort	Ayurvedic
Ceratophyllum demersum	Tuhlub	Coontail, Hornwort	Unani
Ceratophyllum demersum	Pashm vazg	Coontail, Hornwort	Unani
Ceratophyllum demersum	Velampasi	Coontail, Hornwort	Siddha/Tamil
Ceratophyllum demersum	Sivaar	Coontail, Hornwort	Folk
Cereus grandiflorus	Nivadung Paanchkoni	Cereus, Night Blooming Cereus, Sweet Scented Cactus	Folk
Ceriops candolleana	Pavrikutti	Compound Cymed Mangrove	Folk/Tamil
Ceriops candolleana	Balobalarao	Compound Cymed Mangrove	Folk (Trade)
Ceriops candolleana	Pandikutti	Compound Cymed Mangrove	Siddha/Tamil
Ceriops candolleana	Gadera	Compound Cymed Mangrove	Folk/Telugu
Ceriops candolleana	Keraari	Compound Cymed Mangrove	Folk/Kannada
Ceriops candolleana	Chowri	Compound Cymed Mangrove	Folk/Kannada
Ceropegia bulbosa	Khappar-kaddu	Candlestick Ceropegia	Folk
Ceropegia bulbosa	Bhuu-tumbi	Candlestick Ceropegia	Folk
Ceropegia bulbosa	Paataal-Tumbi	Candlestick Ceropegia	Folk
Ceropegia bulbosa	Gilothi	Candlestick Ceropegia	Folk
Ceropegia bulbosa	Galot	Candlestick Ceropegia	Folk
Ceropegia bulbosa	Gilodya	Candlestick Ceropegia	Folk
Ceropegia juncea	Kanvel	Leafless Godlet Flower	Folk
Ceropegia juncea	Vel-khantudi	Leafless Godlet Flower	Folk/Marathi
Cetraria islandica	Shaileya	Cetraria, Iceland Lichen, Liceland Moss	Ayurvedic
Cetraria islandica	Chharela	Cetraria, Iceland Lichen, Liceland Moss	Folk
Cheiranthus cheiri	Tudri	Wall-flower, Gilli Flower	Unani

Table Contd.

Botanical Name	Indian Name	English Name	Medicinal System
Chenopodium album	Vaastuuka	Fat Hen, Lamb's Quarters, White Goosefoot, Wild Spinach, Pigweed	Ayurvedic
Chenopodium album	Bathuaa	Fat Hen, Lamb's Quarters, White Goosefoot, Wild Spinach, Pigweed	Unani
Chenopodium album	Baathu	Fat Hen, Lamb's Quarters, White Goosefoot, Wild Spinach, Pigweed	Unani
Chenopodium album	Paruppukeerai	Fat Hen, Lamb's Quarters, White Goosefoot, Wild Spinach, Pigweed	Siddha/Tamil
Chenopodium album	Chandan Betu	Fat Hen, Lamb's Quarters, White Goosefoot, Wild Spinach, Pigweed	Folk/Bengal
Chenopodium album	Chillika	Fat Hen, Lamb's Quarters, White Goosefoot, Wild Spinach, Pigweed	Ayurvedic
Chenopodium album	Chilli-shaak	Fat Hen, Lamb's Quarters, White Goosefoot, Wild Spinach, Pigweed	Folk
Chenopodium ambrosioides	Sugandh-vaastuuka	Indian Wormseed, Sweet Pigweed, Mexican Tea	Ayurvedic
Chenopodium ambrosioides	Kshetra-vaastuuka	Indian Wormseed, Sweet Pigweed, Mexican Tea	Ayurvedic
Chenopodium ambrosioides	Kattasam-badam	Indian Wormseed, Sweet Pigweed, Mexican Tea	Siddha/Tamil
Chenopodium ambrosioides	Khatuaa	Indian Wormseed, Sweet Pigweed, Mexican Tea	Folk
Chenopodium botrys	Jangaddi	Feather Geramium, Jerusalem-Oak	Folk
Chenopodium botrys	Sahanik	Feather Geramium, Jerusalem-Oak	Folk
Chenopodium botrys	Vaastuuka	Feather Geramium, Jerusalem-Oak	Ayurvedic
Chloris gayana	Rhoolsoohullu	Giant Rhodes, Rhodes-Grass	Folk
Chlorophytum arundinaceum	Mushali Shveta	White Musali	Ayurvedic
Chlorophytum arundinaceum	Musali Safed	White Musali	Unani

Table Contd.

Botanical Name	Indian Name	English Name	Medicinal System
Chlorophytum arundinaceum	Biskandri	White Musali	Unani
Chlorophytum arundinaceum	Vallaimusali	White Musali	Siddha/Tamil
Chlorophytum arundinaceum	Nising	White Musali	Folk
Chlorophytum arundinaceum	Tibbati Ginseng	White Musali	Folk
Chlorophytum tuberosum	Mushali Shveta	White Musali	Ayurvedic
Chlorophytum tuberosum	Dhauli Musali	White Musali	Folk
Chlorophytum tuberosum	Musali	White Musali	Unani
Chlorophytum tuberosum	Vallaimusali	White Musali	Siddha/Tamil
Chloroxylon swietenia	Karumboraju	Indian Satinwood Tree	Siddha/Tamil
Chloroxylon swietenia	Kudavuboraju	Indian Satinwood Tree	Siddha/Tamil
Chloroxylon swietenia	Porashu	Indian Satinwood Tree	Siddha/Tamil
Chloroxylon swietenia	Bheria	Indian Satinwood Tree	Folk
Chloroxylon swietenia	Bherul	Indian Satinwood Tree	Folk
Chloroxylon swietenia	Raktarohidi	Indian Satinwood Tree	Folk
Chondrodendron tomentosum	Paatha	False Pareira Brava	Ayurvedic
Chondrodendron tomentosum	Ambashthaa	False Pareira Brava	Ayurvedic
Chonemorpha macrophylla	Muurvaa	Wood Vine	Ayurvedic
Chrozophora plicata	Suuryaavart	Chrozophora	Ayurvedic
Chrozophora plicata	Nilakanthi	Chrozophora	Folk
Chrysanthemum indicum	Shatapatri	Chrysanthemum	Ayurvedic
Chrysanthemum indicum	Guldaaudi	Chrysanthemum	Unani
Chrysanthemum indicum	Samanthipoo	Chrysanthemum	Siddha/Tamil
Chrysanthemum indicum	Akkarakkaram	Chrysanthemum	Siddha/Tamil
Chukrasia tabularis	Aglay	Bastard Cedar, White Cedar, Indian Red Wood	Siddha/Tamil
Chukrasia tabularis	Melei veppu	Bastard Cedar, White Cedar, Indian Red Wood	Siddha/Tamil
Chukrasia tabularis	Chikrassy	Bastard Cedar, White Cedar, Indian Red Wood	Folk/Bengal
Cicer arietinum	Chanaka	Bengal Gram, Chick Pea	Ayurvedic
Cicer arietinum	Chanakaa	Bengal Gram, Chick Pea	Ayurvedic

Table Contd.

Botanical Name	Indian Name	English Name	Medicinal System
Cicer arietinum	Harimantha	Bengal Gram, Chick Pea	Ayurvedic
Cicer arietinum	Vajimantha	Bengal Gram, Chick Pea	Ayurvedic
Cicer arietinum	Jivan	Bengal Gram, Chick Pea	Ayurvedic
Cicer arietinum	Sakal-priya	Bengal Gram, Chick Pea	Ayurvedic
Cicer arietinum	Nakhud	Bengal Gram, Chick Pea	Unani
Cicer arietinum	Chunda kadalai	Bengal Gram, Chick Pea	Siddha/Tamil
Cicer arietinum	Mookkuk-kadalai	Bengal Gram, Chick Pea	Siddha/Tamil
Cichorium endivia	Kaasani	Succory, Endive	Ayurvedic
Cichorium endivia	Bustaani Kaasani	Succory, Endive	Unani
Cichorium intybus	Hindubaa	Chicory, Indian Endive	Unani
Cichorium intybus	Kaasani Dashti	Chicory, Indian Endive	Unani
Cichorium intybus	Kasinikkeerai	Chicory, Indian Endive	Siddha/Tamil
Cimicifuga racemosa	Cohosh	Black Cohosh Root, Black Snake Root	Folk
Cimicifuga racemosa	Jiuenti	Black Cohosh Root, Black Snake Root	Folk
Cinchona officinalis	Quinine	Crown or Loxa Bark	Ayurvedic
Cinchona officinalis	Al-keenaa	Crown or Loxa Bark	Unani
Cinchona officinalis	Kanakanaa	Crown or Loxa Bark	Unani
Cinnamomum camphora	Karpura	Camphor Tree	Ayurvedic
Cinnamomum camphora	Ghanasaara	Camphor Tree	Ayurvedic
Cinnamomum camphora	Chandra	Camphor Tree	Ayurvedic
Cinnamomum camphora	Chandra Prabhaa	Camphor Tree	Ayurvedic
Cinnamomum camphora	Sitaabhra	Camphor Tree	Ayurvedic
Cinnamomum camphora	Hima-valukaa	Camphor Tree	Ayurvedic
Cinnamomum camphora	Himopala	Camphor Tree	Ayurvedic
Cinnamomum camphora	Himakara	Camphor Tree	Ayurvedic
Cinnamomum camphora	Shashi	Camphor Tree	Ayurvedic
Cinnamomum camphora	Indu	Camphor Tree	Ayurvedic
Cinnamomum camphora	Tushaara	Camphor Tree	Ayurvedic
Cinnamomum camphora	Gandhadravya	Camphor Tree	Ayurvedic
Cinnamomum camphora	Shitalraja	Camphor Tree	Ayurvedic

Table Contd.

Botanical Name	Indian Name	English Name	Medicinal System
Cinnamomum camphora	Kaafoor	Camphor Tree	Unani
Cinnamomum camphora	Indu	Camphor Tree	Siddha/Tamil
Cinnamomum camphora	Karupporam	Camphor Tree	Siddha/Tamil
Cinnamomum cassia	Tvak	Chinese Cinnamon, Cassia bark	Ayurvedic
Cinnamomum cassia	Daalchini	Chinese Cinnamon, Cassia bark	Ayurvedic
Cinnamomum cassia	Elavangapattiri	Chinese Cinnamon, Cassia bark	Siddha/Tamil
Cinnamomum tamala	Tejpatra	Indian Cassia Lignea	Ayurvedic
Cinnamomum tamala	Patra	Indian Cassia Lignea	Ayurvedic
Cinnamomum tamala	Patraka	Indian Cassia Lignea	Ayurvedic
Cinnamomum tamala	Utkat	Indian Cassia Lignea	Ayurvedic
Cinnamomum tamala	Tamaalpatra	Indian Cassia Lignea	Ayurvedic
Cinnamomum tamala	Naalukaa	Indian Cassia Lignea	Ayurvedic
Cinnamomum tamala	Naalikaa	Indian Cassia Lignea	Ayurvedic
Cinnamomum tamala	Saleekhaa	Indian Cassia Lignea	Unani
Cinnamomum tamala	Saazaj Hindi	Indian Cassia Lignea	Unani
Cinnamomum tamala	Talishpattiri	Indian Cassia Lignea	Siddha/Tamil
Cinnamomum tamala	Elavangapattiri	Indian Cassia Lignea	Siddha/Tamil
Cinnamomum tamala	Tejpaata	Indian Cassia Lignea	Folk
Cinnamomum zeylanicum	Tvak	Cinnamon, Ceylon Cinnamon	Ayurvedic
Cinnamomum zeylanicum	Daaruchini	Cinnamon, Ceylon Cinnamon	Ayurvedic
Cinnamomum zeylanicum	Chochaa	Cinnamon, Ceylon Cinnamon	Ayurvedic
Cinnamomum zeylanicum	Choncha	Cinnamon, Ceylon Cinnamon	Ayurvedic
Cinnamomum zeylanicum	Varaanga	Cinnamon, Ceylon Cinnamon	Ayurvedic
Cinnamomum zeylanicum	Utkata	Cinnamon, Ceylon Cinnamon	Ayurvedic
Cinnamomum zeylanicum	Daarusitaa	Cinnamon, Ceylon Cinnamon	Ayurvedic
Cinnamomum zeylanicum	Daarchini	Cinnamon, Ceylon Cinnamon	Unani
Cinnamomum zeylanicum	Elavangappattai	Cinnamon, Ceylon Cinnamon	Siddha/Tamil
Cinnamomum zeylanicum	Taj	Cinnamon, Ceylon Cinnamon	Folk
Cissampelos pareira	Paathaa	Velvet-Leaf Pareira, Pareira Brava	Ayurvedic
Cissampelos pareira	Ambashthaa	Velvet-Leaf Pareira, Pareira Brava	Ayurvedic
Cissampelos pareira	Varatiktaaa	Velvet-Leaf Pareira, Pareira Brava	Ayurvedic

Table Contd.

Botanical Name	Indian Name	English Name	Medicinal System
Cissampelos pareira	Vriki	Velvet-Leaf Pareira, Pareira Brava	Ayurvedic
Cissampelos pareira	Aviddhakarni	Velvet-Leaf Pareira, Pareira Brava	Ayurvedic
Cissampelos pareira	Piluphalaa	Velvet-Leaf Pareira, Pareira Brava	Ayurvedic
Cissampelos pareira	Shreyashi	Velvet-Leaf Pareira, Pareira Brava	Ayurvedic
Cissampelos pareira	Paathaa	Velvet-Leaf Pareira, Pareira Brava	Unani
Cissampelos pareira	Paadak kizhangu	Velvet-Leaf Pareira, Pareira Brava	Siddha/Tamil
Cissampelos pareira	Appattakodi	Velvet-Leaf Pareira, Pareira Brava	Siddha/Tamil
Cissus quadrangula	Asthisamhaari	Square Stalked Vine, Adamant Creeper	Ayurvedic
Cissus quadrangula	Asthisamhrita	Square Stalked Vine, Adamant Creeper	Ayurvedic
Cissus quadrangula	Asthi-samyojaka	Square Stalked Vine, Adamant Creeper	Ayurvedic
Cissus quadrangula	Chaturdhaaraa	Square Stalked Vine, Adamant Creeper	Ayurvedic
Cissus quadrangula	Hadjod	Square Stalked Vine, Adamant Creeper	Unani
Cissus quadrangula	Asthi-shrankhala	Square Stalked Vine, Adamant Creeper	Ayurvedic
Cissus quadrangula	Perandai	Square Stalked Vine, Adamant Creeper	Siddha/Tamil
Citrullus colocynthis	Indravaaruni	Colocynth Bitter Apple	Ayurvedic
Citrullus colocynthis	Indravalli	Colocynth Bitter Apple	Ayurvedic
Citrullus colocynthis	Indravaarunikaa	Colocynth Bitter Apple	Ayurvedic
Citrullus colocynthis	Gavaakshi	Colocynth Bitter Apple	Ayurvedic
Citrullus colocynthis	Chitra	Colocynth Bitter Apple	Ayurvedic
Citrullus colocynthis	Chitraphalaa	Colocynth Bitter Apple	Ayurvedic
Citrullus colocynthis	Indraasuri	Colocynth Bitter Apple	Ayurvedic
Citrullus colocynthis	Mrigadaani	Colocynth Bitter Apple	Ayurvedic
Citrullus colocynthis	Mrigairvaaru	Colocynth Bitter Apple	Ayurvedic
Citrullus colocynthis	Vishaalaa	Colocynth Bitter Apple	Ayurvedic

Table Contd.

Botanical Name	Indian Name	English Name	Medicinal System
Citrullus colocynthis	Aindri	Colocynth Bitter Apple	Ayurvedic
Citrullus colocynthis	Indraayana	Colocynth Bitter Apple	Ayurvedic
Citrullus colocynthis	Hanzal	Colocynth Bitter Apple	Unani
Citrullus colocynthis	Verikkumatti	Colocynth Bitter Apple	Siddha/Tamil
Citrullus vulgaris	Kaalinda	Watermelon	Ayurvedic
Citrullus vulgaris	Tarbuz	Watermelon	Unani
Citrullus vulgaris	Poiychaviral	Watermelon	Siddha/Tamil
Citrullus vulgaris	Tharbuzapalam	Watermelon	Siddha/Tamil
Citrus aurantifolia	Nimbuka	Acid or Sour Lime, Country Lime	Ayurvedic
Citrus aurantifolia	Limu Kaghzi	Acid or Sour Lime, Country Lime	Unani
Citrus aurantifolia	Elummichhan	Acid or Sour Lime, Country Lime	Siddha/Tamil
Citrus aurantifolia	Thurinjippazham	Acid or Sour Lime, Country Lime	Siddha/Tamil
Citrus aurantifolia	Kaagazi Nimbu	Acid or Sour Lime, Country Lime	Folk
Citrus aurantium	Khattaa	Citrus Dulcis, Sour Orange, Sweet Orange	Folk
Citrus aurantium	Naaraththai	Citrus Dulcis, Sour Orange, Sweet Orange	Siddha/Tamil
Citrus limon	Jambira	Lemon	Ayurvedic
Citrus limon	Jambaka	Lemon	Ayurvedic
Citrus limon	Nimbuka	Lemon	Ayurvedic
Citrus limon	Jaamphal	Lemon	Ayurvedic
Citrus limon	Jambir Nimbu	Lemon	Ayurvedic
Citrus limon	Jamiri Nimbu	Lemon	Ayurvedic
Citrus limon	Galgal	Lemon	Folk
Citrus limon	Leemu-e-khaarki	Lemon	Unani
Citrus limon	Dantashatha	Lemon	Ayurvedic
Citrus limon	Airaavata	Lemon	Ayurvedic
Citrus limon	Leemu	Lemon	Unani
Citrus limon	Utraj	Lemon	Unani
Citrus limon	Periya Elumuchhai	Lemon	Siddha/Tamil
Citrus maxima	Madhukarkatikaa	Pummelo, Shaddock	Ayurvedic
Citrus maxima	Chakotra	Pummelo, Shaddock	Unani
Citrus maxima	Pambalimasu	Pummelo, Shaddock	Siddha/Tamil

Table Contd.

Botanical Name	Indian Name	English Name	Medicinal System
Citrus maxima	Mahaa-nibu	Pummelo, Shaddock	Folk
Citrus maxima	Sadaaphal	Pummelo, Shaddock	Folk
Citrus medica	Maatulunga	Citron	Ayurvedic
Citrus medica	Lunga	Citron	Ayurvedic
Citrus medica	Maatulaka	Citron	Ayurvedic
Citrus medica	Mahaalunga	Citron	Ayurvedic
Citrus medica	Bijpuura	Citron	Ayurvedic
Citrus medica	Bijaahva	Citron	Ayurvedic
Citrus medica	Turanj	Citron	Unani
Citrus medica	Kadaranarathai	Citron	Siddha/Tamil
Citrus medica	Naarthankai	Citron	Siddha/Tamil
Citrus medica	Thurinjippazham	Citron	Siddha/Tamil
Citrus medica	Bijoraa	Citron	Folk
Citrus paradisi	Chakotraa	Grapefruit, 'Marsh' Grapefruit	Folk
Citrus paradisi	Chima Bombilimaas	Grapefruit, 'Marsh' Grapefruit	Folk/Tamil
Clausena pentaphylla	Ratanjot	Clausena	Folk
Clausena pentaphylla	Rowana	Clausena	Folk
Claviceps purpurea	Annamaya	Ergot of Rye, Fungus of Rye	Ayurvedic
Claviceps purpurea	Sraavikaa	Ergot of Rye, Fungus of Rye	Ayurvedic
Claviceps purpurea	Dhaanya-ruk	Ergot of Rye, Fungus of Rye	Ayurvedic
Claviceps purpurea	Ergot	Ergot of Rye, Fungus of Rye	Siddha/Tamil
Clematis gouriana	Belkangu	Morvel, Virgin's Bower	Folk
Cleome brachycarpa	Panwaar	Bastard Mustard	Unani
Cleome icosandra	Aadityabhakta	Wild Mustard	Ayurvedic
Cleome icosandra	Tilaparni	Wild Mustard	Ayurvedic
Cleome icosandra	Hurhur	Wild Mustard	Ayurvedic
Cleome icosandra	Panwaar	Wild Mustard	Unani
Cleome icosandra	Halhul	Wild Mustard	Unani
Cleome icosandra	Nayikkadugu	Wild Mustard	Siddha/Tamil
Cleome icosandra	Nalvellai	Wild Mustard	Siddha/Tamil
Clerodendrum indicum	Vaamana-haati	Turk's Turban, Tube-Flower	Ayurvedic
Clerodendrum indicum	Kavalai	Turk's Turban, Tube-Flower	Siddha/Tamil

Table Contd.

Botanical Name	Indian Name	English Name	Medicinal System
Clerodendrum indicum	Narivalai	Turk's Turban, Tube-Flower	Siddha/Tamil
Clerodendrum inerme	Putigandhaa	Smooth Volkameria	Ayurvedic
Clerodendrum inerme	Kundali	Smooth Volkameria	Ayurvedic
Clerodendrum inerme	Vanajai	Smooth Volkameria	Ayurvedic
Clerodendrum inerme	Peenaari	Smooth Volkameria	Siddha/Tamil
Clerodendrum inerme	Sangan-kuppi	Smooth Volkameria	Siddha/Tamil
Clerodendrum inerme	Lanjai	Smooth Volkameria	Folk
Clerodendrum infortunatum	Bhaandira	Glory Bower	Ayurvedic
Clerodendrum infortunatum	Bhaandi	Glory Bower	Ayurvedic
Clerodendrum infortunatum	Kaari	Glory Bower	Ayurvedic
Clerodendrum infortunatum	Karukanni	Glory Bower	Siddha/Tamil
Clerodendrum infortunatum	Perugilai	Glory Bower	Siddha/Tamil
Clerodendrum phlomidis	Agnimantha	Glory Bower	Ayurvedic
Clerodendrum phlomidis	Ganikaarikaa	Glory Bower	Ayurvedic
Clerodendrum phlomidis	Tarkaari	Glory Bower	Ayurvedic
Clerodendrum phlomidis	Vikraantaa	Glory Bower	Ayurvedic
Clerodendrum phlomidis	Jayanti	Glory Bower	Ayurvedic
Clerodendrum phlomidis	Jai	Glory Bower	Ayurvedic
Clerodendrum phlomidis	Jayaa	Glory Bower	Ayurvedic
Clerodendrum phlomidis	Vaijayanti	Glory Bower	Ayurvedic
Clerodendrum phlomidis	Shriparni	Glory Bower	Ayurvedic
Clerodendrum phlomidis	Naadeyi	Glory Bower	Ayurvedic
Clerodendrum phlomidis	Thazhuthaazhai	Glory Bower	Siddha/Tamil
Clerodendrum phlomidis	Laghu Arni	Glory Bower	Folk
Clerodendrum serratum	Bhaargi	Blue-flowered Glory Tree, Beetle Killer	Ayurvedic
Clerodendrum serratum	Bhaarangi	Blue-flowered Glory Tree, Beetle Killer	Ayurvedic
Clerodendrum serratum	Angaarvalli	Blue-flowered Glory Tree, Beetle Killer	Ayurvedic
Clerodendrum serratum	Phanji	Blue-flowered Glory Tree, Beetle Killer	Ayurvedic
Clerodendrum serratum	Braahman-yashtikaa	Blue-flowered Glory Tree, Beetle Killer	Ayurvedic

Table Contd.

Botanical Name	Indian Name	English Name	Medicinal System
Clerodendrum serratum	Kharshaak	Blue-flowered Glory Tree, Beetle Killer	Ayurvedic
Clerodendrum serratum	Padma	Blue-flowered Glory Tree, Beetle Killer	Ayurvedic
Clerodendrum serratum	Bhragubhavaa	Blue-flowered Glory Tree, Beetle Killer	Ayurvedic
Clerodendrum serratum	Vaamanahaati	Blue-flowered Glory Tree, Beetle Killer	Ayurvedic
Clerodendrum serratum	Kandoorbarangi	Blue-flowered Glory Tree, Beetle Killer	Siddha/Tamil
Clerodendrum serratum	Cherutekku	Blue-flowered Glory Tree, Beetle Killer	Siddha/Tamil
Clitoria ternatea	Girikarnikaa	Butterfly Pea, Winged-leaved Clitoria, Mezereon	Ayurvedic
Clitoria ternatea	Aparaajitaa	Butterfly Pea, Winged-leaved Clitoria, Mezereon	Ayurvedic
Clitoria ternatea	Aasphota	Butterfly Pea, Winged-leaved Clitoria, Mezereon	Ayurvedic
Clitoria ternatea	Girimallikaa	Butterfly Pea, Winged-leaved Clitoria, Mezereon	Ayurvedic
Clitoria ternatea	Girikanyaa	Butterfly Pea, Winged-leaved Clitoria, Mezereon	Ayurvedic
Clitoria ternatea	Kokilaa	Butterfly Pea, Winged-leaved Clitoria, Mezereon	Ayurvedic
Clitoria ternatea	Yonipushpaa	Butterfly Pea, Winged-leaved Clitoria, Mezereon	Ayurvedic
Clitoria ternatea	Vishnukraantaa	Butterfly Pea, Winged-leaved Clitoria, Mezereon	Ayurvedic
Clitoria ternatea	Mezereon Hindi	Butterfly Pea, Winged-leaved Clitoria, Mezereon	Unani
Clitoria ternatea	Kaakkanam	Butterfly Pea, Winged-leaved Clitoria, Mezereon	Siddha/Tamil
Clitoria ternatea	Koyal	Butterfly Pea, Winged-leaved Clitoria, Mezereon	Folk
Coccinia indica	Bimbi	Ivy-Gourd	Ayurvedic
Coccinia indica	Tundi	Ivy-Gourd	Ayurvedic
Coccinia indica	Tundikaa	Ivy-Gourd	Ayurvedic
Coccinia indica	Tundikeri	Ivy-Gourd	Ayurvedic
Coccinia indica	Kunduru	Ivy-Gourd	Ayurvedic

Table Contd.

Botanical Name	Indian Name	English Name	Medicinal System
Coccinia indica	Raktaphala	Ivy-Gourd	Ayurvedic
Coccinia indica	Piluparni	Ivy-Gourd	Ayurvedic
Coccinia indica	Dantchhadaa	Ivy-Gourd	Ayurvedic
Coccinia indica	Kanduri	Ivy-Gourd	Unani
Coccinia indica	Kovvai	Ivy-Gourd	Siddha/Tamil
Cocculus hirsutus	Chhilihinta	Broom-Creeper, Ink-Berry	Ayurvedic
Cocculus hirsutus	Paataala-garuda	Broom-Creeper, Ink-Berry	Ayurvedic
Cocculus hirsutus	Mahaamuulaa	Broom-Creeper, Ink-Berry	Ayurvedic
Cocculus hirsutus	Dirghavalli	Broom-Creeper, Ink-Berry	Ayurvedic
Cocculus hirsutus	Jalajamani	Broom-Creeper, Ink-Berry	Ayurvedic
Cocculus hirsutus	Kattukodi	Broom-Creeper, Ink-Berry	Siddha/Tamil
Cochlearia armoracia	Horseradish	Red Cole	Folk
Cochlospermum gossypium	Peelikapaasi	Golden Silk Tree, White Silk Cotton Tree	Folk
Cochlospermum gossypium	Kumbi	Golden Silk Tree, White Silk Cotton Tree	Folk
Cochlospermum gossypium	Kongilavu	Golden Silk Tree, White Silk Cotton Tree	Siddha/Tamil
Cocos nucifera	Naarikela	Coconut Palm	Ayurvedic
Cocos nucifera	Naalikera	Coconut Palm	Ayurvedic
Cocos nucifera	Laangali	Coconut Palm	Ayurvedic
Cocos nucifera	Tunga	Coconut Palm	Ayurvedic
Cocos nucifera	Skandhaphala	Coconut Palm	Ayurvedic
Cocos nucifera	Sadaaphala	Coconut Palm	Ayurvedic
Cocos nucifera	Trnaraaja	Coconut Palm	Ayurvedic
Cocos nucifera	Kuurchshirshaka	Coconut Palm	Ayurvedic
Cocos nucifera	Naarjeel	Coconut Palm	Unani
Cocos nucifera	Naariyal	Coconut Palm	Unani
Cocos nucifera	Tenkai	Coconut Palm	Siddha/Tamil
Cocos nucifera	Kopparai	Coconut Palm	Siddha/Tamil
Coffea arabica	Kahvaa	Arabian Coffee	Unani
Coffea arabica	Kaapi	Arabian Coffee	Siddha/Tamil
Coffea arabica	Bannu	Arabian Coffee	Siddha/Tamil
Coix lacryma-jobi	Gavedhukaa	Job's Tears	Ayurvedic

Table Contd.

Botanical Name	Indian Name	English Name	Medicinal System
Coix lacryma-jobi	Kaatu Kunthumani	Job's Tears	Siddha/Tamil
Coix lacryma-jobi	Garaheduaa	Job's Tears	Folk
Coix lacryma-jobi	Gargari	Job's Tears	Folk
Colchicum luteum	Hiranyatuttha	Hermodactyls, Colchicum, Meadow Saffron, Golden Collyrium	Ayurvedic
Colchicum luteum	Surajaan Talkh	Hermodactyls, Colchicum, Meadow Saffron, Golden Collyrium	Unani
Coleus amboinicus	Parna-yavaani	Indian Borage	Ayurvedic
Coleus amboinicus	Karpoorvalli	Indian Borage	Siddha/Tamil
Coleus amboinicus	Pattaa Ajawaayin	Indian Borage	Folk
Coleus amboinicus	Pattharachuur	Indian Borage	Folk
Coleus barbatus	Gandira	Coleus	Ayurvedic
Coleus barbatus	Garmar	Coleus	Folk
Coleus barbatus	Gurmal	Coleus	Folk
Coleus vettiveroides	Hrivera	Coleus	Ayurvedic
Coleus vettiveroides	Hiruberaka	Coleus	Ayurvedic
Coleus vettiveroides	Ambu	Coleus	Ayurvedic
Coleus vettiveroides	Ambhas	Coleus	Ayurvedic
Coleus vettiveroides	Udaka	Coleus	Ayurvedic
Coleus vettiveroides	Udichya	Coleus	Ayurvedic
Coleus vettiveroides	Jala	Coleus	Ayurvedic
Coleus vettiveroides	Vaari	Coleus	Ayurvedic
Coleus vettiveroides	Toya	Coleus	Ayurvedic
Coleus vettiveroides	Vaalaka	Coleus	Ayurvedic
Coleus vettiveroides	Baalaa	Coleus	Ayurvedic
Coleus vettiveroides	Baalaka	Coleus	Ayurvedic
Coleus vettiveroides	Baala	Coleus	Ayurvedic
Coleus vettiveroides	Kuruver	Coleus	Siddha/Tamil
Coleus vettiveroides	Iruveli	Coleus	Folk
Colocasia esculenta	Pindaaluka	Taro, Edible Yam	Ayurvedic
Colocasia esculenta	Aaluki	Taro, Edible Yam	Ayurvedic

Table Contd.

Botanical Name	Indian Name	English Name	Medicinal System
Colocasia esculenta	Chaembu	Taro, Edible Yam	Siddha/Tamil
Colocasia esculenta	Shaeppam-kizhangu	Taro, Edible Yam	Siddha/Tamil
Colocasia esculenta	Arvi	Taro, Edible Yam	Folk
Colocasia esculenta	Ghuiyaa	Taro, Edible Yam	Folk
Commelina benghalensis	Kanchata	Tropical Spiderwort	Ayurvedic
Commelina benghalensis	Karnamorata	Tropical Spiderwort	Ayurvedic
Commelina benghalensis	Karnasphota	Tropical Spiderwort	Ayurvedic
Commelina benghalensis	Kanavazhai	Tropical Spiderwort	Siddha/Tamil
Commelina benghalensis	Kananagakarai	Tropical Spiderwort	Siddha/Tamil
Commelina benghalensis	Kenaa	Tropical Spiderwort	Folk
Commelina nudiflora	Kanchata	Day Flower, Kenna vegetable	Ayurvedic
Commelina nudiflora	Kenaa	Day Flower, Kenna vegetable	Folk
Commiphora spp.	Guggul/Bol	*C. mukul/C. myrrha*	Ayurvedic/Unani
Conium maculatum	Shaukaraan	Spotted Hemlock, Poison Hemlock	Unani
Conium maculatum	Kuniyun	Spotted Hemlock, Poison Hemlock	Unani
Convolvulus arvensis	Bhadrabalaa	Deer's Foot, Devil's Garters	Ayurvedic
Convolvulus arvensis	Hiranpadi	Deer's Foot, Devil's Garters	Ayurvedic
Convolvulus arvensis	Lablaab	Deer's Foot, Devil's Garters	Ayurvedic
Convolvulus arvensis	Hirankhuri	Deer's Foot, Devil's Garters	Ayurvedic
Convolvulus arvensis	Haranpagaa	Deer's Foot, Devil's Garters	Ayurvedic
Convolvulus pluricaulis	Shankhapushpi	Conch-flowered Bindweed	Ayurvedic
Convolvulus pluricaulis	Shankhaahvaa	Conch-flowered Bindweed	Ayurvedic
Convolvulus pluricaulis	Kshirapushpi	Conch-flowered Bindweed, White-flowered Shankhpushpi	Ayurvedic
Convolvulus pluricaulis	Maangalya Kusuma	Conch-flowered Bindweed, White-flowered Shankhpushpi	Ayurvedic
Convolvulus pluricaulis	Vishnukraanti	Conch-flowered Bindweed, White-flowered Shankhpushpi	Ayurvedic
Convolvulus pluricaulis	Vishnukraantaa	Conch-flowered Bindweed, White-flowered Shankhpushpi	Ayurvedic
Convolvulus pluricaulis	Sankhaahuli	Conch-flowered Bindweed, White-flowered Shankhpushpi	Unani

Table Contd.

Botanical Name	Indian Name	English Name	Medicinal System
Convolvulus pluricaulis	Sivakraandi	Conch-flowered Bindweed, White-flowered Shankhpushpi	Siddha/Tamil
Convolvulus pluricaulis	Vishnukraandi	Conch-flowered Bindweed, White-flowered Shankhpushpi	Siddha/Tamil
Convolvulus scammonia	Saqmunia	Scammony	Unani
Coptis teeta	Mamira	Gold Thread	Ayurvedic
Coptis teeta	Maamiraa	Gold Thread	Ayurvedic
Coptis teeta	Tiktamuulaa	Gold Thread	Ayurvedic
Coptis teeta	Maamisaa	Gold Thread	Ayurvedic
Coptis teeta	Titaa	Gold Thread	Folk
Corallocarpus epigaeus	Shukanaasaa	Indian Bryonia	Ayurvedic
Corallocarpus epigaeus	Nahikaa	Indian Bryonia	Ayurvedic
Corallocarpus epigaeus	Katunaahi	Indian Bryonia	Ayurvedic
Corallocarpus epigaeus	Paataala-garudaa	Indian Bryonia	Ayurvedic
Corallocarpus epigaeus	Kollankovai	Indian Bryonia	Siddha/Tamil
Corallocarpus epigaeus	Aaakaasa-garudan	Indian Bryonia	Siddha/Tamil
Corchorus aestuans	Chunchu	White Jute	Ayurvedic
Corchorus aestuans	Chanchu	White Jute	Ayurvedic
Corchorus aestuans	Chinchaa	White Jute	Ayurvedic
Corchorus aestuans	Chench Shaaka	White Jute	Folk
Corchorus aestuans	Titapat	White Jute	Folk
Corchorus capsularis	Kaala Shaaka	White Jute	Ayurvedic
Corchorus capsularis	Pirattai-keerai	White Jute	Folk/Tamil
Corchorus capsularis	Naadi Shaaka	White Jute	Folk
Corchorus capsularis	Narichaa	White Jute	Folk
Corchorus capsularis	Titapat	White Jute	Folk
Corchorus fascicularis	Chanchuka	Chanchee Vegetable	Ayurvedic
Corchorus fascicularis	Chanchu	Chanchee Vegetable	Ayurvedic
Corchorus fascicularis	Chanchu Shaaka	Chanchee Vegetable	Folk
Corchorus fascicularis	Baaphali	Chanchee Vegetable	Folk
Cordia myxa	Shleshmaataka	Sabestan Plum	Ayurvedic

Table Contd.

Botanical Name	Indian Name	English Name	Medicinal System
Curcuma amada	Karpuraa	Mango-ginger, Wild Turmeric	Ayurvedic
Curcuma amada	Aambaa Haldi	Mango-ginger, Wild Turmeric	Unani
Curcuma amada	Daarchob	Mango-ginger, Wild Turmeric	Unani
Curcuma amada	Mangaiinji	Mango-ginger, Wild Turmeric	Folk/Tamil
Curcuma angustifolia	Tvakshira	East Indian Arrowroot, Travancore Starch	Ayurvedic
Curcuma angustifolia	Tvakshiri	East Indian Arrowroot, Travancore Starch	Ayurvedic
Curcuma angustifolia	Tikhur	East Indian Arrowroot, Travancore Starch	Unani
Curcuma angustifolia	Tabaasheer	East Indian Arrowroot, Travancore Starch	Unani
Curcuma angustifolia	Ararutgaddalu	East Indian Arrowroot, Travancore Starch	Folk/Tamil
Curcuma aromatica	Karpuraa	Wild Turmeric, Yellow Zedoary	Ayurvedic
Curcuma aromatica	Aranya-rajanikanda	Wild Turmeric, Yellow Zedoary	Ayurvedic
Curcuma aromatica	Van Haridraa	Wild Turmeric, Yellow Zedoary	Ayurvedic
Curcuma aromatica	Daarchob	Wild Turmeric, Yellow Zedoary	Unani
Curcuma aromatica	Kastoori Manjal	Wild Turmeric, Yellow Zedoary	Siddha/Tamil
Curcuma caesia	Rajani	Black Zedorary	Ayurvedic
Curcuma caesia	Nishaa	Black Zedorary	Ayurvedic
Curcuma caesia	Nishi	Black Zedorary	Ayurvedic
Curcuma caesia	Raatri	Black Zedorary	Ayurvedic
Curcuma caesia	Kaali Haldi	Black Zedorary	Ayurvedic
Curcuma caesia	Nilkanth	Black Zedorary	Ayurvedic
Curcuma caesia	Narkachura	Black Zedorary	Ayurvedic
Curcuma caesia	Zarambaad	Black Zedorary	Unani
Curcuma caesia	Manupasapu	Black Zedorary	Folk/Telugu
Curcuma longa	Haridraa	Turmeric	Ayurvedic
Curcuma longa	Priyaka	Turmeric	Ayurvedic
Curcuma longa	Haridruma	Turmeric	Ayurvedic
Curcuma longa	Kshanda	Turmeric	Ayurvedic
Curcuma longa	Gauri	Turmeric	Ayurvedic

Table Contd.

Botanical Name	Indian Name	English Name	Medicinal System
Curcuma longa	Kaanchani	Turmeric	Ayurvedic
Curcuma longa	Krimighna	Turmeric	Ayurvedic
Curcuma longa	Varavarnini	Turmeric	Ayurvedic
Curcuma longa	Yoshitapriyaa	Turmeric	Ayurvedic
Curcuma longa	Hattavilaasini	Turmeric	Ayurvedic
Curcuma longa	Naktaahvaa	Turmeric	Ayurvedic
Curcuma longa	Sharvari	Turmeric	Ayurvedic
Curcuma longa	Zard Chob	Turmeric	Unani
Curcuma longa	Manjal	Turmeric	Siddha/Tamil
Curcuma zedoaria	Karchuura	Zedoary, Zerumbet	Ayurvedic
Curcuma zedoaria	Draavida	Zedoary, Zerumbet	Ayurvedic
Curcuma zedoaria	Palaashi	Zedoary, Zerumbet	Ayurvedic
Curcuma zedoaria	Narakachura	Zedoary, Zerumbet	Ayurvedic
Curcuma zedoaria	Gandhmuulaka	Zedoary, Zerumbet	Ayurvedic
Curcuma zedoaria	Shati	Zedoary, Zerumbet	Ayurvedic
Curcuma zedoaria	Zarambaad	Zedoary, Zerumbet	Unani
Curcuma zedoaria	Kichhilik-kizhangu	Zedoary, Zerumbet	Siddha/Tamil
Cuscuta epithymum	Aakaashvalli	Lesser Doddar, Hellweed, Devil's Guts	Ayurvedic
Cuscuta epithymum	Amarvalli	Lesser Doddar, Hellweed, Devil's Guts	Ayurvedic
Cuscuta epithymum	Amarvela	Lesser Doddar, Hellweed, Devil's Guts	Ayurvedic
Cuscuta epithymum	Aftimoon	Lesser Doddar, Hellweed, Devil's Guts	Unani
Cuscuta epithymum	Sitammapogu-nalu	Lesser Doddar, Hellweed, Devil's Guts	Folk/Telugu
Cuscuta reflexa	Amarvalli	Doddar	Ayurvedic
Cuscuta reflexa	Kasoos	Doddar	Unani
Cyamopsis tetragonoloba	Kshudra Shimbi	Cluster Bean, Guar	Ayurvedic
Cyamopsis tetragonoloba	Goraksha-phalini	Cluster Bean, Guar	Ayurvedic
Cyamopsis tetragonoloba	Guaar	Cluster Bean, Guar	Ayurvedic
Cyamopsis tetragonoloba	Gwaalin	Cluster Bean, Guar	Ayurvedic

Table Contd.

Botanical Name	Indian Name	English Name	Medicinal System
Cyamopsis tetragonoloba	Guaar phali	Cluster Bean, Guar	Unani
Cyamopsis tetragonoloba	Kothaveray	Cluster Bean, Guar	Folk/Tamil
Cyclea arnotii	Raaj-Paathaa	Green Jelly Shrub	Folk
Cyclea arnotii	Paathaa (Kerala)	Green Jelly Shrub	Folk
Cydonia oblonga	Amritaphala	Quince Fruit	Ayurvedic
Cydonia oblonga	Paatalaa	Quince Fruit	Ayurvedic
Cydonia oblonga	Simbitikaa	Quince Fruit	Ayurvedic
Cydonia oblonga	Bihi	Quince Fruit	Unani
Cydonia oblonga	Bihidaanaa	Quince Fruit	Unani
Cydonia oblonga	Shimaimathala	Quince Fruit	Siddha/Tamil
Cymbopogon citratus	Bhuutika	Lemongrass	Ayurvedic
Cymbopogon citratus	Bhuutikaa	Lemongrass	Ayurvedic
Cymbopogon jwarancusa	Karna-kusha	Vetiver-scented Grass	Folk/Bengal
Cymbopogon jwarancusa	Laamajjaka	Vetiver-scented Grass	Ayurvedic
Cymbopogon jwarancusa	Laamaajja	Vetiver-scented Grass	Ayurvedic
Cymbopogon jwarancusa	Izkhar	Vetiver-scented Grass	Unani
Cymbopogon jwarancusa	Vilaamichchan	Vetiver-scented Grass	Siddha/Tamil
Cymbopogon martinii	Rohisha-trn	Rosha Grass, Palmarosa	Ayurvedic
Cymbopogon martinii	Dhyaamaka	Rosha Grass, Palmarosa	Ayurvedic
Cymbopogon martinii	Kavathampillu	Rosha Grass, Palmarosa	Folk/Tamil
Cymbopogon nardus	Jambir-trn	Ceylon Citronella Grass	Ayurvedic
Cymbopogon nardus	Kamachipillu	Ceylon Citronella Grass	Folk/Tamil
Cymbopogon schoenanthus	Rohisha	Camel-Hay	Ayurvedic
Cymbopogon schoenanthus	Rusaa Ghaas	Camel-Hay	Unani
Cymbopogon schoenanthus	Izkhar	Camel-Hay	Unani
Cynara scolymus	Harshaf	Globe Artichoke	Unani
Cynodon dactylon	Duurvaa	Bermuda Grass, Bahama Grass, Couch Grass	Ayurvedic
Cynodon dactylon	Bhaargavi	Bermuda Grass, Bahama Grass, Couch Grass	Ayurvedic
Cynodon dactylon	Shatvalli	Bermuda Grass, Bahama Grass, Couch Grass	Ayurvedic
Cynodon dactylon	Shatparvaa	Bermuda Grass, Bahama Grass, Couch Grass	Ayurvedic

Table Contd.

Botanical Name	Indian Name	English Name	Medicinal System
Cynodon dactylon	Tiktaparvaa	Bermuda Grass, Bahama Grass, Couch Grass	Ayurvedic
Cynodon dactylon	Shatviryaa	Bermuda Grass, Bahama Grass, Couch Grass	Ayurvedic
Cynodon dactylon	Sahastravirya	Bermuda Grass, Bahama Grass, Couch Grass	Ayurvedic
Cynodon dactylon	Shitaa	Bermuda Grass, Bahama Grass, Couch Grass	Ayurvedic
Cynodon dactylon	Anantaa	Bermuda Grass, Bahama Grass, Couch Grass	Ayurvedic
Cynodon dactylon	Golomi	Bermuda Grass, Bahama Grass, Couch Grass	Ayurvedic
Cynodon dactylon	Duub	Bermuda Grass, Bahama Grass, Couch Grass	Unani
Cynodon dactylon	Arugampullu	Bermuda Grass, Bahama Grass, Couch Grass	Siddha/Tamil
Cyperus articulatus	Kronchaadana	Guinea Rush, Ardue	Ayurvedic
Cyperus esculentus	Chichoda	Earth Almond, Chufa, Rush Nut, Tiger Nut	Ayurvedic
Cyperus esculentus	Chichodaa	Earth Almond, Chufa, Rush Nut, Tiger Nut	Folk
Cyperus esculentus	Kaseru (Punjab)	Earth Almond, Chufa, Rush Nut, Tiger Nut	Folk
Cyperus rotundus	Musta	Nut Grass	Ayurvedic
Cyperus rotundus	Mustaa	Nut Grass	Ayurvedic
Cyperus rotundus	Mustaka	Nut Grass	Ayurvedic
Cyperus rotundus	Abda	Nut Grass	Ayurvedic
Cyperus rotundus	Ambuda	Nut Grass	Ayurvedic
Cyperus rotundus	Ambhoda	Nut Grass	Ayurvedic
Cyperus rotundus	Ambodhara	Nut Grass	Ayurvedic
Cyperus rotundus	Bhadra	Nut Grass	Ayurvedic
Cyperus rotundus	Bhadraa	Nut Grass	Ayurvedic
Cyperus rotundus	Bhadramusta	Nut Grass	Ayurvedic
Cyperus rotundus	Bhadramustaa	Nut Grass	Ayurvedic
Cyperus rotundus	Bhadramustaka	Nut Grass	Ayurvedic
Cyperus rotundus	Ghana	Nut Grass	Ayurvedic
Cyperus rotundus	Jalada	Nut Grass	Ayurvedic

Table Contd.

Botanical Name	Indian Name	English Name	Medicinal System
Cyperus rotundus	Jaldhara	Nut Grass	Ayurvedic
Cyperus rotundus	Meghaahvaa	Nut Grass	Ayurvedic
Cyperus rotundus	Neerada	Nut Grass	Ayurvedic
Cyperus rotundus	Vaarida	Nut Grass	Ayurvedic
Cyperus rotundus	Vaaridhara	Nut Grass	Ayurvedic
Cyperus rotundus	Payoda	Nut Grass	Ayurvedic
Cyperus rotundus	Vishadhvansi	Nut Grass	Ayurvedic
Cyperus rotundus	Ganda-Duurvaa	Nut Grass	Ayurvedic
Cyperus rotundus	Naagarmothaa	Nut Grass	Unani
Cyperus rotundus	Saad-e-Kufi	Nut Grass	Unani
Cyperus rotundus	Koraikki-zhangu	Nut Grass	Siddha/Tamil
Cyperus rotundus	Tungamustalu	Nut Grass	Folk/Telugu
Cyperus scariosus	Tungae hullar gedde	Nut Grass	Folk/Kannada
Cyperus scariosus	Korakizhangu	Nut Grass	Folk/Malayalam
Cyperus scariosus	Muttanna	Nut Grass	Folk/South
Cyperus scariosus	Naagara-mustaka	Nut Grass	Siddha/Tamil
Cyperus scariosus	Koraikkilangu	Nut Grass	Siddha/Tamil
Cyperus scariosus	Naagara-mothaa	Nut Grass	Unani
Cytisus scoparius	Broom	Broom, Scotch Broom, Yellow Broom	Folk/South
Dactyloctenium aegyptium	Timidaa	Spider Grass	Folk
Dactyloctenium aegyptium	Makaraa	Spider Grass	Folk
Dactyloctenium aegyptium	Makari	Spider Grass	Folk
Dactyloctenium aegyptium	Nrityakaundaka	Spider Grass	Ayurvedic
Dactyloctenium aegyptium	Panchaanguli	Spider Grass	Ayurvedic
Dactyloctenium aegyptium	Takraa	Spider Grass	Ayurvedic
Dactyloctenium aegyptium	Takraahvaa	Spider Grass	Ayurvedic
Daemonorops draco	Damm-ul-Akhwain	East Indian Dragon's Blood	Unani
Daemonorops draco	Heeraadokhi	East Indian Dragon's Blood	Ayurvedic

Table Contd.

Botanical Name	Indian Name	English Name	Medicinal System
Daemonorops draco	Khoon-kharaabaa	East Indian Dragon's Blood	Ayurvedic
Daemonorops draco	Raktaniryaas	East Indian Dragon's Blood	Ayurvedic
Daemonorops jenkinsianus	Vetra	Calamus	Ayurvedic
Dalbergia lanceolaria	Takoli	Takoliwood	Folk
Dalbergia lanceolaria	Bithuaa	Takoliwood	Folk
Dalbergia lanceolaria	Erigai	Takoliwood	Folk/Tamil
Dalbergia lanceolaria	Gorakh	Takoliwood	Folk
Dalbergia lanceolaria	Navelangu	Takoliwood	Folk/Tamil
Dalbergia latifolia	Simsipaa	East Indian Rosewood, Bombay Blackwood	Ayurvedic
Dalbergia latifolia	Kapilaa	East Indian Rosewood, Bombay Blackwood	Ayurvedic
Dalbergia latifolia	Saraa	East Indian Rosewood, Bombay Blackwood	Ayurvedic
Dalbergia latifolia	Karundoroiral	East Indian Rosewood, Bombay Blackwood	Siddha/Tamil
Dalbergia latifolia	Shisam	East Indian Rosewood, Bombay Blackwood	Unani
Dalbergia latifolia	Mandalpatrikaa	East Indian Rosewood, Bombay Blackwood	Ayurvedic
Dalbergia latifolia	Goraksha	East Indian Rosewood, Bombay Blackwood	Ayurvedic
Dalbergia sissoides	Shisam	Malabar Blackwood	Folk
Dalbergia sissoides	Kushimshapaa	Malabar Blackwood	Ayurvedic
Dalbergia sissoides	Vel-itti	Malabar Blackwood	Siddha/Tamil
Dalbergia sissoides	Sisau	Malabar Blackwood	Folk
Dalbergia sissoo	Iupoolai	Sissoo, South Indian Redwood	Siddha/Tamil
Dalbergia sissoo	Krishnashim-shapaa	Sissoo, South Indian Redwood	Ayurvedic
Dalbergia sissoo	Picchilaa	Sissoo, South Indian Redwood	Ayurvedic
Dalbergia sissoo	Shimshapaa	Sissoo, South Indian Redwood	Ayurvedic
Dalbergia sissoo	Shisam	Sissoo, South Indian Redwood	Unani
Dalbergia sympathetica	Pentagul	Pentagul Tree	Folk
Dalbergia sympathetica	Tibali	Pentagul Tree	Folk
Dalbergia volubilis	Bankharaa	Cinnamom-scented Bark Tree	Folk

Table Contd.

Botanical Name	Indian Name	English Name	Medicinal System
Dalbergia volubilis	Bhatiaa	Cinnamom-scented Bark Tree	Folk
Dalbergia volubilis	Gorakhi	Cinnamom-scented Bark Tree	Ayurvedic
Dalbergia volubilis	Punali	Cinnamom-scented Bark Tree	Siddha/Tamil
Daphne oleoides	Kanthan	Mezereon	Folk
Daphne oleoides	Kutilal	Mezereon	Folk
Datisca cannabina	Akal-ber	False Hemp	Folk
Datisca cannabina	Bhang-jala	False Hemp	Folk
Datura alba	Dhattuura	Thornapple	Ayurvedic
Datura alba	Dhaturaa	Thornapple	Unani
Datura innoxia	Dhattuura	Angel's Trumpet, Sacred Datura	Ayurvedic
Datura innoxia	Dhaturaa	Angel's Trumpet, Sacred Datura	Unani
Datura innoxia	Joz Maasil	Angel's Trumpet, Sacred Datura	Unani
Datura metel	Dhastura	Thornapple, Downy Datura	Ayurvedic
Datura metel	Dhattuura	Thornapple, Downy Datura	Ayurvedic
Datura metel	Dhaturaa	Thornapple, Downy Datura	Unani
Datura metel	Dhustuura	Thornapple, Downy Datura	Ayurvedic
Datura metel	Dhustuuraka	Thornapple, Downy Datura	Ayurvedic
Datura metel	Dhuurta	Thornapple, Downy Datura	Ayurvedic
Datura metel	Haatta	Thornapple, Downy Datura	Ayurvedic
Datura metel	Harapriya	Thornapple, Downy Datura	Ayurvedic
Datura metel	Hema	Thornapple, Downy Datura	Ayurvedic
Datura metel	Kanaka	Thornapple, Downy Datura	Ayurvedic
Datura metel	Karuvoomatthai	Thornapple, Downy Datura	Siddha/Tamil
Datura metel	Maatula.	Thornapple, Downy Datura	Ayurvedic
Datura metel	Oomaththai	Thornapple, Downy Datura	Siddha/Tamil
Datura metel	Shivapriya	Thornapple, Downy Datura	Ayurvedic
Datura metel	Unmatta	Thornapple, Downy Datura	Ayurvedic
Datura stramonium	Dhaturaa	Thornapple, Jimsonweed, Stramonium	Unani
Datura stramonium	Dhuurta	Thornapple, Jimsonweed, Stramonium	Ayurvedic
Datura stramonium	Unmatta	Thornapple, Jimsonweed, Stramonium	Ayurvedic

Table Contd.

Botanical Name	Indian Name	English Name	Medicinal System
Datura stramonium	Kitav	Thornapple, Jimsonweed, Stramonium	Ayurvedic
Datura stramonium	Krishna-dhattuura	Thornapple, Jimsonweed, Stramonium	Ayurvedic
Datura stramonium	Maatul	Thornapple, Jimsonweed, Stramonium	Ayurvedic
Datura stramonium	Madan	Thornapple, Jimsonweed, Stramonium	Ayurvedic
Datura stramonium	Tuuri	Thornapple, Jimsonweed, Stramonium	Ayurvedic
Daucus carota	Gaajara	Carrot, Cultivated Carrot, Wild Carrot	Ayurvedic
Daucus carota	Garjara	Carrot, Cultivated Carrot, Wild Carrot	Ayurvedic
Daucus carota	Granjana	Carrot, Cultivated Carrot, Wild Carrot	Ayurvedic
Daucus carota	Gaajar	Carrot, Cultivated Carrot, Wild Carrot	Unani
Decalepis hamiltonii	Desi Ushbaa	Sweet Sarsaparilla	Unani
Decalepis hamiltonii	Mahali kizhangu	Sweet Sarsaparilla	Siddha/Tamil
Delima scandens	Paaniya Valli	Delima	Ayurvedic
Delonix regia	Gulmohar	Flamboyant Flame Tree, Gold Mohur	Ayurvedic
Delonix regia	Vatanarayanan	Flamboyant Flame Tree, Gold Mohur	Folk/Telugu
Delonix regia	Perungondrai	Flamboyant Flame Tree, Gold Mohur	Siddha/Tamil
Delonix regia	Krishna Chudaa	Flamboyant Flame Tree, Gold Mohur	Siddha/Tamil
Delonix regia	White Gulmohar	Flamboyant Flame Tree, Gold Mohur	Folk
Delphinium brunonianum	Sprikkaa	Musk Larkspur	Ayurvedic
Delphinium brunonianum	Prukkaa	Musk Larkspur	Ayurvedic
Delphinium cashmirianum	Larkspur Tagara	Kashmir Larkspur	Ayurvedic
Delphinium consolida	Larkspur	Forking Larkspur, Larkspur, Lark's Claw, Knight's Spur	Folk
Delphinium denudatum	Nirvishi	Larkspur	Ayurvedic
Delphinium denudatum	Jadwaar Khataai	Larkspur	Unani

Table Contd.

Botanical Name	Indian Name	English Name	Medicinal System
Delphinium denudatum	Maatiryaaq	Larkspur	Unani
Delphinium staphisagria	Mulvizaj	Stavesacre	Unani
Delphinium vestitum	Nirvisha	Candle Larkspur, Bee Larkspur	Ayurvedic
Delphinium zalil	Sprikkaa	Zalil Larkspur	Ayurvedic
Delphinium zalil	Asbarga	Zalil Larkspur	Ayurvedic
Delphinium zalil	Zarir	Zalil Larkspur	Unani
Delphinium zalil	Zalil	Zalil Larkspur	Unani
Delphinium zalil	Asbarg	Zalil Larkspur	Unani
Delphinium zalil	Gul-Zalil (flower)	Zalil Larkspur	Unani
Dendrobium ovatum	Jivanti	Pigeon Orchid, Cooktown Orchid	Ayurvedic
Dendrobium ovatum	Nagli	Pigeon Orchid, Cooktown Orchid	Folk
Dendrophthoe falcata	Bandaaka	Mango and Citrus Parasite	Ayurvedic
Dendrophthoe falcata	Vrkshaadani	Mango and Citrus Parasite	Ayurvedic
Dendrophthoe falcata	Vrkshruuhaa	Mango and Citrus Parasite	Ayurvedic
Dendrophthoe falcata	Pulluri	Mango and Citrus Parasite	Siddha/Tamil
Dendrophthoe falcata	Plavithil	Mango and Citrus Parasite	Siddha/Tamil
Dendrophthoe falcata	Baandaa	Mango and Citrus Parasite	Folk
Derris indica	Naktmaal	Indian Beech, Pongamia Oil Tree	Ayurvedic
Derris indica	Guchhpushpak	Indian Beech, Pongamia Oil Tree	Ayurvedic
Derris indica	Ghritpuur	Indian Beech, Pongamia Oil Tree	Ayurvedic
Derris indica	Udkirya	Indian Beech, Pongamia Oil Tree	Ayurvedic
Derris indica	Karanja	Indian Beech, Pongamia Oil Tree	Ayurvedic
Derris indica	Pungu	Indian Beech, Pongamia Oil Tree	Siddha/Tamil
Derris uliginosa	Paan-lataa	Tuba Root	Folk
Derris uliginosa	Kitani	Tuba Root	Folk
Descurainia sophia	Khaakasi	Flix Weed, Flax Weed	Unani
Descurainia sophia	Khuubkalaan	Flix Weed, Flax Weed	Unani
Descurainia sophia	Khubb	Flix Weed, Flax Weed	Unani
Desmodium gangeticum	Shaaliparni	Shaalparni, Beggarweed	Ayurvedic
Desmodium gangeticum	Shaalaparni	Shaalparni, Beggarweed	Ayurvedic
Desmodium gangeticum	Sthiraa	Shaalparni, Beggarweed	Ayurvedic
Desmodium gangeticum	Somyaa	Shaalparni, Beggarweed	Ayurvedic

Table Contd.

Botanical Name	Indian Name	English Name	Medicinal System
Desmodium gangeticum	Guhaa	Shaalparni, Beggarweed	Ayurvedic
Desmodium gangeticum	Triparni	Shaalparni, Beggarweed	Ayurvedic
Desmodium gangeticum	Vidaarigandha	Shaalparni, Beggarweed	Ayurvedic
Desmodium gangeticum	Anshumati	Shaalparni, Beggarweed	Ayurvedic
Desmodium gangeticum	Prshniparni	Shaalparni, Beggarweed (Uraria Picta: also used as Shaalparni)	Ayurvedic
Desmodium gangeticum	Pulladi	Shaalparni, Beggarweed	Siddha/Tamil
Desmodium gangeticum	Sirupulladi Moovilai (root)	Shaalparni, Beggarweed	Siddha/Tamil
Desmodium gangeticum	Sarivan	Shaalparni, Beggarweed	Folk
Desmodium triflorum	Tripaadi	Matty Trefoil	Ayurvedic
Desmodium triflorum	Hamsapaadi	Matty Trefoil	Ayurvedic
Desmodium triflorum	Seruppadi	Matty Trefoil	Siddha/Tamil
Desmodium triflorum	Jangali Methi	Matty Trefoil	Folk
Desmodium triflorum	Ran-methi	Matty Trefoil	Folk
Desmostachya bipinnata	Kusha	Sacrificial Grass	Ayurvedic
Desmostachya bipinnata	Kshurapatra	Sacrificial Grass	Ayurvedic
Desmostachya bipinnata	Suuchyagra	Sacrificial Grass	Ayurvedic
Desmostachya bipinnata	Yagyabhuu-shana	Sacrificial Grass	Ayurvedic
Desmostachya bipinnata	Tharubai	Sacrificial Grass	Siddha/Tamil
Dianthus caryophyllus	Carnation	Carnation, Clove Pink	Folk
Dicentra canadensis	Bhotia-baadaam	Squirrel Corn	Folk
Dichroa febrifuga	Basak	Dichroa Quinine	Folk
Dichrostachys cinerea	Virataru	Chinese Lantern, Kalihari Christmastree	Ayurvedic
Dichrostachys cinerea	Vellantaru	Chinese Lantern, Kalihari Christmastree	Ayurvedic
Dichrostachys cinerea	Viravrksha	Chinese Lantern, Kalihari Christmastree	Ayurvedic
Dichrostachys cinerea	Vidathalai	Chinese Lantern, Kalihari Christmastree	Siddha/Tamil
Dichrostachys cinerea	Varatuli	Chinese Lantern, Kalihari Christmastree	Folk

Table Contd.

Botanical Name	Indian Name	English Name	Medicinal System
Dioscorea esculenta	Suthani	Lesser Yam, Karen Potato	Folk
Dioscorea glabra	Shankhaaluka	Gluey Yam	Ayurvedic
Dioscorea hamiltonii	Vaaraahi (var.)	The Prized Yam	Ayurvedic
Dioscorea hamiltonii	Naagar-kanda	The Prized Yam	Folk
Dioscorea oppositifolia	Amlikaakanda (controversial)	Cylindrical Yam	Ayurvedic
Dioscorea oppositifolia	Aambaalio Kanda	Cylindrical Red Yam	Folk
Dioscorea oppositifolia	Kavala-kodi	Cylindrical Red Yam	Siddha/Tamil
Dioscorea oppositifolia	Venilai Valli	Cylindrical Red Yam	Siddha/Tamil
Dioscorea pentaphylla	Kaantaalu	Cylindrical Brown Yam	Folk
Dioscorea pentaphylla	Vaaraahikanda	Cylindrical Brown Yam	Ayurvedic
Dioscorea prazeri	Neelaalu	Poisonous Black Yam	Ayurvedic
Diospyros ebenum	Aaabnuus	Ebony Persimmon, Malabar Ebony, Ceylon Ebony	Unani
Diospyros ebenum	Acha-Thumbi	Ebony Persimmon, Malabar Ebony, Ceylon Ebony	Siddha/Tamil
Diospyros ebenum	Tinduka	Ebony Persimmon, Malabar Ebony, Ceylon Ebony	Ayurvedic
Diospyros embryopteris	Asitkaaraka	Gaub Persimmon, Riber Ebony	Ayurvedic
Diospyros embryopteris	Kaalaskandha	Gaub Persimmon, Riber Ebony	Ayurvedic
Diospyros embryopteris	Nilasaara	Gaub Persimmon, Riber Ebony	Ayurvedic
Diospyros embryopteris	Sphuurjaka	Gaub Persimmon, Riber Ebony	Ayurvedic
Diospyros embryopteris	Tinduka	Gaub Persimmon, Riber Ebony	Ayurvedic
Diospyros embryopteris	Tinduki	Gaub Persimmon, Riber Ebony	Ayurvedic
Diospyros embryopteris	Tendu	Gaub Persimmon, Riber Ebony	Unani
Diospyros embryopteris	Tumbika	Gaub Persimmon, Riber Ebony	Siddha/Tamil
Diospyros embryopteris	Kattatti	Gaub Persimmon, Riber Ebony	Siddha/Tamil
Diospyros kaki	Tinduka (var.)	Japanese Persimmon	Ayurvedic
Diospyros melanoxylon	Dirghapatrakaa	Coromandel Ebony, Persimmon	Ayurvedic
Diospyros melanoxylon	Tinduka (var.)	Coromandel Ebony, Persimmon	Ayurvedic
Diospyros melanoxylon	Karum Dumbi	Coromandel Ebony, Persimmon	Siddha/Tamil
Diospyros melanoxylon	Thumbi	Coromandel Ebony, Persimmon	Siddha/Tamil
Diospyros melanoxylon	Beedi-elai	Coromandel Ebony, Persimmon	Siddha/Tamil
Diospyros montana	Kaaka-tinduka	Mountain Persimmon	Ayurvedic

Table Contd.

Botanical Name	Indian Name	English Name	Medicinal System
Diospyros montana	Visha-tinduka	Mountain Persimmon	Ayurvedic
Diospyros montana	Vakkanai	Mountain Persimmon	Siddha/Tamil
Diospyros montana	Vakkanatan	Mountain Persimmon	Siddha/Tamil
Diospyros montana	Timru	Mountain Persimmon	Folk
Diospyros tomentosa	Tinduka (var.)	Nepal Ebony Persimmon	Ayurvedic
Diospyros tomentosa	Viralaa	Nepal Ebony Persimmon	Ayurvedic
Diospyros tomentosa	Tumbi	Nepal Ebony Persimmon	Siddha/Tamil
Diospyros tomentosa	Ebony	Nepal Ebony Persimmon	Folk
Dipterocarpus alatus	Ashwakarna	Gurjun	Ayurvedic
Dipterocarpus alatus	Garjan	Gurjun	Ayurvedic
Dipterocarpus alatus	Jarandruma	Gurjun	Ayurvedic
Dipterocarpus alatus	Shveta-Garjan	Gurjun	Ayurvedic
Dipterocarpus turbinatus	Ajakarna	Common Gurjun Tree, Wood Oil Tree	Ayurvedic
Dipterocarpus turbinatus	Ashwakarna	Common Gurjun Tree, Wood Oil Tree	Ayurvedic
Dipterocarpus turbinatus	Chhaagakarna	Common Gurjun Tree, Wood Oil Tree	Ayurvedic
Dipterocarpus turbinatus	Ennei	Common Gurjun Tree, Wood Oil Tree	Siddha/Tamil
Dipterocarpus turbinatus	Kanyong	Common Gurjun Tree, Wood Oil Tree	Folk/ Meghalaya
Dipterocarpus turbinatus	Gurjan	Common Gurjun Tree, Wood Oil Tree	Folk/Gujarat
Dodonaea viscosa	Raasana (Andhra Pradesh)	Jamacia Switch Sorrel	Ayurvedic
Dodonaea viscosa	Aliar	Jamacia Switch Sorrel	Folk
Dodonaea viscosa	Velari	Jamacia Switch Sorrel	Siddha/Tamil
Dolichandrone falcate	Mesha-shringi	Corky-winged-seed Tree	Ayurvedic
Dolichandrone falcate	Vishaanikaa	Corky-winged-seed Tree	Ayurvedic
Dolichandrone falcate	Rishabhaka	Corky-winged-seed Tree	Folk/South
Dolichandrone falcate	Kaddalattai	Corky-winged-seed Tree	Siddha/Tamil
Dolichandrone falcate	Manchingi	Corky-winged-seed Tree	Folk
Dolichos biflorus	Khalva	Horsegram	Ayurvedic
Dolichos biflorus	Kulattha	Horsegram	Ayurvedic

Table Contd.

Botanical Name	Indian Name	English Name	Medicinal System
Dolichos biflorus	Kulittha	Horsegram	Ayurvedic
Dolichos biflorus	Vardhipatraka	Horsegram	Ayurvedic
Dolichos biflorus	Kulthi	Horsegram	Unani
Dolichos biflorus	Kollu	Horsegram	Siddha/Tamil
Dolichos biflorus	Kaanam	Horsegram	Siddha/Tamil
Dolichos falcatus	Kulatthikaa	Kapik	Ayurvedic
Dolichos lablab	Nishpaava	Indian Butter Bean, Lablab Bean, Horsebean	Ayurvedic
Dolichos lablab	Sem	Indian Butter Bean, Lablab Bean, Horsebean	Ayurvedic
Dolichos lablab	Lab Laab	Indian Butter Bean, Lablab Bean, Horsebean	Unani
Dolichos lablab	Semphali	Indian Butter Bean, Lablab Bean, Horsebean	Unani
Dolichos lablab	Avarin (Seed)	Indian Butter Bean, Lablab Bean, Horsebean	Siddha/Tamil
Dorema ammoniacum	Ushaka	Ammoniacum, Gum Ammoniac	Ayurvedic
Dorema ammoniacum	Uushaka	Ammoniacum, Gum Ammoniac	Ayurvedic
Dorema ammoniacum	Ushaq	Ammoniacum, Gum Ammoniac	Unani
Dorema ammoniacum	Ushah	Ammoniacum, Gum Ammoniac	Unani
Dorema ammoniacum	Kandal	Ammoniacum, Gum Ammoniac	Unani
Doronicum hookeri	Daarunaj Aqrabi	Leopard's Bane	Unani
Doronicum pardalianches	Daarunaj Aqrabi	Leopard's Bane	Unani
Doronicum roylei	Daarunaj Aqrabi Hindi	Leopard's Bane	Unani
Dracaena cinnabari	Heeraadokhi	Dragon's Blood	Ayurvedic
Dracaena cinnabari	Khoonkharaabaa	Dragon's Blood	Ayurvedic
Dracaena cinnabari	Dammul-Akhwain	Dragon's Blood	Unani
Dracocephalum moldavica	Raam Tulasi	Dragon's Head	Ayurvedic
Dracocephalum moldavica	Feranjmushk	Dragon's Head	Unani
Dracontium polyphyllum	Kattu Karun-ayikkilangu	Stunk Weed, Poleca Weed	Siddha/Tamil
Dracontium polyphyllum	Jangali Suuran	Stunk Weed, Poleca Weed	Folk
Dregea volubilis	Madhu-maalati	Wattakaka	Ayurvedic
Dregea volubilis	Muurvaa	Wattakaka	Ayurvedic

Table Contd.

Botanical Name	Indian Name	English Name	Medicinal System
Dregea volubilis	Nak-chhikkini	Wattakaka	Ayurvedic
Dregea volubilis	Hemajivanti	Wattakaka	Ayurvedic
Dregea volubilis	Kodippalai	Wattakaka	Siddha/Tamil
Drosera peltata	Brahma-suvarchalaa	Sundew	Ayurvedic
Drosera peltata	Mukhjali	Sundew	Folk
Drynaria quercifolia	Ashvakatri	Drynaria Fern	Ayurvedic
Drynaria quercifolia	Baandar-Baashing	Drynaria Fern	Folk
Dryobalanops camphora	Bhimseni Kapoor	Bornoe or Barus Camphor	Ayurvedic
Dryobalanops camphora	Baraas Kapoor	Bornoe or Barus Camphor	Folk
Dryopteris filix-mas	Sarakhs	Male Fern, Aspidium	Unani
Dryopteris filix-mas	Sarakhs Muzakkar	Male Fern, Aspidium	Unani
Dryopteris filix-mas	Iruvi	Male Fern, Aspidium	Siddha/Tamil
Drypetes roxburghii	Putrajivaka	Putrajiva	Ayurvedic
Drypetes roxburghii	Putrakamanjari	Putrajiva	Ayurvedic
Drypetes roxburghii	Sutajva	Putrajiva	Ayurvedic
Drypetes roxburghii	Karupali	Putrajiva	Siddha/Tamil
Drypetes roxburghii	Irukolli	Putrajiva	Siddha/Tamil
Duranta plumieri	Durantaa	Creeping Skin Flower, Pigeon Berry	Folk
Durio zibethinus	Durio	Durian, Civet Fruit	Folk
Dysoxylum binectariferum	Agunivagil	Termite-resistant Cedar	Siddha/Tamil
Dysoxylum binectariferum	Cembil	Termite-resistant Cedar	Siddha/Tamil
Dysoxylum binectariferum	Lassuni	Termite-resistant Cedar	Folk
Ecballium elaterium	Kantaki Indravaaruni	Squirting Cucumber	Ayurvedic
Ecballium elaterium	Kateri Indryaayana	Squirting Cucumber	Folk
Ecballium elaterium	Kitran	Squirting Cucumber	Folk
Ecbolium linneanum	Nilambari	Blue Fox Tail Nail Dye	Siddha/Tamil
Echinochloa colonum	Varaka	Shama Millet	Ayurvedic
Echinochloa colonum	Jangali sawuk	Shama Millet	Folk
Echinochloa colonum	Shamaa	Shama Millet	Folk

Table Contd.

Botanical Name	Indian Name	English Name	Medicinal System
Echinochloa colonum	Saanvaa	Shama Millet	Folk
Echinochloa colonum	Karumpul	Shama Millet	Siddha/Tamil
Echinochloa colonum	Varsanam-pillu	Shama Millet	Siddha/Tamil
Echinochloa crus-galli	Ambah Shyaamaaka	Barnyard Millet	Ayurvedic
Echinochloa crus-galli	Oathupul	Barnyard Millet	Siddha/Tamil
Echinochloa crus-galli	Samak	Barnyard Millet	Folk
Echinochloa frumentacea	Shyaamaaka	Japanese Barnyard Millet	Ayurvedic
Echinochloa frumentacea	Kudrraivali pillu	Japanese Barnyard Millet	Siddha/Tamil
Echinochloa frumentacea	Shamaa	Japanese Barnyard Millet	Folk
Echinochloa frumentacea	Saanvaa	Japanese Barnyard Millet	Folk
Echinops echinatus	Brahmadandi	Globe-Thistle, Camel's Thistle	Ayurvedic
Echinops echinatus	Utkantaka	Globe-Thistle, Camel's Thistle	Ayurvedic
Echinops echinatus	Uttundaka	Globe-Thistle, Camel's Thistle	Ayurvedic
Echinops echinatus	Uunta-Kateraa	Globe-Thistle, Camel's Thistle	Folk
Eclipta alba	Bhringaraaja	Trailing Eclipta Plant	Ayurvedic
Eclipta alba	Bhringaahva	Trailing Eclipta Plant	Ayurvedic
Eclipta alba	Bhringaja	Trailing Eclipta Plant	Ayurvedic
Eclipta alba	Bhrngaaraka	Trailing Eclipta Plant	Ayurvedic
Eclipta alba	Kesharanjan	Trailing Eclipta Plant	Ayurvedic
Eclipta alba	Kesharaaja	Trailing Eclipta Plant	Ayurvedic
Eclipta alba	Maarka	Trailing Eclipta Plant	Ayurvedic
Eclipta alba	Maarkava	Trailing Eclipta Plant	Ayurvedic
Eclipta alba	Suurya-vallabha	Trailing Eclipta Plant	Unani
Eclipta alba	Karisalaan-kanni	Trailing Eclipta Plant	Siddha/Tamil
Eclipta alba	Bhangaraa	Trailing Eclipta Plant	Folk
Ehretia buxifolia	Kattuvettilai	Carmonia Shrub	Siddha/Tamil
Ehretia buxifolia	Kuruvingi	Carmonia Shrub	Siddha/Tamil
Ehretia buxifolia	Pala	Carmonia Shrub	Folk
Ehretia laevis	Charmi-vrksha	Datrang Tree	Ayurvedic
Ehretia laevis	Addula	Datrang Tree	Siddha/Tamil
Ehretia laevis	Chamror	Datrang Tree	Folk
Ehretia laevis	Kuptaa	Datrang Tree	Folk

Table Contd.

Botanical Name	Indian Name	English Name	Medicinal System
Ehretia laevis	Datarangi	Datrang Tree	Folk
Eichhornia crassipes	Jalakumbhi	Water-Hyacinth, Bengal Terror, Blue Devil, The Million Dollar Weed	Ayurvedic
Eichhornia crassipes	Akasa thammarai	Water-Hyacinth, Bengal Terror, Blue Devil, The Million Dollar Weed	Siddha/Tamil
Elaeocarpus ganitrus	Panch-mukhi	Utrasum Bead Tree	Ayurvedic
Elaeocarpus ganitrus	Rudraaksha	Utrasum Bead Tree	Ayurvedic
Elaeocarpus ganitrus	Rudraaksham	Utrasum Bead Tree	Siddha/Tamil
Elaeocarpus serratus	Rudraaksha (var.)	Wild Olive Tree, Ceylon Olive	Ayurvedic
Elaeocarpus serratus	Uttraccham	Wild Olive Tree, Ceylon Olive	Siddha/Tamil
Elaeocarpus serratus	Ulankarei	Wild Olive Tree, Ceylon Olive	Siddha/Tamil
Elaeocarpus tuberculatus	Rudraaksha (var.)	Western Ghat Olive-Nut Tree	Ayurvedic
Elaeocarpus tuberculatus	Ruthracham	Western Ghat Olive-Nut Tree	Siddha/Tamil
Elaeocarpus tuberculatus	Pagumbar	Western Ghat Olive-Nut Tree	Siddha/Tamil
Elaeocarpus tuberculatus	Rudirak	Western Ghat Olive-Nut Tree	Folk
Elaeocarpus tuberculatus	Bhutali	Western Ghat Olive-Nut Tree	Folk
Elaeodendron glaucum	Krishnamokshaka	Jamrasi Gum Tree	Ayurvedic
Elaeodendron glaucum	Selluppaimaram	Jamrasi Gum Tree	Siddha/Tamil
Elaeodendron glaucum	Kaala-mokhaa	Jamrasi Gum Tree	Folk
Elaeodendron glaucum	Ratangaruur	Jamrasi Gum Tree	Folk
Elaeodendron glaucum	Jamrasi (gum)	Jamrasi Gum Tree	Folk
Eleocharis dulcis	Shringaataka	Chinese Water Chestnut	Ayurvedic
Eleocharis dulcis	Kasheruka	Chinese Water Chestnut	Ayurvedic
Elephantopus scaber	Mayura-shikhaa	Prickly-leaved Elephant's Foot	Ayurvedic
Elephantopus scaber	Gojihvaa	Prickly-leaved Elephant's Foot	Ayurvedic
Elephantopus scaber	Yaanaichhuvadi	Prickly-leaved Elephant's Foot	Siddha/Tamil
Elephantopus scaber	Mayurjuti	Prickly-leaved Elephant's Foot	Folk
Elephantopus scaber	Maaraajuti	Prickly-leaved Elephant's Foot	Folk
Elettaria cardamomum	Elaa	Lesser Cardamom	Ayurvedic
Elettaria cardamomum	Sukshmailaa	Lesser Cardamom	Ayurvedic
Elettaria cardamomum	Kshudrailaa	Lesser Cardamom	Ayurvedic

Table Contd.

Botanical Name	Indian Name	English Name	Medicinal System
Elettaria cardamomum	Bhrngaparnikaa	Lesser Cardamom	Ayurvedic
Elettaria cardamomum	Tutthaa	Lesser Cardamom	Ayurvedic
Elettaria cardamomum	Draavidi	Lesser Cardamom	Ayurvedic
Elettaria cardamomum	Prithvikaa	Lesser Cardamom	Ayurvedic
Elettaria cardamomum	Triputaa	Lesser Cardamom	Ayurvedic
Elettaria cardamomum	Truti	Lesser Cardamom	Ayurvedic
Elettaria cardamomum	Upkunchikaa	Lesser Cardamom	Ayurvedic
Elettaria cardamomum	Heel Khurd	Lesser Cardamom	Unani
Elettaria cardamomum	Elakkaai	Lesser Cardamom	Siddha/Tamil
Elettaria cardamomum	Ilaayachi	Lesser Cardamom	Folk
Eleusine coracana	Madhuuli	Finger Millet, African Millet, Ragi	Ayurvedic
Eleusine coracana	Markatahasta-trna	Finger Millet, African Millet, Ragi	Ayurvedic
Eleusine coracana	Ragi	Finger Millet, African Millet, Ragi	Siddha/Tamil
Eleusine coracana	Kezhvaregu	Finger Millet, African Millet, Ragi	Siddha/Tamil
Eleusine indica	Nandimukha (var.)	Crowfoot Grass, Crab Grass	Ayurvedic
Eleusine indica	Nandiaa	Crowfoot Grass, Crab Grass	Folk
Eleusine indica	Mahaar Naachni	Crowfoot Grass, Crab Grass	Folk
Eleusine indica	Thippa Ragi	Crowfoot Grass, Crab Grass	Folk
Elsholtzia cristata	Ajagandhaa	Himalayan Pseudo-Basil	Ayurvedic
Elsholtzia cristata	Ban-Tulasi	Himalayan Pseudo-Basil	Folk
Elsholtzia cristata	Bovai	Himalayan Pseudo-Basil	Folk
Elsholtzia cristata	Phoot-Kanda	Himalayan Pseudo-Basil	Folk
Elytraria crenata	Dasmori	Dasmori	Folk
Elytraria crenata	Patharchattaa	Dasmori	Folk
Embelia ribes	Vidanga	Embelia	Ayurvedic
Embelia ribes	Amogha	Embelia	Ayurvedic
Embelia ribes	Baobarang	Embelia	Unani
Embelia ribes	Barang Kaabuli	Embelia	Unani
Embelia ribes	Chitratandula	Embelia	Ayurvedic
Embelia ribes	Jantughna	Embelia	Ayurvedic

Table Contd.

Botanical Name	Indian Name	English Name	Medicinal System
Embelia ribes	Jantunaashana	Embelia	Ayurvedic
Embelia ribes	Krmighna	Embelia	Ayurvedic
Embelia ribes	Krmihara	Embelia	Ayurvedic
Embelia ribes	Krmiripu	Embelia	Ayurvedic
Embelia ribes	Vaayuvidangam	Embelia	Siddha/Tamil
Embelia ribes	Vella	Embelia	Ayurvedic
Embelia robusta	Vidanga	Broad-leaved Embelia	Ayurvedic
Embelia robusta	Baayabirang	Broad-leaved Embelia	Folk
Emblica officinalis	Aaamalaki	Embic, Indian Gooseberry	Ayurvedic
Emblica officinalis	Aaamalaka	Embic, Indian Gooseberry	Ayurvedic
Emblica officinalis	Dhaatri	Embic, Indian Gooseberry	Ayurvedic
Emblica officinalis	Kaayasthaa	Embic, Indian Gooseberry	Ayurvedic
Emblica officinalis	Amoghaa	Embic, Indian Gooseberry	Ayurvedic
Emblica officinalis	Amritaphala	Embic, Indian Gooseberry	Ayurvedic
Emblica officinalis	Amla	Embic, Indian Gooseberry	Ayurvedic
Emblica officinalis	Aaamalaa	Embic, Indian Gooseberry	Ayurvedic
Emblica officinalis	Dhaatriphala	Embic, Indian Gooseberry	Ayurvedic
Emblica officinalis	Vayasyaa	Embic, Indian Gooseberry	Ayurvedic
Emblica officinalis	Vrshya	Embic, Indian Gooseberry	Ayurvedic
Emblica officinalis	Shiva	Embic, Indian Gooseberry	Ayurvedic
Emblica officinalis	Hattha	Embic, Indian Gooseberry	Ayurvedic
Emblica officinalis	Aamalaa	Embic, Indian Gooseberry	Unani
Emblica officinalis	Amlaj	Embic, Indian Gooseberry	Unani
Emblica officinalis	Nellikkaai	Embic, Indian Gooseberry	Siddha/Tamil
Emblica officinalis	Nelli	Embic, Indian Gooseberry	Siddha/Tamil
Emilia sonchifolia	Shash-shruti	Emilia Salad	Ayurvedic
Emilia sonchifolia	Hirankhuri	Emilia Salad	Unani
Emilia sonchifolia	Sadamandi	Emilia Salad	Folk
Enhydra fluctuans	Harakuch	Marsh Herb, Water Cress	Folk
Enhydra fluctuans	Hil-mochikaa	Marsh Herb, Water Cress	Ayurvedic
Enicostemma littorale	Chhotaa Chirayataa	Indian Gentian	Folk
Enicostemma littorale	Vellargu	Indian Gentian	Siddha/Tamil

Table Contd.

Botanical Name	Indian Name	English Name	Medicinal System
Enicostemma littorale	Maamajjaka	Indian Gentian	Ayurvedic
Enicostemma littorale	Naagjhvaa	Indian Gentian	Ayurvedic
Enicostemma littorale	Naahi	Indian Gentian	Ayurvedic
Enicostemma littorale	Tikshnapatra	Indian Gentian	Ayurvedic
Enicostemma littorale	Naai	Indian Gentian	Unani
Enicostemma littorale	Naahi	Indian Gentian	Unani
Entada scandens	Gardel	Garbee Bean, Mackay Bean, Elephant Creeper	Folk
Entada scandens	Chillu	Garbee Bean, Mackay Bean, Elephant Creeper	Siddha/Tamil
Entada scandens	Vattavalli	Garbee Bean, Mackay Bean, Elephant Creeper	Siddha/Tamil
Entada scandens	Gil-gaachh	Garbee Bean, Mackay Bean, Elephant Creeper	Folk
Ephedra gerardiana	Soma-valli	Ephedra	Ayurvedic
Ephedra gerardiana	Asmaaniyaa	Ephedra	Folk
Ephedra gerardiana	Asmaaniyaabuuti	Ephedra	Folk
Ephedra gerardiana	Tut-gandhaa	Ephedra	Folk
Ephedra gerardiana	Soma-kalp	Ephedra	Folk
Ephedra gerardiana	Traani	Ephedra	Folk
Equisetum arvense	Ashwa-puchha	Field Horsetail	Ayurvedic
Erigeron canadensis	Jaraayupriya	Canadian Fleabane	Ayurvedic
Erigeron canadensis	Makshikaa-visha	Canadian Fleabane	Ayurvedic
Erigeron canadensis	Palit	Canadian Fleabane	Ayurvedic
Eriobotrya japonica	Lottaaka	Loquat, Japanese Medlar	Ayurvedic
Eriobotrya japonica	Lokaat	Loquat, Japanese Medlar	Unani
Eriobotrya japonica	Ilakotta	Loquat, Japanese Medlar	Siddha/Tamil
Eriobotrya japonica	Nokkotta	Loquat, Japanese Medlar	Siddha/Tamil
Eruca sativa	Tuvari	Rocket-Salad	Ayurvedic
Eruca sativa	Tuvarikaa	Rocket-Salad	Ayurvedic
Eruca sativa	Shveta-sursaa	Rocket-Salad	Ayurvedic
Eruca sativa	Bhuutaghna	Rocket-Salad	Ayurvedic
Eruca sativa	Daradharsha	Rocket-Salad	Ayurvedic
Eruca sativa	Siddaartha	Rocket-Salad	Ayurvedic
Eruca sativa	Jirjeer	Rocket-Salad	Unani

Table Contd.

Botanical Name	Indian Name	English Name	Medicinal System
Eruca sativa	Taraamiraa	Rocket-Salad	Unani
Eruca sativa	Safed Sarson	Rocket-Salad	Folk
Ervataemia coronaria	Nandivriksha	East Indian Rosebay	Ayurvedic
Ervataemia coronaria	Tagar	East Indian Rosebay	Ayurvedic
Ervataemia coronaria	Nandiyaavattam	East Indian Rosebay	Siddha/Tamil
Erycibe paniculata	Unamkodi	Kari Climber (Assam)	Siddha/Tamil
Erycibe paniculata	Ashoka-rohini	Kari Climber (Assam)	Ayurvedic
Eryngium caeruleum	Dudhali	Turnip-shaped Himalayan Carrot	Folk
Eryngium caeruleum	Pahaari Gaajar	Turnip-shaped Himalayan Carrot	Folk
Eryngium caeruleum	Saleli-misri	Turnip-shaped Himalayan Carrot	Folk
Eryngium foetidum	Brahma-Dhaniyaa	Sea Holly	Folk
Eryngium foetidum	Jangali Gaajar *(var.)*	Sea Holly	Folk
Erythraea roxburghii	Kiraat-tikta	Pseudo-Chiretta	Ayurvedic
Erythraea roxburghii	Yavatiktaa	Pseudo-Chiretta	Ayurvedic
Erythraea roxburghii	Khet-chiraayataa	Pseudo-Chiretta	Folk
Erythrina indica	Paaribhadra	Indian Coral Tree	Ayurvedic
Erythrina indica	Paaribhadraka	Indian Coral Tree	Ayurvedic
Erythrina indica	Paarijaataka	Indian Coral Tree	Ayurvedic
Erythrina indica	Mandaara	Indian Coral Tree	Ayurvedic
Erythrina indica	Dadap	Indian Coral Tree	Ayurvedic
Erythrina indica	Kantaki-palaasha	Indian Coral Tree	Ayurvedic
Erythrina indica	Kantkimshuka	Indian Coral Tree	Ayurvedic
Erythrina indica	Raktapushpa	Indian Coral Tree	Ayurvedic
Erythrina indica	Nimbataru	Indian Coral Tree	Ayurvedic
Erythrina indica	Kaliyana-murukkan	Indian Coral Tree	Siddha/Tamil
Erythrina indica	Farhad	Indian Coral Tree	Folk
Erythrina stricta	Muraa	Scarlet-flowered Coral Tree	Ayurvedic
Erythrina stricta	Mullu-murukku	Scarlet-flowered Coral Tree	Siddha/Tamil
Erythroxylum coca	Sivadari	Coca, Cocaine Plant	Siddha/Tamil
Erythroxylum monogynum	Kattuchandanam	Bastard Sandal, Red Cedar	Ayurvedic

Table Contd.

Botanical Name	Indian Name	English Name	Medicinal System
Erythroxylum monogynum	Devadaram	Bastard Sandal, Red Cedar	Siddha/Tamil
Erythroxylum monogynum	Gandh-giri	Bastard Sandal, Red Cedar	Folk
Eucalyptus globulus	Tilaparna	Blue-gum Tree, Australian Gum Tree	Ayurvedic
Eucalyptus globulus	Tailaparna	Blue-gum Tree, Australian Gum Tree	Ayurvedic
Eucalyptus globulus	Sugandhapatra	Blue-gum Tree, Australian Gum Tree	Ayurvedic
Eucalyptus globulus	Neelaniryaasa	Blue-gum Tree, Australian Gum Tree	Ayurvedic
Eucalyptus globulus	Tribhandi	Blue-gum Tree, Australian Gum Tree	Ayurvedic
Eucalyptus globulus	Triputaa	Blue-gum Tree, Australian Gum Tree	Ayurvedic
Eucalyptus globulus	Haritaparna	Blue-gum Tree, Australian Gum Tree	Ayurvedic
Eucalyptus globulus	Suvahaa	Blue-gum Tree, Australian Gum Tree	Ayurvedic
Eucalyptus globulus	Rechani	Blue-gum Tree, Australian Gum Tree	Ayurvedic
Eucalyptus globulus	Nishotraa	Blue-gum Tree, Australian Gum Tree	Ayurvedic
Eucalyptus globulus	Neelgiri Oil	Blue-gum Tree, Australian Gum Tree	Unani
Eucalyptus globulus	Karpooramaram	Blue-gum Tree, Australian Gum Tree	Siddha/Tamil
Eugenia uniflora	Pitaanga	Surinam Cherry	Ayurvedic
Eulaliopsis binata	Balvaja	Baib Grass, Sabai Grass	Ayurvedic
Eulaliopsis binata	Bhaabar	Baib Grass, Sabai Grass	Folk
Eulophia campestris	Amrita	Salep Orchid	Ayurvedic
Eulophia campestris	Munjaataka	Salep Orchid	Ayurvedic
Eulophia campestris	Saalam-misri	Salep Orchid	Ayurvedic
Eulophia campestris	Sudhaa-muuli	Salep Orchid	Ayurvedic
Eulophia herbacea	Munjaataka	Salep Orchid	Ayurvedic
Eulophia herbacea	Saalam-misri	Salep Orchid	Ayurvedic
Eulophia nuda	Amarkanda	Goruma Tuber, Riddhi	Ayurvedic
Eulophia nuda	Baalakanda	Goruma Tuber, Riddhi	Ayurvedic

Table Contd.

Botanical Name	Indian Name	English Name	Medicinal System
Eulophia nuda	Maalaakanda	Goruma Tuber, Riddhi	Ayurvedic
Eulophia nuda	Ambarkanda	Goruma Tuber, Riddhi	Folk
Eulophia pratensis	Sata-vari	Salep (var.)	Folk (Maharashtra)
Euonymus tingens	Bhillotaka	Spindle Wood, Wahoo,	Ayurvedic
Euonymus tingens	Barphali	Spindle Wood, Wahoo,	Folk
Euonymus tingens	Chopra	Spindle Wood, Wahoo,	Folk
Euonymus tingens	Kunku	Spindle Wood, Wahoo,	Folk
Euonymus tingens	Mermahaul	Spindle Wood, Wahoo,	Folk
Eupatorium cannabinum	Bundaar	Hemp Agrimony, Water Hemp, Hemp Eupatorium	Folk
Eupatorium cannabinum	Tongollati	Hemp Agrimony, Water Hemp, Hemp Eupatorium	Folk
Eupatorium triplinerve	Ayaapaana	Ayapana Tea	Ayurvedic
Eupatorium triplinerve	Vishalyakarani	Ayapana Tea	Ayurvedic
Eupatorium triplinerve	Ayapanai	Ayapana Tea	Siddha/Tamil
Eupatorium triplinerve	Ayapani	Ayapana Tea	Folk
Euphorbia antiquorum	Snuhi	Triangular Spurge	Ayurvedic
Euphorbia antiquorum	Vajra-kantaka	Triangular Spurge	Ayurvedic
Euphorbia antiquorum	Vajratundi	Triangular Spurge	Ayurvedic
Euphorbia antiquorum	Chathurakkali	Triangular Spurge	Siddha/Tamil
Euphorbia antiquorum	Tridhaari	Triangular Spurge	Folk
Euphorbia antiquorum	Tidhaaraa Sehunda	Triangular Spurge	Folk
Euphorbia dracunculoides	Charmakashaa	Dragon Spurge	Ayurvedic
Euphorbia dracunculoides	Charmasaahvaa	Dragon Spurge	Ayurvedic
Euphorbia dracunculoides	Saatalaa	Dragon Spurge	Ayurvedic
Euphorbia dracunculoides	Sapralaa	Dragon Spurge	Ayurvedic
Euphorbia dracunculoides	Saptalaa	Dragon Spurge	Ayurvedic
Euphorbia dracunculoides	Viduraa	Dragon Spurge	Ayurvedic
Euphorbia dracunculoides	Thuhar	Dragon Spurge	Unani
Euphorbia dracunculoides	Thusimullai	Dragon Spurge	Siddha/Tamil
Euphorbia dracunculoides	Tillakada	Dragon Spurge	Siddha/Tamil
Euphorbia dracunculoides	Titali	Dragon Spurge	Folk

Table Contd.

Botanical Name	Indian Name	English Name	Medicinal System
Euphorbia hirta	Dudhi	Euphorbia, Australian Asthma Weed, Pill-bearing Spurge	Ayurvedic
Euphorbia hirta	Dudhikaa	Euphorbia, Australian Asthma Weed, Pill-bearing Spurge	Ayurvedic
Euphorbia hirta	Naagaarjuni	Euphorbia, Australian Asthma Weed, Pill-bearing Spurge	Ayurvedic
Euphorbia hirta	Vikshirini	Euphorbia, Australian Asthma Weed, Pill-bearing Spurge	Ayurvedic
Euphorbia hirta	Dudhi Khurd	Euphorbia, Australian Asthma Weed, Pill-bearing Spurge	Unani
Euphorbia hirta	Amman pachharisi	Euphorbia, Australian Asthma Weed, Pill-bearing Spurge	Siddha/Tamil
Euphorbia hypericifolia	Dugdhikaa	Oblong-leaved Spurge	Ayurvedic
Euphorbia neriifolia	Snuhi	Holy Milk Hedge, Dog's Tongue	Ayurvedic
Euphorbia neriifolia	Samant-dugdhaa	Holy Milk Hedge, Dog's Tongue	Ayurvedic
Euphorbia neriifolia	Sehunda	Holy Milk Hedge, Dog's Tongue	Ayurvedic
Euphorbia neriifolia	Singhtunda	Holy Milk Hedge, Dog's Tongue	Ayurvedic
Euphorbia neriifolia	Snuk	Holy Milk Hedge, Dog's Tongue	Ayurvedic
Euphorbia neriifolia	Gudaa	Holy Milk Hedge, Dog's Tongue	Ayurvedic
Euphorbia neriifolia	Sudhaa	Holy Milk Hedge, Dog's Tongue	Ayurvedic
Euphorbia neriifolia	Vajra	Holy Milk Hedge, Dog's Tongue	Ayurvedic
Euphorbia neriifolia	Vajjri	Holy Milk Hedge, Dog's Tongue	Ayurvedic
Euphorbia neriifolia	Vajjradram	Holy Milk Hedge, Dog's Tongue	Ayurvedic
Euphorbia neriifolia	Thuuhar	Holy Milk Hedge, Dog's Tongue	Ayurvedic
Euphorbia neriifolia	Ielaikkali	Holy Milk Hedge, Dog's Tongue	Siddha/Tamil
Euphorbia neriifolia	Perumbukalli	Holy Milk Hedge, Dog's Tongue	Siddha/Tamil
Euphorbia nivulia	Snuhi	Corky-barked Spurge	Ayurvedic
Euphorbia nivulia	Patra-Snuhi	Corky-barked Spurge	Ayurvedic
Euphorbia nivulia	Kalli	Corky-barked Spurge	Siddha/Tamil
Euphorbia nivulia	Naga-kalli	Corky-barked Spurge	Siddha/Tamil
Euphorbia pilosa	Saataka	Fragrant Himalayan Spurge	Ayurvedic
Euphorbia pilosa	Saptalaa	Fragrant Himalayan Spurge	Ayurvedic
Euphorbia resinifera	Farfiyuun	Resin Spurge	Unani
Euphorbia resinifera	Afarbiyuun	Resin Spurge	Unani
Euphorbia royleana	Snuhi	Thor Spurge	Ayurvedic

Table Contd.

Botanical Name	Indian Name	English Name	Medicinal System
Euphorbia royleana	Snuk	Thor Spurge	Ayurvedic
Euphorbia royleana	Sehunda	Thor Spurge	Ayurvedic
Euphorbia royleana	Gudaa	Thor Spurge	Ayurvedic
Euphorbia royleana	Thuuhar	Thor Spurge	Unani
Euphorbia royleana	Surai	Thor Spurge	Folk
Euphorbia thomsoniana	Hiyaavali	Hirvi Spurge	Ayurvedic
Euphorbia thomsoniana	Svarnakshiri	Hirvi Spurge	Ayurvedic
Euphorbia thomsoniana	Kanchanakshiri	Hirvi Spurge	Ayurvedic
Euphorbia thomsoniana	Pitadugdhaa	Hirvi Spurge	Ayurvedic
Euphorbia thomsoniana	Katuparni	Hirvi Spurge	Ayurvedic
Euphorbia thomsoniana	Hiravi	Hirvi Spurge	Folk
Euphorbia thomsoniana	Titari	Hirvi Spurge	Folk
Euphorbia thymifolia	Dudhi	Thyme-leaf Spurge	Ayurvedic
Euphorbia thymifolia	Dugdhikaa	Thyme-leaf Spurge	Ayurvedic
Euphorbia thymifolia	Naagaarjuni	Thyme-leaf Spurge	Ayurvedic
Euphorbia thymifolia	Swaaduparni	Thyme-leaf Spurge	Ayurvedic
Euphorbia thymifolia	Sittrapaladi	Thyme-leaf Spurge	Siddha/Tamil
Euphorbia tirucalli	Saptalaa	Milk-Bush, Milk Hedge, Indian Tree Spurge, Aveloz, Petroleum Plant	Ayurvedic
Euphorbia tirucalli	Saatalaa	Milk-Bush, Milk Hedge, Indian Tree Spurge, Aveloz, Petroleum Plant	Ayurvedic
Euphorbia tirucalli	Tirukalli	Milk-Bush, Milk Hedge, Indian Tree Spurge, Aveloz, Petroleum Plant	Siddha/Tamil
Euphorbia tirucalli	Angulia-thuuhar	Milk-Bush, Milk Hedge, Indian Tree Spurge, Aveloz, Petroleum Plant	Folk
Euphoria longan	Aakshiki	Longan	Ayurvedic
Euphoria longan	Puvatti	Longan	Siddha/Tamil
Euphoria longan	Shempuvan	Longan	Siddha/Tamil
Euphoria longan	Aashaphala	Longan	Folk
Euphoria longan	Naaglichi	Longan	Folk
Euphrasia simplex	Eyebright	Eyebright	Folk
Euryale ferox	Makhaann	Gorgan Nut, Fox Nut	Ayurvedic

Table Contd.

Botanical Name	Indian Name	English Name	Medicinal System
Ferula foetida	Vedhi	Asafoetida	Ayurvedic
Ferula foetida	Hilteet	Asafoetida	Unani
Ferula foetida	Heeng	Asafoetida	Unani
Ferula foetida	Perumkaayam	Asafoetida	Siddha/Tamil
Ferula galbaniflua	Gaosheer	Galbanum	Unani
Ferula galbaniflua	Jawaasheer	Galbanum	Unani
Ferula jaeschkeana	Hingupatri	Kashmiri Ferula	Ayurvedic
Ferula narthex	Hingu (var.)	Narthex Asafoetida	Ayurvedic
Ferula narthex	Hilteet	Narthex Asafoetida	Unani
Ferula narthex	Heeng	Narthex Asafoetida	Unani
Ferula narthex	Perungayam	Narthex Asafoetida	Siddha/Tamil
Ferula persica	Sakbeenaj	Sagapenum	Unani
Ferula persica	Sakbekh	Sagapenum	Unani
Ferula sumbul	Sumbul	Musk Root	Folk
Ferula sumbul	Sambala	Musk Root	Folk
Ficus altissima	Choraka-patra (var.)	Council Tree,Lofty Fig Tree	Ayurvedic
Ficus altissima	Nandi vriksha (var.)	Council Tree,Lofty Fig Tree	Ayurvedic
Ficus altissima	Gadgubar	Council Tree,Lofty Fig Tree	Folk
Ficus arnottiana	Gajapaadapa	Indian Rock Fig	Ayurvedic
Ficus arnottiana	Nandi Vriksha	Indian Rock Fig	Ayurvedic
Ficus arnottiana	Paarasa Pipala	Indian Rock Fig	Ayurvedic
Ficus arnottiana	Prarohi	Indian Rock Fig	Ayurvedic
Ficus arnottiana	Kagoti	Indian Rock Fig	Siddha/Tamil
Ficus asperrima	Kharapatra	Brahma's Banyan, Sandpaper Fig	Ayurvedic
Ficus asperrima	Kal-arasu	Brahma's Banyan, Sandpaper Fig	Siddha/Tamil
Ficus asperrima	Kaala-umar	Brahma's Banyan, Sandpaper Fig	Folk
Ficus beng(h)alensis	Bahupaada	Banyan Tree	Ayurvedic
Ficus beng(h)alensis	Dhruv	Banyan Tree	Ayurvedic
Ficus beng(h)alensis	Nyagrodha	Banyan Tree	Ayurvedic
Ficus beng(h)alensis	Vata	Banyan Tree	Ayurvedic
Ficus beng(h)alensis	Bargad	Banyan Tree	Unani
Ficus beng(h)alensis	Darakht-e-Reesh	Banyan Tree	Unani

Table Contd.

Botanical Name	Indian Name	English Name	Medicinal System
Ficus beng(h)alensis	Aaalamaram	Banyan Tree	Siddha/Tamil
Ficus benjamina	Malai Ichi	Java Fig	Siddha/Tamil
Ficus benjamina	Pon Ichi	Java Fig	Siddha/Tamil
Ficus benjamina	Putrajuvi	Java Fig	Siddha/Tamil
Ficus benjamina	Pimpri	Java Fig	Folk
Ficus carica	Bhadrodumbara	Common Fig	Ayurvedic
Ficus carica	Manjul	Common Fig	Ayurvedic
Ficus carica	Phalgu	Common Fig	Ayurvedic
Ficus carica	Raajodumbara	Common Fig	Ayurvedic
Ficus carica	Anjeer	Common Fig	Unani
Ficus carica	Teen	Common Fig	Unani
Ficus carica	Semaiatti	Common Fig	Siddha/Tamil
Ficus cordifolia	Ashmantaka (var.)	Rumpf's Fig	Ayurvedic
Ficus cordifolia	Ashtaa	Rumpf's Fig	Folk
Ficus cordifolia	Gajanaa	Rumpf's Fig	Folk
Ficus cordifolia	Paakar	Rumpf's Fig	Folk
Ficus cunia	Choraka-patra	Indian Fig	Ayurvedic
Ficus cunia	Laakshaa-vriksha	Indian Fig	Ayurvedic
Ficus cunia	Laghu-udumbara	Indian Fig	Ayurvedic
Ficus cunia	Malayu	Indian Fig	Ayurvedic
Ficus cunia	Taragadu	Indian Fig	Siddha/Tamil
Ficus dalhousiae	Soma-valka	Carica Fig	Ayurvedic
Ficus dalhousiae	Kal Aal	Carica Fig	Siddha/Tamil
Ficus dalhousiae	Pei Aal	Carica Fig	Siddha/Tamil
Ficus heterophylla	Traayamaanaa	Oak-Leaf Fig	Ayurvedic
Ficus heterophylla	Traayanti	Oak-Leaf Fig	Ayurvedic
Ficus heterophylla	Kodi Athi	Oak-Leaf Fig	Siddha/Tamil
Ficus heterophylla	Daantiraa	Oak-Leaf Fig	Folk
Ficus hispida	Kaakodumbara	Devil's Fig, Rough-leaved Fig	Ayurvedic
Ficus hispida	Kaashtodumbara	Devil's Fig, Rough-leaved Fig	Ayurvedic
Ficus hispida	Malapu	Devil's Fig, Rough-leaved Fig	Ayurvedic
Ficus hispida	Malayu	Devil's Fig, Rough-leaved Fig	Ayurvedic

Table Contd.

Botanical Name	Indian Name	English Name	Medicinal System
Ficus hispida	Phalgu	Devil's Fig, Rough-leaved Fig	Ayurvedic
Ficus hispida	Anjir Dashti	Devil's Fig, Rough-leaved Fig	Unani
Ficus hispida	Chona Atthi	Devil's Fig, Rough-leaved Fig	Siddha/Tamil
Ficus hispida	Peyatti	Devil's Fig, Rough-leaved Fig	Siddha/Tamil
Ficus lacor	Karpari	White Fig	Ayurvedic
Ficus lacor	Parkati	White Fig	Ayurvedic
Ficus lacor	Pitana	White Fig	Ayurvedic
Ficus lacor	Plaksha	White Fig	Ayurvedic
Ficus lacor	Ichchi	White Fig	Siddha/Tamil
Ficus lacor	Kallalnaram	White Fig	Siddha/Tamil
Ficus lacor	Kurugu	White Fig	Siddha/Tamil
Ficus microcarpa	Plaksha	Indian Laurel Fig	Ayurvedic
Ficus microcarpa	Kal Ichi	Indian Laurel Fig	Siddha/Tamil
Ficus microcarpa	Itti	Indian Laurel Fig	Folk
Ficus palmata	Anjiri	Indian Fig	Ayurvedic
Ficus palmata	Phalgu	Indian Fig	Ayurvedic
Ficus palmata	Manjimedi	Indian Fig	Folk/Telugu
Ficus racemosa	Hema-daudhaka	Cluster Fig, Country Fig	Ayurvedic
Ficus racemosa	Jantuphala	Cluster Fig, Country Fig	Ayurvedic
Ficus racemosa	Sadaaphala	Cluster Fig, Country Fig	Ayurvedic
Ficus racemosa	Udumbara	Cluster Fig, Country Fig	Ayurvedic
Ficus racemosa	Yagyaanga	Cluster Fig, Country Fig	Ayurvedic
Ficus racemosa	Anjir-e-Aadam	Cluster Fig, Country Fig	Unani
Ficus racemosa	Anjir-e-Ahmak	Cluster Fig, Country Fig	Unani
Ficus racemosa	Gular	Cluster Fig, Country Fig	Unani
Ficus racemosa	Aththi	Cluster Fig, Country Fig	Siddha/Tamil
Ficus religiosa	Ashvattha	Peepal, Bot-tree	Ayurvedic
Ficus religiosa	Bodhidru	Peepal, Bot-tree	Ayurvedic
Ficus religiosa	Bodhivrkisha	Peepal, Bot-tree	Ayurvedic
Ficus religiosa	Sebya	Peepal, Bot-tree	Ayurvedic
Ficus religiosa	Chalapatra	Peepal, Bot-tree	Ayurvedic
Ficus religiosa	Gajabhaksha	Peepal, Bot-tree	Ayurvedic
Ficus religiosa	Kshiradruma	Peepal, Bot-tree	Ayurvedic

Table Contd.

Botanical Name	Indian Name	English Name	Medicinal System
Ficus religiosa	Peepal	Peepal, Bot-tree	Ayurvedic
Ficus religiosa	Peepal	Peepal, Bot-tree	Unani
Ficus religiosa	Arasam	Peepal, Bot-tree	Siddha/Tamil
Ficus religiosa	Ashvatham	Peepal, Bot-tree	Siddha/Tamil
Ficus talboti	Plaksha	Pakar Tree	Ayurvedic
Ficus talboti	Itthi	Pakar Tree	Siddha/Tamil
Ficus talboti	Kal Itthi	Pakar Tree	Siddha/Tamil
Fimbristylis ovata	Ibha-muulaka	Fringe-Rush	Ayurvedic
Flacourtia indica	Vikankata	Ramontchi, Madagascar Plum, Mauritius Plum, Governor's Plum	Ayurvedic
Flacourtia indica	Yajnyavrksha	Ramontchi, Madagascar Plum, Mauritius Plum, Governor's Plum	Ayurvedic
Flacourtia indica	Gopakantaa	Ramontchi, Madagascar Plum, Mauritius Plum, Governor's Plum	Ayurvedic
Flacourtia indica	Sruva-vriksha	Ramontchi, Madagascar Plum, Mauritius Plum, Governor's Plum	Ayurvedic
Flacourtia indica	Sottai-kala	Ramontchi, Madagascar Plum, Mauritius Plum, Governor's Plum	Siddha/Tamil
Flacourtia indica	Katukala	Ramontchi, Madagascar Plum, Mauritius Plum, Governor's Plum	Siddha/Tamil
Flacourtia indica	Poniol	Ramontchi, Madagascar Plum, Mauritius Plum, Governor's Plum	Folk
Flacourtia indica	Kataaya	Ramontchi, Madagascar Plum, Mauritius Plum, Governor's Plum	Folk
Flacourita indica	Kakaiyaa	Ramontchi, Madagascar Plum, Mauritius Plum, Governor's Plum	Folk
Flacourtia jangomas	Praachinaamalaka	Puneala Plum	Ayurvedic
Flacourtia jangomas	Paaniyaamalaka	Puneala Plum	Ayurvedic
Flacourtia jangomas	Taalisfar	Puneala Plum	Unani
Flacourtia jangomas	Nabaq Hindi	Puneala Plum	Unani

Table Contd.

Botanical Name	Indian Name	English Name	Medicinal System
Flacourtia jangomas	Zarnab	Puneala Plum	Unani
Flacourtia jangomas	Saralu	Puneala Plum	Siddha/Tamil
Flacourtia jangomas	Vayangarai	Puneala Plum	Siddha/Tamil
Flacourtia jangomas	Paniyaalaa	Puneala Plum	Folk
Flacourtia sepiaria	Vikankata	Governor's Plum	Ayurvedic
Flacourtia sepiaria	Kinkini	Governor's Plum	Ayurvedic
Flacourtia sepiaria	Kondai	Governor's Plum	Folk
Flacourtia sepiaria	Kondari	Governor's Plum	Folk
Foeniculum vulgare	Mishreyaa	Fennel	Ayurvedic
Foeniculum vulgare	Mishi	Fennel	Ayurvedic
Foeniculum vulgare	Madhurikaa	Fennel	Ayurvedic
Foeniculum vulgare	Madhuraa	Fennel	Ayurvedic
Foeniculum vulgare	Shatapushpaa	Fennel	Ayurvedic
Foeniculum vulgare	Shataahvaa	Fennel	Ayurvedic
Foeniculum vulgare	Baadiyaan	Fennel	Unani
Foeniculum vulgare	Saunf	Fennel	Unani
Foeniculum vulgare	Sombu	Fennel	Siddha/Tamil
Fraxinus hookery	Kum	European Ash, Weeping Ash	Folk
Fraxinus hookery	Sum	European Ash, Weeping Ash	Folk
Fraxinus hookery	Hum	European Ash, Weeping Ash	Folk
Fraxinus hookery	Sinnun	European Ash, Weeping Ash	Folk
Fraxinus ornus	Turanjeen	Flake Manna	Unani
Fritillaria cirrhosa	Yathu	Himalayan Fritillaria Bulb	Folk
Fritillaria imperialis	Fritillary	Crown Imperial, Imperial Fritillary	Folk
Fritillaria roylei	Kshira-Kaakoli	Pei-mu (China), Kakoli	Ayurvedic
Fritillaria roylei	Viraa	Pei-mu (China), Kakoli	Ayurvedic
Fritillaria roylei	Kaayasthikaa	Pei-mu (China), Kakoli	Ayurvedic
Fritillaria roylei	Vaaysoli	Pei-mu (China), Kakoli	Ayurvedic
Fucus vesiculosus	Kelp	Bladderwrack	Folk
Fumaria officinalis	Parpata	Fumitory	Ayurvedic
Fumaria officinalis	Shaahtaraa	Fumitory	Unani
Fumaria parviflora	Parpata	Fumitory	Ayurvedic
Fumaria parviflora	Parpataka	Fumitory	Ayurvedic

Table Contd.

Botanical Name	Indian Name	English Name	Medicinal System
Fumaria parviflora	Varatikta	Fumitory	Ayurvedic
Fumaria parviflora	Renu	Fumitory	Ayurvedic
Fumaria parviflora	Kavacha	Fumitory	Ayurvedic
Fumaria parviflora	Sukshmapatra	Fumitory	Ayurvedic
Fumaria parviflora	Shaahtaraa	Fumitory	Unani
Fumaria parviflora	Thura	Fumitory	Siddha/Tamil
Fumaria parviflora	Pittapaaparaa	Fumitory	Folk
Fumaria vaillantii	Parpata	Yellow Fumitory	Ayurvedic
Fumaria vaillantii	Shaahtaraa	Yellow Fumitory	Unani
Fumaria vaillantii	Pittapaaparaa	Yellow Fumitory	Folk
Galium aparine	Cleaver	Goosegrass, Cleavers	Folk
Galium verum	Cleaver	Lady's Bedstraw, Cheese Rennet	Folk
Garcinia cambogia	Kokam (var.)	Gamboge Tree	Ayurvedic
Garcinia cambogia	Vrkshaamla	Gamboge Tree	Ayurvedic
Garcinia cambogia	Kodakkapuli	Gamboge Tree	Siddha/Tamil
Garcinia cowa	Kowaa	Indo-Malayan Brindleberry	Ayurvedic
Garcinia cowa	Paaraavata	Indo-Malayan Brindleberry	Ayurvedic
Garcinia cowa	Kaphal	Indo-Malayan Brindleberry	Folk
Garcinia cowa	Kujithekera	Indo-Malayan Brindleberry	Folk
Garcinia hanburyi	Kaalakushtha	Siam Gamboge	Ayurvedic
Garcinia hanburyi	Kankushtha	Siam Gamboge	Ayurvedic
Garcinia hanburyi	Tamaala	Siam Gamboge	Ayurvedic
Garcinia hanburyi	Usaar-e-revand	Siam Gamboge	Unani
Garcinia indica	Amlavrikshak	Kokam Butter Tree, Mangosteen Oil Tree	Ayurvedic
Garcinia indica	Amsula	Kokam Butter Tree, Mangosteen Oil Tree	Ayurvedic
Garcinia indica	Chukra	Kokam Butter Tree, Mangosteen Oil Tree	Ayurvedic
Garcinia indica	Kokam	Kokam Butter Tree, Mangosteen Oil Tree	Ayurvedic
Garcinia indica	Tintidika	Kokam Butter Tree, Mangosteen Oil Tree	Ayurvedic
Garcinia indica	Vrkshaamla	Kokam Butter Tree, Mangosteen Oil Tree	Ayurvedic

Table Contd.

Botanical Name	Indian Name	English Name	Medicinal System
Garcinia indica	Murgal	Kokam Butter Tree, Mangosteen Oil Tree	Siddha/Tamil
Garcinia indica	Kokam	Kokam Butter Tree, Mangosteen Oil Tree	Folk
Garcinia mangostana	Mangusta	Mangosteen, Dodol	Siddha/Tamil
Garcinia mangostana	Sulambuli	Mangosteen, Dodol	Siddha/Tamil
Garcinia mangostana	Mangustaan	Mangosteen, Dodol	Folk
Garcinia morella	Kankushtha	Indian Gamboge	Ayurvedic
Garcinia morella	Tamaal	Indian Gamboge	Ayurvedic
Garcinia morella	Taapichha	Indian Gamboge	Ayurvedic
Garcinia morella	Ushaare-revand	Indian Gamboge	Ayurvedic
Garcinia morella	Iravakhinni	Indian Gamboge	Siddha/Tamil
Garcinia pedunculata	Amlavetasa	Bengal Brindleberry	Ayurvedic
Garcinia pedunculata	Vetasaamla	Bengal Brindleberry	Ayurvedic
Garcinia pedunculata	Thaikala	Bengal Brindleberry	Folk
Garcinia xanthochymus	Tamaal (var.)	Egg Tree	Ayurvedic
Garcinia xanthochymus	Vrkshaamla (var.)	Egg Tree	Ayurvedic
Garcinia xanthochymus	Kulavi	Egg Tree	Siddha/Tamil
Garcinia xanthochymus	Malaippachai	Egg Tree	Siddha/Tamil
Garcinia xanthochymus	Mukki	Egg Tree	Siddha/Tamil
Garcinia xanthochymus	Tamalam	Egg Tree	Siddha/Tamil
Garcinia xanthochymus	Amsul	Egg Tree	Folk
Gardenia gummifera	Venupatrikaa	Gummy Cape Jasmine	Ayurvedic
Gardenia gummifera	Naadihingu	Gummy Cape Jasmine	Ayurvedic
Gardenia gummifera	Hingushiva-atikaa	Gummy Cape Jasmine	Ayurvedic
Gardenia gummifera	Hingupatrikaa	Gummy Cape Jasmine	Ayurvedic
Gardenia gummifera	Hingupatri	Gummy Cape Jasmine	Ayurvedic
Gardenia gummifera	Dikaamaali	Gummy Cape Jasmine	Unani
Gardenia gummifera	Dikamalli	Gummy Cape Jasmine	Siddha/Tamil
Gardenia gummifera	Kambil	Gummy Cape Jasmine	Siddha/Tamil
Gardenia gummifera	Sinna Kambil	Gummy Cape Jasmine	Siddha/Tamil
Gardenia jasminoides	Gandharaaja	Cape Jasmine	Ayurvedic
Gardenia jasminoides	Karinga	Cape Jasmine	Siddha/Tamil

Table Contd.

Botanical Name	Indian Name	English Name	Medicinal System
Gardenia latifolia	Parpataki	Boxwood Gardenia	Ayurvedic
Gardenia latifolia	Kumbay	Boxwood Gardenia	Siddha/Tamil
Gardenia latifolia	Perungambil	Boxwood Gardenia	Siddha/Tamil
Gardenia latifolia	Paaparaa	Boxwood Gardenia	Folk
Gardenia latifolia	Ban-pindaalu	Boxwood Gardenia	Folk
Gardenia resinifera	Naadihingu	Brilliant Gardenia, Cambi Resin Tree	Ayurvedic
Gardenia resinifera	Jantuka	Brilliant Gardenia, Cambi Resin Tree	Ayurvedic
Gardenia resinifera	Dikaamaali	Brilliant Gardenia, Cambi Resin Tree	Unani
Gardenia resinifera	Kambil	Brilliant Gardenia, Cambi Resin Tree	Folk/Tamil
Gardenia resinifera	Erubikki	Brilliant Gardenia, Cambi Resin Tree	Folk/Telugu
Gardenia resinifera	Dikkamalli	Brilliant Gardenia, Cambi Resin Tree	Siddha/Tamil
Gardenia turgida	Karahaata	Bharangi Bark Tree	Ayurvedic
Gardenia turgida	Kharahaara	Bharangi Bark Tree	Ayurvedic
Gardenia turgida	Mahaapindi	Bharangi Bark Tree	Ayurvedic
Gardenia turgida	Thanella	Bharangi Bark Tree	Ayurvedic
Gardenia turgida	Nanjundam	Bharangi Bark Tree	Siddha/Tamil
Gardenia turgida	Malangarai	Bharangi Bark Tree	Siddha/Tamil
Garuga pinnata	Paaranki	Grey Downy Balsam	Ayurvedic
Garuga pinnata	Kharpata	Grey Downy Balsam	Ayurvedic
Garuga pinnata	Karre Vembu	Grey Downy Balsam	Siddha/Tamil
Garuga pinnata	Arunelli	Grey Downy Balsam	Siddha/Tamil
Garuga pinnata	Ghogar	Grey Downy Balsam	Folk
Garuga pinnata	Toon	Grey Downy Balsam	Folk
Gaultheria fragrantissima	Gandhapuura	Fragrant Wintergreen, Indian Wintergreen	Ayurvedic
Gaultheria fragrantissima	Gandhapuurna	Fragrant Wintergreen, Indian Wintergreen	Ayurvedic
Gaultheria fragrantissima	Kolakkaai	Fragrant Wintergreen, Indian Wintergreen	Siddha/Tamil
Gelidium amansii	Agar-Agar	Agar Agar, Japanese Isinglass	Folk

Table Contd.

Botanical Name	Indian Name	English Name	Medicinal System
Gentiana kurroo	Traayamaana	Himalayan Gentian, Indian Gentian Root	Ayurvedic
Gentiana kurroo	Traayanti	Himalayan Gentian, Indian Gentian Root	Ayurvedic
Gentiana kurroo	Traayanta	Himalayan Gentian, Indian Gentian Root	Ayurvedic
Gentiana kurroo	Traayantikaa	Himalayan Gentian, Indian Gentian Root	Ayurvedic
Gentiana kurroo	Neelkanthi	Himalayan Gentian, Indian Gentian Root	Ayurvedic
Gentiana kurroo	Anujaa	Himalayan Gentian, Indian Gentian Root	Ayurvedic
Gentiana kurroo	Girijaa	Himalayan Gentian, Indian Gentian Root	Ayurvedic
Gentiana kurroo	Girishaanujaa	Himalayan Gentian, Indian Gentian Root	Ayurvedic
Gentiana kurroo	Balbhra	Himalayan Gentian, Indian Gentian Root	Ayurvedic
Gentiana kurroo	Paalani	Himalayan Gentian, Indian Gentian Root	Ayurvedic
Gentiana kurroo	Ghaafis	Himalayan Gentian, Indian Gentian Root	Unani
Geophila repens	Karintakaali	Corrida, Yerba de guava (US)	Folk
Geranium nepalense	Bhanda	Nepal Geranium, Nepalese Crane's Bill	Ayurvedic
Geranium nepalense	Bhandaa	Nepal Geranium, Nepalese Crane's Bill	Ayurvedic
Geranium nepalense	Cheenitroghaans	Nepal Geranium, Nepalese Crane's Bill	Folk/ Nepalese
Geranium nepalense	Ratanjot (var.)	Nepal Geranium, Nepalese Crane's Bill	Folk
Geranium nepalense	Roel	Nepal Geranium, Nepalese Crane's Bill	Folk
Geranium robertianum	Herb Robert	Herb-Robert Geranium	Folk
Geranium wallichianum	Ratanjot	Wallich Crane's Bill	Ayurvedic
Geranium wallichianum	Laal Jadi	Wallich Crane's Bill	Folk
Geranium wallichianum	Laal Jahri	Wallich Crane's Bill	Folk
Geranium wallichianum	Kaoashund	Wallich Crane's Bill	Folk

Table Contd.

Botanical Name	Indian Name	English Name	Medicinal System
Geum urbanum	Gogji-mul	Avens Root, Herb Bennet, Wood Avens	Folk/Kashmir
Ginkgo biloba	Balkuwari	Maidenhair Tree	Folk
Girardinia heterophylla	Vrishchikaa	Himalayan Nettle	Ayurvedic
Girardinia heterophylla	Bichhuu-booti	Himalayan Nettle	Folk
Girardinia heterophylla	Awaa	Himalayan Nettle	Folk
Girardinia heterophylla	Chikri	Himalayan Nettle	Folk
Gironniera reticulata	Kodaittani	Diancaoxieshu (Chinese)	Siddha/Tamil
Gironniera reticulata	Narakyaa-ood	Diancaoxieshu (Chinese)	Folk
Gisekia pharnaceoides	Baalu-ka-saag	Jisucao (Chinese)	Folk
Gisekia pharnaceoides	Morang	Jisucao (Chinese)	Folk
Gisekia pharnaceoides	Sareli	Jisucao (Chinese)	Folk
Gisekia pharnaceoides	Elavaaluka	Jisucao (Chinese)	Ayurvedic
Glinus lotoides	Siru seruppadai	Lotus Sweetjuice, Damascisa	Siddha/Tamil
Glinus lotoides	Gandhi-buuti	Lotus Sweetjuice, Damascisa	Folk
Gloriosa superba	Laangali	Glory Lily, Super Lily, Tiger's Claws	Ayurvedic
Gloriosa superba	Laangaliki	Glory Lily, Super Lily, Tiger's Claws	Ayurvedic
Gloriosa superba	Laangalaki	Glory Lily, Super Lily, Tiger's Claws	Ayurvedic
Gloriosa superba	Laanglaahva	Glory Lily, Super Lily, Tiger's Claws	Ayurvedic
Gloriosa superba	Indrapushpi	Glory Lily, Super Lily, Tiger's Claws	Ayurvedic
Gloriosa superba	Agnishikhaa	Glory Lily, Super Lily, Tiger's Claws	Ayurvedic
Gloriosa superba	Anantaa	Glory Lily, Super Lily, Tiger's Claws	Ayurvedic
Gloriosa superba	Vishaalyaa	Glory Lily, Super Lily, Tiger's Claws	Ayurvedic
Gloriosa superba	Halini	Glory Lily, Super Lily, Tiger's Claws	Ayurvedic
Gloriosa superba	Sirikramaa	Glory Lily, Super Lily, Tiger's Claws	Ayurvedic
Gloriosa superba	Shukra-pushpikaa	Glory Lily, Super Lily, Tiger's Claws	Ayurvedic

Table Contd.

Botanical Name	Indian Name	English Name	Medicinal System
Gloriosa superba	Vahnimukhi	Glory Lily, Super Lily, Tiger's Claws	Ayurvedic
Gloriosa superba	Garbhanut	Glory Lily, Super Lily, Tiger's Claws	Ayurvedic
Gloriosa superba	Garbhapaatani	Glory Lily, Super Lily, Tiger's Claws	Ayurvedic
Gloriosa superba	Kalihaari	Glory Lily, Super Lily, Tiger's Claws	Ayurvedic
Gloriosa superba	Kalikaari	Glory Lily, Super Lily, Tiger's Claws	Ayurvedic
Gloriosa superba	Kalappanki-zhangu	Glory Lily, Super Lily, Tiger's Claws	Siddha/Tamil
Glossocardia bosvallia	Parpata	Pathari, Seri	Ayurvedic
Glossocardia bosvallia	Parapalanamu	Pathari, Seri	Siddha/Tamil
Glycine max	Soyabean	Soybean, Soya	Folk
Glycine max	Raam Kurthi	Soybean, Soya	Folk
Glycine max	Bhat	Soybean, Soya	Folk
Glycosmis pentaphylla	Vana-nimbuukaa	Orangeberry, Ginberry	Ayurvedic
Glycosmis pentaphylla	Ashwa-shaakhota	Orangeberry, Ginberry	Ayurvedic
Glycosmis pentaphylla	Konji	Orangeberry, Ginberry	Siddha/Tamil
Glycosmis pentaphylla	Amam	Orangeberry, Ginberry	Siddha/Tamil
Glycosmis pentaphylla	Kula-pannai	Orangeberry, Ginberry	Siddha/Tamil
Glycosmis pentaphylla	Bana-Nimbu	Orangeberry, Ginberry	Folk
Glycosmis pentaphylla	Paanal	Orangeberry, Ginberry	Folk
Glycyrrhiza glabra	Yashtimadhu	Licorice, Liquorice	Ayurvedic
Glycyrrhiza glabra	Madhuyash-tyaahvaa	Licorice, Liquorice	Ayurvedic
Glycyrrhiza glabra	Madhuli	Licorice, Liquorice	Ayurvedic
Glycyrrhiza glabra	Madhuyashtikaa	Licorice, Liquorice	Ayurvedic
Glycyrrhiza glabra	Atirasaa	Licorice, Liquorice	Ayurvedic
Glycyrrhiza glabra	Madhurasaa	Licorice, Liquorice	Ayurvedic
Glycyrrhiza glabra	Madhuka	Licorice, Liquorice	Ayurvedic
Glycyrrhiza glabra	Yastikaahva	Licorice, Liquorice	Ayurvedic
Glycyrrhiza glabra	Yashtyaahva	Licorice, Liquorice	Ayurvedic
Glycyrrhiza glabra	Yashti	Licorice, Liquorice	Ayurvedic

Table Contd.

Botanical Name	Indian Name	English Name	Medicinal System
Glycyrrhiza glabra	Yashtika	Licorice, Liquorice	Ayurvedic
Glycyrrhiza glabra	Yashtimadhuka	Licorice, Liquorice	Ayurvedic
Glycyrrhiza glabra	Klitaka	Licorice, Liquorice	Ayurvedic
Glycyrrhiza glabra	Asl-us-soos	Licorice, Liquorice	Unani
Glycyrrhiza glabra	Mulethi	Licorice, Liquorice	Unani
Glycyrrhiza glabra	Rubb-us-soos	Licorice, Liquorice	Unani
Glycyrrhiza glabra	Athimathuram	Licorice, Liquorice	Siddha/Tamil
Gmelina arborea	Gambhaari	Candahar Tree, White Teak	Ayurvedic
Gmelina arborea	Kaashmari	Candahar Tree, White Teak	Ayurvedic
Gmelina arborea	Kaashmarya	Candahar Tree, White Teak	Ayurvedic
Gmelina arborea	Sarvatobhadraa	Candahar Tree, White Teak	Ayurvedic
Gmelina arborea	Bhadra	Candahar Tree, White Teak	Ayurvedic
Gmelina arborea	Mahaabhadraa	Candahar Tree, White Teak	Ayurvedic
Gmelina arborea	Sadaabhadraa	Candahar Tree, White Teak	Ayurvedic
Gmelina arborea	Madhuparnikaa	Candahar Tree, White Teak	Ayurvedic
Gmelina arborea	Sriparni	Candahar Tree, White Teak	Ayurvedic
Gmelina arborea	Pitarohini	Candahar Tree, White Teak	Ayurvedic
Gmelina arborea	Hiraa	Candahar Tree, White Teak	Ayurvedic
Gmelina arborea	Bhadraparni	Candahar Tree, White Teak	Ayurvedic
Gmelina arborea	Trishati	Candahar Tree, White Teak	Ayurvedic
Gmelina arborea	Kattanam	Candahar Tree, White Teak	Siddha/Tamil
Gmelina arborea	Kumizham	Candahar Tree, White Teak	Siddha/Tamil
Gmelina asiatica	Gambhaari	Small Cashmere Tree	Ayurvedic
Gmelina asiatica	Gopabhadra	Small Cashmere Tree	Ayurvedic
Gmelina asiatica	Vikarini	Small Cashmere Tree	Ayurvedic
Gmelina asiatica	Kumizham	Small Cashmere Tree	Siddha/Tamil
Gnaphalium luteo-album	Bal-raksha	Jersey Cudweed, Cotton Weed, Cat's Foot, Everlasting Flower	Folk
Gnetum montanum	Anapendu	Joint Fir	Siddha/Tamil
Gnetum montanum	Peiodal	Joint Fir	Siddha/Tamil
Gordonia obtusa	Miyilai	Loblolly Bay, Grey Laurel	Folk/South
Gordonia obtusa	Atangi	Loblolly Bay, Grey Laurel	Folk/South
Gordonia obtusa	Ola	Loblolly Bay, Grey Laurel	Folk/South

Table Contd.

Botanical Name	Indian Name	English Name	Medicinal System
Gordonia obtusa	Nagette	Loblolly Bay, Grey Laurel	Folk/Nilgiri
Gordonia obtusa	Thorilla	Loblolly Bay, Grey Laurel	Folk/South
Gossypium arboreum	Kaarpaasi	Tree Cotton, Desi Cotton	Ayurvedic
Gossypium arboreum	Semparththi	Tree Cotton, Desi Cotton	Siddha/Tamil
Gossypium arboreum	Sivappuparutthi	Tree Cotton, Desi Cotton	Siddha/Tamil
Gossypium arboreum	Kapaasa	Tree Cotton, Desi Cotton	Folk
Gossypium barbadense	Kaarpaasa	Egyptian Cotton, Sea-Island Cotton	Ayurvedic
Gossypium barbadense	Semparuththi	Egyptian Cotton, Sea-Island Cotton	Siddha/Tamil
Gossypium barbadense	Kapaasa	Egyptian Cotton, Sea-Island Cotton	Folk
Gossypium herbaceum	Kaarpaasa	Asiatic Cotton, Levant Cotton, Uppam Cotton	Ayurvedic
Gossypium herbaceum	Kaarpaasi	Asiatic Cotton, Levant Cotton, Uppam Cotton	Ayurvedic
Gossypium herbaceum	Kaarpaasaka	Asiatic Cotton, Levant Cotton, Uppam Cotton	Ayurvedic
Gossypium herbaceum	Rakta-Kaarpaasa	Asiatic Cotton, Levant Cotton, Uppam Cotton	Ayurvedic
Gossypium herbaceum	Shona-Kaarpaasa	Asiatic Cotton, Levant Cotton, Uppam Cotton	Ayurvedic
Gossypium herbaceum	Samudraantaa	Asiatic Cotton, Levant Cotton, Uppam Cotton	Ayurvedic
Gossypium herbaceum	Tuula	Asiatic Cotton, Levant Cotton, Uppam Cotton	Ayurvedic
Gossypium herbaceum	Pichu	Asiatic Cotton, Levant Cotton, Uppam Cotton	Ayurvedic
Gossypium herbaceum	Bhaaradwaaji	Asiatic Cotton, Levant Cotton, Uppam Cotton	Ayurvedic
Gossypium herbaceum	Tundikeri	Asiatic Cotton, Levant Cotton, Uppam Cotton	Ayurvedic
Gossypium herbaceum	Pambahdaanaa	Asiatic Cotton, Levant Cotton, Uppam Cotton	Unani
Gossypium herbaceum	Paruttikkootam	Asiatic Cotton, Levant Cotton, Uppam Cotton	Siddha/Tamil
Gouania leptostachya	Batvaasi	Soapy Chewing-stick Tree	Folk
Gouania leptostachya	Bitkil-chaand	Soapy Chewing-stick Tree	Folk

Table Contd.

Botanical Name	Indian Name	English Name	Medicinal System
Gracilaria lichenoides	Chinai-ghaas	Ceylon Moss	Folk
Grangea maderaspatana	Aakaarakarabha	Madras Carpet	Ayurvedic
Grangea maderaspatana	Maasipathri	Madras Carpet	Siddha/Tamil
Grangea maderaspatana	Mastaru	Madras Carpet	Folk
Grangea maderaspatana	Mukhatari	Madras Carpet	Folk
Grangea maderaspatana	Maachipatri	Madras Carpet	Folk
Graptophyllum picum	Kaalaa-aduusaa	Caricature Plant, Jamaican Cotton	Folk
Graptophyllum picum	Ysjudemaram	Caricature Plant, Jamaican Cotton	Folk/Tamil
Grewia asiatica	Parushaka	Indian Phalsa	Ayurvedic
Grewia asiatica	Parusha	Indian Phalsa	Ayurvedic
Grewia asiatica	Phaalsaa	Indian Phalsa	Unani
Grewia asiatica	Palisa	Indian Phalsa	Siddha/Tamil
Grewia asiatica	Thadachi	Indian Phalsa	Siddha/Tamil
Grewia hirsuta	Naagabalaa	Veronicalolia, Naagbala	Ayurvedic
Grewia hirsuta	Gud-sharkaraa	Veronicalolia, Naagbala	Ayurvedic
Grewia hirsuta	Gulshakari	Veronicalolia, Naagbala	Folk
Grewia hirsuta	Tavadu	Veronicalolia, Naagbala	Siddha/Tamil
Grewia populifolia	Gaangeru (ki)	Orange-red Phalsa, Tapadi	Ayurvedic
Grewia populifolia	Achhu	Orange-red Phalsa, Tapadi	Siddha/Tamil
Grewia populifolia	Gangeran	Orange-red Phalsa, Tapadi	Folk
Grewia sclerophylla	Parushaka	Bhokota	Ayurvedic
Grewia sclerophylla	Dhanvana	Bhokota	Ayurvedic
Grewia sclerophylla	Kattu Kadali	Bhokota	Siddha/Tamil
Grewia sclerophylla	Jangali Phaalsaa	Bhokota	Folk
Grewia tiliaefolia	Dhanvana	Dhaman	Ayurvedic
Grewia tiliaefolia	Dhanur-vriksha	Dhaman	Ayurvedic
Grewia tiliaefolia	Tarra	Dhaman	Siddha/Tamil
Grewia tiliaefolia	Unnu	Dhaman	Siddha/Tamil
Grewia tiliaefolia	Sadachi	Dhaman	Siddha/Tamil
Grewia tiliaefolia	Dhaamin	Dhaman	Folk
Grewia tiliaefolia	Dhaaman	Dhaman	Folk
Grewia villosa	Kullai	Tamthar	Siddha/Tamil
Grewia villosa	Dhohan	Tamthar	Folk

Table Contd.

Botanical Name	Indian Name	English Name	Medicinal System
Hardwickia binata	Anjana	Copaiba-grade Balsam	Ayurvedic
Hardwickia binata	Katudugu	Copaiba-grade Balsam	Siddha/Tamil
Hardwickia binata	Kodapalai	Copaiba-grade Balsam	Siddha/Tamil
Hedera helix	Maravalai	Common Ivy, Bentwood	Siddha/Tamil
Hedera nepalensis	Baandaa	Nepal Ivy	Folk
Hedera nepalensis	Bandaa	Nepal Ivy	Folk
Hedera nepalensis	Lablab	Nepal Ivy	Folk
Hedychium coronarium	Shati	Ginger Ivy	Ayurvedic
Hedychium spicatum	Shathi	Spiked Ginger Ivy	Ayurvedic
Hedychium spicatum	Shati	Spiked Ginger Ivy	Ayurvedic
Hedychium spicatum	Gandhashathi	Spiked Ginger Ivy	Ayurvedic
Hedychium spicatum	Gandhapalaashi	Spiked Ginger Ivy	Ayurvedic
Hedychium spicatum	Kapuurkachari	Spiked Ginger Ivy	Ayurvedic
Hedychium spicatum	Suvrataa	Spiked Ginger Ivy	Ayurvedic
Hedychium spicatum	Gandhaarikaa	Spiked Ginger Ivy	Ayurvedic
Hedychium spicatum	Gandhavadhuu	Spiked Ginger Ivy	Ayurvedic
Hedychium spicatum	Gandhamuulikaa	Spiked Ginger Ivy	Ayurvedic
Hedychium spicatum	Kapuurkachari	Spiked Ginger Ivy	Unani
Hedychium spicatum	Poolankizangu	Spiked Ginger Ivy	Siddha/Tamil
Hedychium spicatum	Kichilikizangu	Spiked Ginger Ivy	Siddha/Tamil
Hedychium spicatum	Ban-haldi	Spiked Ginger Ivy	Folk
Hedyotis corymbosa	Kshetraparpata	Old World Diamond Flower	Ayurvedic
Helianthus annuus	Suurajmukhi	Sunflower	Ayurvedic
Helianthus annuus	Suuryaavarta	Sunflower	Ayurvedic
Helianthus annuus	Suryakanti	Sunflower	Siddha/Tamil
Helicteres isora	Aavartani	East Indian Screw Tree	Ayurvedic
Helicteres isora	Aavartphalaa	East Indian Screw Tree	Ayurvedic
Helicteres isora	Aavartaki	East Indian Screw Tree	Ayurvedic
Helicteres isora	Marorphali	East Indian Screw Tree	Unani
Helicteres isora	Valampiri	East Indian Screw Tree	Siddha/Tamil
Heliotropium indicum	Hastishundi	Scorpion Tail	Ayurvedic
Heliotropium indicum	Duraalabhaa	Scorpion Tail	Ayurvedic
Heliotropium indicum	Vrischikaali	Scorpion Tail	Ayurvedic

Table Contd.

Botanical Name	Indian Name	English Name	Medicinal System
Heliotropium indicum	Thaelkodukku-ppondu	Scorpion Tail	Siddha/Tamil
Helleborus niger	Khuraasaani Kutaki	Black Hellebore, Christmas Rose	Ayurvedic
Helleborus niger	Kharbaq Siyah	Black Hellebore, Christmas Rose	Unani
Helleborus niger	Khuraasaani Kutaki	Black Hellebore, Christmas Rose	Unani
Hemerocallis fulva	Tiger Lily	Common Yellow Day-lily, Tawny Day-lily, Orange Day-lily	Folk
Hemidesmus indicus	Shveta Saarivaa	Indian Sarsaparilla	Ayurvedic
Hemidesmus indicus	Anantmuula	Indian Sarsaparilla	Ayurvedic
Hemidesmus indicus	Gopi	Indian Sarsaparilla	Ayurvedic
Hemidesmus indicus	Gopaa	Indian Sarsaparilla	Ayurvedic
Hemidesmus indicus	Gopakanyaa	Indian Sarsaparilla	Ayurvedic
Hemidesmus indicus	Gopavalli	Indian Sarsaparilla	Ayurvedic
Hemidesmus indicus	Gopasutaa	Indian Sarsaparilla	Ayurvedic
Hemidesmus indicus	Krishodari	Indian Sarsaparilla	Ayurvedic
Hemidesmus indicus	Sphotaa	Indian Sarsaparilla	Ayurvedic
Hemidesmus indicus	Utpalsaarivaa	Indian Sarsaparilla	Ayurvedic
Hemidesmus indicus	Kapuuri	Indian Sarsaparilla	Ayurvedic
Hemidesmus indicus	Dugdhgarbhaa	Indian Sarsaparilla	Ayurvedic
Hemidesmus indicus	Ushbaa Hindi	Indian Sarsaparilla	Unani
Hemidesmus indicus	Nannaari	Indian Sarsaparilla	Siddha/Tamil
Hemidesmus indicus	Suganthipala	Indian Sarsaparilla	Siddha/Tamil
Hemionitis arifolia	Chakuliya	Male Fern	Folk
Hemionitis arifolia	Raamabaanam	Male Fern	Folk
Heracleum candicans	Kaindal	Cowparsnip	Folk
Heracleum candicans	Gandhraayana	Cowparsnip	Folk
Herniaria glabra	Herniary	Smooth Rupture-Wort	Folk
Heterophragma roxburghii	Waarasa	Karen Wood	Ayurvedic
Heterophragma roxburghii	Barokalagoru	Karen Wood	Siddha/Tamil
Heterophragma roxburghii	Paatang	Karen Wood	Folk
Heterophragma roxburghii	Pullunga	Karen Wood	Folk
Hibiscus abelmoschus	Kasturi-vendai	Musk Seed, Ambette Seed, Muskmallow	Siddha/Tamil

Table Contd.

Botanical Name	Indian Name	English Name	Medicinal System
Hibiscus abelmoschus	Mushkdaanaa	Musk Seed, Ambette Seed, Muskmallow	Unani
Hibiscus abelmoschus	Kattaphala	Musk Seed, Ambette Seed, Muskmallow	Ayurvedic
Hibiscus abelmoschus	Katuka	Musk Seed, Ambette Seed, Muskmallow	Ayurvedic
Hibiscus abelmoschus	Lataakasturi	Musk Seed, Ambette Seed, Muskmallow	Ayurvedic
Hibiscus abelmoschus	Lataakasturikaa	Musk Seed, Ambette Seed, Muskmallow	Ayurvedic
Hibiscus cannabinus	Pulichhai	Bimlipatam Jute, Kenaf, Mesta, Deccan Hemp	Folk/Tamil
Hibiscus cannabinus	Kasini	Bimlipatam Jute, Kenaf, Mesta, Deccan Hemp	Folk/Tamil
Hibiscus cannabinus	Konda-gengura	Bimlipatam Jute, Kenaf, Mesta, Deccan Hemp	Folk/Telugu
Hibiscus cannabinus	Patsan	Bimlipatam Jute, Kenaf, Mesta, Deccan Hemp	Folk
Hibiscus cannabinus	Ambari	Bimlipatam Jute, Kenaf, Mesta, Deccan Hemp	Folk
Hibiscus cannabinus	Ambaadi	Bimlipatam Jute, Kenaf, Mesta, Deccan Hemp	Folk
Hibiscus mutabilis	Sthala-Padam	Cotton-Rose, Chinese-Rose, Confederate Rose	Ayurvedic
Hibiscus mutabilis	Sthal-Kamal	Cotton-Rose, Chinese-Rose, Confederate Rose	Ayurvedic
Hibiscus mutabilis	Irratai-vellai-chembarattam	Cotton-Rose, Chinese-Rose, Confederate Rose	Siddha/Tamil
Hibiscus mutabilis	Sembarattai	Cotton-Rose, Chinese-Rose, Confederate Rose	Siddha/Tamil
Hibiscus rosa-sinensis	Gul-e-Gurhal	Rose-of-China, Shoe-flower, Chinese Hibiscus	Unani
Hibiscus rosa-sinensis	Semparatthai Poo/Elai (Flower/leaf)	Rose-of-China, Shoe-flower, Chinese Hibiscus	Siddha/Tamil
Hibiscus rosa-sinensis	Japaa	Rose-of-China, Shoe-flower, Chinese Hibiscus	Ayurvedic
Hibiscus rosa-sinensis	Javaa	Rose-of-China, Shoe-flower, Chinese Hibiscus	Ayurvedic

Table Contd.

Botanical Name	Indian Name	English Name	Medicinal System
Hibiscus rosa-sinensis	Odrapushpa	Rose-of-China, Shoe-flower, Chinese Hibiscus	Ayurvedic
Hibiscus rosa-sinensis	Rudrapushpa	Rose-of-China, Shoe-flower, Chinese Hibiscus	Ayurvedic
Hibiscus rosa-sinensis	Arunaa	Rose-of-China, Shoe-flower, Chinese Hibiscus	Ayurvedic
Hibiscus sabdariffa	Ambashtthaki	Roselle, Jamaican Sorrel, Natal Sorrel, Red Sorrel	Ayurvedic
Hibiscus sabdariffa	Sivappu kashmakki	Roselle, Jamaican Sorrel, Natal Sorrel, Red Sorrel	Siddha/Tamil
Hibiscus sabdariffa	Pulichai-keerai	Roselle, Jamaican Sorrel, Natal Sorrel, Red Sorrel	Siddha/Tamil
Hibiscus sabdariffa	Ettagonguru	Roselle, Jamaican Sorrel, Natal Sorrel, Red Sorrel	Folk/Telugu
Hibiscus sabdariffa	Seemai kasuru	Roselle, Jamaican Sorrel, Natal Sorrel, Red Sorrel	Siddha/Tamil
Hibiscus sabdariffa	Laal-ambaari	Roselle, Jamaican Sorrel, Natal Sorrel, Red Sorrel	Folk
Hibiscus sabdariffa	Patavaa	Roselle, Jamaican Sorrel, Natal Sorrel, Red Sorrel	Folk
Hibiscus sabdariffa	Patsan	Roselle, Jamaican Sorrel, Natal Sorrel, Red Sorrel	Folk
Hibiscus surattensis	Ran Bhindi	Wild Sour, Bush Sorrel	Ayurvedic
Hibiscus surattensis	Kishli-keerai	Wild Sour, Bush Sorrel	Siddha/Tamil
Hippophae rhamnoides	Dhurchuk	Seabuckthorn, Sand Thorn	Folk
Hippophae rhamnoides	Chumaa	Seabuckthorn, Sand Thorn	Folk
Hippophae rhamnoides	Tarwaa	Seabuckthorn, Sand Thorn	Folk
Hippophae rhamnoides	Sirmaa	Seabuckthorn, Sand Thorn	Folk
Hiptage benghalensis	Atimukta	Hiptage	Ayurvedic
Hiptage benghalensis	Atimuktaka	Hiptage	Ayurvedic
Hiptage benghalensis	Maadhavi	Hiptage	Ayurvedic
Hiptage benghalensis	Vaasanti	Hiptage	Ayurvedic
Hiptage benghalensis	Pundrika	Hiptage	Ayurvedic
Hiptage benghalensis	Mandaka	Hiptage	Ayurvedic
Hiptage benghalensis	Vimukta	Hiptage	Ayurvedic
Hiptage benghalensis	Kaamuka	Hiptage	Ayurvedic
Hiptage benghalensis	Maadhavi	Hiptage	Siddha/Tamil

Table Contd.

Botanical Name	Indian Name	English Name	Medicinal System
Hiptage benghalensis	Vasandagala-malligai	Hiptage	Siddha/Tamil
Holarrhena antidysenterica	Kutaja	Easter Tree, Ivory Tree, Tellicherry Bark	Ayurvedic
Holarrhena antidysenterica	Girimallikaa	Easter Tree, Ivory Tree, Tellicherry Bark	Ayurvedic
Holarrhena antidysenterica	Kaalinga	Easter Tree, Ivory Tree, Tellicherry Bark	Ayurvedic
Holarrhena antidysenterica	Kalingaka	Easter Tree, Ivory Tree, Tellicherry Bark	Ayurvedic
Holarrhena antidysenterica	Indravriksha	Easter Tree, Ivory Tree, Tellicherry	Ayurvedic
Holarrhena antidysenterica	Shakra	Easter Tree, Ivory Tree, Tellicherry	Ayurvedic
Holarrhena antidysenterica	Vatsa	Easter Tree, Ivory Tree, Tellicherry	Ayurvedic
Holarrhena antidysenterica	Vatsaka	Easter Tree, Ivory Tree, Tellicherry	Ayurvedic
Holarrhena antidysenterica	Shakraahvya	Easter Tree, Ivory Tree, Tellicherry	Ayurvedic
Holarrhena antidysenterica	Indrayava (Seed)	Easter Tree, Ivory Tree, Tellicherry	Ayurvedic
Holarrhena antidysenterica	Indrabija (Seed)	Easter Tree, Ivory Tree, Tellicherry	Ayurvedic
Holarrhena antidysenterica	Vatsabija (Seed)	Easter Tree, Ivory Tree, Tellicherry	Ayurvedic
Holarrhena antidysenterica	Kurchi (Bark)	Easter Tree, Ivory Tree, Tellicherry	Ayurvedic
Holarrhena antidysenterica	Inderjo Talkh (Seed)	Easter Tree, Ivory Tree, Tellicherry	Unani
Holarrhena antidysenterica	Teewaaj-e-Khataai	Easter Tree, Ivory Tree, Tellicherry	Unani
Holarrhena antidysenterica	Kudasappaalai-pattai (Bark)	Easter Tree, Ivory Tree, Tellicherry	Siddha/Tamil
Holarrhena antidysenterica	Kudasappaalai-vidai (Seed)	Easter Tree, Ivory Tree, Tellicherry	Siddha/Tamil
Holoptelea integrifolia	Chirbilva	Indian Elm, Kanju Wood	Ayurvedic
Holoptelea integrifolia	Putika	Indian Elm, Kanju Wood	Ayurvedic
Holoptelea integrifolia	Prakirya	Indian Elm, Kanju Wood	Ayurvedic

Table Contd.

Botanical Name	Indian Name	English Name	Medicinal System
Holoptelea integrifolia	Avil thol	Indian Elm, Kanju Wood	Folk/Tamil
Holoptelea integrifolia	Ayil pattai (bark)	Indian Elm, Kanju Wood	Folk/Tamil
Holostemma annularis	Ark-pushpi	Holostemma Creeper	Ayurvedic
Holostemma annularis	Palay-keerai	Holostemma Creeper	Folk/Tamil
Homonoia riparia	Paashaana-bheda	Willow-leaved Water Croton	Ayurvedic
Homonoia riparia	Kshudra Paashaana-bheda	Willow-leaved Water Croton	Ayurvedic
Homonoia riparia	Kattu alari	Willow-leaved Water Croton	Siddha/Tamil
Hordeum vulgare	Yava	Barley	Ayurvedic
Hordeum vulgare	Hayeshtha	Barley	Ayurvedic
Hordeum vulgare	Hayapriya	Barley	Ayurvedic
Hordeum vulgare	Shuka-dhaanya	Barley	Ayurvedic
Hordeum vulgare	Tikshnashuka	Barley	Ayurvedic
Hordeum vulgare	Barley	Barley	Unani
Hordeum vulgare	Jao Shaeer	Barley	Unani
Hordeum vulgare	Yavam	Barley	Folk/Tamil
Hordeum vulgare	Saambaluppu (ash)	Barley	Siddha/Tamil
Hovenia dulcis	Sikkaa	Japanese Raisin Tree, Coral Tree	Folk
Hugonia mystax	Kaakibeeraa	Climbing Flax	Folk
Hugonia mystax	Kansamaara	Climbing Flax	Folk
Hugonia mystax	Agori	Climbing Flax	Siddha/Tamil
Hugonia mystax	Motirakkanni	Climbing Flax	Siddha/Tamil
Humulus lupulus	Hashish-ut-Dinaar	Hops	Unani
Hura crepitans	Mullarasanam	Sandbox Tree, Monkey Dinner-bell	Siddha/Tamil
Hydnocarpus kurzii	Tuvaraka	Chalmogra	Ayurvedic
Hydnocarpus kurzii	Chaalmograa	Chalmogra	Unani
Hydnocarpus kurzii	Tukhm-e-Biranj Mograa	Chalmogra	Unani
Hydnocarpus kurzii	Niradi-muththu	Chalmogra	Siddha/Tamil
Hydnocarpus laurifolia	Tuvaraka	Soorty Oil Tree	Ayurvedic
Hydnocarpus laurifolia	Katu-Kapittha	Soorty Oil Tree	Ayurvedic
Hydnocarpus laurifolia	Kushtavairi	Soorty Oil Tree	Ayurvedic

Table Contd.

Botanical Name	Indian Name	English Name	Medicinal System
Hydnocarpus laurifolia	Garudaphala	Soorty Oil Tree	Ayurvedic
Hydnocarpus laurifolia	Chaalmograa	Soorty Oil Tree	Ayurvedic
Hydnocarpus laurifolia	Chaalmograa	Soorty Oil Tree	Unani
Hydnocarpus laurifolia	Tukhm-e-Biranj Mograa	Soorty Oil Tree	Unani
Hydnocarpus laurifolia	Niradi-muttu	Soorty Oil Tree	Siddha/Tamil
Hydnocarpus laurifolia	Maravattai	Soorty Oil Tree	Siddha/Tamil
Hydrocotyle javanica	Manduukaparni	Java Pennywort	Folk
Hydrocotyle javanica	Brahma-manduuki	Java Pennywort	Folk
Hydrolea zeylanica	Laangali (Kerala)	Ceylon Hydrolea	Ayurvedic
Hygrophila auriculata	Kokilaaksha	Indian Swampweed	Ayurvedic
Hygrophila auriculata	Kokilaakshi	Indian Swampweed	Ayurvedic
Hygrophila auriculata	Ikshuraka	Indian Swampweed	Ayurvedic
Hygrophila auriculata	Ikshura	Indian Swampweed	Ayurvedic
Hygrophila auriculata	Kshuraka	Indian Swampweed	Ayurvedic
Hygrophila auriculata	Bikshu	Indian Swampweed	Ayurvedic
Hygrophila auriculata	Kaakekshu	Indian Swampweed	Ayurvedic
Hygrophila auriculata	Taalmakhaanaa	Indian Swampweed	Unani
Hygrophila auriculata	Neermulli	Indian Swampweed	Siddha/Tamil
Hymenodictyon excelsum	Bhramar-chhalikaa	Bridal Couch Tree	Ayurvedic
Hymenodictyon excelsum	Ugragandhaa	Bridal Couch Tree	Ayurvedic
Hymenodictyon excelsum	Bhringa-vriksha	Bridal Couch Tree	Ayurvedic
Hymenodictyon excelsum	Sagappu	Bridal Couch Tree	Siddha/Tamil
Hymenodictyon excelsum	Vellei Kadambu	Bridal Couch Tree	Siddha/Tamil
Hymenodictyon excelsum	Peranjoli	Bridal Couch Tree	Siddha/Tamil
Hymenodictyon excelsum	Bhaulan	Bridal Couch Tree	Folk
Hymenodictyon excelsum	Bhramarchhali	Bridal Couch Tree	Folk
Hymenodictyon excelsum	Bhuurkunda	Bridal Couch Tree	Folk
Hyoscyamus muticus	Paarsika-yavaani	Egyptian Henbane	Ayurvedic
Hyoscyamus muticus	Turushkaa	Egyptian Henbane	Ayurvedic

Table Contd.

Botanical Name	Indian Name	English Name	Medicinal System
Hyoscyamus muticus	Ajwaayin Khuraasaani	Egyptian Henbane	Unani
Hyoscyamus muticus	Shuukraan	Egyptian Henbane	Unani
Hyoscyamus muticus	Tukhm-bang	Egyptian Henbane	Unani
Hyoscyamus muticus	Vajra-bhang	Egyptian Henbane	Folk
Hyoscyamus niger	Paarsika-yavaani	Indian Henbane, Black Henbane	Ayurvedic
Hyoscyamus niger	Yavaani	Indian Henbane, Black Henbane	Ayurvedic
Hyoscyamus niger	Madkaarini	Indian Henbane, Black Henbane	Ayurvedic
Hyoscyamus niger	Turushkaa	Indian Henbane, Black Henbane	Ayurvedic
Hyoscyamus niger	Khuraashaanikaa	Indian Henbane, Black Henbane	Ayurvedic
Hyoscyamus niger	Khuraasaani Ajwaayin	Indian Henbane, Black Henbane	Ayurvedic
Hyoscyamus niger	Barz-ul-Banj	Indian Henbane, Black Henbane	Unani
Hyoscyamus niger	Khuraasaani Ajwaayin	Indian Henbane, Black Henbane	Unani
Hyoscyamus niger	Paarseeka yavaani	Indian Henbane, Black Henbane	Siddha/Tamil
Hyoscyamus niger	Khurasani Omam	Indian Henbane, Black Henbane	Siddha/Tamil
Hypecoum leptocarpum	Zirgulaki	Waziri Opium Herb	Folk
Hypecoum leptocarpum	Waziri	Waziri Opium Herb	Folk
Hypericum perforatum	Heufaariqoon	Common St. John's Wort	Unani
Hypericum perforatum	Bassant	Common St. John's Wort	Unani
Hypericum perforatum	Balsaan	Common St. John's Wort	Unani
Hyptis suaveolens	Tumbaaka	American Mint, American Patchouli	Ayurvedic
Hyptis suaveolens	Gangaa Tulasi	American Mint, American Patchouli	Folk
Hyptis suaveolens	Vilaayati Tulasi	American Mint, American Patchouli	Folk
Hyptis suaveolens	Bhunsari	American Mint, American Patchouli	Folk
Hyssopus officinalis	Dayaa-kunji	Hyssop	Ayurvedic
Hyssopus officinalis	Zuufaa	Hyssop	Unani
Hyssopus officinalis	Zuufaa Yaabis	Hyssop	Unani
Hyssopus officinalis	Diyaanku	Hyssop	Folk

Table Contd.

Botanical Name	Indian Name	English Name	Medicinal System
Iberis amara	Candy-tuft	Rocket Candy-tuft, Clown's Mustard	Folk
Ichnocarpus frutescens	Gopavalli	Black Creeper	Ayurvedic
Ichnocarpus frutescens	Krishna Saarivaa (var.)	Black Creeper	Ayurvedic
Ichnocarpus frutescens	Krishna-muuli	Black Creeper	Ayurvedic
Ichnocarpus frutescens	Shyaamalataa	Black Creeper	Ayurvedic
Ichnocarpus frutescens	Karunannari	Black Creeper	Siddha/Tamil
Ichnocarpus frutescens	Makalikilanzhu	Black Creeper	Siddha/Tamil
Ichnocarpus frutescens	Kaalisar	Black Creeper	Folk
Ichnocarpus frutescens	Karantaa	Black Creeper	Folk
Ilex aquifolium	Holly	English Holly, Common Holly	Folk
Ilex paraguariensis	Mate Tea	Mate Tea, Yerba Mate, Paraguay Tea	Folk
Illicium anisatum	Baadiyaan	Star Anise	Unani
Illicium verum	Baadyaan Khataai	Star Anise, Chinese Anise, Aniseed Stars	Unani
Illicium verum	Takkola	Star Anise, Chinese Anise, Aniseed Stars	Ayurvedic
Illicium verum	Anasippo	Star Anise, Chinese Anise, Aniseed Stars	Siddha/Tamil
Illicium verum	Anasphal	Star Anise, Chinese Anise, Aniseed Stars	Folk
Impatiens balsamina	Tarini	Garden Balsam	Ayurvedic
Impatiens balsamina	Gul-menhdi	Garden Balsam	Unani
Impatiens balsamina	Kasittumbai	Garden Balsam	Siddha/Tamil
Imperata cylindrica	Darbha	Thatch Grass	Ayurvedic
Imperata cylindrica	Suuchyagra	Thatch Grass	Ayurvedic
Imperata cylindrica	Yagnika	Thatch Grass	Ayurvedic
Imperata cylindrica	Yagyabhuushana	Thatch Grass	Ayurvedic
Imperata cylindrica	Bahir	Thatch Grass	Ayurvedic
Imperata cylindrica	Dharba	Thatch Grass	Siddha/Tamil
Imperata cylindrica	Daabh	Thatch Grass	Folk
Indigofera arrecta	Nili	Natal Indigo, Java Indigo, Bengal Indigo	Ayurvedic

Table Contd.

Botanical Name	Indian Name	English Name	Medicinal System
Indigofera articulata	Nili	Egyptian Indigo, Arabian Indigo, Wild Indigo, Surat Indigo	Ayurvedic
Indigofera articulata	Aaramuri	Egyptian Indigo, Arabian Indigo, Wild Indigo, Surat Indigo	Siddha/Tamil
Indigofera articulata	Iruppumuri	Egyptian Indigo, Arabian Indigo, Wild Indigo, Surat Indigo	Siddha/Tamil
Indigofera articulata	Kattavuri	Egyptian Indigo, Arabian Indigo, Wild Indigo, Surat Indigo	Siddha/Tamil
Indigofera articulata	Surmai Nila	Egyptian Indigo, Arabian Indigo, Wild Indigo, Surat Indigo	Folk
Indigofera aspalathoides	Nili	Wiry Indigo	Ayurvedic
Indigofera aspalathoides	Shivanimba	Wiry Indigo	Ayurvedic
Indigofera aspalathoides	Sivanaarvembu	Wiry Indigo	Siddha/Tamil
Indigofera aspalathoides	Iraivanvembu	Wiry Indigo	Siddha/Tamil
Indigofera aspalathoides	Shivanimba	Wiry Indigo	Folk
Indigofera enneaphylla	Vaasukaa	Trailing Indigo	Ayurvedic
Indigofera enneaphylla	Cheppunerinjil	Trailing Indigo	Siddha/Tamil
Indigofera enneaphylla	Hanumaan-buuti	Trailing Indigo	Folk
Indigofera enneaphylla	Bhui-nila	Trailing Indigo	Folk
Indigofera oblongifolia	Bana-Nila	Wild Indigo, Mysore Panicled Indigo	Ayurvedic
Indigofera oblongifolia	Dill	Wild Indigo, Mysore Panicled Indigo	Ayurvedic
Indigofera oblongifolia	Jhill	Wild Indigo, Mysore Panicled Indigo	Ayurvedic
Indigofera oblongifolia	Vasmaa	Wild Indigo, Mysore Panicled Indigo	Unani
Indigofera oblongifolia	Kattukkar-chammathi	Wild Indigo, Mysore Panicled Indigo	Siddha/Tamil
Indigofera oblongifolia	Nili	Wild Indigo, Mysore Panicled Indigo	Folk
Indigofera pulchella	Nili	Cassia Indigo	Ayurvedic
Indigofera pulchella	Nirinji	Cassia Indigo	Siddha/Tamil
Indigofera tinctoria	Nilikaa	Indigo	Ayurvedic
Indigofera tinctoria	Gramyaa	Indigo	Ayurvedic
Indigofera tinctoria	Shriphalaa	Indigo	Ayurvedic

Table Contd.

Botanical Name	Indian Name	English Name	Medicinal System
Ipomoea marginata	Tirutaalli	Purple Heart Morning Glory	Folk
Ipomoea muricata	Krishnabija	Traveller's Midnight Lilies	Ayurvedic
Ipomoea muricata	Kattu talai	Traveller's Midnight Lilies	Folk/Tamil
Ipomoea muricata	Michaai	Traveller's Midnight Lilies	Folk
Ipomoea nil	Antah-kotarpushpi	Pharbitis Seeds	Ayurvedic
Ipomoea nil	Kaalaanjani	Pharbitis Seeds	Ayurvedic
Ipomoea nil	Krishnabija	Pharbitis Seeds	Ayurvedic
Ipomoea nil	Kaalaadaanaa	Pharbitis Seeds	Ayurvedic
Ipomoea nil	Shyaamabija	Pharbitis Seeds	Ayurvedic
Ipomoea nil	Shankhani	Pharbitis Seeds	Ayurvedic
Ipomoea nil	Jhaaramaaricha	Pharbitis Seeds	Ayurvedic
Ipomoea nil	Kaalaadaanaa	Pharbitis Seeds	Unani
Ipomoea nil	Kaakkattan	Pharbitis Seeds	Folk/Tamil
Ipomoea pes-caprae	Chhagalaantri	Goat's Foot Creeper	Ayurvedic
Ipomoea pes-caprae	Maryaada-valli	Goat's Foot Creeper	Ayurvedic
Ipomoea pes-caprae	Adambu	Goat's Foot Creeper	Siddha/Tamil
Ipomoea pes-caprae	Attukkal	Goat's Foot Creeper	Folk/Tamil
Ipomoea pes-caprae	Musattalai	Goat's Foot Creeper	Folk/Tamil
Ipomoea petaloidea	Shyaamaa	False Jalap, Hawaii Morning Glory	Ayurvedic
Ipomoea petaloidea	Chhaagalaantri	False Jalap, Hawaii Morning Glory	Ayurvedic
Ipomoea petaloidea	Vriddhadaaraka	False Jalap, Hawaii Morning Glory	Ayurvedic
Ipomoea petaloidea	Vriddhadaaru	False Jalap, Hawaii Morning Glory	Ayurvedic
Ipomoea petaloidea	Shaaraf	False Jalap, Hawaii Morning Glory	Unani
Ipomoea petaloidea	Nilapoosani	False Jalap, Hawaii Morning Glory	Siddha/Tamil
Ipomoea petaloidea	Bidhaaraa	False Jalap, Hawaii Morning Glory	Folk
Ipomoea petaloidea	Nishoth (black var.)	False Jalap, Hawaii Morning Glory	Folk
Ipomoea purga	Jalaapaa	Jalap	Folk

Table Contd.

Botanical Name	Indian Name	English Name	Medicinal System
Ipomoea purpurea	Karakatiyaa (Seeds)	Tall Morning-Glory	Folk
Ipomoea quamoclit	Kaamalataa	Cypress Vine, Indian Pink	Ayurvedic
Ipomoea quamoclit	Kembumalligai	Cypress Vine, Indian Pink	Siddha/Tamil
Ipomoea quamoclit	Mayirmanikkam	Cypress Vine, Indian Pink	Siddha/Tamil
Ipomoea quamoclit	Sitaakesh	Cypress Vine, Indian Pink	Folk
Ipomoea reniformis	Aakhuparni	Mouse-ear Shrub	Ayurvedic
Ipomoea reniformis	Aakhuparnika	Mouse-ear Shrub	Ayurvedic
Ipomoea reniformis	Muusaakarni	Mouse-ear Shrub	Ayurvedic
Ipomoea reniformis	Aakhukarni	Mouse-ear Shrub	Ayurvedic
Ipomoea reniformis	Undurukarnikaa	Mouse-ear Shrub	Ayurvedic
Ipomoea reniformis	Yelikkaad-hukeerai	Mouse-ear Shrub	Siddha/Tamil
Ipomoea reniformis	Perettaikkirai	Mouse-ear Shrub	Siddha/Tamil
Ipomoea sepiaria	Banakalami	Big-flowered Morning Glory	Ayurvedic
Ipomoea sepiaria	Hanumaan-Vel	Big-flowered Morning Glory	Ayurvedic
Ipomoea sepiaria	Manjika	Big-flowered Morning Glory	Ayurvedic
Ipomoea sepiaria	Thaalikeerai	Big-flowered Morning Glory	Siddha/Tamil
Ipomoea vitifolia	Nauli	Funnei-flowered Twiner	Folk
Ipomoea vitifolia	Nawal	Funnei-flowered Twiner	Folk
Iris ensata	Paarseeka Vachaa	Japanese Iris	Ayurvedic
Iris ensata	Haimavati	Japanese Iris	Ayurvedic
Iris ensata	Shveta Vachaa	Japanese Iris	Ayurvedic
Iris ensata	Baalbach	Japanese Iris	Ayurvedic
Iris ensata	Irsaa	Japanese Iris	Unani
Iris ensata	Sosan	Japanese Iris	Unani
Iris ensata	Iris	Japanese Iris	Unani
Iris ensata	Marjal	Japanese Iris	Folk
Iris ensata	Unarjal	Japanese Iris	Folk
Iris germanica	Paarseeka Vachaa	Orris, Iridis Rhizome, German Iris	Ayurvedic
Iris germanica	Haimavati	Orris, Iridis Rhizome, German Iris	Ayurvedic
Iris germanica	Shveta Vachaa	Orris, Iridis Rhizome, German Iris	Ayurvedic
Iris germanica	Baal-bach	Orris, Iridis Rhizome, German Iris	Ayurvedic

Table Contd.

Botanical Name	Indian Name	English Name	Medicinal System
Iris kumaonensis	Karkar	Kumaon Iris	Folk
Iris kumaonensis	Tezma	Kumaon Iris	Folk
Iris nepalensis	Paarseeka Vachaa	Nepal Iris	Ayurvedic
Iris nepalensis	Sosan	Nepal Iris	Folk
Iris nepalensis	Shoti	Nepal Iris	Folk
Iris nepalensis	Chalnundar	Nepal Iris	Folk
Iris nepalensis	Chiluchi	Nepal Iris	Folk
Iris pseudacorus	Paashaanabheda	Yellow Flag	Folk
Iris versicolour	Haimavati Vachaa	Blue Flag Root, Liver Lity	Ayurvedic
Isatis tinctoria	Woad	German Indigo	Folk
Ixora coccinea	Bandhuka	Jungleflame Ixora	Ayurvedic
Ixora coccinea	Paaranti	Jungleflame Ixora	Ayurvedic
Ixora coccinea	Vetchi	Jungleflame Ixora	Siddha/Tamil
Ixora coccinea	Kullai	Jungleflame Ixora	Folk/Tamil
Ixora coccinea	Rukmini	Jungleflame Ixora	Folk
Ixora coccinea	Rangan	Jungleflame Ixora	Folk
Ixora parviflora	Nevari	Torchwood Tree	Ayurvedic
Ixora parviflora	Nevali	Torchwood Tree	Ayurvedic
Ixora parviflora	Ishwara	Torchwood Tree	Ayurvedic
Ixora parviflora	Rangan	Torchwood Tree	Ayurvedic
Ixora parviflora	Shulundu-kora	Torchwood Tree	Siddha/Tamil
Ixora parviflora	Korivi	Torchwood Tree	Folk/Tamil
Jacaranda acutifolia	Nili-gulmohar	Brazil Rosewood, Green Ebony	Folk
Jasminum angustifolium	Aasphotaa	Wild Jasmine	Ayurvedic
Jasminum angustifolium	Bana-mallikaa	Wild Jasmine	Ayurvedic
Jasminum angustifolium	Vana-malli	Wild Jasmine	Ayurvedic
Jasminum angustifolium	Kaanan-mallikaa	Wild Jasmine	Ayurvedic
Jasminum angustifolium	Kaatumalli	Wild Jasmine	Siddha/Tamil
Jasminum arborescens	Nava-mallikaa	Tree Jasmine	Ayurvedic
Jasminum arborescens	Chameli (var.)	Tree Jasmine	Folk
Jasminum arborescens	Maalati (var.)	Tree Jasmine	Folk

Table Contd.

Botanical Name	Indian Name	English Name	Medicinal System
Jasminum arborescens	Nagamalli	Tree Jasmine	Siddha/Tamil
Jasminum auriculatum	Juuhi	Cultivated Jasmine	Folk
Jasminum auriculatum	Usimalligai	Cultivated Jasmine	Siddha/Tamil
Jasminum auriculatum	Mugdhee	Cultivated Jasmine	Ayurvedic
Jasminum auriculatum	Yuuthi	Cultivated Jasmine	Ayurvedic
Jasminum auriculatum	Yuuthikaa	Cultivated Jasmine	Ayurvedic
Jasminum flexile	Chameli (var.)	Jasmine, Juhi	Folk
Jasminum flexile	Maalati (var.)	Jasmine, Juhi	Ayurvedic
Jasminum flexile	Ramabanam mullai	Jasmine, Juhi	Siddha/Tamil
Jasminum heterophyllum	Svarna-yuuthikaa (var.)	Yellow Jasmine	Ayurvedic
Jasminum heterophyllum	Juuhi (yellow var.)	Yellow Jasmine	Folk
Jasminum humile	Hemapushpikaa	Yellow Jasmine, Nepal Jasmine, Italian Jasmine	Ayurvedic
Jasminum humile	Svarnajaati	Yellow Jasmine, Nepal Jasmine, Italian Jasmine	Ayurvedic
Jasminum humile	Svarna-yuuthikaa	Yellow Jasmine, Nepal Jasmine, Italian Jasmine	Ayurvedic
Jasminum humile	Vaasanti	Yellow Jasmine, Nepal Jasmine, Italian Jasmine	Ayurvedic
Jasminum humile	Semmalligai	Yellow Jasmine, Nepal Jasmine, Italian Jasmine	Siddha/Tamil
Jasminum humile	Juuhi (yellow var.)	Yellow Jasmine, Nepal Jasmine, Italian Jasmine	Folk
Jasminum malabaricum	Mudgara	Climbing Mogara	Ayurvedic
Jasminum malabaricum	Mogaraa	Climbing Mogara	Folk
Jasminum malabaricum	Ran-mogaraa	Climbing Mogara	Folk
Jasminum multiflorum	Kasturi Mogaraa	Downy Jasmine	Ayurvedic
Jasminum multiflorum	Kunda	Downy Jasmine	Ayurvedic
Jasminum multiflorum	Magarandam	Downy Jasmine	Siddha/Tamil
Jasminum multiflorum	Malli	Downy Jasmine	Siddha/Tamil
Jasminum multiflorum	Kasturi Mogaraa	Downy Jasmine	Folk
Jasminum officinale	Jaati	Spanish Jasmine	Ayurvedic

Table Contd.

Botanical Name	Indian Name	English Name	Medicinal System
Jasminum officinale	Jaatikaa	Spanish Jasmine	Ayurvedic
Jasminum officinale	Jaatimalli	Spanish Jasmine	Ayurvedic
Jasminum officinale	Pravaaljaati	Spanish Jasmine	Ayurvedic
Jasminum officinale	Saumana-syaayani	Spanish Jasmine	Ayurvedic
Jasminum officinale	Sumanaa	Spanish Jasmine	Ayurvedic
Jasminum officinale	Chetikaa	Spanish Jasmine	Ayurvedic
Jasminum officinale	Hriddgandhaa	Spanish Jasmine	Ayurvedic
Jasminum officinale	Maalati	Spanish Jasmine	Ayurvedic
Jasminum officinale	Chameli	Spanish Jasmine	Ayurvedic
Jasminum officinale	Yaasmin	Spanish Jasmine	Unani
Jasminum officinale	Manmadabanam	Spanish Jasmine	Siddha/Tamil
Jasminum officinale	Malli	Spanish Jasmine	Siddha/Tamil
Jasminum officinale	Padar-malligai	Spanish Jasmine	Siddha/Tamil
Jasminum officinale	Pichi	Spanish Jasmine	Siddha/Tamil
Jasminum rottlerianum	Vana-mallikaa	Wild jasmine (Western Ghats)	Ayurvedic
Jasminum rottlerianum	Erumaimullai	Wild jasmine (Western Ghats)	Siddha/Tamil
Jasminum rottlerianum	Kattumalligei	Wild jasmine (Western Ghats)	Siddha/Tamil
Jasminum rottlerianum	Uyyakondan	Wild jasmine (Western Ghats)	Siddha/Tamil
Jasminum sambac	Mallikaa	Arabian Jasmine, Tuscan Jasmine, Double Jasmine	Ayurvedic
Jasminum sambac	Madayanti	Arabian Jasmine, Tuscan Jasmine, Double Jasmine	Ayurvedic
Jasminum sambac	Madyantikaa	Arabian Jasmine, Tuscan Jasmine, Double Jasmine	Ayurvedic
Jasminum sambac	Nava-Mallikaa	Arabian Jasmine, Tuscan Jasmine, Double Jasmine	Ayurvedic
Jasminum sambac	Shita-bhiru	Arabian Jasmine, Tuscan Jasmine, Double Jasmine	Ayurvedic
Jasminum sambac	Vaarshiki	Arabian Jasmine, Tuscan Jasmine, Double Jasmine	Ayurvedic
Jasminum sambac	Malligai	Arabian Jasmine, Tuscan Jasmine, Double Jasmine	Siddha/Tamil
Jasminum sambac	Mograa	Arabian Jasmine, Tuscan Jasmine, Double Jasmine	Unani
Jasminum sambac	Ban-mallikaa	Arabian Jasmine, Tuscan Jasmine, Double Jasmine	Folk

Table Contd.

Botanical Name	Indian Name	English Name	Medicinal System
Jasminum sambac	Belaa	Arabian Jasmine, Tuscan Jasmine, Double Jasmine	Folk
Jasminum sambac	Motiaabelaa	Arabian Jasmine, Tuscan Jasmine, Double Jasmine	Folk
Jateorhiza palmata	Kalambaka	Calumba, Colombo	Ayurvedic
Jateorhiza palmata	Kolumbu	Calumba, Colombo	Siddha/Tamil
Jatropha curcas	Bagharenda (var.)	Physic Nut, Purging Nut	Folk
Jatropha curcas	Kattu Amanaku	Physic Nut, Purging Nut	Siddha/Tamil
Jatropha curcas	Vyaaghrairanda	Physic Nut, Purging Nut	Ayurvedic
Jatropha curcas	Sthula-eranda	Physic Nut, Purging Nut	Ayurvedic
Jatropha curcas	Kaanan-eranda	Physic Nut, Purging Nut	Ayurvedic
Jatropha glandulifera	Vyaaghrairanda	Jatropha (South India)	Ayurvedic
Jatropha glandulifera	Adalai	Jatropha (South India)	Siddha/Tamil
Jatropha glandulifera	Eliyamanakku	Jatropha (South India)	Siddha/Tamil
Jatropha glandulifera	Bagharenda	Jatropha (South India)	Folk
Jatropha glandulifera	Jangali-erandi	Jatropha (South India)	Folk
Jatropha gossypifolia	Rakta-Vyaaghrairanda	Physic Nut, Purging Nut	Ayurvedic
Jatropha gossypifolia	Stalai	Physic Nut, Purging Nut	Siddha/Tamil
Jatropha gossypifolia	Laal Bagharenda	Physic Nut, Purging Nut	Folk
Jatropha multifida	Brihat-Danti	Coral Plant, Physic Nut	Ayurvedic
Jatropha multifida	Danti	Coral Plant, Physic Nut	Folk
Juglans regia	Akshoda	Walnut Tree	Ayurvedic
Juglans regia	Akshodaka	Walnut Tree	Ayurvedic
Juglans regia	Akshota	Walnut Tree	Ayurvedic
Juglans regia	Shailbhava	Walnut Tree	Ayurvedic
Juglans regia	Pilu	Walnut Tree	Ayurvedic
Juglans regia	Karparaal	Walnut Tree	Ayurvedic
Juglans regia	Vrantphala	Walnut Tree	Ayurvedic
Juglans regia	Akhrot	Walnut Tree	Unani
Juglans regia	Akrottu	Walnut Tree	Siddha/Tamil
Juncus effusus	Rush	Rush, Matting Rush	Folk
Juniperus communis	Hapushaa	Common Juniper	Ayurvedic

Table Contd.

Botanical Name	Indian Name	English Name	Medicinal System
Kalanchoe laciniata	Malakalli	Christmastree Plant	Siddha/Tamil
Kalanchoe laciniata	Hemsaagar	Christmastree Plant	Folk
Kalanchoe pinnata	Parnabija	Christmastree Plant	Ayurvedic
Kalanchoe pinnata	Pattharchuur	Christmastree Plant	Ayurvedic
Kalanchoe pinnata	Pattharchat	Christmastree Plant	Ayurvedic
Kalanchoe pinnata	Hemsaagar	Christmastree Plant	Ayurvedic
Kalanchoe pinnata	Zakhm-e-Hayaat	Christmastree Plant	Unani
Kalanchoe pinnata	Runakalli	Christmastree Plant	Siddha/Tamil
Kandelia rheedii	Thuvar kandan	Backwater Kandal Tree	Siddha/Tamil
Kandelia rheedii	Rasunia	Backwater Kandal Tree	Folk
Kandelia rheedii	Guria	Backwater Kandal Tree	Folk
Kedrostis foetidissima	Appakovay	Lobed-leaf Foetid Plant	Folk
Kedrostis foetidissima	Kukumadona	Lobed-leaf Foetid Plant	Folk
Kedrostis foetidissima	Nagadonda	Lobed-leaf Foetid Plant	Folk
Kedrostis foetidissima	Nurakvel	Lobed-leaf Foetid Plant	Folk
Khaya senegalensis	Nigerian Mahogany	African Mahogany	Folk
Kigelia pinnata	Jhaar Phaanuus	Common Sausage Tree	Folk
Kingiodendron pinnatum	Samparni	Piney	Ayurvedic
Kingiodendron pinnatum	Kodapalai	Piney	Siddha/Tamil
Kingiodendron pinnatum	Madayansambrani	Piney	Siddha/Tamil
Kirganelia reticulata	Kaamboji	Black-berried Featherfoil	Ayurvedic
Kirganelia reticulata	Panjuli	Black-berried Featherfoil	Folk
Kleinhovia hospita	Bol	Crowned Bol Tree	Folk
Kleinhovia hospita	Panuitteku	Crowned Bol Tree	Folk
Knema angustifolia	Motaa-pasuti	Pseudo-Redsander Tree	Folk
Knema angustifolia	Ramguwaa	Pseudo-Redsander Tree	Folk
Kochia indica	Bui-chholi	Kochia Weed	Folk
Kochia indica	Kauraro	Kochia Weed	Folk
Krameria triandra	Rhatany	Peruvian Rhatany, Krameria	Folk
Kydia calycina	Pola	Pula Tree	Folk
Kydia calycina	Pulu	Pula Tree	Folk
Kydia calycina	Pula	Pula Tree	Folk
Kydia calycina	Polao	Pula Tree	Folk

Table Contd.

Botanical Name	Indian Name	English Name	Medicinal System
Kydia calycina	Vendi	Pula Tree	Folk
Kydia calycina	Potri	Pula Tree	Folk
Kydia calycina	Konda Potari	Pula Tree	Folk
Kydia calycina	Pandiki	Pula Tree	Folk
Kydia calycina	Pachabotuka	Pula Tree	Folk
Kydia calycina	Velukku	Pula Tree	Folk
Kydia calycina	Venta	Pula Tree	Folk
Kydia calycina	Nedunar	Pula Tree	Folk
Kyllinga triceps	Nirvishaa (var.)	Spikesedge, The Sedge of Jamaica	Ayurvedic
Kyllinga triceps	Mustaka (var.)	Spikesedge, The Sedge of Jamaica	Ayurvedic
Kyllinga triceps	Apivisha	Spikesedge, The Sedge of Jamaica	Ayurvedic
Kyllinga triceps	Mustu	Spikesedge, The Sedge of Jamaica	Folk
Lactuca runcinata	Undir-chaa-kaan	Wild Lettuce	Folk
Lactuca sativa	Kaahuu Bustaani	Garden Lettuce	Unani
Lactuca sativa	Salaad Pattaa	Garden Lettuce	Unani
Lactuca sativa	Salaad Baaghi	Garden Lettuce	Unani
Lactuca sativa	Salattu	Garden Lettuce	Siddha/Tamil
Lactuca serriola	Salaad	Wild Lettuce, Prickly Lettuce	Ayurvedic
Lactuca serriola	Vanya-Kaahuu	Wild Lettuce, Prickly Lettuce	Ayurvedic
Lactuca serriola	Kaahuu Sahrai	Wild Lettuce, Prickly Lettuce	Unani
Lactuca serriola	Kaahuu Barri	Wild Lettuce, Prickly Lettuce	Unani
Lactuca serriola	Salattu	Wild Lettuce, Prickly Lettuce	Siddha/Tamil
Lactuca virosa	Kaahuu Barri (var.)	Bitter Lettuce, Wild Lettuce	Unani
Lactuca virosa	Kaahuu Sahrai (var.)	Bitter Lettuce, Wild Lettuce	Unani
Lagenaria siceraria	Ikshavaaku	Bitter Bottle-Gourd	Ayurvedic
Lagenaria siceraria	Katu-tumbi	Bitter Bottle-Gourd	Ayurvedic
Lagenaria siceraria	Pindaphalaa	Bitter Bottle-Gourd	Ayurvedic
Lagenaria siceraria	Tiktaalaavu	Bitter Bottle-Gourd	Ayurvedic
Lagenaria siceraria	Tumbini	Bitter Bottle-Gourd	Ayurvedic

Table Contd.

Botanical Name	Indian Name	English Name	Medicinal System
Lagenaria siceraria	Kaddu-e-talkh	Bitter Bottle-Gourd	Unani
Lagenaria siceraria	Suraikai	Bitter Bottle-Gourd	Siddha/Tamil
Lagerstroemia flos-reginae	Kadalai	Pride of India, Queen's Flowers, Queen Crape Myrtle	Folk/Tamil
Lagerstroemia flos-reginae	Pumaruttu	Pride of India, Queen's Flowers, Queen Crape Myrtle	Folk/Tamil
Lagerstroemia flos-reginae	Jaarul	Pride of India, Queen's Flowers, Queen Crape Myrtle	Folk
Lagerstroemia indica	Pavalak-kurinji	Common Crape Myrtle	Folk/Tamil
Lagerstroemia indica	Sinappu	Common Crape Myrtle	Folk/Tamil
Lagerstroemia indica	Saavani	Common Crape Myrtle	Folk
Lagerstroemia indica	Faraash	Common Crape Myrtle	Folk
Lagerstroemia parviflora	Siddhaka	Lendi, Benteak	Ayurvedic
Lagerstroemia parviflora	Siddha	Lendi, Benteak	Ayurvedic
Lagerstroemia parviflora	Syandana	Lendi, Benteak	Ayurvedic
Lagerstroemia parviflora	Dhauraa	Lendi, Benteak	Folk
Lagerstroemia parviflora	Bakli	Lendi, Benteak	Folk
Lagerstroemia parviflora	Chungi	Lendi, Benteak	Folk
Lagerstroemia parviflora	Lendira (trade)	Lendi, Benteak	Folk
Laggera alata	Amadok	False Tobacco	Folk
Lallemantia royleana	Baalango	Balanga Seed	Unani
Lallemantia royleana	Tukhm-e-Baalango	Balanga Seed	Unani
Lallemantia royleana	Tuut-malangaa	Balanga Seed	Folk
Lamium album	Lamia	White Dead Nettle, Archangel	Folk
Laminum amplexicaule	Titpaati	Henbit Dead Nettle	Folk
Laminum amplexicaule	Jipachi	Henbit Dead Nettle	Folk
Lamprachaenium microcephalum	Ajadandi	Purple-flowered Brahmadandi	Folk
Lamprachaenium microcephalum	Brahmdandi	Purple-flowered Brahmadandi	Folk
Lamprachaenium microcephalum	Baramdandi	Purple-flowered Brahmadandi	Unani
Lannea coromandelica	Jingini	Jhingan	Ayurvedic
Lannea coromandelica	Jhingan	Jhingan	Ayurvedic

Table Contd.

Botanical Name	Indian Name	English Name	Medicinal System
Lannea coromandelica	Gudamanjari	Jhingan	Ayurvedic
Lannea coromandelica	Kalasan	Jhingan	Siddha/Tamil
Lannea coromandelica	Anaikkarai	Jhingan	Siddha/Tamil
Lannea coromandelica	Odiyan	Jhingan	Folk/Tamil
Lansium domesticum	Duku	Langsat Fruit, Dockoa	Folk
Lantana camara	Chaturaangi	Lantana, Wild Sage, Surinam Tea Plant	Ayurvedic
Lantana camara	Vanachchhedi	Lantana, Wild Sage, Surinam Tea Plant	Ayurvedic
Lantana camara	Ghaaneri	Lantana, Wild Sage, Surinam Tea Plant	Folk
Lantana camara	Unnichedi	Lantana, Wild Sage, Surinam Tea Plant	Siddha/Tamil
Laportea crenulata	Perunkanchori	Devil Nettle, Fever Nettle	Siddha/Tamil
Laportea crenulata	Chorpaat	Devil Nettle, Fever Nettle	Folk
Laportea crenulata	Utigun	Devil Nettle, Fever Nettle	Folk
Larix griffithiana	Boargasella	Himalayan Larch, Sikkim Larch	Folk
Larix griffithiana	Binyi	Himalayan Larch, Sikkim Larch	Folk
Lasia spinosa	Kantaka-choramu	Prickly Lasia	Folk/Tamil
Lasia spinosa	Mulasari	Prickly Lasia	Siddha/Tamil
Lasia spinosa	Kantakachu	Prickly Lasia	Folk
Lasia spinosa	Kaantaasaru	Prickly Lasia	Folk
Lasiosiphon eriocephalus	Nachinaai	Wooly-headed Gnidia	Siddha/Tamil
Lasiosiphon eriocephalus	Raamethaa	Wooly-headed Gnidia	Folk
Lathyrus sativus	Khesaari	Chickling Vetch, Grass Pea	Folk
Lathyrus sativus	Latari	Chickling Vetch, Grass Pea	Folk
Lathyrus sativus	Kalaaya	Chickling Vetch, Grass Pea	Folk
Launaea mucronata	Dudh-phaad	Yellow Amrour	Folk
Launaea pinnatifida	Gojihvaa	Bhonpatri	Ayurvedic
Launaea pinnatifida	Golomikaa	Bhonpatri	Ayurvedic
Launaea pinnatifida	Vana-gobhi	Bhonpatri	Folk
Launaea pinnatifida	Paathri	Bhonpatri	Folk
Laurus nobilis	Habb-ul-Ghaar	Laurel, Sweet Bay	Unani
Laurus nobilis	Daphni	Laurel, Sweet Bay	Unani

Table Contd.

Botanical Name	Indian Name	English Name	Medicinal System
Lavandula angustifolia	Lavender	Lavender	Unani
Lavandula bipinnata	Shankhapushpi	Wild Lavender	Ayurvedic
Lavandula stoechas	Ustukhuddus	Arabian or French Lavender	Unani
Lavandula stoechas	Alfaajan	Arabian or French Lavender	Unani
Lavandula stoechas	Dhaaru	Arabian or French Lavender	Folk
Lawsonia inermis	Madayanti	Henna	Ayurvedic
Lawsonia inermis	Madayantikaa	Henna	Ayurvedic
Lawsonia inermis	Mendika	Henna	Ayurvedic
Lawsonia inermis	Ranjaka	Henna	Ayurvedic
Lawsonia inermis	Hinaa	Henna	Unani
Lawsonia inermis	Mehndi	Henna	Unani
Lawsonia inermis	Azhavanam	Henna	Siddha/Tamil
Lawsonia inermis	Marudhonri	Henna	Siddha/Tamil
Leea aequata	Kaakajanghaa	Black-berry Holly	Ayurvedic
Leea aequata	Nadikaantaa	Black-berry Holly	Ayurvedic
Leea aequata	Sulomaasha	Black-berry Holly	Ayurvedic
Leea aequata	Paaraavatapaadi	Black-berry Holly	Ayurvedic
Leea aequata	Surapadi	Black-berry Holly	Folk
Leea crispa	Banachelt	Grey-berry Holly	Folk
Leea crispa	Banachalit	Grey-berry Holly	Folk
Leea crispa	Nalugu	Grey-berry Holly	Folk
Leea crispa	Nellu	Grey-berry Holly	Folk
Leea indica	Chhatri	Purple-berry Holly	Ayurvedic
Leea indica	Karkatajihvaa	Purple-berry Holly	Ayurvedic
Leea indica	Kukurjihvaa	Purple-berry Holly	Ayurvedic
Leea indica	Nalava	Purple-berry Holly	Folk/Tamil
Leea indica	Nyekki	Purple-berry Holly	Folk/Tamil
Leea indica	Ottanali	Purple-berry Holly	Folk/Tamil
Leea indica	Karkani	Purple-berry Holly	Folk
Leea macrophylla	Hastikanda	Tuberous Holly	Ayurvedic
Leea macrophylla	Hasti-karna Falaasha	Tuberous Holly	Ayurvedic
Leea macrophylla	Kekidandaa	Tuberous Holly	Ayurvedic

Table Contd.

Botanical Name	Indian Name	English Name	Medicinal System
Leea macrophylla	Hatkan	Tuberous Holly	Folk
Leea macrophylla	Dholsamudra	Tuberous Holly	Folk
Leea macrophylla	Haath	Tuberous Holly	Folk
Leea macrophylla	Kaan	Tuberous Holly	Folk
Lens culinaris	Masura	Lentil	Ayurvedic
Lens culinaris	Masurikaa	Lentil	Ayurvedic
Lens culinaris	Mangalyaa	Lentil	Ayurvedic
Lens culinaris	Mangalyak	Lentil	Ayurvedic
Lens culinaris	Adaasa	Lentil	Ayurvedic
Lens culinaris	Masoor	Lentil	Unani
Lens culinaris	Misurpurpu	Lentil	Folk/Tamil
Leonotis nepetaefolia	Granthiparni	Christmas Candlestick, Jonny Collins, Lion's Ear, Lion's Tail	Ayurvedic
Leonotis nepetaefolia	Kaakapuchha	Christmas Candlestick, Jonny Collins, Lion's Ear, Lion's Tail	Ayurvedic
Leonotis nepetaefolia	Gathivan	Christmas Candlestick, Jonny Collins, Lion's Ear, Lion's Tail	Folk
Leonotis nepetaefolia	Deepamaal	Christmas Candlestick, Jonny Collins, Lion's Ear, Lion's Tail	Folk
Leonurus cardiaca	Baranjaasif	Common Motherwort	Unani
Lepidagathis cristata	Safed Raasnaa	Spotted White-flowered Pluchea	Folk
Lepidagathis cristata	Hiran-chaaro	Spotted White-flowered Pluchea	Folk
Lepidagathis cristata	Paniru	Spotted White-flowered Pluchea	Folk
Lepidium iberis	Bazr-ul-khumkhum	Peppercress	Unani
Lepidium iberis	Todari	Peppercress	Unani
Lepidium latifolium	Gonyuch	Peppercress	Folk
Lepidium sativum	Chandrashuura	Gardencress, Tongue Grass	Ayurvedic
Lepidium sativum	Chandrikaa	Gardencress, Tongue Grass	Ayurvedic
Lepidium sativum	Vaas-pushpaa	Gardencress, Tongue Grass	Ayurvedic
Lepidium sativum	Pashumehan-kaarika	Gardencress, Tongue Grass	Ayurvedic
Lepidium sativum	Nandini	Gardencress, Tongue Grass	Ayurvedic

Table Contd.

Botanical Name	Indian Name	English Name	Medicinal System
Limnophila aromatica	Aamragandha Karpuur	Turpentine Spinach	Folk
Limnophila aromatica	Karpuur	Turpentine Spinach	Folk
Limnophila aromatica	Ambuli	Turpentine Spinach	Folk
Limnophila aromatica	Manganari	Turpentine Spinach	Folk
Limnophila aromatica	Kuttra	Turpentine Spinach	Folk
Limnophila indica	Kuttra	Oil-of-lemons Spinach	Folk
Limnophila indica	Karpuur	Oil-of-lemons Spinach	Folk
Limnophila indica	Ambuli	Oil-of-lemons Spinach	Folk
Limnophila indica	Manganari	Oil-of-lemons Spinach	Folk
Limonia crenulata	Bilvaparni	Naringi, Beli	Ayurvedic
Limonia crenulata	Nayvila	Naringi, Beli	Siddha/Tamil
Limonia crenulata	Ran-limbu	Naringi, Beli	Folk
Limonia crenulata	Naringi	Naringi, Beli	Folk
Limonia crenulata	Tondsha	Naringi, Beli	Folk
Limonia crenulata	Beli	Naringi, Beli	Folk
Limonia crenulata	Binthaa	Naringi, Beli	Folk
Lindenbergia indica	Haldi Basanto	Nettle-leaved Lindenbergia	Folk
Lindenbergia indica	Dhol	Nettle-leaved Lindenbergia	Folk
Lindenbergia indica	Patthar-chatti	Nettle-leaved Lindenbergia	Folk
Lindenbergia indica	Bheet-chatti	Nettle-leaved Lindenbergia	Folk
Lindera neesiana	Gandha-daaru	Spicebush, Benjamin Bush	Folk
Lindera neesiana	Siltimur	Spicebush, Benjamin Bush	Folk
Linum usitatissimum	Atasi	Linseed, Flax	Ayurvedic
Linum usitatissimum	Umaa	Linseed, Flax	Ayurvedic
Linum usitatissimum	Masrnaa	Linseed, Flax	Ayurvedic
Linum usitatissimum	Nilapushpi	Linseed, Flax	Ayurvedic
Linum usitatissimum	Kshumaa	Linseed, Flax	Ayurvedic
Linum usitatissimum	Kattan	Linseed, Flax	Unani
Linum usitatissimum	Ali-virail	Linseed, Flax	Siddha/Tamil
Linum usitatissimum	Sirrali (Seed)	Linseed, Flax	Siddha/Tamil
Lipasis rostrata	Jivaka-Rshabhaka	Jivak Orchid	Ayurvedic
Lippia geminata	Basula	Melissa Lipia	Folk

Table Contd.

Botanical Name	Indian Name	English Name	Medicinal System
Lippia geminata	Naagaa-aiari	Melissa Lipia	Folk
Lippia nodiflora	Jalapippali	Wild Sage	Ayurvedic
Lippia nodiflora	Shaaradi	Wild Sage	Ayurvedic
Lippia nodiflora	Shakulaadani	Wild Sage	Ayurvedic
Lippia nodiflora	Jalakarnaa	Wild Sage	Ayurvedic
Lippia nodiflora	Matsyagandhaa	Wild Sage	Ayurvedic
Lippia nodiflora	Laangali	Wild Sage	Ayurvedic
Lippia nodiflora	Bukkum Booti	Wild Sage	Unani
Lippia nodiflora	Paduthalai	Wild Sage	Siddha/Tamil
Liquidambar formosana	Silhak (var.)	Fragrant Maple	Ayurvedic
Liquidambar formosana	Silaaras (var.)	Fragrant Maple	Unani
Liquidambar orientalis	Turushka	Storax, Oriental Sweet Gum	Ayurvedic
Liquidambar orientalis	Silhaka	Storax, Oriental Sweet Gum	Ayurvedic
Liquidambar orientalis	Kapitaila	Storax, Oriental Sweet Gum	Ayurvedic
Liquidambar orientalis	Ambar Saayil	Storax, Oriental Sweet Gum	Unani
Liquidambar orientalis	Silaaras	Storax, Oriental Sweet Gum	Unani
Liquidambar orientalis	Neri-arishippal	Storax, Oriental Sweet Gum	Siddha/Tamil
Liriodendron tulipifera	Canary Tree	Tulip Tree	Folk
Litchi chinensis	Lichi	Litchi, Lychee	Folk
Lithospermum officinale	Lubis firmun	Corn Gromwell	Folk
Litsea glutinosa	Medaasaka	Common Tallow Lowrel	Ayurvedic
Litsea glutinosa	Maidaa-lakdi	Common Tallow Lowrel	Unani
Litsea glutinosa	Maghaase-Hindi	Common Tallow Lowrel	Unani
Litsea glutinosa	Mushaippeyetti	Common Tallow Lowrel	Siddha/Tamil
Litsea glutinosa	Elumpurukki	Common Tallow Lowrel	Siddha/Tamil
Litsea glutinosa	Uralli	Common Tallow Lowrel	Siddha/Tamil
Litsea monopetala	Maidaa-lakdi (var.)	Yati	Ayurvedic
Litsea monopetala	Maidalagadil	Yati	Siddha/Tamil
Litsea monopetala	Picinpattai	Yati	Siddha/Tamil
Litsea stocksii	Posha	Yati	Folk
Litsea stocksii	Pisi	Yati	Folk
Lobelia inflata	Devanala	Indian Tabacco, Pukeweed	Ayurvedic

Table Contd.

Botanical Name	Indian Name	English Name	Medicinal System
Lygodium flexuosum	Bhuuta-bhairavi	Wolfberry, Scrambling Fern	Folk
Lygodium flexuosum	Bhuuta-raaj	Wolfberry, Scrambling Fern	Folk
Lygodium flexuosum	Kalzhaa	Wolfberry, Scrambling Fern	Folk
Lyonia ovalifolia	Angyaar	Oval-leaved Staggerbush	Folk
Lyonia ovalifolia	Arwan	Oval-leaved Staggerbush	Folk
Lyonia ovalifolia	Angeri	Oval-leaved Staggerbush	Siddha/Tamil
Maba nigrescens	Ragat-Rohido	Karuti Ebony	Folk
Maba nigrescens	Rakta-Rohido	Karuti Ebony	Folk
Madhuca butyracea	Madhuuka	Phulwara, Indian Butter Tree	Ayurvedic
Madhuca butyracea	Maakhaniaa Mahuaa	Phulwara, Indian Butter Tree	Folk
Madhuca butyracea	Phulwaaraa	Phulwara, Indian Butter Tree	Folk
Madhuca indica	Madhuuka	Mahua Tree, Moha	Ayurvedic
Madhuca indica	Madhupushpa	Mahua Tree, Moha	Ayurvedic
Madhuca indica	Madhusrav	Mahua Tree, Moha	Ayurvedic
Madhuca indica	Gudapushpa	Mahua Tree, Moha	Ayurvedic
Madhuca indica	Mahuaa	Mahua Tree, Moha	Unani
Madhuca indica	Ieluppai	Mahua Tree, Moha	Siddha/Tamil
Madhuca longifolia	Illupei	South Indian Mahua	Siddha/Tamil
Madhuca longifolia	Elupa	South Indian Mahua	Siddha/Tamil
Madhuca longifolia	Naatu Iluppai	South Indian Mahua	Siddha/Tamil
Madhuca longifolia	Iruppai	South Indian Mahua	Siddha/Tamil
Madhuca longifolia	Jala-Madhuuka	South Indian Mahua	Folk
Madhuca longifolia	Jala-Mahuaa	South Indian Mahua	Folk
Madhuca longifolia	Madhuulaka	South Indian Mahua	Folk
Maerua arenaria	Morata	Desert Maerua, Hemkand	Ayurvedic
Maerua arenaria	Piluparni	Desert Maerua, Hemkand	Ayurvedic
Maerua arenaria	Madhusravaa	Desert Maerua, Hemkand	Ayurvedic
Maerua arenaria	Bhumichakkarai	Desert Maerua, Hemkand	Siddha/Tamil
Maerua arenaria	Murhari	Desert Maerua, Hemkand	Folk
Magnolia grandiflora	Him-Champaa	Bull Bay, Great Laurel Magnolia, Southern Magnolia	Ayurvedic
Mahonia nepaulensis	Chhatri	Holly Leaved Berberry	Folk
Mahonia nepualensis	Haldia	Holly Leaved Berberry	Folk

Table Contd.

Botanical Name	Indian Name	English Name	Medicinal System
Mallotus philippensis	Kampillaka	Kamala Tree, Monkey Face Tree	Ayurvedic
Mallotus philippensis	Kampilla	Kamala Tree, Monkey Face Tree	Ayurvedic
Mallotus philippensis	Karkash	Kamala Tree, Monkey Face Tree	Ayurvedic
Mallotus philippensis	Raktaanga	Kamala Tree, Monkey Face Tree	Ayurvedic
Mallotus philippensis	Rechan	Kamala Tree, Monkey Face Tree	Ayurvedic
Mallotus philippensis	Chandra	Kamala Tree, Monkey Face Tree	Ayurvedic
Mallotus philippensis	Kamilla	Kamala Tree, Monkey Face Tree	Unani
Mallotus philippensis	Kambilaa	Kamala Tree, Monkey Face Tree	Unani
Mallotus philippensis	Kaplila	Kamala Tree, Monkey Face Tree	Siddha/Tamil
Mallotus philippensis	Kalupatti	Kamala Tree, Monkey Face Tree	Siddha/Tamil
Malpighia glabra	Acerola	Barbados Cherry, Acerola	Folk
Malpighia punicifolia	Vallari	West Indian Cherry	Folk
Malpighia punicifolia	Simeyaranelli	West Indian Cherry	Folk
Malus pumila	Sinchitikaa	Cultivated Apple	Ayurvedic
Malus pumila	Seb	Cultivated Apple	Folk
Malus pumila	Sev	Cultivated Apple	Folk
Malva rotundifolia	Suvarchalaa	Round-leaved Mallow, Drawf Mallow, Cheese Cake Flower	Ayurvedic
Malva rotundifolia	Khubhaazi	Round-leaved Mallow, Drawf Mallow, Cheese Cake Flower	Unani
Malva rotundifolia	Gul-Khair	Round-leaved Mallow, Drawf Mallow, Cheese Cake Flower	Unani
Malva sylvestris	Suvarchalaa (var.)	Common Mallow, Blue Mallow, High Mallow	Ayurvedic
Malva sylvestris	Khubbaazi	Common Mallow, Blue Mallow, High Mallow	Unani
Malva sylvestris	Bhubhaazi	Common Mallow, Blue Mallow, High Mallow	Unani
Malva sylvestris	Gul-Khair	Common Mallow, Blue Mallow, High Mallow	Unani
Mandragora autumnalis	Lakshmanaa	Mandrake	Ayurvedic
Mangifera indica	Aamra	Mango	Ayurvedic
Mangifera indica	Aamrakeshi	Mango	Ayurvedic
Mangifera indica	Rasaal	Mango	Ayurvedic
Mangifera indica	Sahakaara	Mango	Ayurvedic
Mangifera indica	Pikavallabha	Mango	Ayurvedic

Table Contd.

Botanical Name	Indian Name	English Name	Medicinal System
Mangifera indica	Madhudoot	Mango	Ayurvedic
Mangifera indica	Atisaurabha	Mango	Ayurvedic
Mangifera indica	Chuta	Mango	Ayurvedic
Mangifera indica	Aam	Mango	Unani
Mangifera indica	Ambaj	Mango	Unani
Mangifera indica	Manga	Mango	Folk/Tamil
Mangifera indica	Maa	Mango	Folk/Tamil
Mangifera indica	Mamaram (bark)	Mango	Siddha/Tamil
Mangifera indica	Mangottai Paruppu	Mango	Siddha/Tamil
Manihot esculenta	Maravalli kizhangu	Manioc, Tapioca, Cassava	Siddha/Tamil
Manihot esculenta	Ezhalai kizhangu	Manioc, Tapioca, Cassava	Siddha/Tamil
Manihot esculenta	Tapioca	Manioc, Tapioca, Cassava	Folk
Manilkara kauki	Khirni	Kauki	Ayurvedic
Manilkara kauki	Palai	Kauki	Siddha/Tamil
Maranta arundinacea	Koovaikizhangu	Arrowroot	Siddha/Tamil
Maranta arundinacea	Kookaineer	Arrowroot	Siddha/Tamil
Marrubium vulgare	Faraasiyun	Horehound	Unani
Marsdenia roylei	Muurvaa (var.)	Marua Vine	Ayurvedic
Marsdenia roylei	Maruaa-bel	Marua Vine	Folk
Marsdenia roylei	Khaarchu	Marua Vine	Folk
Marsdenia tenacissima	Muurvaa	White Turpeth	Ayurvedic
Marsdenia tenacissima	Atirasaa	White Turpeth	Ayurvedic
Marsdenia tenacissima	Madhurasaa	White Turpeth	Ayurvedic
Marsdenia tenacissima	Gokarni	White Turpeth	Ayurvedic
Marsdenia tenacissima	Morataa	White Turpeth	Ayurvedic
Marsdenia tenacissima	Madhulikaa	White Turpeth	Ayurvedic
Marsdenia tenacissima	Suvaa	White Turpeth	Ayurvedic
Marsdenia tenacissima	Devi	White Turpeth	Ayurvedic
Marsdenia tenacissima	Tejani	White Turpeth	Ayurvedic
Marsdenia tenacissima	Tiktavalli	White Turpeth	Ayurvedic
Marsdenia tenacissima	Perunkurinjan	White Turpeth	Siddha/Tamil
Marsdenia tenacissima	Maruaa-bel	White Turpeth	Folk

Table Contd.

Botanical Name	Indian Name	English Name	Medicinal System
Marsilea minuta	Sunishannaka	Dwarf Waterclover, Pepperwort	Ayurvedic
Marsilea minuta	Parnaka	Dwarf Waterclover, Pepperwort	Ayurvedic
Marsilea minuta	Vastika-parnika	Dwarf Waterclover, Pepperwort	Ayurvedic
Marsilea minuta	Swastika	Dwarf Waterclover, Pepperwort	Ayurvedic
Marsilea minuta	Chatushpatri	Dwarf Waterclover, Pepperwort	Ayurvedic
Marsilea minuta	Susunishaak	Dwarf Waterclover, Pepperwort	Ayurvedic
Marsilea minuta	Chaupaitra	Dwarf Waterclover, Pepperwort	Ayurvedic
Martynia annua	Kaakanaasikaa	Devil's Claw, Tiger Claw	Ayurvedic
Martynia annua	Kaakaangi	Devil's Claw, Tiger Claw	Ayurvedic
Martynia annua	Shirobal	Devil's Claw, Tiger Claw	Ayurvedic
Martynia annua	Kakatundi	Devil's Claw, Tiger Claw	Siddha/Tamil
Martynia annua	Thelkodukkukai	Devil's Claw, Tiger Claw	Siddha/Tamil
Martynia annua	Hathajori	Devil's Claw, Tiger Claw	Folk
Martynia annua	Bichhuu	Devil's Claw, Tiger Claw	Folk
Matricaria chamomilla	Baabunaa	German Chamomile, Chamomile	Unani
Matthiola incana	Tudri Safed	Stock, Gilli-flower	Unani
Meconopsis aculeata	Gul-e-Nilum	Blue Poppy	Folk
Meconopsis aculeata	Gudi	Blue Poppy	Folk
Meconopsis aculeata	Kunda	Blue Poppy	Folk
Meconopsis aculeata	Kanderi	Blue Poppy	Folk
Meconopsis aculeata	Kalihaari	Blue Poppy	Folk
Medicago sativa	Alfalfa	Alfalfa, Lucerne	Ayurvedic
Medicago sativa	Vilaayati-gawuth	Alfalfa, Lucerne	Ayurvedic
Medicago sativa	Lasunghaas	Alfalfa, Lucerne	Ayurvedic
Medicago sativa	Lusan	Alfalfa, Lucerne	Ayurvedic
Medicago sativa	Barsem	Alfalfa, Lucerne	Unani
Melaleuca leucadendron	Kaayaaputi	Cajeput Tree, Swamp Tea Tree, White Tea Tree	Folk
Melastoma malabathricum	Laakheri	Indian Rhododendron	Folk
Melastoma malabathricum	Paalorey	Indian Rhododendron	Folk
Melastoma malabathricum	Tulasi	Indian Rhododendron	Folk
Melastoma malabathricum	Nakkukappan	Indian Rhododendron	Folk
Melastoma malabathricum	Phutuka	Indian Rhododendron	Folk

Table Contd.

Botanical Name	Indian Name	English Name	Medicinal System
Melia azedarach	Mahaanimba	Persian Lilac, Pride of India	Ayurvedic
Melia azedarach	Ramyaka	Persian Lilac, Pride of India	Ayurvedic
Melia azedarach	Dreka	Persian Lilac, Pride of India	Ayurvedic
Melia azedarach	Bakaayan	Persian Lilac, Pride of India	Unani
Melia azedarach	Malai vembu	Persian Lilac, Pride of India	Siddha/Tamil
Melia composita	Arangaka	Hill Neem, Malabar Neem, Common Bead Tree	Ayurvedic
Melia composita	Malaivembu	Hill Neem, Malabar Neem, Common Bead Tree	Folk
Melilotus alba	Ilkil-ul-Malik	White Sweet Clover	Unani
Melilotus alba	Naakhunaa	White Sweet Clover	Unani
Melilotus indica	Vana-methikaa	Sweet Clover, Annual Yellow Sweet Clover, Small-flowered Melilot	Ayurvedic
Melilotus indica	Ilkil-ul-Malik	Sweet Clover, Annual Yellow Sweet Clover, Small-flowered Melilot	Unani
Melilotus indica	Ban-Methi	Sweet Clover, Annual Yellow Sweet Clover, Small-flowered Melilot	Folk
Melilotus indica	Senji	Sweet Clover, Annual Yellow Sweet Clover, Small-flowered Melilot	Folk
Melilotus officinalis	Asaab-ul-Malik	Yellow Sweet Clover, Melilot	Unani
Melilotus officinalis	Iklil-ul-Malik	Yellow Sweet Clover, Melilot	Unani
Melilotus officinalis	Naakhunaa	Yellow Sweet Clover, Melilot	Unani
Melissa axillaris	Billilotan	Lemon Balm	Unani
Melissa officinalis	Baadranjboyaa	Mountain Balm, Sweet or Lemon Balm	Unani
Melissa officinalis	Billilotan	Mountain Balm, Sweet or Lemon Balm	Unani
Melochia corchorifolia	Pinnakkuppundu	Chocolate-Weed	Siddha/Tamil
Melochia corchorifolia	Chunch	Chocolate-Weed	Folk
Melochia corchorifolia	Bilpat	Chocolate-Weed	Folk
Melothria maderaspatana	Ahilekhana	Rough Bryony	Ayurvedic
Melothria maderaspatana	Trikoshaki	Rough Bryony	Ayurvedic
Melothria maderaspatana	Musumsukkai	Rough Bryony	Siddha/Tamil

Table Contd.

Botanical Name	Indian Name	English Name	Medicinal System
Melothria maderaspatana	Agmaki	Rough Bryony	Folk
Memecylon edule	Anjani	Iron Wood	Ayurvedic
Memecylon edule	Kasai	Iron Wood	Siddha/Tamil
Memecylon edule	Anjani	Iron Wood	Siddha/Tamil
Memecylon edule	Yaalki	Iron Wood	Folk
Memecylon edule	Lokhandi	Iron Wood	Folk
Mentha aquatica	Pudinaa Nahari	Water Mint, Wild Mint	Unani
Mentha arvensis	Naanaa	Japanese Mint	Unani
Mentha longifolia	Pudinaa-Barri	English Horsemint	Unani
Mentha longifolia	Jangali Pudinaa	English Horsemint	Unani
Mentha piperita	Vilaayati Pudinaa	Peppermint, Brandy Mint	Ayurvedic
Mentha spicata	Pudinaa	Spearmint, Garden Mint	Ayurvedic
Mentha spicata	Podinaka	Spearmint, Garden Mint	Ayurvedic
Mentha spicata	Puutihaa	Spearmint, Garden Mint	Ayurvedic
Mentha spicata	Rochini	Spearmint, Garden Mint	Ayurvedic
Mentha spicata	Nanaa	Spearmint, Garden Mint	Unani
Mentha spicata	Pudinaa Kohi	Spearmint, Garden Mint	Unani
Menyanthes trifoliata	Buckbean	Bogbean, Buckbean, Goat's Bean, Marsh Trefoil	Folk
Merremia quinquefolia	Prasaarini	Five-fingered Morning Glory, Rock Rosemary	Ayurvedic
Merremia tridentata	Tala-nili	Woodrose, Merremia	Ayurvedic
Merremia tridentata	Mudiyaak-koonthal	Woodrose, Merremia	Siddha/Tamil
Mesua ferrea	Naagakeshara	Iron-wood, Mesu	Ayurvedic
Mesua ferrea	Naagapushpa	Iron-wood, Mesu	Ayurvedic
Mesua ferrea	Chaampeya	Iron-wood, Mesu	Ayurvedic
Mesua ferrea	Naaga	Iron-wood, Mesu	Ayurvedic
Mesua ferrea	Naagakinjalika	Iron-wood, Mesu	Ayurvedic
Mesua ferrea	Ahipushpa	Iron-wood, Mesu	Ayurvedic
Mesua ferrea	Naarmushk	Iron-wood, Mesu	Unani
Mesua ferrea	Sirunagappo	Iron-wood, Mesu	Siddha/Tamil
Mesua ferrea	Naagakeshram	Iron-wood, Mesu	Siddha/Tamil

Table Contd.

Botanical Name	Indian Name	English Name	Medicinal System
Meyna laxiflora	Pinditaka	Muyna	Ayurvedic
Meyna laxiflora	Muyna	Muyna	Folk
Meyna laxiflora	Moyna	Muyna	Folk
Meyna laxiflora	Muduna	Muyna	Folk
Meyna laxiflora	Manakkarai	Muyna	Siddha/Tamil
Michelia champaca	Champaka	Champak, Golden Champa	Ayurvedic
Michelia champaca	Svarna Champaka	Champak, Golden Champa	Ayurvedic
Michelia champaca	Hemapushpa	Champak, Golden Champa	Ayurvedic
Michelia champaca	Chaampeya	Champak, Golden Champa	Ayurvedic
Michelia champaca	Sanbagam	Champak, Golden Champa	Siddha/Tamil
Microcos paniculata	Asar	Kadamb	Folk
Microcos paniculata	Thengpren-keorong	Kadamb	Folk/Assam
Microcos paniculata	Kadambu	Kadamb	Folk/Tamil
Microcos paniculata	Visalam	Kadamb	Folk/Tamil
Microcos paniculata	Kottei	Kadamb	Folk/Tamil
Microcos paniculata	Abhrangu	Kadamb	Folk
Micromeria capitellata	Pudinaa (var.)	Pseudo-Mint	Folk
Microstylis musifera	Jivaka	Jivaka	Ayurvedic
Microstylis musifera	Madhura	Jivaka	Ayurvedic
Microstylis musifera	Shranga	Jivaka	Ayurvedic
Microstylis musifera	Hriswaanga	Jivaka	Ayurvedic
Microstylis musifera	Kurcha	Jivaka	Ayurvedic
Microstylis musifera	Shirraka	Jivaka	Ayurvedic
Microstylis wallichii	Rshabhaka	Rshabhaka	Ayurvedic
Microstylis wallichii	Rshabha	Rshabhaka	Ayurvedic
Microstylis wallichii	Rshabham	Rshabhaka	Ayurvedic
Microstylis wallichii	Vrishabh	Rshabhaka	Ayurvedic
Microstylis wallichii	Dhira	Rshabhaka	Ayurvedic
Microstylis wallichii	Vishani	Rshabhaka	Ayurvedic
Mikania cordata	Mikaaniaa	Heartleaf Hempvine	Folk
Miliusa velutina	Rshiyaproktaa	Sal-Forest Miliusa	Ayurvedic
Miliusa velutina	Gandha-Palaasa	Sal-Forest Miliusa	Folk

Table Contd.

Botanical Name	Indian Name	English Name	Medicinal System
Miliusa velutina	Kaari	Sal-Forest Miliusa	Folk
Millettia auriculata	Godaar	Evergreen Wisteria	Folk
Millettia racemosa	Godaar	Evergreen Wisteria	Folk
Millingtonia hortensis	Maramalli	Indian Cork Tree	Siddha/Tamil
Millingtonia hortensis	Aakaasha Neem	Indian Cork Tree	Folk
Millingtonia hortensis	Neem-Chameli	Indian Cork Tree	Folk
Mimosa pudica	Lajjaalu	Sensitive-plant, Humble-Plant	Ayurvedic
Mimosa pudica	Laajavanti	Sensitive-plant, Humble-Plant	Ayurvedic
Mimosa pudica	Namaskaari	Sensitive-plant, Humble-Plant	Ayurvedic
Mimosa pudica	Samangaa	Sensitive-plant, Humble-Plant	Ayurvedic
Mimosa pudica	Sankochini	Sensitive-plant, Humble-Plant	Ayurvedic
Mimosa pudica	Shamipatraa	Sensitive-plant, Humble-Plant	Ayurvedic
Mimosa pudica	Khadirkaa	Sensitive-plant, Humble-Plant	Ayurvedic
Mimosa pudica	Raktapaadi	Sensitive-plant, Humble-Plant	Ayurvedic
Mimosa pudica	Chhuimui	Sensitive-plant, Humble-Plant	Unani
Mimosa pudica	Sharmili	Sensitive-plant, Humble-Plant	Unani
Mimosa pudica	Laajwanti	Sensitive-plant, Humble-Plant	Unani
Mimosa pudica	Thottalsurungi	Sensitive-plant, Humble-Plant	Siddha/Tamil
Mimusops elengi	Bakula	Spanish-Cherry, West Indian Medlar, Bullet Wood	Ayurvedic
Mimusops elengi	Keshara	Spanish-Cherry, West Indian Medlar, Bullet Wood	Ayurvedic
Mimusops elengi	Simhakeshara	Spanish-Cherry, West Indian Medlar, Bullet Wood	Ayurvedic
Mimusops elengi	Sthiraa	Spanish-Cherry, West Indian Medlar, Bullet Wood	Ayurvedic
Mimusops elengi	Sthirapushpa	Spanish-Cherry, West Indian Medlar, Bullet Wood	Ayurvedic
Mimusops elengi	Vishaarada	Spanish-Cherry, West Indian Medlar, Bullet Wood	Ayurvedic
Mimusops elengi	Dhanvi	Spanish-Cherry, West Indian Medlar, Bullet Wood	Ayurvedic
Mimusops elengi	Madhupushpa	Spanish-Cherry, West Indian Medlar, Bullet Wood	Ayurvedic
Mimusops elengi	Madhugandha	Spanish-Cherry, West Indian Medlar, Bullet Wood	Ayurvedic

Table Contd.

Botanical Name	Indian Name	English Name	Medicinal System
Monochoria vaginalis	Nirkancha	Oval-leaved Pondweed, Pickerel Weed	Ayurvedic
Monochoria vaginalis	Senkzhuneer-kizhangu	Oval-leaved Pondweed, Pickerel Weed	Siddha/Tamil
Monochoria vaginalis	Nukha	Oval-leaved Pondweed, Pickerel Weed	Folk
Monochoria vaginalis	Nanda	Oval-leaved Pondweed, Pickerel Weed	Folk
Monotropa uniflora	Him-Paadapa	Indian Pipe, Ice Plant	Folk
Morinda citrifolia	Ashyuka	Indian Mulberry	Ayurvedic
Morinda citrifolia	Akshi	Indian Mulberry	Ayurvedic
Morinda citrifolia	Atchy	Indian Mulberry	Ayurvedic
Morinda citrifolia	Nunaa	Indian Mulberry	Siddha/Tamil
Morinda citrifolia	Togaru	Indian Mulberry	Siddha/Tamil
Moringa concanensis	Shigru (Red var.)	Drumstick, Horse-Radish	Ayurvedic
Moringa concanensis	Kaatumurungai	Drumstick, Horse-Radish	Siddha/Tamil
Moringa pterygosperma	Shigru (white var.)	Drumstick, Horse-Radish	Ayurvedic
Moringa pterygosperma	Madhu Shigru	Drumstick, Horse-Radish	Ayurvedic
Moringa pterygosperma	Sigra	Drumstick, Horse-Radish	Ayurvedic
Moringa pterygosperma	Shobhaanjana	Drumstick, Horse-Radish	Ayurvedic
Moringa pterygosperma	Haritashaaka	Drumstick, Horse-Radish	Ayurvedic
Moringa pterygosperma	Raktaka	Drumstick, Horse-Radish	Ayurvedic
Moringa pterygosperma	Murangi	Drumstick, Horse-Radish	Ayurvedic
Moringa pterygosperma	Mochaka	Drumstick, Horse-Radish	Ayurvedic
Moringa pterygosperma	Akshiva	Drumstick, Horse-Radish	Ayurvedic
Moringa pterygosperma	Tikshnagandhaa	Drumstick, Horse-Radish	Ayurvedic
Moringa pterygosperma	Sahajan	Drumstick, Horse-Radish	Unani
Moringa pterygosperma	Murungai	Drumstick, Horse-Radish	Siddha/Tamil
Morus alba	Shahtuut	Chinese White-Mulberry	Unani
Morus alba	Tuut	Chinese White-Mulberry	Unani
Morus nigra	Tuut Siyaah	Black Mulberry	Unani
Mucuna monosperma	Kaakaandolaa	Negro Bean	Ayurvedic
Mucuna monosperma	Periyattalargai	Negro Bean	Siddha/Tamil

Table Contd.

Botanical Name	Indian Name	English Name	Medicinal System
Mucuna monosperma	Kaagadolia	Negro Bean	Folk
Mucuna prurita	Aatmaguptaa	Cowhage, Horse-eye Bean	Ayurvedic
Mucuna prurita	Kapikacchuu	Cowhage, Horse-eye Bean	Ayurvedic
Mucuna prurita	Rshabhi	Cowhage, Horse-eye Bean	Ayurvedic
Mucuna prurita	Adhigandhaa	Cowhage, Horse-eye Bean	Ayurvedic
Mucuna prurita	Ajadaaa	Cowhage, Horse-eye Bean	Ayurvedic
Mucuna prurita	Kacchuraa	Cowhage, Horse-eye Bean	Ayurvedic
Mucuna prurita	Laanguli	Cowhage, Horse-eye Bean	Ayurvedic
Mucuna prurita	Rshyaproktaa	Cowhage, Horse-eye Bean	Ayurvedic
Mucuna prurita	Swaguptaa	Cowhage, Horse-eye Bean	Ayurvedic
Mucuna prurita	Shyaamguptaa	Cowhage, Horse-eye Bean	Ayurvedic
Mucuna prurita	Markati	Cowhage, Horse-eye Bean	Ayurvedic
Mucuna prurita	Kanduraa	Cowhage, Horse-eye Bean	Ayurvedic
Mucuna prurita	Kevaanch	Cowhage, Horse-eye Bean	Ayurvedic
Mucuna prurita	Shuukashimbi	Cowhage, Horse-eye Bean	Ayurvedic
Mucuna prurita	Konchh	Cowhage, Horse-eye Bean	Unani
Mucuna prurita	Poonaikkaali	Cowhage, Horse-eye Bean	Siddha/Tamil
Murdannia nudiflora	Koshapushpi	Nakedstem Dewflower	Ayurvedic
Murdannia nudiflora	Kanshura	Nakedstem Dewflower	Folk
Murdannia scapiflora	Siyaah Musli	Few-flowered Dewflower	Siddha/Tamil
Murdannia scapiflora	Sismulia	Few-flowered Dewflower	Folk
Murdannia scapiflora	Kureli	Few-flowered Dewflower	Folk
Murraya exotica	Konji	Chinese Boxwood, Andaman Satinwood	Siddha/Tamil
Murraya exotica	Kaamini	Chinese Boxwood, Andaman Satinwood	Folk
Murraya exotica	Aanthil	Chinese Boxwood, Andaman Satinwood	Folk
Murraya koenigii	Surabhini-nimba	Curry-Leaf Tree	Ayurvedic
Murraya koenigii	Karipattaa	Curry-Leaf Tree	Unani
Murraya koenigii	Karuveppilai	Curry-Leaf Tree	Siddha/Tamil
Murraya koenigii	Karivempu	Curry-Leaf Tree	Siddha/Tamil
Murraya koenigii	Kattuveppilai	Curry-Leaf Tree	Siddha/Tamil
Murraya koenigii	Mithaa Neem	Curry-Leaf Tree	Folk

Table Contd.

Botanical Name	Indian Name	English Name	Medicinal System
Murraya koenigii	Kathneem	Curry-Leaf Tree	Folk
Murraya koenigii	Gandhela	Curry-Leaf Tree	Folk
Murraya koenigii	Barsanga	Curry-Leaf Tree	Folk
Musa paradisiaca	Kadali	Banana, Plantain	Ayurvedic
Musa paradisiaca	Rambhaa	Banana, Plantain	Ayurvedic
Musa paradisiaca	Sakrtphala	Banana, Plantain	Ayurvedic
Musa paradisiaca	Vaaranaa	Banana, Plantain	Ayurvedic
Musa paradisiaca	Mochaa	Banana, Plantain	Ayurvedic
Musa paradisiaca	Ambusaara	Banana, Plantain	Ayurvedic
Musa paradisiaca	Anshumatiphal	Banana, Plantain	Ayurvedic
Musa paradisiaca	Kelaa	Banana, Plantain	Unani
Musa paradisiaca	Mouz	Banana, Plantain	Unani
Musa paradisiaca	Vaazhai	Banana, Plantain	Siddha/Tamil
Mussaenda frondosa	Shrivati	White Lady, White Rag Plant	Ayurvedic
Mussaenda frondosa	Vellai-yilai	White Lady, White Rag Plant	Siddha/Tamil
Mussaenda frondosa	Velli-madandai	White Lady, White Rag Plant	Siddha/Tamil
Mussaenda frondosa	Shrivara	White Lady, White Rag Plant	Folk
Mussaenda frondosa	Bedina	White Lady, White Rag Plant	Folk
Mussaenda frondosa	Bebina	White Lady, White Rag Plant	Folk
Mussaenda frondosa	Bhutakesha	White Lady, White Rag Plant	Folk
Mussaenda frondosa	Naagaballi	White Lady, White Rag Plant	Folk
Mycrotomia benthami	Dimok	Pseudo-Ratanjot	Folk
Mycrotomia benthami	Ratanjot	Pseudo-Ratanjot	Folk
Myrica nagi	Katphala	Box Myrtle	Ayurvedic
Myrica nagi	Kushbhikaa	Box Myrtle	Ayurvedic
Myrica nagi	Shriparnikaa	Box Myrtle	Ayurvedic
Myrica nagi	Mahaavalkal	Box Myrtle	Ayurvedic
Myrica nagi	Bhadraa	Box Myrtle	Ayurvedic
Myrica nagi	Bhadravati	Box Myrtle	Ayurvedic
Myrica nagi	Kaayaphal	Box Myrtle	Unani
Myrica nagi	Marudam	Box Myrtle	Siddha/Tamil
Myristica fragrans	Jaatiphala	Nutmeg	Ayurvedic
Myristica fragrans	Jaatishasya	Nutmeg	Ayurvedic

Table Contd.

Botanical Name	Indian Name	English Name	Medicinal System
Myristica fragrans	Maalatiphala	Nutmeg	Ayurvedic
Myristica fragrans	Jaatipatri	Nutmeg	Ayurvedic
Myristica fragrans	Jaatipatra	Nutmeg	Ayurvedic
Myristica fragrans	Jaatipatraka	Nutmeg	Ayurvedic
Myristica fragrans	Jaatikosha (Mace)	Nutmeg	Ayurvedic
Myristica fragrans	Jauzbuwaa (Seed)	Nutmeg	Unani
Myristica fragrans	Bisbaasaa (Mace)	Nutmeg	Unani
Myristica fragrans	Jaathikkai	Nutmeg	Siddha/Tamil
Myristica fragrans	Saadikai	Nutmeg	Siddha/Tamil
Myristica fragrans	Saadippatthiri (Mace)	Nutmeg	Siddha/Tamil
Myristica fragrans	Jaadippatiri (Mace)	Nutmeg	Siddha/Tamil
Myristica malabarica	Paashikaa	Malabar Nutmeg, False Nutmeg, Bombay Nutmeg, Bombay Mace	Ayurvedic
Myristica malabarica	Raamapatri	Malabar Nutmeg, False Nutmeg, Bombay Nutmeg, Bombay Mace	Ayurvedic
Myristica malabarica	Ku-Jaavitri	Malabar Nutmeg, False Nutmeg, Bombay Nutmeg, Bombay Mace	Ayurvedic
Myristica malabarica	Pashupaashi	Malabar Nutmeg, False Nutmeg, Bombay Nutmeg, Bombay Mace	Ayurvedic
Myristica malabarica	Pathiri	Malabar Nutmeg, False Nutmeg, Bombay Nutmeg, Bombay Mace	Siddha/Tamil
Myristica malabarica	Kattu Jhadi	Malabar Nutmeg, False Nutmeg, Bombay Nutmeg, Bombay Mace	Siddha/Tamil
Myroxylon balsamum	Balsam	Tolu Balsam Tree	Unani
Myrsine africana	Vaayavidanga	Pseudo-Embelia	Ayurvedic
Myrsine africana	Bebrang	Pseudo-Embelia	Folk
Myrsine africana	Kakhum	Pseudo-Embelia	Folk
Myrsine africana	Shamshaad	Pseudo-Embelia	Folk

Table Contd.

Botanical Name	Indian Name	English Name	Medicinal System
Nepeta hindostana	Baadranjbuuyaa	Catnip, Catnep, Catmint	Unani
Nepeta hindostana	Billilotan	Catnip, Catnep, Catmint	Unani
Neptunia oleracea	Lajjaalu (var.)	Sensitive Plant	Ayurvedic
Neptunia oleracea	Alambushaa	Sensitive Plant	Ayurvedic
Neptunia oleracea	Sadai	Sensitive Plant	Siddha/Tamil
Neptunia oleracea	Sundaikkirai	Sensitive Plant	Siddha/Tamil
Neptunia oleracea	Paani-lajak	Sensitive Plant	Folk
Nerium indicum	Karaveera	Indian Oleander, White Oleander	Ayurvedic
Nerium indicum	Viraka	Indian Oleander, White Oleander	Ayurvedic
Nerium indicum	Ashvamaaraka	Indian Oleander, White Oleander	Ayurvedic
Nerium indicum	Hayamaaraka	Indian Oleander, White Oleander	Ayurvedic
Nerium indicum	Gauripushpa	Indian Oleander, White Oleander	Ayurvedic
Nerium indicum	Divyapushpa	Indian Oleander, White Oleander	Ayurvedic
Nerium indicum	Shatakumbhak	Indian Oleander, White Oleander	Ayurvedic
Nerium indicum	Siddhapushpa	Indian Oleander, White Oleander	Ayurvedic
Nerium indicum	Ravipriya	Indian Oleander, White Oleander	Ayurvedic
Nerium indicum	Kaner Safed	Indian Oleander, White Oleander	Unani
Nerium indicum	Diflaa	Indian Oleander, White Oleander	Unani
Nerium indicum	Samm-ul-maar	Indian Oleander, White Oleander	Unani
Nerium indicum	Khar-zaharah	Indian Oleander, White Oleander	Unani
Nerium indicum	Arali	Indian Oleander, White Oleander	Siddha/Tamil
Nerium indicum	Genneru	Indian Oleander, White Oleander	Folk/Telugu
Nerium indicum	Karaviram	Indian Oleander, White Oleander	Siddha/Tamil

Table Contd.

Botanical Name	Indian Name	English Name	Medicinal System
Nerium oleander	Karaveeraka	Indian Oleander, White Oleander	Siddha/Tamil
Nerium oleander	Raktapushpa	Indian Oleander, White Oleander	Ayurvedic
Nerium oleander	Raktaprasava	Indian Oleander, White Oleander	Ayurvedic
Nerium oleander	Surkh Kaner	Red Oleander, Rose Bay	Unani
Nervilia aragoana	Padmachaarini	Tall Shield Orchid	Ayurvedic
Nervilia aragoana	Shankhaaluka	Tall Shield Orchid	Ayurvedic
Neuracanthus sphaerostachyus	Ganther	Pin Cushion Plant	Folk
Neuracanthus sphaerostachyus	Ghosa-vel	Pin Cushion Plant	Folk
Nicotiana tabacum	Taamraparna	Tobacco	Ayurvedic
Nicotiana tabacum	Dhuumrapatraa	Tobacco	Ayurvedic
Nicotiana tabacum	Tambaakhu	Tobacco	Unani
Nigella damascena	Upakunchikaa (var.)	Love-in-a-mist	Ayurvedic
Nigella damascena	Karumchee-rakam	Love-in-a-mist	Siddha/Tamil
Nigella sativa	Kaalaajaaji	Black Cumin, Small Fennel	Ayurvedic
Nigella sativa	Kalikaa	Black Cumin, Small Fennel	Ayurvedic
Nigella sativa	Prthvikaa	Black Cumin, Small Fennel	Ayurvedic
Nigella sativa	Sthulajiraka	Black Cumin, Small Fennel	Ayurvedic
Nigella sativa	Sushavi	Black Cumin, Small Fennel	Ayurvedic
Nigella sativa	Upkunchikaa	Black Cumin, Small Fennel	Ayurvedic
Nigella sativa	Kalonji	Black Cumin, Small Fennel	Unani
Nigella sativa	Kamaazaruus	Black Cumin, Small Fennel	Unani
Nigella sativa	Karuncheerakam Seeragm	Black Cumin, Small Fennel	Siddha/Tamil
Nilgirianthus ciliatus	Sahachara	Kurunji	Ayurvedic
Nilgirianthus ciliatus	Kurinji	Kurunji	Siddha/Tamil
Nilgirianthus ciliatus	Sinnangurinji	Kurunji	Siddha/Tamil
Nothosaerva brachiata	Dhaulaa-findauri	Grains of Selim	Folk
Notonia grandiflora	Mosakathuthalai	Common Fleshy Rag-weed	Siddha/Tamil

Table Contd.

Botanical Name	Indian Name	English Name	Medicinal System
Notonia grandiflora	Waandar-Roti	Common Fleshy Rag-weed	Folk
Notonia grandiflora	Gaidar	Common Fleshy Rag-weed	Folk
Nyctanthes arbor-tristis	Paarijaata	Tree of Sorrow, Night Jasmine, Coral Jasmine	Ayurvedic
Nyctanthes arbor-tristis	Shephaali	Tree of Sorrow, Night Jasmine, Coral Jasmine	Ayurvedic
Nyctanthes arbor-tristis	Shephaalikaa	Tree of Sorrow, Night Jasmine, Coral Jasmine	Ayurvedic
Nyctanthes arbor-tristis	Mandaara	Tree of Sorrow, Night Jasmine, Coral Jasmine	Ayurvedic
Nyctanthes arbor-tristis	Harasingaar	Tree of Sorrow, Night Jasmine, Coral Jasmine	Unani
Nyctanthes arbor-tristis	Pavazha mattigai	Tree of Sorrow, Night Jasmine, Coral Jasmine	Folk/Tamil
Nymphaea alba	Kumuda	European White Water-lily	Ayurvedic
Nymphaea alba	Utpala	European White Water-lily	Ayurvedic
Nymphaea alba	Nilofar	European White Water-lily	Unani
Nymphaea alba	Alli	European White Water-lily	Siddha/Tamil
Nymphaea rubra	Kumuda	Indian Red Water-lily	Ayurvedic
Nymphaea rubra	Utpala	Indian Red Water-lily	Ayurvedic
Nymphaea rubra	Alli-tamarai	Indian Red Water-lily	Folk/Tamil
Nymphaea rubra	Vellambal	Indian Red Water-lily	Folk/Tamil
Nymphaea stellata	Nilotpala	Indian Blue Water-lily	Ayurvedic
Nymphaea stellata	Nilofar	Indian Blue Water-lily	Unani
Nymphaea stellata	Neelothpalam	Indian Blue Water-lily	Siddha/Tamil
Nymphoides macrospermum	Granthik Tagar	Tagar	Folk
Ochna jabotapita	Chilanti	Bird's Eye Bush	Folk/Tamil
Ochna jabotapita	Sherundi	Bird's Eye Bush	Folk/Tamil
Ochna jabotapita	Kanaka Champaa	Bird's Eye Bush	Folk
Ochrocarpus longifolius	Surapunnaaga	Red-dye-flowerbud, Pseudo-Mesua ferra	Ayurvedic
Ochrocarpus longifolius	Nagappu	Red-dye-flowerbud, Pseudo-Mesua ferra	Folk/Tamil
Ochrocarpus longifolius	Nagesarpu	Red-dye-flowerbud, Pseudo-Mesua ferra	Folk/Tamil
Ochrocarpus longifolius	Laal-Naagakeshar	Red-dye-flowerbud, Pseudo-Mesua ferra	Folk

Table Contd.

Botanical Name	Indian Name	English Name	Medicinal System
Ochrocarpus longifolius	Surangi	Red-dye-flowerbud, Pseudo-Mesua ferra	Folk
Ocimum basilicum	Barbari	Sweet Basil, Basil Herb	Ayurvedic
Ocimum basilicum	Tuvari	Sweet Basil, Basil Herb	Ayurvedic
Ocimum basilicum	Tungi	Sweet Basil, Basil Herb	Ayurvedic
Ocimum basilicum	Kharpushpa	Sweet Basil, Basil Herb	Ayurvedic
Ocimum basilicum	Ajgandhikaa	Sweet Basil, Basil Herb	Ayurvedic
Ocimum basilicum	Baabui Tulasi	Sweet Basil, Basil Herb	Ayurvedic
Ocimum basilicum	Faranjmishk	Sweet Basil, Basil Herb	Unani
Ocimum basilicum	Raihan	Sweet Basil, Basil Herb	Unani
Ocimum basilicum	Tiruneetrup-pachhilai	Sweet Basil, Basil Herb	Siddha/Tamil
Ocimum basilicum	Bana-Tulasi	Sweet Basil, Basil Herb	Folk
Ocimum basilicum	Sabzaa	Sweet Basil, Basil Herb	Folk
Ocimum canum	Kaali Tulasi	Hoary Basil	Ayurvedic
Ocimum canum	Vana-Tulasi	Hoary Basil	Ayurvedic
Ocimum canum	Ganjamkorai	Hoary Basil	Folk/Tamil
Ocimum canum	Nayi-Tulasi	Hoary Basil	Folk/Tamil
Ocimum gratissimum	Vriddha Tulasi	Shrubby Basil	Ayurvedic
Ocimum gratissimum	Raam-Tulasi	Shrubby Basil	Ayurvedic
Ocimum gratissimum	Raan-Tulasi	Shrubby Basil	Ayurvedic
Ocimum gratissimum	Elumicham-Tulasi	Shrubby Basil	Folk/Tamil
Ocimum gratissimum	Peria-Tulasi	Shrubby Basil	Folk/Tamil
Ocimum kilimandscharicum	Karpura Tulasi	Camphor Basil	Ayurvedic
Ocimum sanctum	Tulasi	Holy Basil, Sacred Basil	Ayurvedic
Ocimum sanctum	Surasaa	Holy Basil, Sacred Basil	Ayurvedic
Ocimum sanctum	Surasa	Holy Basil, Sacred Basil	Ayurvedic
Ocimum sanctum	Bhuutaghni	Holy Basil, Sacred Basil	Ayurvedic
Ocimum sanctum	Suravalli	Holy Basil, Sacred Basil	Ayurvedic
Ocimum sanctum	Sulabhaa	Holy Basil, Sacred Basil	Ayurvedic
Ocimum sanctum	Manjarikaa	Holy Basil, Sacred Basil	Ayurvedic
Ocimum sanctum	Bahumanjari	Holy Basil, Sacred Basil	Ayurvedic
Ocimum sanctum	Deva-dundhubhi	Holy Basil, Sacred Basil	Ayurvedic

Table Contd.

Botanical Name	Indian Name	English Name	Medicinal System
Ocimum sanctum	Apet-raakshasi	Holy Basil, Sacred Basil	Ayurvedic
Ocimum sanctum	Shuulaghni	Holy Basil, Sacred Basil	Ayurvedic
Ocimum sanctum	Graamya	Holy Basil, Sacred Basil	Ayurvedic
Ocimum sanctum	Tulasi	Holy Basil, Sacred Basil	Unani
Ocimum sanctum	Tulasi	Holy Basil, Sacred Basil	Siddha/Tamil
Ocimum sanctum	Nalla-Tulasi	Holy Basil, Sacred Basil	Siddha/Tamil
Ocimum viride	Taap-maari Tulasi	Fever Plant of Sierra Leone	Folk
Oenanthe javanica	Jateraa	Water Dropwort	Folk
Oenanthe javanica	Panturasi	Water Dropwort	Folk
Oenothera odorata	Evening Primrose	Evening Primrose (var.), Sundrop (var.)	Folk
Olax scandens	Dheniaani	Olax	Ayurvedic
Olax scandens	Karbudaar	Olax	Ayurvedic
Olax scandens	Malliveppam	Olax	Folk/Tamil
Olax scandens	Kadalranchi	Olax	Folk/Tamil
Olax scandens	Rimil-beeri	Olax	Folk
Oldenlandia umbellata	Inbooral	Indian Madder, Chay-Root	Siddha/Tamil
Oldenlandia umbellata	Chiraval	Indian Madder, Chay-Root	Folk
Olea europaea	Zaitoon	Olive	Unani
Onosma bracteatum	Gojihvaa	Borage	Ayurvedic
Onosma bracteatum	Kharpatraa	Borage	Ayurvedic
Onosma bracteatum	Darvipatraa	Borage	Ayurvedic
Onosma bracteatum	Vrishjihvaa	Borage	Ayurvedic
Onosma bracteatum	Gaozabaan	Borage	Unani
Onosma bracteatum	Ununjil	Borage	Siddha/Tamil
Onosma echioides	Ratanjot	Goldendrop, Red-dye Onosma	Unani
Operculina turpethum	Trivrta	Indian Jalap, Turpeth	Ayurvedic
Operculina turpethum	Tribhandi	Indian Jalap, Turpeth	Ayurvedic
Operculina turpethum	Triputaa	Indian Jalap, Turpeth	Ayurvedic
Operculina turpethum	Saralaa	Indian Jalap, Turpeth	Ayurvedic
Operculina turpethum	Suvahaa	Indian Jalap, Turpeth	Ayurvedic
Operculina turpethum	Rechani	Indian Jalap, Turpeth	Ayurvedic

Table Contd.

Botanical Name	Indian Name	English Name	Medicinal System
Operculina turpethum	Nishotra	Indian Jalap, Turpeth	Ayurvedic
Operculina turpethum	Kumbha	Indian Jalap, Turpeth	Ayurvedic
Operculina turpethum	Kaalameshi	Indian Jalap, Turpeth	Ayurvedic
Operculina turpethum	Sushenaa	Indian Jalap, Turpeth	Ayurvedic
Operculina turpethum	Shyaamaa	Indian Jalap, Turpeth	Ayurvedic
Operculina turpethum	Turbud	Indian Jalap, Turpeth	Unani
Operculina turpethum	Nishoth	Indian Jalap, Turpeth	Unani
Operculina turpethum	Karunchivadai	Indian Jalap, Turpeth	Siddha/Tamil
Ophioglossum vulgatum	Sarpachhada	English Adder's Tongue, Serpant's Tongue	Folk
Ophiorrhiza mungos	Sarpaakshi	Mongoose Plant	Ayurvedic
Ophiorrhiza mungos	Keerippundu	Mongoose Plant	Folk/Tamil
Ophiorrhiza mungos	Sarahati	Mongoose Plant	Folk
Ophiorrhiza mungos	Mungus-vel	Mongoose Plant	Folk
Opuntia cochinellifera	Puchikalli	Cochineal Cactus	Siddha/Tamil
Opuntia dillenii	Naagaphani	Prickly Pear, Slipper Thorn	Ayurvedic
Opuntia dillenii	Kanthaari	Prickly Pear, Slipper Thorn	Ayurvedic
Opuntia dillenii	Naagaphani	Prickly Pear, Slipper Thorn	Unani
Opuntia dillenii	Sappathikalli	Prickly Pear, Slipper Thorn	Folk/Tamil
Opuntia dillenii	Nagathali	Prickly Pear, Slipper Thorn	Folk/Tamil
Opuntia vulgaris	Naagaphani (var.)	Prickly Pear	Ayurvedic
Orchis latifolia	Munjaataka	Orchis, Salep	Ayurvedic
Orchis latifolia	Saalam-misri	Orchis, Salep	Ayurvedic
Orchis latifolia	Saalam-panjaa	Orchis, Salep	Ayurvedic
Orchis latifolia	Saaleb	Orchis, Salep	Unani
Orchis latifolia	Khusyaat-us-Saalab	Orchis, Salep	Unani
Orchis latifolia	Saalab Misri	Orchis, Salep	Unani
Orchis latifolia	Silamishri	Orchis, Salep	Siddha/Tamil
Origanum majorana	Sukhaatmaka	Sweet Marjoram	Ayurvedic
Origanum majorana	Marubaka	Sweet Marjoram	Ayurvedic
Origanum majorana	Phanijjaka	Sweet Marjoram	Ayurvedic
Origanum majorana	Marzanjosh	Sweet Marjoram	Unani

Table Contd.

Botanical Name	Indian Name	English Name	Medicinal System
Origanum majorana	Maruvu	Sweet Marjoram	Siddha/Tamil
Origanum majorana	Santhraa	Sweet Marjoram	Folk
Origanum majorana	Jangali Maruaa	Sweet Marjoram	Folk
Oroxylum indicum	Shyonaaka	Indian Trumpet Flower	Ayurvedic
Oroxylum indicum	Shoshana	Indian Trumpet Flower	Ayurvedic
Oroxylum indicum	Tuntuka	Indian Trumpet Flower	Ayurvedic
Oroxylum indicum	Kutannata	Indian Trumpet Flower	Ayurvedic
Oroxylum indicum	Madhukparna	Indian Trumpet Flower	Ayurvedic
Oroxylum indicum	Patrorna	Indian Trumpet Flower	Ayurvedic
Oroxylum indicum	Bhalluka	Indian Trumpet Flower	Ayurvedic
Oroxylum indicum	Prthushimba	Indian Trumpet Flower	Ayurvedic
Oroxylum indicum	Aralu	Indian Trumpet Flower	Ayurvedic
Oroxylum indicum	Peruvaagai	Indian Trumpet Flower	Siddha/Tamil
Oroxylum indicum	Sonaa-paathaa	Indian Trumpet Flower	Folk
Orthosiphon grandiflorus	Mutri-Tulasi	Kidney Tea Plant, Java Tea	Folk
Orthosiphon tomentosus	Prataanikaa	Cat's Whiskers	Ayurvedic
Orthosiphon tomentosus	Tulasi (var.)	Cat's Whiskers	Folk
Orthosiphon tomentosus	Kattu-thrithava	Cat's Whiskers	Folk
Oryza sativa	Shaali	Rice	Ayurvedic
Oryza sativa	Vrihidhaanya	Rice	Ayurvedic
Oryza sativa	Tandula	Rice	Ayurvedic
Oryza sativa	Nivara	Rice	Ayurvedic
Oryza sativa	Biranj Saathi	Rice	Unani
Oryza sativa	Nell	Rice	Siddha/Tamil
Osbeckia chinensis	Bhui-lukham	Chinese Osbeckia	Folk
Osmanthus fragrans	Vasuka	Sweet Olive Tree	Ayurvedic
Osmanthus fragrans	Bakula	Sweet Olive Tree	Folk
Osmanthus fragrans	Silingi	Sweet Olive Tree	Folk
Osmanthus fragrans	Bagahul	Sweet Olive Tree	Folk
Osmanthus fragrans	Buuk	Sweet Olive Tree	Folk
Osyris wightiana	Popli	African Sandalwood, Zanzibar Lawa Wood	Folk
Osyris wightiana	Paral	African Sandalwood, Zanzibar Lawa Wood	Folk

Table Contd.

Botanical Name	Indian Name	English Name	Medicinal System
Osyris wightiana	Jhuri	African Sandalwood, Zanzibar Lawa Wood	Folk
Osyris wightiana	Dalmi	African Sandalwood, Zanzibar Lawa Wood	Folk
Osyris wightiana	Dalmia	African Sandalwood, Zanzibar Lawa Wood	Folk
Ougeinia dalbergioides	Tinishaa	Chariot Tree, Punjab Kino	Ayurvedic
Ougeinia dalbergioides	Tinisha	Chariot Tree, Punjab Kino	Ayurvedic
Ougeinia dalbergioides	Syandana	Chariot Tree, Punjab Kino	Ayurvedic
Ougeinia dalbergioides	Nemi	Chariot Tree, Punjab Kino	Ayurvedic
Ougeinia dalbergioides	Sarvasaara	Chariot Tree, Punjab Kino	Ayurvedic
Ougeinia dalbergioides	Ashmagarbhaka	Chariot Tree, Punjab Kino	Ayurvedic
Ougeinia dalbergioides	Vajjala	Chariot Tree, Punjab Kino	Ayurvedic
Ougeinia dalbergioides	Chitrakrt	Chariot Tree, Punjab Kino	Ayurvedic
Ougeinia dalbergioides	Narivengai	Chariot Tree, Punjab Kino	Folk/Tamil
Ougeinia dalbergioides	Saanan	Chariot Tree, Punjab Kino	Folk
Oxalis acetosella	Chaangeri	Common Wood-Sorrel	Ayurvedic
Oxalis acetosella	Tinpatiyaa	Common Wood-Sorrel	Folk
Oxalis acetosella	Amrul	Common Wood-Sorrel	Folk
Oxalis corniculata	Chaangeri	Indian Sorrel	Ayurvedic
Oxalis corniculata	Amlapatrikaa	Indian Sorrel	Ayurvedic
Oxalis corniculata	Amlikaa	Indian Sorrel	Ayurvedic
Oxalis corniculata	Chukraa	Indian Sorrel	Ayurvedic
Oxalis corniculata	Chukrikaa	Indian Sorrel	Ayurvedic
Oxalis corniculata	Chhatraamlikaa	Indian Sorrel	Ayurvedic
Oxalis corniculata	Ambutaa Bhaaji	Indian Sorrel	Unani
Oxalis corniculata	Amutaa Saag	Indian Sorrel	Unani
Oxalis corniculata	Puliyaarai	Indian Sorrel	Siddha/Tamil
Oxalis corniculata	Tinpatiyaa	Indian Sorrel	Folk
Oxalis corniculata	Ambilonaa	Indian Sorrel	Folk
Oxyria digyna	Choh-hanka	Mountain Sorrel, Alpine Sorrel	Siddha/Tamil
Oxyria digyna	Amlu	Mountain Sorrel, Alpine Sorrel	Folk
Oxyria digyna	Kailaashi	Mountain Sorrel, Alpine Sorrel	Folk
Oxystelma secamone	Dugdhikaa	Dudhni, Chamuuk plaa lot (Thai)	Ayurvedic

Table Contd.

Botanical Name	Indian Name	English Name	Medicinal System
Oxystelma secamone	Duudhilataa	Dudhni, Chamuuk plaa lot (Thai)	Ayurvedic
Oxystelma secamone	Usippalai	Dudhni,Chamuuk plaa lot (Thai)	Folk/Tamil
Oxystelma secamone	Usipallai	Dudhni,Chamuuk plaa lot (Thai)	Folk
Oxystelma secamone	Dudhani	Dudhni,Chamuuk plaa lot (Thai)	Folk
Oxystelma secamone	Jaladudhi	Dudhni,Chamuuk plaa lot (Thai)	Folk
Paederia foetida	Prasaarini	Skunk Vine	Ayurvedic
Paederia foetida	Gandha-prasaarini	Skunk Vine	Ayurvedic
Paederia foetida	Gandhali	Skunk Vine	Folk
Paederia foetida	Hiran-vel	Skunk Vine	Folk
Paederia foetida	Penarisangai	Skunk Vine	Siddha/Tamil
Paederia foetida	Gandhabhaaduli	Skunk Vine	Folk
Paeonia emodi	Ood Saleeb	Himalayan Paeony	Unani
Paeonia emodi	Ood Gharqi	Himalayan Paeony	Unani
Paeonia emodi	Phaavaaniaa	Himalayan Paeony	Unani
Paeonia officinalis	Ood Gharqi	European Paeony	Unani
Paeonia officinalis	Ood Saleeb	European Paeony	Unani
Panax pseudoginseng	Indian Ginseng	Indian Pseudoginseng	Ayurvedic
Pandanus fascicularis	Ketaka	Screw Pine	Ayurvedic
Pandanus fascicularis	Ketaki	Screw Pine	Ayurvedic
Pandanus fascicularis	Suuchikaa pushpaa	Screw Pine	Ayurvedic
Pandanus fascicularis	Jambuka	Screw Pine	Ayurvedic
Pandanus fascicularis	Trinshunya	Screw Pine	Ayurvedic
Pandanus fascicularis	Ketakark	Screw Pine	Ayurvedic
Pandanus fascicularis	Krakchachhada	Screw Pine	Ayurvedic
Pandanus fascicularis	Keoraa	Screw Pine	Unani
Pandanus fascicularis	Thazhai	Screw Pine	Folk/Tamil
Pandanus fascicularis	Thalay	Screw Pine	Folk/Tamil
Pandanus utilis	Ketaki	Stilt-rooted Screw Pine	Ayurvedic

Table Contd.

Botanical Name	Indian Name	English Name	Medicinal System
Panicum miliaceum	Chinaaka	Common Millet, Proso Millet, Hog Millet	Ayurvedic
Panicum miliaceum	Cheenaa	Common Millet, Proso Millet, Hog Millet	Ayurvedic
Panicum miliaceum	Chinaa Ghaas	Common Millet, Proso Millet, Hog Millet	Unani
Panicum miliaceum	Faaluudaa	Common Millet, Proso Millet, Hog Millet	Unani
Panicum miliaceum	Panivaragu	Common Millet, Proso Millet, Hog Millet	Folk/Tamil
Panicum miliaceum	Kadukanni	Common Millet, Proso Millet, Hog Millet	Folk/Tamil
Panicum miliaceum	Chenaa	Common Millet, Proso Millet, Hog Millet	Folk
Papaver rhoeas	Rakta Posta	Corn Poppy, Red Poppy	Ayurvedic
Papaver rhoeas	Sivappu	Corn Poppy, Red Poppy	Siddha/Tamil
Papaver rhoeas	Kasakasa	Corn Poppy, Red Poppy	Siddha/Tamil
Papaver rhoeas	Laal Posta	Corn Poppy, Red Poppy	Folk
Papaver rhoeas	Laal Kaskas	Corn Poppy, Red Poppy	Folk
Papaver somniferum	Ahiphena	Opium	Ayurvedic
Papaver somniferum	Aaphuuka	Opium Poppy	Ayurvedic
Papaver somniferum	Post-daanaa (seed)	Opium Poppy	Ayurvedic
Papaver somniferum	Afyum	Opium	Unani
Papaver somniferum	Tukhm-e-khashkhaash	Opium Poppy	Unani
Papaver somniferum	Kasakasa (Seeds)	Opium Poppy	Siddha/Tamil
Papaver somniferum	Abini	Opium	Siddha/Tamil
Paris polyphylla	Haimavati	Herb Paris, Tingling Rootstock Plant	Ayurvedic
Paris polyphylla	Shveta-vachaa	Herb Paris, Tingling Rootstock Plant	Ayurvedic
Paris polyphylla	Baal-bach	Herb Paris, Tingling Rootstock Plant	Folk
Parmelia perlata	Shaileya	Parmelia Lichen	Ayurvedic
Parmelia perlata	Shaileyaka	Parmelia Lichen	Ayurvedic
Parmelia perlata	Shilaapushpa	Parmelia Lichen	Ayurvedic

Table Contd.

Botanical Name	Indian Name	English Name	Medicinal System
Pedalium murex	Gokantaka	Caltrops (bigger var.)	Ayurvedic
Pedalium murex	Swaadukantaka	Caltrops (bigger var.)	Ayurvedic
Pedalium murex	Khaar-e-khasak Kalaan	Caltrops (bigger var.)	Unani
Pedalium murex	Gokharu Kalaan	Caltrops (bigger var.)	Unani
Pedalium murex	Aanai nerunchil	Caltrops (bigger var.)	Siddha/Tamil
Pedicularis pectinata	Mishran	Lousewort	Folk/Punjab
Pedicularis pectinata	Michren	Lousewort	Folk
Pedicularis pectinata	Lugro-maarpro	Lousewort	Folk/Kashmir
Pedilanthus tithymaloides	Vilaayati-sher	Slipper Plant, Bird-Cactus	Folk
Pedilanthus tithymaloides	Naagaphani	Slipper Plant, Bird-Cactus	Folk
Pedilanthus tithymaloides	Naagadaman	Slipper Plant, Bird-Cactus	Folk
Peganum harmala	Haramal	Wild Rue, Foreign Henna, Syrian Rue	Ayurvedic
Peganum harmala	Isband	Wild Rue, Foreign Henna, Syrian Rue	Ayurvedic
Peganum harmala	Isband-laahauri	Wild Rue, Foreign Henna, Syrian Rue	Folk
Peganum harmala	Simaiyalavinai	Wild Rue, Foreign Henna, Syrian Rue	Siddha/Tamil
Pelargonium graveolens	Algerian Geranium	Geranium	Folk
Peltophorum pterocarpum	Kondachinta	Copper Pod, Rusty Shield-Bearer	Folk/Telugu
Peltophorum pterocarpum	Perungondrai	Copper Pod, Rusty Shield-Bearer	Siddha/Tamil
Pentapetes phoenicea	Bandhujiva	Midday Flower, Copper Cup, Scarlet Mallow, Florimpia	Ayurvedic
Pentapetes phoenicea	Bandhuuka	Midday Flower, Copper Cup, Scarlet Mallow, Florimpia	Ayurvedic
Pentapetes phoenicea	Arkavallabha	Midday Flower, Copper Cup, Scarlet Mallow, Florimpia	Ayurvedic
Pentapetes phoenicea	Gul-dupahariaa	Midday Flower, Copper Cup, Scarlet Mallow, Florimpia	Folk
Pentatropis microphylla	Kaakanaasaa	Ambervel, Beak-shaped Elliptic Flower	Ayurvedic
Pentatropis microphylla	Kaakanaasikaa	Ambervel, Beak-shaped Elliptic Flower	Ayurvedic

Table Contd.

Botanical Name	Indian Name	English Name	Medicinal System
Pentatropis microphylla	Kaakaangi	Ambervel, Beak-shaped Elliptic Flower	Ayurvedic
Pentatropis microphylla	Kaaktundphalaa	Ambervel, Beak-shaped Elliptic Flower	Ayurvedic
Pentatropis microphylla	Shringiritti	Ambervel, Beak-shaped Elliptic Flower	Ayurvedic
Pentatropis microphylla	Uppilankodi	Ambervel, Beak-shaped Elliptic Flower	Siddha/Tamil
Pentatropis microphylla	Singarauti	Ambervel, Beak-shaped Elliptic Flower	Folk
Pentatropis microphylla	Amarvel	Ambervel, Beak-shaped Elliptic Flower	Folk
Pentatropis spiralis	Kaakanaasaa	Ambervel	Ayurvedic
Pentatropis spiralis	Ambarvel	Ambervel	Folk
Pentatropis spiralis	Vanaveri	Ambervel	Folk
Pergularia extensa	Uttamaarani	Hairknot Plant, Whitlow Plant	Ayurvedic
Pergularia extensa	Vrischikaali	Hairknot Plant, Whitlow Plant	Ayurvedic
Pergularia extensa	Vishaanikaa	Hairknot Plant, Whitlow Plant	Ayurvedic
Pergularia extensa	Phalakantaka	Hairknot Plant, Whitlow Plant	Ayurvedic
Pergularia extensa	Uththaamani	Hairknot Plant, Whitlow Plant	Siddha/Tamil
Pergularia extensa	Veli-paruthi	Hairknot Plant, Whitlow Plant	Folk/Tamil
Pergularia extensa	Utaran	Hairknot Plant, Whitlow Plant	Folk
Pericampylus glaucus	Baarak-kaant	Broad-leaved Moonseed	Folk
Pericampylus glaucus	Goriaa-loti	Broad-leaved Moonseed	Folk
Perilepta auriculata	Kurinji	Pandai	Siddha/Tamil
Perilepta auriculata	Pandadi	Pandai	Folk
Perilla frutescens	Ban-Jiraa	Perilla, Wild Coleus	Folk
Perilla frutescens	Ban-tulasi	Perilla, Wild Coleus	Folk
Perilla frutescens	Bhanjeer	Perilla, Wild Coleus	Folk
Perilla frutescens	Bhasindi	Perilla, Wild Coleus	Folk
Periploca aphylla	Barri	Milk Broom	Folk
Periploca calophylla	Krishna Saarivaa	Ging she teng (Chinese)	Ayurvedic
Peristrophe bicalyculata	Nadikaantaa	Panicled Peristrophe	Ayurvedic
Peristrophe bicalyculata	Praachibalaa	Panicled Peristrophe	Ayurvedic
Peristrophe bicalyculata	Sulomshaa	Panicled Peristrophe	Ayurvedic

Table Contd.

Botanical Name	Indian Name	English Name	Medicinal System
Peristrophe bicalyculata	Kaakatikta	Panicled Peristrophe	Ayurvedic
Peristrophe bicalyculata	Kaakajanghaa	Panicled Peristrophe	Ayurvedic
Peristrophe bicalyculata	Chebisa	Panicled Peristrophe	Siddha/Tamil
Peristrophe bicalyculata	Masi	Panicled Peristrophe	Folk
Persea americana	Makkhan Phal	Avacado, Alligator Pear	Folk
Persea americana	Kulu Naaspaati	Avacado, Alligator Pear	Folk
Persea macrantha	Picchita-taru	Machilus	Folk
Persea macrantha	Kshudra-aamra	Machilus	Folk
Petroselinum crispum	Fitraasaaliyum	Parsley	Unani
Petroselinum crispum	Karafs-e-Kohi	Parsley	Unani
Peucedanum grande	Baaphali	Wild Carrot	Folk
Peucedanum grande	Duku	Wild Carrot	Folk
Phaseolus aconitifolius	Makushtha	Aconite-Bean, Moth	Ayurvedic
Phaseolus aconitifolius	Moth	Aconite-Bean, Moth	Ayurvedic
Phaseolus aconitifolius	Tulukkapayir	Aconite-Bean, Moth	Siddha/Tamil
Phaseolus adenanthus	Aranya-mudga	South American Snail Vine	Ayurvedic
Phaseolus adenanthus	Mudgaparni	South American Snail Vine	Ayurvedic
Phaseolus adenanthus	Kattupayaru	South American Snail Vine	Siddha/Tamil
Phaseolus lunatus	Shimbi	Double Bean, Lima Bean, Burma Bean	Ayurvedic
Phaseolus lunatus	Lobiyaa	Double Bean, Lima Bean, Burma Bean	Unani
Phaseolus lunatus	Sem	Double Bean, Lima Bean, Burma Bean	Unani
Phaseolus mungo	Maasha	Kidney Bean, Black Gram	Ayurvedic
Phaseolus mungo	Urd-Siyaah	Kidney Bean, Black Gram	Unani
Phaseolus mungo	Ulunthu	Kidney Bean, Black Gram	Siddha/Tamil
Phaseolus radiatus	Mudga	Greengram, Golden Gram	Ayurvedic
Phaseolus radiatus	Mungalya	Greengram, Golden Gram	Ayurvedic
Phaseolus radiatus	Moong	Greengram, Golden Gram	Unani
Phaseolus radiatus	Pattishai-payaru	Greengram, Golden Gram	Siddha/Tamil
Phaseolus trilobus	Mudgaparni	Wild Gram	Ayurvedic
Phaseolus trilobus	Kaakaparni	Wild Gram	Ayurvedic
Phaseolus trilobus	Suuryaparni	Wild Gram	Ayurvedic

Table Contd.

Botanical Name	Indian Name	English Name	Medicinal System
Phaseolus trilobus	Alpikaa	Wild Gram	Ayurvedic
Phaseolus trilobus	Sahaa	Wild Gram	Ayurvedic
Phaseolus trilobus	Kaakamudraa	Wild Gram	Ayurvedic
Phaseolus trilobus	Maarjaar-gandhikaa	Wild Gram	Ayurvedic
Phaseolus trilobus	Kaatupayaru	Wild Gram	Siddha/Tamil
Phaseolus trilobus	Jangali Moong	Wild Gram	Folk
Phaseolus trilobus	Mugavan	Wild Gram	Folk
Phaseolus vulgaris	Raajmah (seed)	Kidney Bean, French Bean, Haricot Bean	Unani
Phaseolus vulgaris	Lobia	Kidney Bean	Unani
Phaseolus vulgaris	Frashbean	Kidney Bean, French Bean, Haricot Bean	Unani
Phlogacanthus thyrsiflorus	Dieng-soh kajut	Nongmangkha, Banheka	Folk
Phlogacanthus thyrsiflorus	Chuhai	Nongmangkha, Banheka	Folk
Phlogacanthus thyrsiflorus	Titaaphul	Nongmangkha, Banheka	Folk
Phoenix dactylifera	Kharjuura	Date Palm	Ayurvedic
Phoenix dactylifera	Kharjuuraka	Date Palm	Ayurvedic
Phoenix dactylifera	Kharjuurikaa	Date Palm	Ayurvedic
Phoenix dactylifera	Pindakhar-juurikaa	Date Palm	Ayurvedic
Phoenix dactylifera	Chhuhaaraa (dry date)	Date Palm	Ayurvedic
Phoenix dactylifera	Khurmaa	Date Palm	Unani
Phoenix dactylifera	Khajuur	Date Palm	Unani
Phoenix dactylifera	Chhuharaa	Date Palm	Unani
Phoenix dactylifera	Pereecham/ pazham (Fruit)	Date Palm	Siddha/Tamil
Phoenix dactylifera	Ita	Date Palm	Siddha/Tamil
Phoenix paludosa	Hintala	Bengal Palm	Ayurvedic
Phoenix paludosa	Hintalamu	Bengal Palm	Folk
Phoenix paludosa	Hital	Bengal Palm	Folk
Phoenix pusilla	Parushaka	Wild Coromandel Palm	Ayurvedic
Phoenix pusilla	Kalangu	Wild Coromandel Palm	Siddha/Tamil
Phoenix pusilla	Ithi	Wild Coromandel Palm	Folk/Tamil

Table Contd.

Botanical Name	Indian Name	English Name	Medicinal System
Phoenix pusilla	Chitti-ita	Wild Coromandel Palm	Folk/Telugu
Phoenix sylvestris	Kharjuuri	Wild Date Palm	Ayurvedic
Phoenix sylvestris	Pedda-ita	Wild Date Palm	Folk/Telugu
Phoenix sylvestris	Periyaitcham	Wild Date Palm	Folk/Tamil
Phoenix sylvestris	Sulemaani Khajuur	Wild Date Palm	Folk
Phoenix sylvestris	Khajuur Desi	Wild Date Palm	Folk
Pholidota articulata	Jivanti	Coelogyne Orchid	Ayurvedic
Phragmites communis	Dil	Common Reed	Folk/Punjab
Phragmites communis	Dambu	Common Reed	Folk/Punjab
Phragmites karka	Nala	Common Reed-grass	Ayurvedic
Phragmites karka	Narakul	Common Reed-grass	Folk
Phragmites karka	Perunanal	Common Reed-grass	Siddha/Tamil
Phyla nodiflora	Jalapippali	Fogfruit, Sawtooth Fogfruit	Ayurvedic
Phyla nodiflora	Laangali	Fogfruit, Sawtooth Fogfruit	Ayurvedic
Phyla nodiflora	Matsyaadani	Fogfruit, Sawtooth Fogfruit	Ayurvedic
Phyla nodiflora	Matsyagandhaa	Fogfruit, Sawtooth Fogfruit	Ayurvedic
Phyla nodiflora	Shaaradi	Fogfruit, Sawtooth Fogfruit	Ayurvedic
Phyla nodiflora	Shakulaadani	Fogfruit, Sawtooth Fogfruit	Ayurvedic
Phyla nodiflora	Vashiraa	Fogfruit, Sawtooth Fogfruit	Ayurvedic
Phyla nodiflora	Poduthalai	Fogfruit, Sawtooth Fogfruit	Siddha/Tamil
Phyllanthus amarus	Bahupatri	Indian Chanca Piedra	Ayurvedic
Phyllanthus amarus	Bahuphalaa	Indian Chanca Piedra	Ayurvedic
Phyllanthus amarus	Bhuudhaatri	Indian Chanca Piedra	Ayurvedic
Phyllanthus amarus	Bhuumya-amalaki	Indian Chanca Piedra	Ayurvedic
Phyllanthus amarus	Taamalaki	Indian Chanca Piedra	Ayurvedic
Phyllanthus amarus	Bhui Aaamalaa	Indian Chanca Piedra	Unani
Phyllanthus amarus	Keezh Kai Nelli	Indian Chanca Piedra	Siddha/Tamil
Phyllanthus distichus	Lavali-phala	Country Gooseberry	Ayurvedic
Phyllanthus distichus	Lowani Hariphala	Country Gooseberry	Ayurvedic
Phyllanthus distichus	Arunelli	Country Gooseberry	Siddha/Tamil
Phyllanthus maderaspatensis	Isfahaan Marv	Kanocha Seed	Unani

Table Contd.

Botanical Name	Indian Name	English Name	Medicinal System
Phyllanthus maderaspatensis	Kanochaa	Kanocha Seed	Unani
Phyllanthus maderaspatensis	Mela-nelli	Kanocha Seed	Siddha/Tamil
Phyllanthus niruri	Bhuumyaa-malaki	Chanca Piedra	Ayurvedic
Phyllanthus simplex	Bhumyaa-malaki (var.)	Wild Chanca Piedra	Ayurvedic
Phyllanthus simplex	Mothi-bhuiaamvali	Wild Chanca Piedra	Folk
Phyllanthus urinaria	Bhuumyaa-malaki (var.)	Cultivated Field Chanca Piedra	Ayurvedic
Phyllanthus urinaria	Hazaar-mani	Cultivated Field Chanca Piedra	Folk
Phyllanthus urinaria	Laal-bhui-aamlaa	Cultivated Field Chanca Piedra	Folk
Phyllanthus urinaria	Senkeezhnelli	Cultivated Field Chanca Piedra	Siddha/Tamil
Phyllanthus urinaria	Taamravalli	Cultivated Field Chanca Piedra	Ayurvedic
Physalis alkekengi	Kaaknaj	Strawberry Tomato, Winter Cherry	Unani
Physalis alkekengi	Raajaputrikaa	Strawberry Tomato, Winter Cherry	Ayurvedic
Physalis minima	Tankaari	Sun-berry	Ayurvedic
Physalis minima	Parpotikaa	Sun-berry	Ayurvedic
Physalis minima	Chirapotikaa	Sun-berry	Ayurvedic
Physalis minima	Sodakku Thakkali	Sun-berry	Siddha/Tamil
Physalis peruviana	Parpoti (var.)	Cape Gooseberry	Ayurvedic
Physalis peruviana	Perungunni	Cape Gooseberry	Siddha/Tamil
Physalis peruviana	Pottipallam	Cape Gooseberry	Siddha/Tamil
Physalis peruviana	Rasbhari	Cape Gooseberry	Folk
Physalis peruviana	Mako	Cape Gooseberry	Folk
Physochlaina praealta	Bajarbang	Hyoscyamine Plant	Folk
Physochlaina praealta	Daturaa	Hyoscyamine Plant	Folk
Physochlaina praealta	Laangtaan	Hyoscyamine Plant	Folk
Physochlaina praealta	Sholar	Hyoscyamine Plant	Folk
Picea smithiana	Roi	West Himalayan Spruce	Folk
Picea smithiana	Rhai	West Himalayan Spruce	Folk
Picea smithiana	Raghaa	West Himalayan Spruce	Folk

Table Contd.

Botanical Name	Indian Name	English Name	Medicinal System
Picea smithiana	Kathela	West Himalayan Spruce	Folk
Picea smithiana	Kandre	West Himalayan Spruce	Folk
Picea smithiana	Morindaa	West Himalayan Spruce	Folk
Picea smithiana	Spruce (trade)	West Himalayan Spruce	Folk
Picrasma quassioides	Bhurangi	Quassia	Ayurvedic
Picrasma quassioides	Nimbi	Quassia	Ayurvedic
Picrasma quassioides	Nimatotaa	Quassia	Folk
Picrorhiza kurroa	Katukaa	Picrorhiza	Ayurvedic
Picrorhiza kurroa	Katurohini	Picrorhiza	Ayurvedic
Picrorhiza kurroa	Kattarohini	Picrorhiza	Ayurvedic
Picrorhiza kurroa	Katuki	Picrorhiza	Ayurvedic
Picrorhiza kurroa	Katukikaa	Picrorhiza	Ayurvedic
Picrorhiza kurroa	Krishnabhedaa	Picrorhiza	Ayurvedic
Picrorhiza kurroa	Kaandaruhaa	Picrorhiza	Ayurvedic
Picrorhiza kurroa	Matsyashakalaa	Picrorhiza	Ayurvedic
Picrorhiza kurroa	Chakraangi	Picrorhiza	Ayurvedic
Picrorhiza kurroa	Shatparvaa	Picrorhiza	Ayurvedic
Picrorhiza kurroa	Arishta	Picrorhiza	Ayurvedic
Picrorhiza kurroa	Ashokarohinya	Picrorhiza	Ayurvedic
Picrorhiza kurroa	Shakuldaani	Picrorhiza	Ayurvedic
Picrorhiza kurroa	Kutki	Picrorhiza	Unani
Picrorhiza kurroa	Kharbaq-e-Hindi	Picrorhiza	Unani
Picrorhiza kurroa	Kaduguragini	Picrorhiza	Siddha/Tamil
Pilocarpus microphyllus	Jaborandi	Jaborandi	Folk
Pimenta dioica	Pimento	Allspice Tree, Jamaica Pepper Tree, Pimento Tree	Folk
Pimpinella anisum	Anisoon	Anise, Aniseed	Unani
Pimpinella anisum	Baadiyaan-roomi	Anise, Aniseed	Unani
Pimpinella saxifraga	Bekh-e-Baadiyaan	Burnet Saxifrage Root, Pimpinella Root	Folk
Pinus excelsa	Chillaa	Indian Blue Pine, Bhutan Pine, Five-leaved Pine	Folk
Pinus excelsa	Sarala	Indian Blue Pine, Bhutan Pine, Five-leaved Pine	Ayurvedic

Table Contd.

Botanical Name	Indian Name	English Name	Medicinal System
Pinus gerardiana	Nikochaka	Neosia Pine, Edible Pine, Chilgoza Pine	Ayurvedic
Pinus gerardiana	Chilgozaa	Neosia Pine, Edible Pine, Chilgoza Pine	Unani
Pinus khasya	Sarala var.	Khasi Pine	Ayurvedic
Pinus khasya	Digsaa	Khasi Pine	Folk
Pinus roxburghii	Sarala	Long-leaved Pine, Three-leaved Pine, Chir Pine	Ayurvedic
Pinus roxburghii	Pita-vriksha	Long-leaved Pine, Three-leaved Pine, Chir Pine	Ayurvedic
Pinus roxburghii	Surabhidaaruka	Long-leaved Pine, Three-leaved Pine, Chir Pine	Ayurvedic
Pinus roxburghii	Dhuupavriksha	Long-leaved Pine, Three-leaved Pine, Chir Pine	Ayurvedic
Pinus roxburghii	Namasu	Long-leaved Pine, Three-leaved Pine, Chir Pine	Ayurvedic
Pinus roxburghii	Shriveshtaka (Oleo-resin)	Long-leaved Pine, Three-leaved Pine, Chir Pine	Ayurvedic
Pinus roxburghii	Ghandh-Birojaa	Long-leaved Pine, Three-leaved Pine, Chir Pine	Ayurvedic
Pinus roxburghii	Sanobar-ul-Hindi	Long-leaved Pine, Three-leaved Pine, Chir Pine	Unani
Pinus roxburghii	Gandh-Bihrojaa (Oleo-resin)	Long-leaved Pine, Three-leaved Pine, Chir Pine	Unani
Pinus roxburghii	Qinn	Long-leaved Pine, Three-leaved Pine, Chir Pine	Unani
Pinus roxburghii	Berzad	Long-leaved Pine, Three-leaved Pine, Chir Pine	Unani
Pinus roxburghii	Simaidevadaru	Long-leaved Pine, Three-leaved Pine, Chir Pine	Siddha/Tamil
Pinus succinifera	Ambar	Baltic Amber, Succinite	Unani
Pinus succinifera	Kahruubaa	Baltic Amber, Succinite	Unani
Piper attenuatum	Kattumilaaku	Oval-leaved Pepper Plant	Siddha/Tamil
Piper betle	Taambula	Betel Pepper	Ayurvedic
Piper betle	Naagvallari	Betel Pepper	Ayurvedic
Piper betle	Naagini	Betel Pepper	Ayurvedic
Piper betle	Taambulvalli	Betel Pepper	Ayurvedic
Piper betle	Saptashiraa	Betel Pepper	Ayurvedic

Table Contd.

Botanical Name	Indian Name	English Name	Medicinal System
Piper betle	Bhujangalataa	Betel Pepper	Ayurvedic
Piper betle	Paan	Betel Pepper	Unani
Piper betle	Tambool	Betel Pepper	Unani
Piper betle	Vetrilai	Betel Pepper	Siddha/Tamil
Piper betle	Nagavalli	Betel Pepper	Folk
Piper betle	Paataalavaasini	Betel Pepper	Folk
Piper chaba	Chavika	Java Long Pepper	Ayurvedic
Piper chaba	Chavya	Java Long Pepper	Ayurvedic
Piper chaba	Gajapippali	Java Long Pepper	Ayurvedic
Piper chaba	Milagu	Java Long Pepper	Siddha/Tamil
Piper cubeba	Kankola	Cubeb, Tailed Pepper	Ayurvedic
Piper cubeba	Kakkola	Cubeb, Tailed Pepper	Ayurvedic
Piper cubeba	Kankolaka	Cubeb, Tailed Pepper	Ayurvedic
Piper cubeba	Takkola	Cubeb, Tailed Pepper	Ayurvedic
Piper cubeba	Koraka	Cubeb, Tailed Pepper	Ayurvedic
Piper cubeba	Kolaka	Cubeb, Tailed Pepper	Ayurvedic
Piper cubeba	Kashphala	Cubeb, Tailed Pepper	Ayurvedic
Piper cubeba	Sheetalchini	Cubeb, Tailed Pepper	Ayurvedic
Piper cubeba	Chinoshana	Cubeb, Tailed Pepper	Ayurvedic
Piper cubeba	Kabaabchini	Cubeb, Tailed Pepper	Unani
Piper cubeba	Habb-ul-uruus	Cubeb, Tailed Pepper	Unani
Piper cubeba	Vaalmilagu	Cubeb, Tailed Pepper	Siddha/Tamil
Piper hamiltonii	Jangali Paan	Wild Pepper	Folk
Piper longum	Pippali	Indian Long Pepper, Joborandi	Ayurvedic
Piper longum	Maagadhi	Indian Long Pepper, Joborandi	Ayurvedic
Piper longum	Maagadha	Indian Long Pepper, Joborandi	Ayurvedic
Piper longum	Maagadhaa	Indian Long Pepper, Joborandi	Ayurvedic
Piper longum	Maagadhikaa	Indian Long Pepper, Joborandi	Ayurvedic
Piper longum	Magadho-dbhavaa	Indian Long Pepper, Joborandi	Ayurvedic
Piper longum	Vaidehi	Indian Long Pepper, Joborandi	Ayurvedic
Piper longum	Upkulyaa	Indian Long Pepper, Joborandi	Ayurvedic
Piper longum	Pippalikam	Indian Long Pepper, Joborandi	Ayurvedic

Table Contd.

Botanical Name	Indian Name	English Name	Medicinal System
Piper longum	Chapalaa	Indian Long Pepper, Joborandi	Ayurvedic
Piper longum	Kanaa	Indian Long Pepper, Joborandi	Ayurvedic
Piper longum	Krishnaa	Indian Long Pepper, Joborandi	Ayurvedic
Piper longum	Uushnaa	Indian Long Pepper, Joborandi	Ayurvedic
Piper longum	Shaundi	Indian Long Pepper, Joborandi	Ayurvedic
Piper longum	Kolaa	Indian Long Pepper, Joborandi	Ayurvedic
Piper longum	Tikshna-tandulaa	Indian Long Pepper, Joborandi	Ayurvedic
Piper longum	Filfil Daraaz	Indian Long Pepper, Joborandi	Unani
Piper longum	Daarfilfil	Indian Long Pepper, Joborandi	Unani
Piper longum	Thippili	Indian Long Pepper, Joborandi	Siddha/Tamil
Piper longum	Arisi thippili	Indian Long Pepper, Joborandi	Siddha/Tamil
Piper longum	Thippili ver (root)	Indian Long Pepper, Joborandi	Siddha/Tamil
Piper nigrum	Maricha	Black Pepper	Ayurvedic
Piper nigrum	Vellaja	Black Pepper	Ayurvedic
Piper nigrum	Uushna	Black Pepper	Ayurvedic
Piper nigrum	Suvrrita	Black Pepper	Ayurvedic
Piper nigrum	Krishnaa	Black Pepper	Ayurvedic
Piper nigrum	Filfil Siyaah	Black Pepper	Unani
Piper nigrum	Filfil Safed	White Pepper	Unani
Piper nigrum	Milagu	Black Pepper	Siddha/Tamil
Piper nigrum	Milagu ver (root)	Black Pepper	Siddha/Tamil
Piper schmidtii	Nilgiri Pepper	Nilgiri Pepper	Folk
Piper sylvaticum	Vana-Pippali	Mountain Long Pepper	Ayurvedic
Piper sylvaticum	Pahaari Peepal	Mountain Long Pepper	Folk
Piper thomsoni	Jangali Paan	Sikkim Betel	Folk
Piper wallichii	Kaattu-milagu	Nepal Pepper	Siddha/Tamil
Piper wallichii	Sambhaaluka	Nepal Pepper	Ayurvedic
Piscidia piscipula	Kukkur-kaashtha	Jamaica Dogwood	Folk
Pisonia aculeata	Baghachuur	Devil's Claw	Folk
Pisonia aculeata	Karindu	Devil's Claw	Siddha/Tamil
Pisonia grandis	Vilaayati Salet	Grand Devil's Claws	Folk

Table Contd.

Botanical Name	Indian Name	English Name	Medicinal System
Pisonia grandis	Leechai kottai keerai	Grand Devil's Claws	Siddha/Tamil
Pisonia grandis	Chinai Salit	Grand Devil's Claws	Folk
Pistacia integerrima	Karkatashringi	Horn-shaped Gall Tree, Kakra Gall Tree	Ayurvedic
Pistacia integerrima	Shringi	Horn-shaped Gall Tree, Kakra Gall Tree	Ayurvedic
Pistacia integerrima	Karkatash-ringikaa	Horn-shaped Gall Tree, Kakra Gall Tree	Ayurvedic
Pistacia integerrima	Karkata	Horn-shaped Gall Tree, Kakra Gall Tree	Ayurvedic
Pistacia integerrima	Karkataakhya	Horn-shaped Gall Tree, Kakra Gall Tree	Ayurvedic
Pistacia integerrima	Kulirashring-aaya	Horn-shaped Gall Tree, Kakra Gall Tree	Ayurvedic
Pistacia integerrima	Kuliravish-aanikaa	Horn-shaped Gall Tree, Kakra Gall Tree	Ayurvedic
Pistacia integerrima	Vakraa	Horn-shaped Gall Tree, Kakra Gall Tree	Ayurvedic
Pistacia integerrima	Vishaani	Horn-shaped Gall Tree, Kakra Gall Tree	Ayurvedic
Pistacia integerrima	Ajashringi	Horn-shaped Gall Tree, Kakra Gall Tree	Ayurvedic
Pistacia integerrima	Kaakraasingi	Horn-shaped Gall Tree, Kakra Gall Tree	Unani
Pistacia integerrima	Kakar	Horn-shaped Gall Tree, Kakra Gall Tree	Unani
Pistacia integerrima	Kaduka poo (Gall)	Horn-shaped Gall Tree, Kakra Gall Tree	Siddha/Tamil
Pistacia lentiscus	Mastagi	Mastic Tree	Unani
Pistacia lentiscus	Mastaki	Mastic Tree	Unani
Pistacia lentiscus	Roomi Mastagi	Mastic Tree	Unani
Pistacia lentiscus	Ponnuikan kungiliyam	Mastic Tree	Siddha/Tamil
Pistacia vera	Mukuulaka	Pistachio, Green Almond	Ayurvedic
Pistacia vera	Ilk-ul-Ambaat (resin)	Pistachio, Green Almond	Unani
Pistacia vera	Pistaa (Kernel)	Pistachio, Green Almond	Unani

Table Contd.

Botanical Name	Indian Name	English Name	Medicinal System
Pistia stratiotes	Jalakumbhi	Water Lettuce, Tropical Duckweed	Ayurvedic
Pistia stratiotes	Vaariparni	Water Lettuce, Tropical Duckweed	Ayurvedic
Pistia stratiotes	Vaarimuuli	Water Lettuce, Tropical Duckweed	Ayurvedic
Pistia stratiotes	Agasatamarai	Water Lettuce, Tropical Duckweed	Ayurvedic
Pithecellobium dulce	Dakhini Babool	Minila Tamarind, Madras Thorn, Quamachil	Folk
Pithecellobium dulce	Vilaayati Imli	Minila Tamarind, Madras Thorn, Quamachil	Folk
Pithecellobium dulce	Kodukkaa Puli	Minila Tamarind, Madras Thorn, Quamachil	Siddha/Tamil
Pithecellobium dulce	Karapilly	Minila Tamarind, Madras Thorn, Quamachil	Siddha/Tamil
Pithecellobium monadelphum	Kachloraa	Grasshopper Tree	Folk
Pithecellobium monadelphum	Kalpakku	Grasshopper Tree	Siddha/Tamil
Pittosporum dasycaulon	Boogri	Pittosporum Cheesewood	Folk
Pittosporum dasycaulon	Gapasundi	Pittosporum Cheesewood	Folk
Pittosporum floribundum	Kattu Sampangi	Ginger-bark Pittosporum	Siddha/Tamil
Pittosporum floribundum	Tumari	Ginger-bark Pittosporum	Folk
Pittosporum floribundum	Vekhali	Ginger-bark Pittosporum	Folk
Pittosporum floribundum	Vikhaari	Ginger-bark Pittosporum	Folk
Plantago amplexicaulis	Aspaghol	Brown Ispaghula	Unani
Plantago lanceolata	Aspaghol	Rib Grass, Ribwort Plantain, English Plantain, Buckhorn Plantain	Unani
Plantago lanceolata	Baartang	Rib Grass, Ribwort Plantain, English Plantain, Buckhorn Plantain	Unani
Plantago lanceolata	Balatang	Rib Grass, Ribwort Plantain, English Plantain, Buckhorn Plantain	Folk
Plantago major	Ashvagola (var.)	Broadleaf Plantain	Ayurvedic
Plantago major	Isabgol	Broadleaf Plantain	Folk

Table Contd.

Botanical Name	Indian Name	English Name	Medicinal System
Plantago ovata	Ashvagola	Ispaghula, Spogel Seeds, Blond Psyllium	Ayurvedic
Plantago ovata	Ashwakarna	Ispaghula, Spogel Seeds, Blond Psyllium	Ayurvedic
Plantago ovata	Aspaghol	Ispaghula, Spogel Seeds, Blond Psyllium	Unani
Plantago ovata	Isapppa	Ispaghula, Spogel Seeds, Blond Psyllium	Siddha/Tamil
Plantago ovata	Isabgol	Ispaghula, Spogel Seeds, Blond Psyllium	Folk
Platanus orientalis	Buin	Oriental Plane, Oriental Sycamore, European Plane Tree	Folk
Platanus orientalis	Chinaar	Oriental Plane, Oriental Sycamore, European Plane Tree	Siddha/Tamil
Platycodon grandiflorum	Chinese Balloon Plant	Balloon Flower Plant, Chinese Bell Flower Plant, "Lung-Herb"	Folk
Plectranthus mollis	Laal-Aghaadaa	Country Borage	Folk
Plesmonium margaritiferum	Vajrakanda	Kharhar Tuber	Ayurvedic
Plesmonium margaritiferum	Kharhar	Kharhar Tuber	Folk
Pluchea indica	Kukarondh	Indian Fleabane	Folk
Pluchea indica	Manjurukh	Indian Fleabane	Folk
Pluchea lanceolata	Raasnaa	Rasana Shrub	Ayurvedic
Pluchea lanceolata	Rasanaa	Rasana Shrub	Ayurvedic
Pluchea lanceolata	Raasnikaa	Rasana Shrub	Ayurvedic
Pluchea lanceolata	Rasaa	Rasana Shrub	Ayurvedic
Pluchea lanceolata	Yuktaa	Rasana Shrub	Ayurvedic
Pluchea lanceolata	Yuktrasaa	Rasana Shrub	Ayurvedic
Pluchea lanceolata	Suvahaa	Rasana Shrub	Ayurvedic
Pluchea lanceolata	Elaaparni	Rasana Shrub	Ayurvedic
Pluchea lanceolata	Vaaya-surai	Rasana Shrub	Folk
Pluchea lanceolata	Raayasan	Rasana Shrub	Folk
Plumbago capensis	Nila-chitraka	South African Leadwort	Ayurvedic
Plumbago indica	Senkoduveri	Rose-coloured Leadwort	Siddha/Tamil
Plumbago indica	Rakta-chitraka	Rose-coloured Leadwort	Ayurvedic
Plumbago zeylanica	Agni	Ceylon Leadwort	Ayurvedic
Plumbago zeylanica	Chitraka	Ceylon Leadwort	Ayurvedic

Table Contd.

Botanical Name	Indian Name	English Name	Medicinal System
Plumbago zeylanica	Vahni	Ceylon Leadwort	Ayurvedic
Plumbago zeylanica	Jvalanaakhya	Ceylon Leadwort	Ayurvedic
Plumbago zeylanica	Krshaanu	Ceylon Leadwort	Ayurvedic
Plumbago zeylanica	Hutaasha	Ceylon Leadwort	Ayurvedic
Plumbago zeylanica	Dahana	Ceylon Leadwort	Ayurvedic
Plumbago zeylanica	Sikhi	Ceylon Leadwort	Ayurvedic
Plumbago zeylanica	Sheetraj Hindi	Ceylon Leadwort	Unani
Plumbago zeylanica	Chittramoolam	Ceylon Leadwort	Siddha/Tamil
Plumeria acuminata	Kshira Champaa	Pagoda Tree	Ayurvedic
Plumeria alba	Kshira Champaka	White Champaka	Ayurvedic
Plumeria alba	Perumal Arali	White Champaka	Siddha/Tamil
Plumeria alba	Vella Champakam	White Champaka	Folk/ Malayalam
Plumeria rubra	Kshira Champaka	Red Jasmine	Ayurvedic
Podophyllum hexandrum	Giriparpata	Indian Podophyllum	Ayurvedic
Podophyllum hexandrum	Bana-kakari	Indian Podophyllum	Folk
Podophyllum hexandrum	Venivel	Indian Podophyllum	Folk
Podophyllum hexandrum	Patvel	Indian Podophyllum	Folk
Podophyllum hexandrum	Paapraa	Indian Podophyllum	Folk
Podophyllum hexandrum	Paapri	Indian Podophyllum	Folk
Podophyllum sikkimensis	Paapraa (var.)	Sikkim Podophyllum	Folk
Pogostemon benghalensis	Ishwar-jataa	Bengal Pogostemon	Folk
Pogostemon benghalensis	Jui-lataa	Bengal Pogostemon	Folk
Pogostemon benghalensis	Phaangalaa	Bengal Pogostemon	Folk
Pogostemon cablin	Paachi	Patchouli	Ayurvedic
Pogostemon cablin	Paanari	Patchouli	Folk
Pogostemon parviflorus	Phaangalaa	Orissa Pogostemon	Folk
Pogostemon patchouli	Paachi	Patchouli	Ayurvedic
Pogostemon patchouli	Pancholi	Patchouli	Ayurvedic
Pogostemon patchouli	Kadir Pachai	Patchouli	Siddha/Tamil
Pogostemon patchouli	Paanch	Patchouli	Folk

Table Contd.

Botanical Name	Indian Name	English Name	Medicinal System
Rauvolfia serpentina	Naakuli	Rauvolfia Root, Serpentina Root, Indian Snakeroot	Ayurvedic
Rauvolfia serpentina	Davaa-e-junoon	Rauvolfia Root, Serpentina Root, Indian Snakeroot	Unani
Rauvolfia serpentina	Dhaval-baruaa	Rauvolfia Root, Serpentina Root, Indian Snakeroot	Folk
Rauvolfia serpentina	Chhotaa Chand	Rauvolfia Root, Serpentina Root, Indian Snakeroot	Folk
Rauvolfia serpentina	Amalpori, Chivan amelpodi	Rauvolfia Root, Serpentina Root, Indian Snakeroot	Siddha/Tamil
Rauvolfia tetraphylla	Badaa Chaand	Wild Snakeroot	Folk
Reinwardtia indica	Abai	Winter-Flax, Yellow Flax	Folk
Reinwardtia indica	Baasanti	Winter-Flax, Yellow Flax	Ayurvedic
Reissantia grahamii	Danshir	Pristimera Root	Folk
Reissantia grahamii	Daushir	Pristimera Root	Folk
Reissantia grahamii	Lokhandi	Pristimera Root	Folk
Reissantia grahamii	Yesti	Pristimera Root	Folk
Reissantia grahamii	Zerwati	Pristimera Root	Folk
Reissantia indica	Atari-lataa	Atari Vine	Folk
Reissantia indica	Kathapahaariaa	Atari Vine	Folk
Reissantia indica	Kazurati	Atari Vine	Folk
Reissantia indica	Lokhandi	Atari Vine	Folk
Reissantia indica	Tirruli	Atari Vine	Folk
Reissantia indica	Odangod	Atari Vine	Siddha/Tamil
Remusatia vivipara	Maanakand	Hitch-hiker Elephant Ear	Folk
Remusatia vivipara	Rukhaalu	Hitch-hiker Elephant Ear	Folk
Reseda luteola	Pita-Ranjak Padapa	Dyer's Rocket, Weld	Folk
Rhamnus procumbens	Buckthorn	Buckthorn	Folk
Rhamnus purshiana	Buckthorn	Buckthorn, Cascara Sagrada, Sacred Bark	Folk
Rhamnus virgata	Chadolaa	Indian Buckthorn	Folk
Rhamnus virgata	Chhaduaa	Indian Buckthorn	Folk
Rhamnus virgata	Tadru	Indian Buckthorn	Folk
Rhamnus wightii	Rakta-Rohidaa	Bitter Ragtrora	Ayurvedic

Table Contd.

Botanical Name	Indian Name	English Name	Medicinal System
Rhaphidophora laciniata	Aaanaiittippili	Pathos, Silver Vine	Folk
Rhaphidophora laciniata	Ganesh-kand	Pathos, Silver Vine	Folk
Rheum emodi	Gandhini Revatikaa	Indian Rhubarb, Himalayan Rhubarb	Ayurvedic
Rheum emodi	Amlaparni	Indian Rhubarb, Himalayan Rhubarb	Ayurvedic
Rheum emodi	Pitamuuli	Indian Rhubarb, Himalayan Rhubarb	Ayurvedic
Rheum emodi	Revandachini	Indian Rhubarb, Himalayan Rhubarb	Ayurvedic
Rheum emodi	Revandchini	Indian Rhubarb, Himalayan Rhubarb	Unani
Rheum emodi	Revalchinikattai	Indian Rhubarb, Himalayan Rhubarb	Siddha/Tamil
Rheum emodi	Nattirevaichini	Indian Rhubarb, Himalayan Rhubarb	Siddha/Tamil
Rheum nobile	Tehuka	Rhubarb	Folk
Rheum officinale	Usaare Rewand	Rhubarb	Unani
Rheum webbianum	Archa	Himalayan Rhubarb	Folk
Rhinacanthus nasuta	Gul-baglaa	Snake Jasmine	Unani
Rhinacanthus nasuta	Nagamalli	Snake Jasmine	Siddha/Tamil
Rhinacanthus nasuta	Paalaka-Juuhi	Snake Jasmine	Ayurvedic
Rhinacanthus nasuta	Yuuthikaparni	Snake Jasmine	Ayurvedic
Rhinacanthus nasuta	Yuuthiparni	Snake Jasmine	Ayurvedic
Rhizophora mucronata	Kamo	True Mangrove	Folk
Rhizophora mucronata	Kandal	True Mangrove	Folk
Rhizophora mucronata	Kandal	True Mangrove	Siddha/Tamil
Rhizophora mucronata	Peykkandal	True Mangrove	Siddha/Tamil
Rhizophora mucronata	Sorapinnai	True Mangrove	Siddha/Tamil
Rhododendron anthopogon	Taalis-faz	Anyhopogon Azalea	Folk
Rhododendron anthopogon	Taalish	Anyhopogon Azalea	Folk
Rhododendron anthopogon	Taalisri	Anyhopogon Azalea	Folk
Rhododendron anthopogon	Tazaktsum	Anyhopogon Azalea	Folk
Rhododendron arboreum	Burans	Tree-Rhododendron, Rose-Tree	Folk
Rhododendron arboreum	Kurbak	Tree-Rhododendron, Rose-Tree	Folk

Table Contd.

Botanical Name	Indian Name	English Name	Medicinal System
Rhododendron arboreum	Pullaas	Tree-Rhododendron, Rose-Tree	Folk
Rhododendron barbatum	Chimal	Giantblood Rhododendron	Folk
Rhododendron barbatum	Guraans	Giantblood Rhododendron	Folk
Rhododendron barbatum	Kurbak	Giantblood Rhododendron	Folk
Rhododendron campanulatum	Cherailu	Paper-bark Azalea	Folk
Rhododendron campanulatum	Chimal	Paper-bark Azalea	Folk
Rhododendron campanulatum	Gagger vurmi	Paper-bark Azalea	Folk
Rhododendron campanulatum	Nichnai	Paper-bark Azalea	Folk
Rhododendron campanulatum	Taalis-far	Paper-bark Azalea	Folk
Rhododendron cinnabarinum	Balu	Cinnamom-red flowered Azalea	Folk
Rhododendron cinnabarinum	Chimal	Cinnamom-red flowered Azalea	Folk
Rhododendron cinnabarinum	Sanu	Cinnamom-red flowered Azalea	Folk
Rhus chinensis	Arkhar	Chinese-Gall Rhus Tree	Folk
Rhus chinensis	Tatri	Chinese-Gall Rhus Tree	Folk
Rhus coriaria	Sumaaq	European or Sicilian Sumach	Unani
Rhus coriaria	Taatraak	European or Sicilian Sumach	Unani
Rhus parviflora	Tintidi	Sumach	Ayurvedic
Rhus parviflora	Tintindeeka	Sumach	Ayurvedic
Rhus parviflora	Sumaaq	Sumach	Unani
Rhus parviflora	Raitung	Sumach	Folk
Rhus parviflora	Tung	Sumach	Folk
Rhus succedanea	Karkatash-ringee	Japanese Wax Tree, Wild Varnish Tree	Ayurvedic
Rhus succedanea	Kaakraasingi	Japanese Wax Tree, Wild Varnish Tree	Unani
Rhus succedanea	Karkata-kasringi	Japanese Wax Tree, Wild Varnish Tree	Siddha/Tamil
Rhus succedanea	Kadukapoo (galls)	Japanese Wax Tree, Wild Varnish Tree	Siddha/Tamil

Table Contd.

Botanical Name	Indian Name	English Name	Medicinal System
Rhynchosia minima	Chittavarai	Rhynchosia	Folk
Rhynchosia minima	Jhinki	Rhynchosia	Folk
Rhynchosia minima	Kammervel	Rhynchosia	Folk
Rhynchosia minima	Raan-ghevaraa	Rhynchosia	Folk
Ribes nigrum	Nabar	European Black Currant	Folk
Ricinus communis	Eranda	Castor Seed	Ayurvedic
Ricinus communis	Chitrabija	Castor Seed	Ayurvedic
Ricinus communis	Triputi	Castor Seed	Ayurvedic
Ricinus communis	Vaataari	Castor Seed	Ayurvedic
Ricinus communis	Chanchu	Castor Seed	Ayurvedic
Ricinus communis	Manda	Castor Seed	Ayurvedic
Ricinus communis	Uruvaka	Castor Seed	Ayurvedic
Ricinus communis	Gandharva-hastaa	Castor Seed	Ayurvedic
Ricinus communis	Panchaangula	Castor Seed	Ayurvedic
Ricinus communis	Vardhamaana	Castor Seed	Ayurvedic
Ricinus communis	Uttaanpatraka	Castor Seed	Ayurvedic
Ricinus communis	Vyaaghrapuchha	Castor Seed	Ayurvedic
Ricinus communis	Chitraa	Castor Seed	Ayurvedic
Ricinus communis	Bedanjeer	Castor Seed	Unani
Ricinus communis	Arand	Castor Seed	Unani
Ricinus communis	Ammanakku	Castor Seed	Siddha/Tamil
Rivea corymbosa	Ololiuqui	Ololiuqui, Snake Plant	Folk
Rivea hypocrateriformis	Musuttai	Midnapore Creeper	Siddha/Tamil
Rivea hypocrateriformis	Kalmi-lataa	Midnapore Creeper	Folk
Rivea hypocrateriformis	Phaang	Midnapore Creeper	Folk
Rivea hypocrateriformis	Phanji	Midnapore Creeper	Ayurvedic
Rivea ornate	Phanji (var.)	Oliliuqui	Ayurvedic
Rivea ornate	Machuttai	Oliliuqui	Siddha/Tamil
Rivea ornate	Phaang	Oliliuqui	Folk
Rivea ornate	Baravat	Oliliuqui	Folk
Rivina humilis	Rivinaa	Baby Pepper, Dog Blood, Blood Berry, Rouge-Plant	Folk

Table Contd.

Botanical Name	Indian Name	English Name	Medicinal System
Robinia pseudoacacia	Black Locust	Locust Tree, Robinia, False Acacia, Black Locust	Folk
Rorippa dufia	Khoobkalaan	Field Cress	Unani
Rorippa dufia	Kattu-kadugu	Field Cress	Siddha/Tamil
Rosa alba	Sevati	Common English Dog Rose, White Cottage Rose	Ayurvedic
Rosa alba	Shveta Taruni	Common English Dog Rose, White Cottage Rose	Ayurvedic
Rosa alba	Sevati	Common English Dog Rose, White Cottage Rose	Unani
Rosa alba	Gul-safed Bustaani	Common English Dog Rose, White Cottage Rose	Unani
Rosa alba	Vard Abyaz	Common English Dog Rose, White Cottage Rose	Unani
Rosa alba	Gul-safed Sahraai	Common English Dog Rose, White Cottage Rose	Unani
Rosa alba	Vard Abyaz Barri	Common English Dog Rose, White Cottage Rose	Unani
Rosa bourboniana	Taruni	Bourbon Rose	Ayurvedic
Rosa bourboniana	Kubajaka	Bourbon Rose	Ayurvedic
Rosa bourboniana	Baaraamaasi	Bourbon Rose	Ayurvedic
Rosa bourboniana	Cheenia-Gulaab	Bourbon Rose	Ayurvedic
Rosa bourboniana	Desi Gulab	Bourbon Rose	Folk
Rosa centifolia	Shatapatri	Cabbage Rose, Provence Rose, Hundred-leaved Rose	Ayurvedic
Rosa centifolia	Shatpatrikaa	Cabbage Rose, Provence Rose, Hundred-leaved Rose	Ayurvedic
Rosa centifolia	Taruni	Cabbage Rose, Provence Rose, Hundred-leaved Rose	Ayurvedic
Rosa centifolia	Devataruni	Cabbage Rose, Provence Rose, Hundred-leaved Rose	Ayurvedic
Rosa centifolia	Karnikaa	Cabbage Rose, Provence Rose, Hundred-leaved Rose	Ayurvedic
Rosa centifolia	Chaarukesharaa	Cabbage Rose, Provence Rose, Hundred-leaved Rose	Ayurvedic
Rosa centifolia	Laakshaa	Cabbage Rose, Provence Rose, Hundred-leaved Rose	Ayurvedic
Rosa centifolia	Gandhaaddhyaa	Cabbage Rose, Provence Rose, Hundred-leaved Rose	Ayurvedic

Table Contd.

Botanical Name	Indian Name	English Name	Medicinal System
Rosa centifolia	Gul-e-Surkh	Cabbage Rose, Provence Rose, Hundred-leaved Rose	Unani
Rosa centifolia	Rajapoo	Cabbage Rose, Provence Rose, Hundred-leaved Rose	Folk/Tamil
Rosa chinensis	Taruni-Kantaka	Bengal Rose, Monthly Rose	Ayurvedic
Rosa chinensis	Chini Gulaab	Bengal Rose, Monthly Rose	Unani
Rosa chinensis	Kaantaa-Gulaab	Bengal Rose, Monthly Rose	Folk
Rosa damascena	Taruni	Damask Rose	Ayurvedic
Rosa damascena	Gul-e-Surkh	Damask Rose	Unani
Rosa damascena	Vard	Damask Rose	Unani
Rosa damascena	Vard-e-Ahmar	Damask Rose	Unani
Rosa damascena	Zard-e-Vard (Stamens)	Damask Rose	Unani
Rosa damascena	Daleek (Fruit)	Damask Rose	Unani
Rosa damascena	Samar-ul-Vard	Damask Rose	Unani
Rosa damascena	Smar-e-Gul	Damask Rose	Unani
Rosa damascena	Irosa	Damask Rose	Siddha/Tamil
Rosa damascena	Fasali Gulaab	Damask Rose	Folk
Rosa macrophylla	Ban-gulaab	Himalayan Rose	Folk
Rosa macrophylla	Vanya Taruni	Himalayan Rose	Ayurvedic
Rosa moschata	Kubjaka	Himalayan Musk Rose	Ayurvedic
Rosa moschata	Kujai	Himalayan Musk Rose	Folk
Rosa moschata	Kuujaa	Himalayan Musk Rose	Folk
Rosa multiflora	Gulaab	Japanese Rose, Seven Sister's Rose, Baby Rose	Folk
Rosa multiflora	Rakta-Taruni	Japanese Rose, Seven Sister's Rose, Baby Rose	Ayurvedic
Rosa rubra	Rakta-Taruni	French Rose	Ayurvedic
Rosa rubra	Gulaab	French Rose	Ayurvedic
Rosa sericea	Jangali Gulaab	Mountain Rose	Folk
Rosa webbiana	Laddaakhi-Sevati	Webb's Rose	Ayurvedic
Roscoea procera	Kaakoli	Kaakoli	Ayurvedic
Roscoea procera	Kshira-Kaakoli	Kaakoli	Ayurvedic
Rosmarinus officinalis	Rusmari	Rosemary	Folk

Table Contd.

Botanical Name	Indian Name	English Name	Medicinal System
Rumex vesicarius	Chuko	Bladder-Dock, Country Sorrel	Ayurvedic
Rumex vesicarius	Hammaaz	Bladder-Dock, Country Sorrel	Unani
Rumex vesicarius	Shakkankeerai	Bladder-Dock, Country Sorrel	Siddha/Tamil
Rungia pectinata	Parpata	Matheran Wild Flower	Ayurvedic
Rungia pectinata	Punakapundu	Matheran Wild Flower	Siddha/Tamil
Rungia repens	Kharmor	Creeping Rungia	Folk
Rungia repens	Kodaga-saleh	Creeping Rungia	Siddha/Tamil
Rungia repens	Parpata	Creeping Rungia	Ayurvedic
Ruscus aculeatus	Butcher's Broom	Butcher's Broom, Jew's Myrtle	Folk
Ruta chalepensis	Aruvadam-chedi	Fringed Rue	Siddha/Tamil
Ruta chalepensis	Aruvada	Fringed Rue	Siddha/Tamil
Ruta chalepensis	Jangali Sudaab	Fringed Rue	Unani
Ruta graveolens	Aruvada	Garden Rue	Siddha/Tamil
Ruta graveolens	Sudaab	Garden Rue	Unani
Ruta graveolens	Suddaab	Garden Rue	Unani
Sabal palmetto	Sabal	Cabbage Palm Indian Sawpalmatto (Fruit)	Folk
Saccharum munja	Munja	Munja Culms	Ayurvedic
Saccharum munja	Bhadramuja	Munja Culms	Ayurvedic
Saccharum munja	Vaana	Munja Culms	Ayurvedic
Saccharum munja	Shara	Munja Culms	Ayurvedic
Saccharum munja	Sara	Munja Culms	Ayurvedic
Saccharum munja	Raamshara	Munja Culms	Ayurvedic
Saccharum munja	Munjipul	Munja Culms	Siddha/Tamil
Saccharum munja	Munjappullu	Munja Culms	Siddha/Tamil
Saccharum munja	Sarpata	Munja Culms	Folk
Saccharum officinarum	Ikshu	Gannaa, Naishakar	Ayurvedic
Saccharum officinarum	Dirgha-chhada	Gannaa, Naishakar	Ayurvedic
Saccharum officinarum	Bhuurirasa	Gannaa, Naishakar	Ayurvedic
Saccharum officinarum	Morata	Gannaa, Naishakar	Ayurvedic
Saccharum officinarum	Asipatra	Gannaa, Naishakar	Ayurvedic
Saccharum officinarum	Madhutrna	Gannaa, Naishakar	Ayurvedic
Saccharum officinarum	Gudamuula	Gannaa, Naishakar	Ayurvedic

Table Contd.

Botanical Name	Indian Name	English Name	Medicinal System
Saccharum officinarum	Trnarasa	Gannaa, Naishakar	Ayurvedic
Saccharum officinarum	Gannaa	Gannaa, Naishakar	Unani
Saccharum officinarum	Naishakar	Gannaa, Naishakar	Unani
Saccharum officinarum	Karumbu	Gannaa, Naishakar	Siddha/Tamil
Saccharum officinarum	Nanal	Gannaa, Naishakar	Siddha/Tamil
Saccharum spontaneum	Kaasha	Thatch Grass, Wild Sugarcane	Ayurvedic
Saccharum spontaneum	Kandekshu	Thatch Grass, Wild Sugarcane	Ayurvedic
Saccharum spontaneum	Shveta-chaamara	Thatch Grass, Wild Sugarcane	Ayurvedic
Saccharum spontaneum	Naanal	Thatch Grass, Wild Sugarcane	Siddha/Tamil
Saccharum spontaneum	Pai Karumbu	Thatch Grass, Wild Sugarcane	Siddha/Tamil
Saccolabium papillosum	Naakuli	Small Warty Acampe	Ayurvedic
Saccolabium papillosum	Vrkshaadani (var.)	Small Warty Acampe	Ayurvedic
Saccolabium papillosum	Raasanaa	Small Warty Acampe	Folk
Saccolabium papillosum	Naakuli	Small Warty Acampe	Folk
Saccolabium papillosum	Gandhalataa	Small Warty Acampe	Folk
Sagittaria trifolia	Chhotaa Kuuta	Old World Arrowhead	Folk
Sagittaria trifolia	Muyaa	Old World Arrowhead	Folk
Salacia chinensis	Nerani	Chinese Salacia	Folk/South
Salacia chinensis	Ingali	Chinese Salacia	Folk
Salacia chinensis	Modhuphal	Chinese Salacia	Folk
Salacia chinensis	Saptachakraa	Chinese Salacia	Ayurvedic
Salacia chinensis	Saptarangi	Chinese Salacia	Ayurvedic
Salacia chinensis	Swarnmuula	Chinese Salacia	Ayurvedic
Salacia macrosperma	Anakoranti	Saptrangi	Folk
Salacia macrosperma	Lendaphala	Saptrangi	Folk
Salacia oblonga	Chundan	Saptrangi	Folk
Salacia oblonga	Ponkoranti	Saptrangi	Folk
Salacia reticulata	Anukudu-chettu	Saptrangi	Folk/South
Salacia reticulata	Ekanyakam	Saptrangi	Folk
Salacia reticulata	Koranti	Saptrangi	Folk/South
Salicornia brachiata	Kohlu	Glasswort,Pickleweed, Marsh Samphire	Folk

Table Contd.

Botanical Name	Indian Name	English Name	Medicinal System
Salix acmophylla	Jala-vetasa	Wild Weeping Willow	Ayurvedic
Salix alba	Bed Saadaa	White Willow, European Willow	Unani
Salix alba	Jalavetasa	White Willow, European Willow	Ayurvedic
Salix alba	Vivir	White Willow, European Willow	Folk
Salix babylonica	Aatru Paalai	Weeping Willow	Siddha/Tamil
Salix babylonica	Giur	Weeping Willow	Folk
Salix babylonica	Bed	Weeping Willow	Folk
Salix caprea	Vetasa	Sallow, Goat Willow, Common Willow	Ayurvedic
Salix caprea	Vaanira	Sallow, Goat Willow, Common Willow	Ayurvedic
Salix caprea	Naadeya	Sallow, Goat Willow, Common Willow	Ayurvedic
Salix caprea	Vanjula	Sallow, Goat Willow, Common Willow	Ayurvedic
Salix caprea	Meghapushpa	Sallow, Goat Willow, Common Willow	Ayurvedic
Salix caprea	Bed Mushk	Sallow, Goat Willow, Common Willow	Unani
Salix fragilis	Tilachaang	Crack Willow, Kashmir Willow	Folk (Himachal)
Salix nigra	Bed-Siyaah	Black Willow	Unani
Salix tetrasperma	Jalavetasa	Indian Willow	Ayurvedic
Salix tetrasperma	Naadeya	Indian Willow	Ayurvedic
Salix tetrasperma	Niketan	Indian Willow	Ayurvedic
Salix tetrasperma	Baishi	Indian Willow	Ayurvedic
Salix tetrasperma	Attupalai	Indian Willow	Siddha/Tamil
Salix tetrasperma	Vaanira	Indian Willow	Folk
Salix tetrasperma	Vaalunja	Indian Willow	Folk
Salmalia malabarica	Shaalmali	Silk Cotton Tree, Semul Tree	Ayurvedic
Salmalia malabarica	Mochaa	Silk Cotton Tree, Semul Tree	Ayurvedic
Salmalia malabarica	Mochaahva	Silk Cotton Tree, Semul Tree	Ayurvedic
Salmalia malabarica	Pichhila	Silk Cotton Tree, Semul Tree	Ayurvedic
Salmalia malabarica	Raktapushpa	Silk Cotton Tree, Semul Tree	Ayurvedic

Table Contd.

Botanical Name	Indian Name	English Name	Medicinal System
Salmalia malabarica	Sthiraayu	Silk Cotton Tree, Semul Tree	Ayurvedic
Salmalia malabarica	Kankataadhya	Silk Cotton Tree, Semul Tree	Ayurvedic
Salmalia malabarica	Tuulini	Silk Cotton Tree, Semul Tree	Ayurvedic
Salmalia malabarica	Shaalmali-veshtaka	Silk Cotton Tree, Semul Tree	Ayurvedic
Salmalia malabarica	Semal	Silk Cotton Tree, Semul Tree	Unani
Salmalia malabarica	Mochras (gum)	Silk Cotton Tree, Semul Tree	Unani
Salmalia malabarica	Mull Ilavam	Silk Cotton Tree, Semul Tree	Siddha/Tamil
Salmalia malabarica	Ielavampisin (gum)	Silk Cotton Tree, Semul Tree	Siddha/Tamil
Salmalia malabarica	Semar	Silk Cotton Tree, Semul Tree	Folk
Salsola kali	Sarjikaa	Glass-Wort, Russian Thistle, Prickly-Saltwort	Ayurvedic
Salsola kali	Katol	Glass-Wort, Russian Thistle, Prickly-Saltwort	Ayurvedic
Salsola kali	Laanaa-buuti	Glass-Wort, Russian Thistle, Prickly-Saltwort	Ayurvedic
Salsola kali	Sajji-buuti	Glass-Wort, Russian Thistle, Prickly-Saltwort	Ayurvedic
Salsola kali	Ushnaan	Glass-Wort, Russian Thistle, Prickly-Saltwort	Unani
Salsola kali	Ghaajuraan	Glass-Wort, Russian Thistle, Prickly-Saltwort	Unani
Salsola kali	Barilla	Glass-Wort, Russian Thistle, Prickly-Saltwort	Folk
Salvadora oleoides	Kalawa	Mustard Tree, Salt Bush Tree, Tooth Brush Tree	Siddha/Tamil
Salvadora oleoides	Pilu	Mustard Tree, Salt Bush Tree, Tooth Brush Tree	Ayurvedic
Salvadora persica	Pilu	Mustard Tree, Salt Bush Tree, Tooth Brush Tree	Ayurvedic
Salvadora persica	Pilukaa	Mustard Tree, Salt Bush Tree, Tooth Brush Tree	Ayurvedic
Salvadora persica	Sransi	Mustard Tree, Salt Bush Tree, Tooth Brush Tree	Ayurvedic
Salvadora persica	Angaahva	Mustard Tree, Salt Bush Tree, Tooth Brush Tree	Ayurvedic
Salvadora persica	Tikshnavriksha	Mustard Tree, Salt Bush Tree, Tooth Brush Tree	Ayurvedic

Table Contd.

Botanical Name	Indian Name	English Name	Medicinal System
Salvadora persica	Miswaak	Mustard Tree, Salt Bush Tree, Tooth Brush Tree	Unani
Salvadora persica	Araak	Mustard Tree, Salt Bush Tree, Tooth Brush Tree	Unani
Salvadora persica	Perungoli	Mustard Tree, Salt Bush Tree, Tooth Brush Tree	Siddha/Tamil
Salvia aegyptiaca	Tukhm-Malangaa	Egyptian Sage	Unani
Salvia coccinea	Samudrashosha (var.)	Red Sage, Texas Sage	Ayurvedic
Salvia haematodes	Behman Surkh	Blood-veined Sage	Unani
Salvia lanata	Kuuthan-Kali	Scarlet Sage	Folk
Salvia moorcroftiana	Kaali-jarri	Wild Sage	Folk
Salvia officinalis	Salvia Sefakuss	Common Sage	Folk
Salvia plebeia	Bhuu-Tulasi	Common Sage	Folk
Salvia plebeia	Kamarkasa (Seed)	Common Sage	Ayurvedic
Salvia plebeia	Samudrashosha	Common Sage	Ayurvedic
Salvia spinosa	Kanochaa	Wrinkled-leaf Sage	Unani
Salvia spinosa	Marv	Wrinkled-leaf Sage	Unani
Salvia spinosa	Seeds—Tukhm Kanochaa	Wrinkled-leaf Sage	Unani
Salvia spinosa	Tukhm Marv	Wrinkled-leaf Sage	Unani
Salvinia cucullata	Aakhukarni	Asian Watermoss	Ayurvedic
Sambucus ebulus	Khamaan Saghir	Dwarf Elder	Unani
Sambucus ebulus	Khamaan-ul-Arzaa	Dwarf Elder	Unani
Sambucus ebulus	Khamaan	Dwarf Elder	Unani
Sambucus ebulus	Mushkiyaara	Dwarf Elder	Siddha/Tamil
Sambucus ebulus	Khamman	Dwarf Elder	Siddha/Tamil
Sambucus ebulus	Gunhulaa	Dwarf Elder	Siddha/Tamil
Sambucus nigra	Khamaan Kabir	European Elder, Black Elder	Unani
Sandoricum indicum	Sevai	European Elder	Siddha/Tamil
Sandoricum indicum	Sayai	European Elder	Siddha/Tamil
Sanicula europaea	Sanikle	Wood Sanicle	Folk

Table Contd.

Botanical Name	Indian Name	English Name	Medicinal System
Sansevieria hyacinthoides	Naagadamani	Ceylon Bowstring Hemp	Ayurvedic
Sansevieria hyacinthoides	Marul	Ceylon Bowstring Hemp	Siddha/Tamil
Sansevieria hyacinthoides	Motta manji	Ceylon Bowstring Hemp	Siddha/Tamil
Sansevieria roxburghiana	Naagadamani	Indian Bowstring Hemp	Ayurvedic
Sansevieria roxburghiana	Takshaki	Indian Bowstring Hemp	Ayurvedic
Sansevieria roxburghiana	Marul	Indian Bowstring Hemp	Siddha/Tamil
Sansevieria roxburghiana	Motta manji	Indian Bowstring Hemp	Siddha/Tamil
Santalum album	Chandana	White Sandalwood	Ayurvedic
Santalum album	Shvetachandana	White Sandalwood	Ayurvedic
Santalum album	Shrikhanda	White Sandalwood	Ayurvedic
Santalum album	Bhadra-Shree	White Sandalwood	Ayurvedic
Santalum album	Gandhsaara	White Sandalwood	Ayurvedic
Santalum album	Malayaja	White Sandalwood	Ayurvedic
Santalum album	Hima	White Sandalwood	Ayurvedic
Santalum album	Ekaangi	White Sandalwood	Ayurvedic
Santalum album	Sandal Safed	White Sandalwood	Unani
Santalum album	Sandal-e-Abyaz	White Sandalwood	Unani
Santalum album	Chandanam	White Sandalwood	Siddha/Tamil
Santalum album	Sandana	White Sandalwood	Siddha/Tamil
Santalum album	Ingam	White Sandalwood	Siddha/Tamil
Santolina chamaecyparissus	"Lemon Queen"	Lavender Cotton	Folk
Sapindus laurifolius	Arishtaka	Soapnut Tree of South India	Ayurvedic
Sapindus laurifolius	Phenila	Soapnut Tree of South India	Ayurvedic
Sapindus laurifolius	Raktabeeja	Soapnut Tree of South India	Ayurvedic
Sapindus laurifolius	Reethaakaranja	Soapnut Tree of South India	Ayurvedic
Sapindus laurifolius	Garbhapaatana	Soapnut Tree of South India	Ayurvedic
Sapindus laurifolius	Reethaa	Soapnut Tree of South India	Unani
Sapindus laurifolius	Puvamkottai	Soapnut Tree of South India	Siddha/Tamil
Sapindus laurifolius	Manipungu	Soapnut Tree of South India	Siddha/Tamil
Sapindus mukorossi	Arishtaka	Chinese Soap Berry, Soap Nut Tree of North India	Ayurvedic
Sapindus mukorossi	Phenila	Chinese Soap Berry, Soap Nut Tree of North India	Ayurvedic

Table Contd.

Botanical Name	Indian Name	English Name	Medicinal System
Sapindus mukorossi	Reethaa	Chinese Soap Berry, Soap Nut Tree of North India	Folk
Sapium indicum	Pencolum	Tallow Tree	Siddha/Tamil
Sapium indicum	Hurnaa	Tallow Tree	Folk
Sapium sebiferum	Tayapippali	Chinese Tallow Tree	Folk
Sapium sebiferum	Vilaayati Shisham	Chinese Tallow Tree	Folk
Sapium sebiferum	Mom-China	Chinese Tallow Tree	Folk
Saponaria officinalis	Saabuni	Bouncing Bet, Fuller's Herb	Folk
Saponaria vaccaria	Musna	Soapwort, Cowcokle	Folk
Saponaria vaccaria	Saabuni	Soapwort, Cowcokle	Folk
Saraca asoca	Ashoka	Ashoka Tree	Ayurvedic
Saraca asoca	Ashoku	Ashoka Tree	Ayurvedic
Saraca asoca	Hempushpa	Ashoka Tree	Ayurvedic
Saraca asoca	Taamrapallava	Ashoka Tree	Ayurvedic
Saraca asoca	Pindapushpa	Ashoka Tree	Ayurvedic
Saraca asoca	Gandhapushpa	Ashoka Tree	Ayurvedic
Saraca asoca	Ashoka	Ashoka Tree	Unani
Saraca asoca	Asokam	Ashoka Tree	Siddha/Tamil
Sarcococca saligna	Geru	Christmas Box	Folk
Sarcococca saligna	Tiliari	Christmas Box	Folk
Sarcococca saligna	Sukatsing	Christmas Box	Folk
Sarcostemma brevistigma	Somavalli	Moon Plant, Soma Plant	Ayurvedic
Sarcostemma brevistigma	Somalataa	Moon Plant, Soma Plant	Ayurvedic
Sarcostemma brevistigma	Somakshiri	Moon Plant, Soma Plant	Ayurvedic
Sarcostemma brevistigma	Saumyaa	Moon Plant, Soma Plant	Ayurvedic
Sarcostemma brevistigma	Dwijpriyaa	Moon Plant, Soma Plant	Ayurvedic
Sarcostemma brevistigma	Somamum	Moon Plant, Soma Plant	Siddha/Tamil
Sarcostemma brevistigma	Somavalli	Moon Plant, Soma Plant	Siddha/Tamil
Sarcostigma kleinii	Ingudi	Ingudi	Ayurvedic
Sarcostigma kleinii	Odal	Ingudi	Folk/Tamil
Sassafras albidum	Sassafras	Ague Tree	Unani
Satureja hortensis	Indian Mint	Summary Savory	Folk

Table Contd.

Botanical Name	Indian Name	English Name	Medicinal System
Sauropus androgynus	Thavasai murungai	Star Goose Berry	Siddha/Tamil
Saussurea affinis	Ganga-muula	East Asian Saw-wort	Folk
Saussurea gossypiphora	Ghuggi	Himalayan Saw-wort	Folk/Garhwal
Saussurea gossypiphora	Jogi Paashaah	Himalayan Saw-wort	Folk/Kashmir
Saussurea gossypiphora	Phen-kamal	Himalayan Saw-wort	Folk
Saussurea heteromalla	Batula	Snow Lotus	Folk
Saussurea heteromalla	Kaaliziri (Seed)	Snow Lotus	Folk
Saussurea hypoleuca	Kushtha	Himalayan Saw-wort	Ayurvedic
Saussurea hypoleuca	Uplet	Himalayan Saw-wort	Folk
Saussurea lappa	Kushtha	Kuth, Costus	Ayurvedic
Saussurea lappa	Kusht	Kuth, Costus	Ayurvedic
Saussurea lappa	Vaapya	Kuth, Costus	Ayurvedic
Saussurea lappa	Kaashmira	Kuth, Costus	Ayurvedic
Saussurea lappa	Gada	Kuth, Costus	Ayurvedic
Saussurea lappa	Rug	Kuth, Costus	Ayurvedic
Saussurea lappa	Ruk	Kuth, Costus	Ayurvedic
Saussurea lappa	Aamaya	Kuth, Costus	Ayurvedic
Saussurea lappa	Paalaka	Kuth, Costus	Ayurvedic
Saussurea lappa	Qust	Kuth, Costus	Unani
Saussurea lappa	Kostum	Kuth, Costus	Siddha/Tamil
Saussurea lappa	Kottam	Kuth, Costus	Siddha/Tamil
Saussurea lappa	Sugandha-Kuutth	Kuth, Costus	Folk
Saussurea obvallata	Birm-kanwal	Sah du goh ghoo (Chinese)	Folk
Saussurea obvallata	Brahma-kamal	Sah du goh ghoo (Chinese)	Folk
Saussurea sacra	Ghuggi	Yogiraj Plant, Sacred Saussurea	Folk/Garhwal
Saussurea sacra	Jogi-paadshaah	Yogiraj Plant, Sacred Saussurea	Folk/Kashmir
Scaevola frutescens	Vella-muttangam	Fan Flower, Malay Rice Paper Plant	Siddha/Tamil
Scaevola frutescens	Bhadraka	Fan Flower, Malay Rice Paper Plant	Folk
Scaevola frutescens	Bhadraaksha	Fan Flower, Malay Rice Paper Plant	Folk
Schima wallichii	Chilauni	Chilauni Needle Wood	Folk

Table Contd.

Botanical Name	Indian Name	English Name	Medicinal System
Schima wallichii	Makria	Chilauni Needle Wood	Folk
Schizachyrium exile	Sprk	Fakara Beardgrass	Ayurvedic
Schizachyrium exile	Sprkaa	Fakara Beardgrass	Ayurvedic
Schleichera oleosa	Koshaamra	Lac Tree, Macassar Oil Tree, Honey Tree, Ceylon Oak	Ayurvedic
Schleichera oleosa	Kshudraamra	Lac Tree, Macassar Oil Tree, Honey Tree, Ceylon Oak	Ayurvedic
Schleichera oleosa	Lakshaa vrksha	Lac Tree, Macassar Oil Tree, Honey Tree, Ceylon Oak	Ayurvedic
Schleichera oleosa	Ghanaskandha	Lac Tree, Macassar Oil Tree, Honey Tree, Ceylon Oak	Ayurvedic
Schleichera oleosa	Puvathipuvam	Lac Tree, Macassar Oil Tree, Honey Tree, Ceylon Oak	Siddha/Tamil
Schleichera oleosa	Pulaachi	Lac Tree, Macassar Oil Tree, Honey Tree, Ceylon Oak	Siddha/Tamil
Schrebera swietenioides	Muskakaa	Weaver's Beam Tree	Ayurvedic
Schrebera swietenioides	Mogalingum	Weaver's Beam Tree	Siddha/Tamil
Schweinfurthia sphaerocarpa	Nepaal-Nimba	Nepal Neem	Ayurvedic
Schweinfurthia sphaerocarpa	Saannipaat	Nepal Neem	Folk
Scilla indica	Korikanda	South Indian Squill	Ayurvedic
Scilla indica	Vana-Palaandu	South Indian Squill	Ayurvedic
Scilla indica	Jangli Piyaz	South Indian Squill	Unani
Scilla indica	Kattu velvengayam	South Indian Squill	Siddha/Tamil
Scindapsus officinalis	Aanaitippili	Sal Forest Pepper	Siddha/Tamil
Scindapsus officinalis	Gajakrishna	Sal Forest Pepper	Ayurvedic
Scindapsus officinalis	Gajapippali	Sal Forest Pepper	Ayurvedic
Scindapsus officinalis	Hastipippali	Sal Forest Pepper	Ayurvedic
Scirpus articulatus	Chichodaa	Paddyfield Club-Rush	Folk
Scirpus articulatus	Laghu Kasheruka	Paddyfield Club-Rush	Ayurvedic
Scirpus corymbosus	Kronchaadana	Water Sedge	Ayurvedic
Scirpus kysoor	Gundatigagaddi	Kaseru Tuber	Siddha/Tamil
Scirpus kysoor	Karundan	Kaseru Tuber	Siddha/Tamil
Scirpus kysoor	Kaseru	Kaseru Tuber	Folk
Scirpus kysoor	Kasheru	Kaseru Tuber	Ayurvedic

Table Contd.

Botanical Name	Indian Name	English Name	Medicinal System
Scirpus kysoor	Kasheruka	Kaseru Tuber	Ayurvedic
Scirpus tuberosus	Raaj Kasheruka	Sea Clubrush	Ayurvedic
Scleria lithosperma	Razor Grass	Slender Nutrush	Folk
Scoparia dulcis	Ghodaa-tulasi	Sweet Broomweed	Folk
Scoparia dulcis	Jastimadhu	Sweet Broomweed	Folk
Scoparia dulcis	Madhukam	Sweet Broomweed	Folk
Scopolia anomala	Scopola	Russian Belladonna, Belladonna Scopola	Folk
Scutellaria galericulata	Skullcap	Scurvey Grass, Marsh Skullcap	Folk
Scutia myrtina	Cheemaat	Chimat Fruit	Folk
Scutia myrtina	Gariki	Chimat Fruit	Folk
Scutia myrtina	Tuvadi	Chimat Fruit	Folk
Sebastiana chamaelea	Bhui-erendi	Snake's Tongue	Folk
Secale cereale	Rye	Rye Grass	Folk
Securinega suffruticosa	Dalme	Securinega	Folk
Securinega suffruticosa	Kodarsi	Securinega	Folk
Securinega suffruticosa	Pandharphali	Securinega	Folk
Securinega suffruticosa	Vellaippula	Securinega	Siddha/Tamil
Selaginella involvens	Hatthaa jodi	Spike Moss	Folk
Selaginella involvens	Kara-jodi-kanda	Spike Moss	Ayurvedic
Selaginella rupestris	Hatthaajodi	Little Clubmoss, Rock Spike-Moss	Folk
Selaginella rupestris	Kara-jodi-kanda	Little Clubmoss, Rock Spike-Moss	Ayurvedic
Selenicereus grandiflorus	Visarpin	Night-Blooming Cereus, Sweet-scented Cactus	Ayurvedic
Selenicereus grandiflorus	Mahaapushpa	Night-Blooming Cereus, Sweet-scented Cactus	Ayurvedic
Selenicereus grandiflorus	Raatripraphulla	Night-Blooming Cereus, Sweet-scented Cactus	Ayurvedic
Selinum monnieri	Muraa (var.)	Snake's Bed	Folk
Selinum tenuifolium	Muraa	Cow Parsley	Ayurvedic
Selinum tenuifolium	Surabhi	Cow Parsley	Ayurvedic
Selinum tenuifolium	Daitya	Cow Parsley	Ayurvedic

Table Contd.

Botanical Name	Indian Name	English Name	Medicinal System
Selinum tenuifolium	Gandhakuti	Cow Parsley	Ayurvedic
Selinum tenuifolium	Gandhavati	Cow Parsley	Ayurvedic
Selinum tenuifolium	Mural	Cow Parsley	Siddha/Tamil
Selinum tenuifolium	Bhuutakeshi	Cow Parsley	Folk
Selinum tenuifolium	Murr	Cow Parsley	Folk
Selinum vaginatum	Rochanaa-Tagara	Tang-kuen	Ayurvedic
Selinum vaginatum	Peshaavari-Bhuutakeshi	Tang-kuen	Folk
Selinum vaginatum	Taggar	Tang-kuen	Folk
Semecarpus anacardium	Bhallaataka	Marking-Nut	Ayurvedic
Semecarpus anacardium	Bhallata	Marking-Nut	Ayurvedic
Semecarpus anacardium	Arushkara	Marking-Nut	Ayurvedic
Semecarpus anacardium	Agnik	Marking-Nut	Ayurvedic
Semecarpus anacardium	Agnimukha	Marking-Nut	Ayurvedic
Semecarpus anacardium	Sophkrit	Marking-Nut	Ayurvedic
Semecarpus anacardium	Viravrksha	Marking-Nut	Ayurvedic
Semecarpus anacardium	Balaadur	Marking-Nut	Unani
Semecarpus anacardium	Bhilaayan	Marking-Nut	Unani
Semecarpus anacardium	Bhilaavaan	Marking-Nut	Unani
Semecarpus anacardium	Seraan kottai	Marking-Nut	Siddha/Tamil
Semecarpus anacardium	Erimugi	Marking-Nut	Siddha/Tamil
Semecarpus anacardium	Bhilaavaan	Marking-Nut	Folk
Sempervivum tectorum	Houseleek	Houseleek	Folk
Senecio jacquemontianus	Hatermuula	Jacquemont's Senecio	Folk
Senecio jacquemontianus	Poshkar	Jacquemont's Senecio	Folk
Senecio vulgaris	Groundsel	Groundsel, Chicken Weed, Bindseed	Folk
Sesamum indicum	Tila	Sesame, Gingelly	Ayurvedic
Sesamum indicum	Snehphala	Sesame, Gingelly	Ayurvedic
Sesamum indicum	Kunjad	Sesame, Gingelly	Unani
Sesamum indicum	Til	Sesame, Gingelly	Unani
Sesamum indicum	Ellu (Oil)	Sesame, Gingelly	Siddha/Tamil
Sesamum indicum	Nallennai (Seed)	Sesame, Gingelly	Siddha/Tamil

Table Contd.

Botanical Name	Indian Name	English Name	Medicinal System
Sesbania bispinosa	Jayanti (var.)	Prickly Sesban, Dhaincha	Ayurvedic
Sesbania bispinosa	Itkata (var.)	Prickly Sesban, Dhaincha	Ayurvedic
Sesbania bispinosa	Mudchembai	Prickly Sesban, Dhaincha	Siddha/Tamil
Sesbania grandiflora	Agastya	Agati Sesban, Swamp Pea	Ayurvedic
Sesbania grandiflora	Agasti	Agati Sesban, Swamp Pea	Ayurvedic
Sesbania grandiflora	Munidrum	Agati Sesban, Swamp Pea	Ayurvedic
Sesbania grandiflora	Munitaru	Agati Sesban, Swamp Pea	Ayurvedic
Sesbania grandiflora	Muni	Agati Sesban, Swamp Pea	Ayurvedic
Sesbania grandiflora	Vangasena	Agati Sesban, Swamp Pea	Ayurvedic
Sesbania grandiflora	Vakrapushpa	Agati Sesban, Swamp Pea	Ayurvedic
Sesbania grandiflora	Kumbha	Agati Sesban, Swamp Pea	Ayurvedic
Sesbania grandiflora	Agaththi	Agati Sesban, Swamp Pea	Siddha/Tamil
Sesbania sesban	Jayantikaa	Common Sesban	Ayurvedic
Sesbania sesban	Jayanti	Common Sesban	Ayurvedic
Sesbania sesban	jayaa	Common Sesban	Ayurvedic
Sesbania sesban	Jwaalaamukhi	Common Sesban	Ayurvedic
Sesbania sesban	Suukshma-muulaa	Common Sesban	Ayurvedic
Sesbania sesban	Suukshma-patraa	Common Sesban	Ayurvedic
Sesbania sesban	Keshruuhaa	Common Sesban	Ayurvedic
Sesbania sesban	Balaamotaa	Common Sesban	Ayurvedic
Sesbania sesban	Sembai	Common Sesban	Siddha/Tamil
Sesbania sesban	Karum-sumbai (leaf)	Common Sesban	Siddha/Tamil
Sesbania sesban	Jainta	Common Sesban	Folk
Seseli indicum	Vanya-yamaani	Wild Seseli	Ayurvedic
Seseli sibiricum	Bhuutakeshi	Himalayan Seseli	Ayurvedic
Setaria italica	Kangu	Italian Millet, Fox-tail Millet	Ayurvedic
Setaria italica	Kanguni	Italian Millet, Fox-tail Millet	Ayurvedic
Setaria italica	Kangunikaa	Italian Millet, Fox-tail Millet	Ayurvedic
Setaria italica	Priyangu Dhaanya (Millet)	Italian Millet, Fox-tail Millet	Ayurvedic
Setaria italica	Tenai	Italian Millet, Fox-tail Millet	Siddha/Tamil

Table Contd.

Botanical Name	Indian Name	English Name	Medicinal System
Shorea robusta	Dhuupa-vriksha	Sal Tree	Ayurvedic
Shorea robusta	Saalasaara	Sal Tree	Ayurvedic
Shorea robusta	Shaala	Sal Tree	Ayurvedic
Shorea robusta	Kungiliyam	Sal Tree	Siddha/Tamil
Shorea robusta	Venkungiliyam (resin)	Sal Tree	Siddha/Tamil
Sibbaldia parviflora	Bajradanti	Sibbaldia	Ayurvedic
Sida acuta	Balaa	Hornbeam-Leaved Sida	Ayurvedic
Sida acuta	Jangali Methi	Hornbeam-Leaved Sida	Folk
Sida cordifolia	Balaa	Country Mallow	Ayurvedic
Sida cordifolia	Sumanganaa	Country Mallow	Ayurvedic
Sida cordifolia	Khara-yashtikaa	Country Mallow	Ayurvedic
Sida cordifolia	Balini	Country Mallow	Ayurvedic
Sida cordifolia	Bhadrabalaa	Country Mallow	Ayurvedic
Sida cordifolia	Bhadraudani	Country Mallow	Ayurvedic
Sida cordifolia	Vaatyaalikaa	Country Mallow	Ayurvedic
Sida cordifolia	Bariyaara	Country Mallow	Unani
Sida cordifolia	Khirhati	Country Mallow	Unani
Sida cordifolia	Khireti	Country Mallow	Unani
Sida cordifolia	Kunayi	Country Mallow	Unani
Sida cordifolia	Kurunthotti	Country Mallow	Siddha/Tamil
Sida rhombifolia	Mahaabalaa	Red-flowered Mallow	Ayurvedic
Sida rhombifolia	Mahaasamangaa	Red-flowered Mallow	Ayurvedic
Sida rhombifolia	Sahadevaa	Red-flowered Mallow	Ayurvedic
Sida rhombifolia	Kshetrabalaa	Red-flowered Mallow	Ayurvedic
Sida rhombifolia	Bariyaara	Red-flowered Mallow	Unani
Sida rhombifolia	Athi Bala-chedi	Red-flowered Mallow	Siddha/Tamil
Sida rhombifolia	Chitrmutti	Red-flowered Mallow	Siddha/Tamil
Sida rhombifolia	Tennacham	Red-flowered Mallow	Siddha/Tamil
Sida spinosa	Arivalmanai-poondu	Prickly Mallow	Siddha/Tamil
Sida spinosa	Balaa-kantakini	Prickly Mallow	Ayurvedic
Sida spinosa	Gangaati	Prickly Mallow	Ayurvedic

Table Contd.

Botanical Name	Indian Name	English Name	Medicinal System
Sida spinosa	Naagabalaa	Prickly Mallow	Ayurvedic
Sida spinosa	Gulasakari	Prickly Mallow	Folk
Sida spinosa	Jangali-methi	Prickly Mallow	Folk
Sida spinosa	Gangeti	Prickly Mallow	Folk
Sida veronicaefolia	Raajabalaa	Prostrate Mallow	Ayurvedic
Sida veronicaefolia	Bhumibalaa	Prostrate Mallow	Ayurvedic
Sida veronicaefolia	Prasaarini	Prostrate Mallow	Ayurvedic
Sida veronicaefolia	Suprasaraa	Prostrate Mallow	Ayurvedic
Sida veronicaefolia	Palampasi	Prostrate Mallow	Siddha/Tamil
Sida veronicaefolia	Farid-booti	Prostrate Mallow	Folk
Siegesbeckia orientalis	Kadambu	The Holy Herb, Sieges-beckia	Siddha/Tamil
Siegesbeckia orientalis	Katampam	The Holy Herb, Sieges-beckia	Siddha/Tamil
Siegesbeckia orientalis	Lat-latiaa	The Holy Herb, Sieges-beckia	Folk
Siegesbeckia orientalis	Lichkuraa	The Holy Herb, Sieges-beckia	Folk
Siegesbeckia orientalis	Pili-badkadi	The Holy Herb, Sieges-beckia	Folk
Silybum marianum	Milk Thistle	Holy Thistle, Milk Thistle	Folk
Sisymbrium irio	Khaaksi	London Rocket	Ayurvedic
Sisymbrium irio	Khuubkalaan	London Rocket	Unani
Smilax aristolochiaefolia	Ushbaa Maghrabi	Mexican Sarsaparilla	Unani
Smilax aspera	Saarivaa (var.)	Italian Sarsaparilla	Ayurvedic
Smilax china	Chobachini	China Root	Ayurvedic
Smilax china	Chopachini	China Root	Ayurvedic
Smilax china	Dweepaantar-Vachaa	China Root	Ayurvedic
Smilax china	Madhusnuhi	China Root	Ayurvedic
Smilax china	Hriddhaatri	China Root	Ayurvedic
Smilax china	Chobchini	China Root	Unani
Smilax china	Parangi chchakkai	China Root	Siddha/Tamil
Smilax glabra	Dweepaantara-Vachaa	Bulbous China Root	Ayurvedic
Smilax glabra	Chobachini (bigger var.)	Bulbous China Root	Ayurvedic

Table Contd.

Botanical Name	Indian Name	English Name	Medicinal System
Smilax lanceifolia	Hindi Chobachini	Himalayan China Root	Ayurvedic
Smilax lanceifolia	Shukchin	Himalayan China Root	Folk
Smilax lanceifolia	Hariaa	Himalayan China Root	Folk
Smilax ornata	Ushbaa	Jamaica Sarsaparilla	Unani
Smilax ovalifolia	Maitri	Wild China Root	Ayurvedic
Smilax ovalifolia	Ushbaa	Wild China Root	Unani
Smilax ovalifolia	Ghot-vel	Wild China Root	Folk
Smilax zeylanica	Malai-thaamara	Indian China Root	Siddha/Tamil
Smilax zeylanica	Jangali Ushbaa	Indian China Root	Unani
Solanum Aculeatissimum	Brihati	Cockroach Berry, Indian Love Apple, Devil's Apple	Ayurvedic
Solanum albicaule	Brihati	Narkanta Prikly Shrub	Ayurvedic
Solanum albicaule	Narkanta	Narkanta Prikly Shrub	Folk
Solanum aviculare	Kantakaari	Kashmir Poison Berry	Ayurvedic
Solanum dabium	Kantakaari	Dubium Seeds	Ayurvedic
Solanum dulcamara	Kaakamaachi-vishesha	Woody Night Shade, Bittersweet, Bitter Nightshade, Felonwort	Ayurvedic
Solanum dulcamara	Valli-kantakaarikaa	Woody Night Shade, Bittersweet, Bitter Nightshade, Felonwort	Ayurvedic
Solanum dulcamara	Mako (red var.)	Woody Night Shade, Bittersweet, Bitter Nightshade, Felonwort	Unani
Solanum elaeagnifolium	Mako	Silverleaf Nightshade	Folk
Solanum erianthum	Chundai	Mullen Nightshade	Folk
Solanum erianthum	Rasagadimaanu	Mullen Nightshade	Folk
Solanum erianthum	Sowdangigida	Mullen Nightshade	Folk
Solanum erianthum	Kadusinde	Mullen Nightshade	Folk
Solanum erianthum	Kutri	Mullen Nightshade	Folk
Solanum ferox	Brihati	Poison-Berry	Ayurvedic
Solanum ferox	Brihatikaa	Poison-Berry	Ayurvedic
Solanum ferox	Mahati	Poison-Berry	Ayurvedic
Solanum ferox	Hinguli	Poison-Berry	Ayurvedic
Solanum ferox	Prasaha	Poison-Berry	Ayurvedic
Solanum ferox	Vartaki	Poison-Berry	Ayurvedic

Table Contd.

Botanical Name	Indian Name	English Name	Medicinal System
Solanum ferox	Kaantaa	Poison-Berry	Ayurvedic
Solanum ferox	Kshudra-bhantaki	Poison-Berry	Ayurvedic
Solanum ferox	Simhi	Poison-Berry	Ayurvedic
Solanum ferox	Bana-bhantaa	Poison-Berry	Ayurvedic
Solanum ferox	Kateri (bigger var.)	Poison-Berry	Ayurvedic
Solanum ferox	Katai Kalaan	Poison-Berry	Unani
Solanum ferox	Mulli	Poison-Berry	Siddha/Tamil
Solanum ferox	Pappara-mulli	Poison-Berry	Siddha/Tamil
Solanum ferox	Karimulli	Poison-Berry	Siddha/Tamil
Solanum ferox	Raam-begun	Poison-Berry	Folk
Solanum indicum	Brihati	Poison Berry	Ayurvedic
Solanum indicum	Kshudra-bhantaaki	Poison Berry	Ayurvedic
Solanum indicum	Kateri (bigger var.)	Poison Berry	Ayurvedic
Solanum indicum	Hadaq	Poison Berry	Unani
Solanum indicum	Kataai Kalaan	Poison Berry	Unani
Solanum indicum	Mulkatri	Poison Berry	Siddha/Tamil
Solanum indicum	Vazhuthunai (root)	Poison Berry	Siddha/Tamil
Solanum indicum	Barahantaa	Poison Berry	Folk
Solanum melongena	Bhantaki	Eggplant, Brinjal	Ayurvedic
Solanum melongena	Bhantaa	Eggplant, Brinjal	Ayurvedic
Solanum melongena	Vaartaaka	Eggplant, Brinjal	Ayurvedic
Solanum melongena	Vaartaaku	Eggplant, Brinjal	Ayurvedic
Solanum melongena	Vaartaakini	Eggplant, Brinjal	Ayurvedic
Solanum melongena	Vrintaaka	Eggplant, Brinjal	Ayurvedic
Solanum melongena	Baingan	Eggplant, Brinjal	Unani
Solanum melongena	Kathirikai	Eggplant, Brinjal	Siddha/Tamil
Solanum melongena	Baingan	Eggplant, Brinjal	Folk
Solanum melongena	Bhantaa	Eggplant, Brinjal	Folk
Solanum nigrum	Kaakamaachi	Black Nightshade	Ayurvedic
Solanum nigrum	Kaakaahya	Black Nightshade	Ayurvedic

Table Contd.

Botanical Name	Indian Name	English Name	Medicinal System
Solanum nigrum	Kaakamaataa	Black Nightshade	Ayurvedic
Solanum nigrum	Dhvanksha-maachi	Black Nightshade	Ayurvedic
Solanum nigrum	Mako	Black Nightshade	Unani
Solanum nigrum	Manithakkali	Black Nightshade	Siddha/Tamil
Solanum torvum	Brihati	West Indian Turkey Berry	Ayurvedic
Solanum torvum	Goshtha-vaartaaku	West Indian Turkey Berry	Ayurvedic
Solanum torvum	Chundai	West Indian Turkey Berry	Siddha/Tamil
Solanum torvum	Ran-Baingan	West Indian Turkey Berry	Folk
Solanum torvum	Goth-begun	West Indian Turkey Berry	Folk
Solanum trilobatum	Alarka	Climbing Brinjal	Ayurvedic
Solanum trilobatum	Kantakaari-lataa	Climbing Brinjal	Ayurvedic
Solanum trilobatum	Valli-kantakaarikaa	Climbing Brinjal	Ayurvedic
Solanum trilobatum	Tooduvalai	Climbing Brinjal	Siddha/Tamil
Solanum tuberosum	Aaluka	Potato	Ayurvedic
Solanum tuberosum	Aaruka	Potato	Ayurvedic
Solanum tuberosum	Golaalu	Potato	Ayurvedic
Solanum tuberosum	Aaluu	Potato	Folk
Solanum xanthocarpum	Kantakaari	Wild Eggplant, Yellow-Berried Nightshade	Ayurvedic
Solanum xanthocarpum	Kantakaarikaa	Wild Eggplant, Yellow-Berried Nightshade	Ayurvedic
Solanum xanthocarpum	Vyaaghri	Wild Eggplant, Yellow-Berried Nightshade	Ayurvedic
Solanum xanthocarpum	Nidigdhikaa	Wild Eggplant, Yellow-Berried Nightshade	Ayurvedic
Solanum xanthocarpum	Nidigdhaa	Wild Eggplant, Yellow-Berried Nightshade	Ayurvedic
Solanum xanthocarpum	Duhsparshaa	Wild Eggplant, Yellow-Berried Nightshade	Ayurvedic
Solanum xanthocarpum	Dhaavani	Wild Eggplant, Yellow-Berried Nightshade	Ayurvedic
Solanum xanthocarpum	Kshudraa	Wild Eggplant, Yellow-Berried Nightshade	Ayurvedic

Table Contd.

Botanical Name	Indian Name	English Name	Medicinal System
Solanum xanthocarpum	Keteri (smaller var.)	Wild Eggplant, Yellow-Berried Nightshade	Ayurvedic
Solanum xanthocarpum	Bhatakataiyaa	Wild Eggplant, Yellow-Berried Nightshade	Ayurvedic
Solanum xanthocarpum	Kataai Khurd	Wild Eggplant, Yellow-Berried Nightshade	Unani
Solanum xanthocarpum	Hadaq	Wild Eggplant, Yellow-Berried Nightshade	Unani
Solanum xanthocarpum	Kandankatthiri	Wild Eggplant, Yellow-Berried Nightshade	Siddha/Tamil
Solidago virgaurea	Golden-rod	European Goldenrod, Woundwort	Folk
Sonchus arvensis	Sahadevi (bigger var.)	Corn Sow Thistle	Ayurvedic
Sonchus asper	Sahadevi (bigger var.)	Spinyleaved Sow Thistle	Ayurvedic
Sonchus asper	Didhi	Spinyleaved Sow Thistle	Folk
Sonchus asper	Mhaataaraa	Spinyleaved Sow Thistle	Folk
Sonchus oleraceus	Duudhi	Milk Thistle	Folk
Sonchus oleraceus	Dodaka	Milk Thistle	Folk
Sonchus oleraceus	Dudhaali	Milk Thistle	Folk
Sonneratia caseolaris	Orchaa	Berembang, Mangrove Apple	Folk
Sonneratia caseolaris	Tivar	Berembang, Mangrove Apple	Folk
Sonneratia caseolaris	Chipi	Berembang, Mangrove Apple	Folk
Sophora japonica	Pagoda Tree	Japanese Pagoda Tree, Chinese Scholar Tree, Umbrella Tree	Folk
Sophora mollis	Khumani	Himalayan Laburnum, Low Mountain Laurel	Folk/Kumaun
Sophora mollis	Pahargungri	Himalayan Laburnum, Low Mountain Laurel	Folk/Kumaun
Sopubia delphinifolia	Dudhaali	Sopubia Root-Parasite	Folk
Sorbus aucuparia	Battal	European Mountain Ash, Rowan Tree, Mountain Ash Berry	Folk
Sorbus aucuparia	Syaar	European Mountain Ash, Rowan Tree, Mountain Ash Berry	Folk
Sorghum vulgare	Yaava-naala	Sorghum, Broomcorn	Ayurvedic

Table Contd.

Botanical Name	Indian Name	English Name	Medicinal System
Stellaria media	Safed Fulki	Common Chickweed	Folk
Stellaria media	Buchbuchaa	Common Chickweed	Folk
Stephania glabra	Paathaa	Indian Tape Vine	Ayurvedic
Stephania glabra	Gidaangu	Indian Tape Vine	Folk
Stephania glabra	Paahraa	Indian Tape Vine	Folk
Stephania hernandiifolia	Raaj-Paathaa (South)	Japanese Tape Vine	Ayurvedic
Sterculia foetida	Kudirai Pidukku	Kola Seeds, Gurru Nuts	Siddha/Tamil
Sterculia foetida	Pinari	Kola Seeds, Gurru Nuts	Siddha/Tamil
Sterculia foetida	Jangali Baadaam	Kola Seeds, Gurru Nuts	Folk
Sterculia urens	Gond Kateeraa	Bissy Nuts, Karaya Gum	Unani
Sterculia urens	Kavalam	Bissy Nuts, Karaya Gum	Siddha/Tamil
Sterculia urens	Karai	Bissy Nuts, Karaya Gum	Folk
Sterculia urens	Kandol	Bissy Nuts, Karaya Gum	Folk
Stereospermum personatum	Paatalaa	Trumpet Flower, Yellow Snake Tree	Ayurvedic
Stereospermum personatum	Paatali	Trumpet Flower, Yellow Snake Tree	Ayurvedic
Stereospermum personatum	Paadhal	Trumpet Flower, Yellow Snake Tree	Ayurvedic
Stereospermum personatum	Krishna-vrantaa	Trumpet Flower, Yellow Snake Tree	Ayurvedic
Stereospermum personatum	Madhu-duuti	Trumpet Flower, Yellow Snake Tree	Ayurvedic
Stereospermum personatum	Kaama-duuti	Trumpet Flower, Yellow Snake Tree	Ayurvedic
Stereospermum personatum	Ativallabhaa	Trumpet Flower, Yellow Snake Tree	Ayurvedic
Stereospermum personatum	Taamrapushpi	Trumpet Flower, Yellow Snake Tree	Ayurvedic
Stereospermum personatum	Kuberaakshi	Trumpet Flower, Yellow Snake Tree	Ayurvedic
Stereospermum personatum	Amoghaa	Trumpet Flower, Yellow Snake Tree	Ayurvedic
Stereospermum personatum	Kumbhipushpi	Trumpet Flower, Yellow Snake Tree	Ayurvedic
Stereospermum personatum	Ambuvaasini	Trumpet Flower, Yellow Snake Tree	Ayurvedic

Table Contd.

Botanical Name	Indian Name	English Name	Medicinal System
Stereospermum personatum	Paadiri	Trumpet Flower, Yellow Snake Tree	Siddha/Tamil
Streblus asper	Shaakhotaka	Siamese Rough Brush	Ayurvedic
Streblus asper	Shaakhota	Siamese Rough Brush	Ayurvedic
Streblus asper	Pitaphalaka	Siamese Rough Brush	Ayurvedic
Streblus asper	Bhuutavaasa	Siamese Rough Brush	Ayurvedic
Streblus asper	Kharachhada	Siamese Rough Brush	Ayurvedic
Streblus asper	Piraayan	Siamese Rough Brush	Siddha/Tamil
Streblus asper	Kharaoli	Siamese Rough Brush	Folk
Streblus asper	Sihoraa	Siamese Rough Brush	Folk
Striga asiatica	Agnivriksha	Witchweed	Ayurvedic
Striga asiatica	Kuranti	Witchweed	Ayurvedic
Striga asiatica	Pallipundu	Witchweed	Siddha/Tamil
Striga asiatica	Agiyaa	Witchweed	Folk
Striga gesneroides	Laal-giyaa	Cowpea Witchweed	Folk
Strobilanthes callosus	Maruaa-daanaa	Carvia Callosa	Folk
Strobilanthes callosus	Kaarvi	Carvia Callosa	Folk
Strobilanthes flaccidifolius	Khumaa	Assam Indigo	Folk
Strobilanthes flaccidifolius	Raampat	Assam Indigo	Folk
Strobilanthes flaccidifolius	Ruum	Assam Indigo	Folk
Strophanthus kombe	Kombe	Kombe Arrow Poison, Large-leaved Poison Rope	Folk
Strychnos colubrina	Kuchilaa-lataa	Trumpet Wood	Ayurvedic
Strychnos colubrina	Kupilu-lataa	Trumpet Wood	Ayurvedic
Strychnos colubrina	Kaajar-vel	Trumpet Wood	Folk
Strychnos ignatii	Kayappankottai	Ignatus Beans	Siddha/Tamil
Strychnos ignatii	Papitaa Vilaayati	Ignatus Beans	Unani
Strychnos nux-vomica	Kapilu	Nux Vomica	Ayurvedic
Strychnos nux-vomica	Kaakatinduka	Nux Vomica	Ayurvedic
Strychnos nux-vomica	Kaakendu	Nux Vomica	Ayurvedic
Strychnos nux-vomica	Kaakapiluka	Nux Vomica	Ayurvedic
Strychnos nux-vomica	Vishamushtikaa	Nux Vomica	Ayurvedic
Strychnos nux-vomica	Vishamushti	Nux Vomica	Ayurvedic

Table Contd.

Botanical Name	Indian Name	English Name	Medicinal System
Strychnos nux-vomica	Vishatinduka	Nux Vomica	Ayurvedic
Strychnos nux-vomica	Kuchilaa	Nux Vomica	Ayurvedic
Strychnos nux-vomica	Ksuchalaa	Nux Vomica	Ayurvedic
Strychnos nux-vomica	Azaraaqi	Nux Vomica	Unani
Strychnos nux-vomica	Kuchlaa	Nux Vomica	Unani
Strychnos nux-vomica	Yettikkottai	Nux Vomica	Siddha/Tamil
Strychnos potatorum	Kataka	Clearing Nut Tree	Ayurvedic
Strychnos potatorum	Katakaphala	Clearing Nut Tree	Ayurvedic
Strychnos potatorum	Payah-prasaadi	Clearing Nut Tree	Ayurvedic
Strychnos potatorum	Chakshushya	Clearing Nut Tree	Ayurvedic
Strychnos potatorum	Nirmali	Clearing Nut Tree	Ayurvedic
Strychnos potatorum	Thettran	Clearing Nut Tree	Siddha/Tamil
Strychnos potatorum	Thetrankottai	Clearing Nut Tree	Siddha/Tamil
Strychnos rheedei	Valli Kanjiram	Snakewood	Siddha/Tamil
Styrax benzoin	Saambiraani	True Gum Benzoin, Sumatra Benzoin or Gum Benjamin	Siddha/Tamil
Styrax benzoin	Lobaan	True Gum Benzoin, Sumatra Benzoin or Gum Benjamin	Unani
Styrax officinale	Silhaka	The True Storax Tree	Ayurvedic
Styrax officinale	Silaarasa	The True Storax Tree	Ayurvedic
Styrax officinale	Turushka	The True Storax Tree	Ayurvedic
Styrax officinale	Kapitaila	The True Storax Tree	Ayurvedic
Styrax officinale	Yavandeshaja	The True Storax Tree	Ayurvedic
Styrax officinale	Usturak	The True Storax Tree	Folk
Styrax officinale	Silaajit	The True Storax Tree	Folk
Sutherlandia frutescens	Sutherlandia	Bladdersenna, Cancerwort, Cape Baloon Pea	Folk
Swertia affinis	Kiraatatikta	Hill Chiretta	Ayurvedic
Swertia angustifolia	Kiraata (sweet var.)	Hill Chiretta	Ayurvedic
Swertia angustifolia	Pahaari Kiretta	Hill Chiretta	Folk
Swertia angustifolia	Mithaa (sweet) Kiryaat	Hill Chiretta	Folk
Swertia chirayita	Kiraata	Chiretta	Ayurvedic
Swertia chirayita	Kairaata	Chiretta	Ayurvedic

Table Contd.

Botanical Name	Indian Name	English Name	Medicinal System
Swertia chirayita	Kiraataka	Chiretta	Ayurvedic
Swertia chirayita	Kandatikta	Chiretta	Ayurvedic
Swertia chirayita	Kiraatatikta	Chiretta	Ayurvedic
Swertia chirayita	Kiraatatiktaka	Chiretta	Ayurvedic
Swertia chirayita	Katutikta	Chiretta	Ayurvedic
Swertia chirayita	Trinnimba	Chiretta	Ayurvedic
Swertia chirayita	Bhuunimba	Chiretta	Ayurvedic
Swertia chirayita	Aranyatikta	Chiretta	Ayurvedic
Swertia chirayita	Raamasenaka	Chiretta	Ayurvedic
Swertia chirayita	Chiraitaa	Chiretta	Unani
Swertia chirayita	Nilavembu	Chiretta	Siddha/Tamil
Swertia ciliata	Shailaja	Black Chiretta	Ayurvedic
Swertia ciliata	Kiraatatikta	Black Chiretta	Ayurvedic
Swertia densifolia	Shailaja	Dense-leaved Chiretta	Ayurvedic
Swertia densifolia	Kiraatatikta	Dense-leaved Chiretta	Ayurvedic
Swertia lawii	Kiraatatikta	Western Ghat Chiretta	Ayurvedic
Swietenia mahagoni	Ciminukku	West Indian Mahogany	Siddha/Tamil
Swietenia mahagoni	Mahaagani	West Indian Mahogany	Folk
Symphorema involucratum	Surudu	Bhingri	Folk
Symphorema involucratum	Konatekkali	Bhingri	Folk
Symphorema involucratum	Gubbadaara	Bhingri	Folk
Symphytum officinale	Sankuutan	Comfrey, Knitbone	Folk
Symplocos paniculata	Lodhra-Pattikaa	Sapphire Berry	Ayurvedic
Symplocos paniculata	Lodh Pathaanı	Sapphire Berry	Unani
Symplocos racemosa	Lodhra	Lodh Tree, Sapphire Berry	Ayurvedic
Symplocos racemosa	Rodhra	Lodh Tree, Sapphire Berry	Ayurvedic
Symplocos racemosa	Shaavara	Lodh Tree, Sapphire Berry	Ayurvedic
Symplocos racemosa	Sthulavalkal	Lodh Tree, Sapphire Berry	Ayurvedic
Symplocos racemosa	Trita	Lodh Tree, Sapphire Berry	Ayurvedic
Symplocos racemosa	Pattikaa Lodhra	Lodh Tree, Sapphire Berry	Ayurvedic
Symplocos racemosa	Shaabara Lodhra	Lodh Tree, Sapphire Berry	Ayurvedic

Table Contd.

Botanical Name	Indian Name	English Name	Medicinal System
Symplocos racemosa	Lodh Pathaani	Lodh Tree, Sapphire Berry	Unani
Symplocos racemosa	Velliloththiram pattai (Bark)	Lodh Tree, Sapphire Berry	Siddha/Tamil
Symplocos racemosa	Velliloththiram	Lodh Tree, Sapphire Berry	Siddha/Tamil
Syringa vulgaris	Lilac	Common Lilac	Folk
Syzygium aromaticum	Lavanga	Clove	Ayurvedic
Syzygium aromaticum	Devakusum	Clove	Ayurvedic
Syzygium aromaticum	Devapushpa	Clove	Ayurvedic
Syzygium aromaticum	Shrisangya	Clove	Ayurvedic
Syzygium aromaticum	Shriprasuunaka	Clove	Ayurvedic
Syzygium aromaticum	Qaranful	Clove	Unani
Syzygium aromaticum	Laung	Clove	Unani
Syzygium aromaticum	Kiraambu	Clove	Siddha/Tamil
Syzygium aromaticum	Lavangam	Clove	Siddha/Tamil
Syzygium cerasoideum	Bhumi Jambu	Piaman Tree	Ayurvedic
Syzygium cerasoideum	Rai Jaamun	Piaman Tree	Folk
Syzygium cerasoideum	Dugdugiaa	Piaman Tree	Folk
Syzygium cerasoideum	Topaakudaa	Piaman Tree	Folk
Syzygium cerasoideum	Peeta-jaam	Piaman Tree	Folk
Syzygium cuminii	Jambu	Java Plum, Jambolan, Black Plum	Ayurvedic
Syzygium cuminii	Mahaaphalaa	Java Plum, Jambolan, Black Plum	Ayurvedic
Syzygium cuminii	Phalendraa	Java Plum, Jambolan, Black Plum	Ayurvedic
Syzygium cuminii	Surabhipatra	Java Plum, Jambolan, Black Plum	Ayurvedic
Syzygium cuminii	Jaamun	Java Plum, Jambolan, Black Plum	Unani
Syzygium cuminii	Naaval	Java Plum, Jambolan, Black Plum	Siddha/Tamil
Syzygium hemisphericum	Vellai Naval	Jambosa	Siddha/Tamil
Syzygium jambos	Peru Navel	Rose Apple	Siddha/Tamil
Syzygium jambos	Raaj-Jambu	Rose Apple	Ayurvedic
Syzygium jambos	Gulaabjaamun	Rose Apple	Folk

Table Contd.

Botanical Name	Indian Name	English Name	Medicinal System
Syzygium malaccense	Malay Jaamun	Malay Apple, Mountain Apple	Folk
Syzygium zeylanicum	Marungi	Sumaich (Cambodia)	Siddha/Tamil
Syzygium zeylanicum	Bhedas	Sumaich (Cambodia)	Folk
Tabernaemontana coronaria	Tagar	East Indian Rosebay	Ayurvedic
Tabernaemontana coronaria	Nandivriksha	East Indian Rosebay	Ayurvedic
Tabernaemontana coronaria	Nandi Pushpa	East Indian Rosebay	Ayurvedic
Tabernaemontana coronaria	Nandiyavattam	East Indian Rosebay	Siddha/Tamil
Tabernaemontana coronaria	Tengari	East Indian Rosebay	Folk
Tabernaemontana coronaria	Chaandani	East Indian Rosebay	Folk
Tabernaemontana dichotoma	Kandalaippalai	Eve's Apple, Forbidden Fruit	Siddha/Tamil
Tabernaemontana dichotoma	Kattalari-palai	Eve's Apple, Forbidden Fruit	Siddha/Tamil
Tabernaemontana dichotoma	Tengari (var.)	Eve's Apple, Forbidden Fruit	Folk
Tacca aspera	Vaaraahikanda	Wild-Bore Tuber	Ayurvedic
Tacca aspera	Vaaraahi	Wild-Bore Tuber	Ayurvedic
Tacca aspera	Duukarkand	Wild-Bore Tuber	Folk
Tacca pinnatifida	Suurana	Fiji Arrowroot, Tahiti Arrowroot	Ayurvedic
Tacca pinnatifida	Karachunai	Fiji Arrowroot, Tahiti Arrowroot	Siddha/Tamil
Tagetes erecta	Jhandu	Big Marigold, Aztec or African Marigold	Ayurvedic
Tagetes erecta	Gendaa	Big Marigold, Aztec or African Marigold	Ayurvedic
Tagetes erecta	Gul-hazaaraa	Big Marigold, Aztec or African Marigold	Unani
Tagetes erecta	Gul-jaafari	Big Marigold, Aztec or African Marigold	Unani
Tagetes erecta	Sadbarg	Big Marigold, Aztec or African Marigold	Unani
Tagetes erecta	Thuruksaamanthi	Big Marigold, Aztec or African Marigold	Siddha/Tamil
Talinum triangulare	Pasali	Ceylon Spinach, Surinam Purslane, Flame Flower, Sweet Heart, Water Leaf, Ceylon Spinach	Folk/Tamil
Talinum triangulare	Cylon-keerai	Ceylon Spinach, Surinam Purslane, Flame Flower, Sweet Heart, Water Leaf, Ceylon Spinach	Folk/Tamil

Table Contd.

Botanical Name	Indian Name	English Name	Medicinal System
Tamarindus indica	Amli	Tamarind Tree	Ayurvedic
Tamarindus indica	Amlikaa	Tamarind Tree	Ayurvedic
Tamarindus indica	Suktaa	Tamarind Tree	Ayurvedic
Tamarindus indica	Chukraa	Tamarind Tree	Ayurvedic
Tamarindus indica	Chukrikaa	Tamarind Tree	Ayurvedic
Tamarindus indica	Chinchaa	Tamarind Tree	Ayurvedic
Tamarindus indica	Chandikaa	Tamarind Tree	Ayurvedic
Tamarindus indica	Tintidika	Tamarind Tree	Ayurvedic
Tamarindus indica	Tamar Hindi	Tamarind Tree	Unani
Tamarindus indica	Puli	Tamarind Tree	Siddha/Tamil
Tamarindus indica	Aanvilam	Tamarind Tree	Siddha/Tamil
Tamarix aphylla	Maacheeka	Athel, Tamarisk	Ayurvedic
Tamarix aphylla	Maachikaa	Athel, Tamarisk	Ayurvedic
Tamarix aphylla	Maayin Khurd	Athel, Tamarisk	Unani
Tamarix aphylla	Sivappattus-havukku	Athel, Tamarisk	Siddha/Tamil
Tamarix aphylla	Laal Jhaau	Athel, Tamarisk	Folk
Tamarix aphylla	Galls—Chhoti-Maayin	Athel, Tamarisk	Folk
Tamarix dioica	Maachikaa	Tamarisk	Ayurvedic
Tamarix dioica	Nirumari	Tamarisk	Siddha/Tamil
Tamarix dioica	Jhaau	Tamarisk	Folk
Tamarix dioica	Galls-Maayin	Tamarisk	Folk
Tamarix ericoides	Maachika	Tamarisk Mucronta	Ayurvedic
Tamarix ericoides	Jhaau	Tamarisk Mucronta	Folk
Tamarix indica	Jhaavuka	Takut Galls	Ayurvedic
Tamarix indica	Bahugranthikaa	Takut Galls	Ayurvedic
Tamarix indica	Shaavaka	Takut Galls	Ayurvedic
Tamarix indica	Maayeen Kalaan	Takut Galls	Unani
Tamarix indica	Maayeen Khurd	Takut Galls	Unani
Tamarix indica	Sirusavakku	Takut Galls	Siddha/Tamil
Tamarix indica	Jhaau	Takut Galls	Folk

Table Contd.

Botanical Name	Indian Name	English Name	Medicinal System
Tanacetum longifolium	Akarkaraa	Long-leaved Tansy	Unani
Tanacetum umbelliferum	Akarkaraa Sweet var.	Sweet Pellitory	Unani
Tanacetum umbelliferum	Buujidaan	Sweet Pellitory	Unani
Taraktogenos kurzii	Chaalmogra	Kalawa Tree	Folk
Taraxacum officinale	Dugdh-pheni	Common Dandelion	Ayurvedic
Taraxacum officinale	Luutaari	Common Dandelion	Ayurvedic
Taraxacum officinale	Payaswani	Common Dandelion	Ayurvedic
Taraxacum officinale	Kaanful	Common Dandelion	Unani
Taraxacum officinale	Kaasani Dashti	Common Dandelion	Unani
Taraxacum officinale	Kaasani Sahraayi	Common Dandelion	Unani
Taraxacum officinale	Hind-baa-al-Barri	Common Dandelion	Unani
Taraxacum officinale	Dudhli	Common Dandelion	Folk
Taraxacum officinale	Dudhal	Common Dandelion	Folk
Tarenna asiatica	Kuraa	Komi Tree	Folk
Taverniera cuneifolia	Jethi-madh	East Indian Moneywort	Folk
Taxus baccata	Dhaatri-patra	European Yew	Ayurvedic
Taxus baccata	Shukapushpa	European Yew	Ayurvedic
Taxus baccata	Sthauneya	European Yew	Ayurvedic
Taxus baccata	Sthauneyaka	European Yew	Ayurvedic
Taxus baccata	Thunera	European Yew	Ayurvedic
Taxus baccata	Vikarna	European Yew	Ayurvedic
Taxus baccata	Zarnab	European Yew	Unani
Taxus baccata	Taaleespatri Bhedam	European Yew	Siddha/Tamil
Taxus baccata	Birmi	European Yew	Folk
Taxus baccata	Thuno	European Yew	Folk
Tecoma stans	Sonapaati	Yellow Elder, Yellow Bells	Siddha/Tamil
Tecoma stans	Thanga arali	Yellow Elder, Yellow Bells	Siddha/Tamil
Tecoma stans	Naga sambagam	Yellow Elder, Yellow Bells	Siddha/Tamil
Tecomella undulata	Rohitaka	Rohida Tree	Ayurvedic
Tecomella undulata	Rohi	Rohida Tree	Ayurvedic

Table Contd.

Botanical Name	Indian Name	English Name	Medicinal System
Tecomella undulata	Daadim-pushpaka	Rohida Tree	Ayurvedic
Tecomella undulata	Daadimchhada	Rohida Tree	Ayurvedic
Tecomella undulata	Plihaghna	Rohida Tree	Ayurvedic
Tectona grandis	Shaaka	Teak Tree	Ayurvedic
Tectona grandis	Bhuumisaha	Teak Tree	Ayurvedic
Tectona grandis	Dwaaradaaru	Teak Tree	Ayurvedic
Tectona grandis	Varadaaru	Teak Tree	Ayurvedic
Tectona grandis	Kharachada	Teak Tree	Ayurvedic
Tectona grandis	Saagawaan	Teak Tree	Ayurvedic
Tectona grandis	Saagauna	Teak Tree	Ayurvedic
Tectona grandis	Thekku	Teak Tree	Siddha/Tamil
Tephrosia purpurea	Sharapunkhaa	Purple Tephrosia, Wild Indigo	Ayurvedic
Tephrosia purpurea	Vishikha-punkhaa	Purple Tephrosia, Wild Indigo	Ayurvedic
Tephrosia purpurea	Sarphokaa	Purple Tephrosia, Wild Indigo	Ayurvedic
Tephrosia purpurea	Sarponkhaa	Purple Tephrosia, Wild Indigo	Unani
Tephrosia purpurea	Sarphukaa	Purple Tephrosia, Wild Indigo	Unani
Tephrosia purpurea	Kolunchi	Purple Tephrosia, Wild Indigo	Folk/Tamil
Tephrosia purpurea	Kollukkaivelai	Purple Tephrosia, Wild Indigo	Folk/Tamil
Tephrosia purpurea	Paavali	Purple Tephrosia, Wild Indigo	Folk/Tamil
Tephrosia purpurea	Mollukkay	Purple Tephrosia, Wild Indigo	Folk/Tamil
Tephrosia purpurea	Kollukkayvelai	Purple Tephrosia, Wild Indigo	Siddha/Tamil
Teramnus labialis	Kattuulandu	Blue Wiss	Siddha/Tamil
Teramnus labialis	Maashaparni	Blue Wiss	Ayurvedic
Teramnus labialis	Mahaasahaa	Blue Wiss	Ayurvedic
Teramnus labialis	Suuryaasani	Blue Wiss	Ayurvedic
Teramnus labialis	Lomash-parni	Blue Wiss	Ayurvedic
Teramnus labialis	Kaamboja	Blue Wiss	Ayurvedic
Teramnus labialis	Krishna-vrintaa	Blue Wiss	Ayurvedic
Terminalia arjuna	Arjuna	Arjun Terminalia	Ayurvedic
Terminalia arjuna	Dhananjaya	Arjun Terminalia	Ayurvedic
Terminalia arjuna	Indravriksha	Arjun Terminalia	Ayurvedic
Terminalia arjuna	Kakubha	Arjun Terminalia	Ayurvedic

Table Contd.

Botanical Name	Indian Name	English Name	Medicinal System
Terminalia arjuna	Kaakubha	Arjun Terminalia	Ayurvedic
Terminalia arjuna	Paartha	Arjun Terminalia	Ayurvedic
Terminalia arjuna	Virataru	Arjun Terminalia	Ayurvedic
Terminalia arjuna	Viravriksha	Arjun Terminalia	Ayurvedic
Terminalia arjuna	Aartagala	Arjun Terminalia	Ayurvedic
Terminalia arjuna	Arjun	Arjun Terminalia	Unani
Terminalia arjuna	Marudam	Arjun Terminalia	Siddha/Tamil
Terminalia bellirica	Bibhitaka	Belleric Myrobalan, Bastard Myrobalan	Ayurvedic
Terminalia bellirica	Vibhitaka	Belleric Myrobalan, Bastard Myrobalan	Ayurvedic
Terminalia bellirica	Bibhitaki	Belleric Myrobalan, Bastard Myrobalan	Ayurvedic
Terminalia bellirica	Bibhita	Belleric Myrobalan, Bastard Myrobalan	Ayurvedic
Terminalia bellirica	Baibhita	Belleric Myrobalan, Bastard Myrobalan	Ayurvedic
Terminalia bellirica	Aksha	Belleric Myrobalan, Bastard Myrobalan	Ayurvedic
Terminalia bellirica	Akshaka	Belleric Myrobalan, Bastard Myrobalan	Ayurvedic
Terminalia bellirica	Kaamaghna	Belleric Myrobalan, Bastard Myrobalan	Ayurvedic
Terminalia bellirica	Kalidrum	Belleric Myrobalan, Bastard Myrobalan	Ayurvedic
Terminalia bellirica	Karshaphala	Belleric Myrobalan, Bastard Myrobalan	Ayurvedic
Terminalia bellirica	Balelaa	Belleric Myrobalan, Bastard Myrobalan	Unani
Terminalia bellirica	Baheraa	Belleric Myrobalan, Bastard Myrobalan	Unani
Terminalia bellirica	Thaanrikkaai	Belleric Myrobalan, Bastard Myrobalan	Siddha/Tamil
Terminalia bellirica	Thandri	Belleric Myrobalan, Bastard Myrobalan	Siddha/Tamil
Terminalia bialata	Chuglam	Andamans Ash, Silver Grey Wood	Folk
Terminalia catappa	Natuvadom	Indian Almond, Tropical Almond	Siddha/Tamil

Table Contd.

Botanical Name	Indian Name	English Name	Medicinal System
Terminalia catappa	Jangali Baadaam	Indian Almond, Tropical Almond	Folk
Terminalia catappa	Desi Baadaam	Indian Almond, Tropical Almond	Folk
Terminalia chebula	Haritaki	Chebulic Myrobalan, Black Myrobalan	Ayurvedic
Terminalia chebula	Kaayasthaa	Chebulic Myrobalan, Black Myrobalan	Ayurvedic
Terminalia chebula	Pathyaa	Chebulic Myrobalan, Black Myrobalan	Ayurvedic
Terminalia chebula	Shreyasi	Chebulic Myrobalan, Black Myrobalan	Ayurvedic
Terminalia chebula	Shivaa	Chebulic Myrobalan, Black Myrobalan	Ayurvedic
Terminalia chebula	Harad	Chebulic Myrobalan, Black Myrobalan	Unani
Terminalia chebula	Halelaa Siyaah	Chebulic Myrobalan, Black Myrobalan	Unani
Terminalia chebula	Halelaa Zard	Chebulic Myrobalan, Black Myrobalan	Unani
Terminalia chebula	Halelaa Kaabuli	Chebulic Myrobalan, Black Myrobalan	Unani
Terminalia chebula	Kadukkaai	Chebulic Myrobalan, Black Myrobalan	Siddha/Tamil
Terminalia citrina	Haritaki	Bengal Myrobalan	Folk/Bengal
Terminalia citrina	Suravaari Harad	Bengal Myrobalan	Folk
Terminalia citrina	Monalu	Bengal Myrobalan	Folk/Assam
Terminalia coriacea	Tani	Leathery Murdah	Folk
Terminalia myriocarpa	Kakubha	Hollock	Ayurvedic
Terminalia paniculata	Kinjal	Flowering Murdah	Folk
Terminalia paniculata	Nimiri	Flowering Murdah	Folk
Terminalia paniculata	Pekadukkai	Flowering Murdah	Folk/Tamil
Terminalia paniculata	Marudu	Flowering Murdah	Folk/Tamil
Terminalia paniculata	Maruva	Flowering Murdah	Folk
Terminalia paniculata	Kindal (trade)	Flowering Murdah	Folk
Terminalia tomentosa	Asan	Laurel (trade)	Folk/Bengal

Table Contd.

Botanical Name	Indian Name	English Name	Medicinal System
Terminalia tomentosa	Karramarda	Laurel (trade)	Folk/Tamil
Terminalia tomentosa	Sarj	Laurel (trade)	Folk
Terminalia tomentosa	Saaj	Laurel (trade)	Folk
Terminalia tomentosa	Sain	Laurel (trade)	Folk
Tetracera laevis	Anaittichal	Sandpaper-Vine	Siddha/Tamil
Tetragonia expansa	Chikesoppu	New Zealand Spinach	Folk/Karnataka
Tetrastigma serrulatum	Charchari	Lizard Plant	Folk/Nepal
Teucrium chamaedrys	Kamaazariuus	Germander, Wall Germander	Unani
Teucrium chamaedrys	Usqurdiyun	Germander, Wall Germander	Unani
Teucrium scordium	Germander	Water-Germander	Folk/Kashmir
Thalictrum foliolosum	Pitamuulikaa	Meadow Rue	Ayurvedic
Thalictrum foliolosum	Pitarangaa	Meadow Rue	Ayurvedic
Thalictrum foliolosum	Piyaaraangaa	Meadow Rue	Ayurvedic
Thalictrum foliolosum	Mamiri	Meadow Rue	Unani
Themeda arundinacea	Sarkharaa	Ulla Grass	Folk
Themeda arundinacea	Kapoor Ghass	Ulla Grass	Folk
Theobroma cacao	Cocoa	Cocoa, Theobroma, Chocolate Tree	Folk
Thespesia lampas	Tundikera	Indian Hemp	Ayurvedic
Thespesia lampas	Bana-Kapaasi	Indian Hemp	Folk
Thespesia lampas	Raan-bhendi	Indian Hemp	Folk
Thespesia populnea	Paarisha	Portia Tree, Tulip Tree, Umbrella Tree, False Rosewood	Ayurvedic
Thespesia populnea	Kapitana	Portia Tree, Tulip Tree, Umbrella Tree, False Rosewood	Ayurvedic
Thespesia populnea	Paarshvpippala	Portia Tree, Tulip Tree, Umbrella Tree, False Rosewood	Ayurvedic
Thespesia populnea	Gardabhaanda	Portia Tree, Tulip Tree, Umbrella Tree, False Rosewood	Ayurvedic
Thespesia populnea	Poovarsu	Portia Tree, Tulip Tree, Umbrella Tree, False Rosewood	Siddha/Tamil
Thevetia peruviana	Pita-Karavira	Yellow Oleander	Ayurvedic

Table Contd.

Botanical Name	Indian Name	English Name	Medicinal System
Thevetia peruviana	Ashvaghna	Yellow Oleander	Ayurvedic
Thevetia peruviana	Divyapushpa	Yellow Oleander	Ayurvedic
Thevetia peruviana	Pachiyalari	Yellow Oleander	Siddha/Tamil
Thlaspi arvense	Drekaa	Pennycress, Fanweed	Folk
Thuja orientalis	Morepankhi	Oriental Arbor-Vitae	Folk
Thymus serphyllum	Ajagandhaa	Mother-of-thyme, Wild Thyme	Ayurvedic
Thymus serphyllum	Vana-Yavaani	Mother-of-thyme, Wild Thyme	Ayurvedic
Thymus serphyllum	Haashaa	Mother-of-thyme, Wild Thyme	Unani
Thymus serphyllum	Jangali Pudinaa	Mother-of-thyme, Wild Thyme	Unani
Thysanolaena agrostis	Juurnaa	Bouquet-Grass, Broom-Grass, Tiger-Grass, Amliso	Ayurvedic
Thysanolaena agrostis	Juurnaahv	Bouquet-Grass, Broom-Grass, Tiger-Grass, Amliso	Ayurvedic
Thysanolaena agrostis	Junaar	Bouquet-Grass, Broom-Grass, Tiger-Grass, Amliso	Folk
Thysanolaena agrostis	Pirlu	Bouquet-Grass, Broom-Grass, Tiger-Grass, Amliso	Folk
Tilia cordata	Tilia	Small-leaved Lime, Linden, Basswood	Folk
Tiliacora acuminata	Kodaparuavalli	Bega Climber	Siddha/Tamil
Tiliacora acuminata	Tiliyaa-koraa	Bega Climber	Folk/Bengal
Tinospora cordifolia	Guduuchi	Heart-leaved Tinospora	Ayurvedic
Tinospora cordifolia	Guduuchikaa	Heart-leaved Tinospora	Ayurvedic
Tinospora cordifolia	Guluuchi	Heart-leaved Tinospora	Ayurvedic
Tinospora cordifolia	Jivanti	Heart-leaved Tinospora	Ayurvedic
Tinospora cordifolia	Amritaa	Heart-leaved Tinospora	Ayurvedic
Tinospora cordifolia	Amritalataa	Heart-leaved Tinospora	Ayurvedic
Tinospora cordifolia	Amritavallari	Heart-leaved Tinospora	Ayurvedic
Tinospora cordifolia	Chinnaruuhaa	Heart-leaved Tinospora	Ayurvedic
Tinospora cordifolia	Chinnodbhavaa	Heart-leaved Tinospora	Ayurvedic
Tinospora cordifolia	Madhuparni	Heart-leaved Tinospora	Ayurvedic
Tinospora cordifolia	Vatsaadani	Heart-leaved Tinospora	Ayurvedic
Tinospora cordifolia	Tantrikaa	Heart-leaved Tinospora	Ayurvedic
Tinospora cordifolia	Kundalini	Heart-leaved Tinospora	Ayurvedic

Table Contd.

Botanical Name	Indian Name	English Name	Medicinal System
Tinospora cordifolia	Gilo	Heart-leaved Tinospora	Unani
Tinospora cordifolia	Gulancha	Heart-leaved Tinospora	Unani
Tinospora cordifolia	Sat-e-Gilo (Starch)	Heart-leaved Tinospora	Unani
Tinospora cordifolia	Seendil	Heart-leaved Tinospora	Siddha/Tamil
Tinospora cordifolia	Amrida-valli	Heart-leaved Tinospora	Folk/Tamil
Tinospora cordifolia	Giloya	Heart-leaved Tinospora	Folk
Tinospora crispa	Guduuchi	Tinospora	Ayurvedic
Tinospora malabarica	Kandodbhava-guduchi	Tinospora	Ayurvedic
Tinospora malabarica	Padma-Guduuchi	Tinospora	Ayurvedic
Tinospora malabarica	Vatsaadani	Tinospora	Ayurvedic
Tinospora malabarica	Gurch	Tinospora	Folk
Toddalia asiatica	Kanchana	Wild Orange Tree, Forest Pepper	Ayurvedic
Toddalia asiatica	Kattu Milagu	Wild Orange Tree, Forest Pepper	Siddha/Tamil
Toddalia asiatica	Milakaranai	Wild Orange Tree, Forest Pepper	Siddha/Tamil
Toddalia asiatica	Jangali Kaali-mirch	Wild Orange Tree, Forest Pepper	Folk
Toddalia asiatica	Kanja	Wild Orange Tree, Forest Pepper	Folk
Torenia travancorica	Kakapu	Wishbone Flower	Folk
Trachelospermum fragrans	Duudhi	Japanese Star-Jasmine	Folk
Trachelospermum fragrans	Akhaahi-lataa	Japanese Star-Jasmine	Folk
Trachyspermum ammi	Yavaani	Ammi, Lovage, Carum, Ajowan	Ayurvedic
Trachyspermum ammi	Yamaani	Ammi, Lovage, Carum, Ajowan	Ayurvedic
Trachyspermum ammi	Yavaanikaa	Ammi, Lovage, Carum, Ajowan	Ayurvedic
Trachyspermum ammi	Yamaanikaa	Ammi, Lovage, Carum, Ajowan	Ayurvedic
Trachyspermum ammi	Dipyaka	Ammi, Lovage, Carum, Ajowan	Ayurvedic
Trachyspermum ammi	Nankhwaah	Ammi, Lovage, Carum, Ajowan	Unani
Trachyspermum ammi	Desi Ajawaayin	Ammi, Lovage, Carum, Ajowan	Unani
Trachyspermum ammi	Omam	Ammi, Lovage, Carum, Ajowan	Siddha/Tamil

Table Contd.

Botanical Name	Indian Name	English Name	Medicinal System
Trachyspermum roxburghianum	Ajamodaa	Ajmud	Ayurvedic
Trachyspermum roxburghianum	Ajmoja	Ajmud	Ayurvedic
Trachyspermum roxburghianum	Ajamoda	Ajmud	Ayurvedic
Trachyspermum roxburghianum	Ayamoda	Ajmud	Ayurvedic
Trachyspermum roxburghianum	Dipyaka	Ajmud	Ayurvedic
Trachyspermum roxburghianum	Karafs-e-Hindi	Ajmud	Unani
Trachyspermum roxburghianum	Ashamtagam	Ajmud	Siddha/Tamil
Tragia involucrata	Vrishchhikaali	Indian Stinging-Nettle	Ayurvedic
Tragia involucrata	Vrishchhika-patrikaa	Indian Stinging-Nettle	Ayurvedic
Tragia involucrata	Poonai kaanchori	Indian Stinging-Nettle	Siddha/Tamil
Tragia involucrata	Sirrukaanchori	Indian Stinging-Nettle	Siddha/Tamil
Tragopogon porrifolius	Oyster-root	Salify, Vegetable-Oyster, Purple Goat's Beard, Oyster Plant	Folk
Trapa bispinosa	Shrngaataka	Water Chestnut	Ayurvedic
Trapa bispinosa	Shrngaata	Water Chestnut	Ayurvedic
Trapa bispinosa	Shrngamuula	Water Chestnut	Ayurvedic
Trapa bispinosa	Trikota	Water Chestnut	Ayurvedic
Trapa bispinosa	Jalaphala	Water Chestnut	Ayurvedic
Trapa bispinosa	Trikonaphala	Water Chestnut	Ayurvedic
Trapa bispinosa	Paaniyaphala	Water Chestnut	Ayurvedic
Trapa bispinosa	Jalkanda	Water Chestnut	Ayurvedic
Trapa bispinosa	Trikona	Water Chestnut	Ayurvedic
Trapa bispinosa	Trika	Water Chestnut	Ayurvedic
Trapa bispinosa	Singhaaraa	Water Chestnut	Unani
Trapa bispinosa	Singara	Water Chestnut	Siddha/Tamil
Trema orientalis	Ambaratthi	Charcoal Tree, Indian Nettle Tree	Siddha/Tamil
Trema orientalis	Jivanti	Charcoal Tree, Indian Nettle Tree	Ayurvedic

Table Contd.

Botanical Name	Indian Name	English Name	Medicinal System
Trema orientalis	Gio	Charcoal Tree, Indian Nettle Tree	Folk
Trewia nudiflora	Gambhaari	False White Teak, Gutel	Ayurvedic
Trewia nudiflora	Tumri	False White Teak, Gutel	Ayurvedic
Trewia nudiflora	Pindaara	False White Teak, Gutel	Ayurvedic
Trewia nudiflora	Attarasu	False White Teak, Gutel	Folk/Tamil
Trewia nudiflora	Nay Kumil	False White Teak, Gutel	Folk/Tamil
Trianthema decandra	Varshaabhu	Horse Purslane	Ayurvedic
Trianthema decandra	Vellai saaranai	Horse Purslane	Siddha/Tamil
Trianthema decandra	Bisakhaparaa	Horse Purslane	Folk
Trianthema govindia	Varshaabhu	Horse Purslane	Ayurvedic
Trianthema portulacastrum	Varshaabhu	Horse Purslane	Ayurvedic
Trianthema portulacastrum	Vrshchira	Horse Purslane	Ayurvedic
Trianthema portulacastrum	Vishakhar-parikaa	Horse Purslane	Ayurvedic
Trianthema portulacastrum	Shilaatikaa	Horse Purslane	Ayurvedic
Trianthema portulacastrum	Shothaghni	Horse Purslane	Ayurvedic
Trianthema portulacastrum	Kshdra	Horse Purslane	Ayurvedic
Trianthema portulacastrum	Shveta-punarnavaa	Horse Purslane	Ayurvedic
Trianthema portulacastrum	Upothaki	Horse Purslane	Ayurvedic
Trianthema portulacastrum	Biskhaparaa	Horse Purslane	Unani
Trianthema portulacastrum	Sharunai	Horse Purslane	Siddha/Tamil
Tribulus alatus	Gokshura	Winged Caltrops	Ayurvedic
Tribulus alatus	Gokharu-kalaan	Winged Caltrops	Unani
Tribulus alatus	Desi Gokharu	Winged Caltrops	Folk
Tribulus alatus	Aakharaa	Winged Caltrops	Folk
Tribulus alatus	Hasaka	Winged Caltrops	Folk
Tribulus terrestris	Gokshura	Land-Caltrops, Puncture Vine	Ayurvedic
Tribulus terrestris	Gokshuraka	Land-Caltrops, Puncture Vine	Ayurvedic
Tribulus terrestris	Kshudra Gokharu	Land-Caltrops, Puncture Vine	Ayurvedic
Tribulus terrestris	Shvadamshtraa	Land-Caltrops, Puncture Vine	Ayurvedic

Table Contd.

Botanical Name	Indian Name	English Name	Medicinal System
Tribulus terrestris	Swaadu-kantaka	Land-Caltrops, Puncture Vine	Ayurvedic
Tribulus terrestris	Trikanta	Land-Caltrops, Puncture Vine	Ayurvedic
Tribulus terrestris	Trikantaka	Land-Caltrops, Puncture Vine	Ayurvedic
Tribulus terrestris	Khar-e-Khasak Khurd	Land-Caltrops, Puncture Vine	Unani
Tribulus terrestris	Sirunerunchil	Land-Caltrops, Puncture Vine	Siddha/Tamil
Tribulus terrestris	Nerunjil	Land-Caltrops, Puncture Vine	Folk/Tamil
Trichodesma indicum	Adah-pushpi	Indian Borage	Ayurvedic
Trichodesma indicum	Adhomukha	Indian Borage	Ayurvedic
Trichodesma indicum	Gandha-pushpika	Indian Borage	Ayurvedic
Trichodesma indicum	Andhaka	Indian Borage	Ayurvedic
Trichodesma indicum	Kalhudaitumbai	Indian Borage	Siddha/Tamil
Trichodesma indicum	Andhaahuli	Indian Borage	Folk
Trichodesma zeylanicum	Adah-pushpi	Ajovan	Ayurvedic
Trichodesma zeylanicum	Jhingi	Ajovan	Ayurvedic
Trichodesma zeylanicum	Hetenuriyaa	Ajovan	Folk
Trichodesma zeylanicum	Jinghini	Ajovan	Folk
Trichodesma zeylanicum	Jalasirasa	Ajovan	Folk
Tricholepis angustifolia	Uuntakataaraa	Camel's Thistle	Folk
Tricholepis angustifolia	Brahmadandi	Camel's Thistle	Ayurvedic
Tricholepis glaberrima	Brahmadandi	Smooth Tricholepis	Ayurvedic
Trichosanthes anguina	Dadhipushpi	Snake-Gourd	Ayurvedic
Trichosanthes anguina	Chichinda	Snake-Gourd	Ayurvedic
Trichosanthes anguina	Shvetaraaji	Snake-Gourd	Ayurvedic
Trichosanthes anguina	Ahiphala	Snake-Gourd	Ayurvedic
Trichosanthes anguina	Pudal	Snake-Gourd	Siddha/Tamil
Trichosanthes anguina	Pudvali	Snake-Gourd	Folk
Trichosanthes anguina	Chikondaa	Snake-Gourd	Folk
Trichosanthes bracteata	Indravaaruni (red var.)	Redball Snakegourd	Ayurvedic
Trichosanthes bracteata	Vishaalaa	Redball Snakegourd	Ayurvedic
Trichosanthes bracteata	Mahaakaala	Redball Snakegourd	Ayurvedic

Table Contd.

Botanical Name	Indian Name	English Name	Medicinal System
Trichosanthes bracteata	Mahendra-vaaruni	Redball Snakegourd	Ayurvedic
Trichosanthes bracteata	Korattai	Redball Snakegourd	Siddha/Tamil
Trichosanthes bracteata	Mahkaar	Redball Snakegourd	Folk
Trichosanthes bracteata	Maakaal	Redball Snakegourd	Folk
Trichosanthes bracteata	Laal Indraayana	Redball Snakegourd	Folk
Trichosanthes bracteata	Kondal	Redball Snakegourd	Folk
Trichosanthes cordata	Bhuumi-kushmaanda	Snake-Gourd	Ayurvedic
Trichosanthes cordata	Patola	Snake-Gourd	Ayurvedic
Trichosanthes cordata	Vidaari (var.)	Snake-Gourd	Ayurvedic/ Bengal
Trichosanthes cordata	Bhui-kumhraa	Snake-Gourd	Folk
Trichosanthes cucumerina	Kattu Pey Pudal	Coiled Snakegourd	Siddha/Tamil
Trichosanthes cucumerina	Tikta-Patoli	Coiled Snakegourd	Ayurvedic
Trichosanthes cucumerina	Vana-Patota	Coiled Snakegourd	Ayurvedic
Trichosanthes cucumerina	Amritaphala	Coiled Snakegourd	Ayurvedic
Trichosanthes dioica	Patola	Patol, Pointed Gourd	Ayurvedic
Trichosanthes dioica	Kulaka	Patol, Pointed Gourd	Ayurvedic
Trichosanthes dioica	Raajiphala	Patol, Pointed Gourd	Ayurvedic
Trichosanthes dioica	Karkashchhada	Patol, Pointed Gourd	Ayurvedic
Trichosanthes dioica	Karkasha	Patol, Pointed Gourd	Ayurvedic
Trichosanthes dioica	Bijagarbha	Patol, Pointed Gourd	Ayurvedic
Trichosanthes dioica	Parwal	Patol, Pointed Gourd	Unani
Trichosanthes dioica	Peyppudal	Patol, Pointed Gourd	Siddha/Tamil
Trichosanthes nervifolia	Patoli	Bitter Chinese Cucumber	Ayurvedic
Trichosanthes nervifolia	Kombu Pudalai	Bitter Chinese Cucumber	Siddha/Tamil
Tridax procumbens	Jayanti	Mexican Daisy	Ayurvedic
Tridax procumbens	Vettukkaaya-thalai	Mexican Daisy	Siddha/Tamil
Tridax procumbens	Akala Kohadi	Mexican Daisy	Folk
Trifolium pratense	Ispast	Red Clover	Unani
Trifolium pratense	Berseem	Red Clover	Unani
Trifolium pratense	Clover	Red Clover	Unani

Table Contd.

Botanical Name	Indian Name	English Name	Medicinal System
Typha elephantina	Gundraa	Elephant Grass, Indian Reed-Mace, Bulrush	Ayurvedic
Typha elephantina	Gundraka	Elephant Grass, Indian Reed-Mace, Bulrush	Ayurvedic
Typha elephantina	Potagala	Elephant Grass, Indian Reed-Mace, Bulrush	Ayurvedic
Typha elephantina	Airakaa	Elephant Grass, Indian Reed-Mace, Bulrush	Ayurvedic
Typha elephantina	Anaikkarai	Elephant Grass, Indian Reed-Mace, Bulrush	Siddha/Tamil
Typha elephantina	Gondapateraa	Elephant Grass, Indian Reed-Mace, Bulrush	Folk
Typha laxmannii	Pizh	Scented Flag	Folk/Kashmir
Typha laxmannii	Airakaa	Scented Flag	Ayurvedic
Typhonium trilobatum	Pidikarunai	Bengal Arum	Siddha/Tamil
Typhonium trilobatum	Karu Karunai Kizhangu	Bengal Arum	Folk/Tamil
Ulmus wallichiana	Hemar	Himalayan Elm	Folk
Ulmus wallichiana	Kitamaara	Himalayan Elm	Folk
Uncaria gambier	Khadira	Pale Catechu, Gambier	Ayurvedic
Uncaria gambier	Chinai Katthaa	Pale Catechu, Gambier	Folk
Uncaria gambier	Kaththakkaambu	Pale Catechu, Gambier	Siddha/Tamil
Uraria alopecuroides	Prishniparni	Jackal's Tail	Ayurvedic
Uraria crinita	Prishniparni	Ekor Kuching, Cat's Tail	Ayurvedic
Uraria lagopoides	Prishniparni	Trailing Uraria	Ayurvedic
Uraria lagopoides	Moovilai (Root)	Trailing Uraria	Siddha/Tamil
Uraria picta	Prishniparni	Trailing Uraria	Ayurvedic
Uraria picta	Prithakparni	Trailing Uraria	Ayurvedic
Uraria picta	Simhapushpi	Trailing Uraria	Ayurvedic
Uraria picta	Kalashi	Trailing Uraria	Ayurvedic
Uraria picta	Dhaavani	Trailing Uraria	Ayurvedic
Uraria picta	Guhaa	Trailing Uraria	Ayurvedic
Uraria picta	Chitraparni	Trailing Uraria	Ayurvedic
Uraria picta	Sittirappaladai	Trailing Uraria	Siddha/Tamil
Urena lobata	Naagabalaa	Pink Chinese Burr, Burr Mallow	Ayurvedic

Table Contd.

Botanical Name	Indian Name	English Name	Medicinal System
Urena lobata	Ottatti	Pink Chinese Burr, Burr Mallow	Folk/Tamil
Urena lobata	Van-bhendi	Pink Chinese Burr, Burr Mallow	Folk
Urena lobata	Lot-loti	Pink Chinese Burr, Burr Mallow	Folk
Urena lobata	Kunjuyaa	Pink Chinese Burr, Burr Mallow	Folk
Urginea indica	Vana-palaandu	Indian Squill, Sea Onion (red and white varieties)	Ayurvedic
Urginea indica	Kolakanda	Indian Squill, Sea Onion (red and white varieties)	Ayurvedic
Urginea indica	Vajrakanda	Indian Squill, Sea Onion (red and white varieties)	Ayurvedic
Urginea indica	Unsul-e-Hindi	Indian Squill, Sea Onion (red and white varieties)	Unani
Urginea indica	Piyaaz-Dasti	Indian Squill, Sea Onion (red and white varieties)	Unani
Urginea indica	Piyaaz-Sahraayi	Indian Squill, Sea Onion (red and white varieties)	Unani
Urginea indica	Isqueel-e-Hindi	Indian Squill, Sea Onion (red and white varieties)	Unani
Urginea indica	Jangali Piyaaz	Indian Squill, Sea Onion (red and white varieties)	Unani
Urginea indica	Narivengayam	Indian Squill, Sea Onion (red and white varieties)	Siddha/Tamil
Urtica dioica	Vrishchhiyaa-shaaka	Stinging Nettle	Ayurvedic
Urtica dioica	Anjuraa	Stinging Nettle	Unani
Urtica dioica	Bicchuu-buuti	Stinging Nettle	Folk
Urtica parviflora	Vrishchhiyaa-shaaka	Hill Nettle	Ayurvedic
Urtica parviflora	Shisuun	Hill Nettle	Folk
Urtica pilulifera	Vrishchiyaa-shaaka	Roman Nettle	Ayurvedic
Urtica pilulifera	Anjuraa	Roman Nettle	Unani
Usnea longissima	Ushnaa	Lichen	Unani
Utricularia bifida	Jhangi (smaller var.)	Bladder Wort	Folk

Table Contd.

Botanical Name	Indian Name	English Name	Medicinal System
Uvaria narum	Pulichan	Cinnamon-leaved Uvaria	Siddha/Tamil
Vaccaria pyramidata	Musna	Soapwort, Cow Herb	Folk
Vaccaria pyramidata	Saabuni	Soapwort, Cow Herb	Folk
Vaccinium symplocifolium	Kilapalam	Indian Bilberry, Blueberry	Folk
Valeriana dubia	Abhramaansi	Common Valerian	Ayurvedic
Valeriana hardwickii	Sugandha-baalaa	Himalayan Valerian	Folk
Valeriana hardwickii	Taggar-ganthodaa	Himalayan Valerian	Folk
Valeriana hardwickii	Tagger	Himalayan Valerian	Folk
Valeriana hardwickii	Asaarun	Himalayan Valerian	Folk
Valeriana leschenaultii	Sugandhabaalaa	Nilgiri Valerian	Folk
Valeriana leschenaultii	Taggar	Nilgiri Valerian	Folk
Valeriana leschenaultii	Baalaka	Nilgiri Valerian	Folk
Valeriana leschenaultii	Tagara	Nilgiri Valerian	Ayurvedic
Valeriana officinalis	Tagara	Valerian, Garden Heliotrope, Common Valerian	Ayurvedic
Valeriana officinalis	Nata	Valerian, Garden Heliotrope, Common Valerian	Ayurvedic
Valeriana officinalis	Baalaka	Valerian, Garden Heliotrope, Common Valerian	Ayurvedic
Valeriana officinalis	Sugandha-baalaa	Valerian, Garden Heliotrope, Common Valerian	Folk
Valeriana officinalis	Taggar	Valerian, Garden Heliotrope, Common Valerian	Folk
Valeriana pyrolaefolia	Dhyaamaka	Smaller-rhizome Jatamansi	Ayurvedic
Valeriana pyrolaefolia	Sugandhabaalaa	Smaller-rhizome Jatamansi	Folk
Valeriana wallichii	Tagara	Indian Valerian	Ayurvedic
Valeriana wallichii	Sugandhabaalaa	Indian Valerian	Ayurvedic
Valeriana wallichii	Kaalaanusaari	Indian Valerian	Ayurvedic
Valeriana wallichii	Kaalaanu-saarikaa	Indian Valerian	Ayurvedic
Valeriana wallichii	Nata	Indian Valerian	Ayurvedic
Valeriana wallichii	Asaarun	Indian Valerian	Unani
Valeriana wallichii	Tagar Reshewaalaa	Indian Valerian	Unani

Table Contd.

Botanical Name	Indian Name	English Name	Medicinal System
Valeriana wallichii	Tagaram	Indian Valerian	Siddha/Tamil
Valeriana wallichii	Taggar	Indian Valerian	Folk
Valeriana wallichii	Baalaka	Indian Valerian	Folk
Valeriana wallichii	Mushkbaalaa	Indian Valerian	Folk
Valeriana wallichii	Asaarun	Indian Valerian	Folk
Valeriana wallichii	Tagar-ganthodaa	Indian Valerian	Folk
Vallaris solanacea	Aasphotaa	Bread Flower	Ayurvedic
Vallaris solanacea	Asphuka	Bread Flower	Ayurvedic
Vallaris solanacea	Bhadravalli	Bread Flower	Ayurvedic
Vallaris solanacea	Saarivaa-utpala	Bread Flower	Ayurvedic
Vallaris solanacea	Haaphara-maali var	Bread Flower	Folk
Vallaris solanacea	Dudhi-bel	Bread Flower	Folk
Vallisneria spiralis	Shaivaala	Eel-Grass, Tape Grass, Wild Celery	Ayurvedic
Vallisneria spiralis	Jallil	Eel-Grass, Tape Grass, Wild Celery	Ayurvedic
Vallisneria spiralis	Sevaar	Eel-Grass, Tape Grass, Wild Celery	Folk
Vanda roxburghii	Raasnaa	Tassellata	Ayurvedic
Vanda roxburghii	Vandaka Raasnaa	Tassellata	Folk
Vanda spathulata	Ponnam-pomaraiva	Plantain Tree, Tree-top Plantain	Folk/South
Vanda spathulata	Svarna-pushpa Bandaa	Plantain Tree, Tree-top Plantain	Ayurvedic
Vanda spathulata	Baandaa	Plantain Tree, Tree-top Plantain	Ayurvedic
Vandellia pedunculata	Gadaga-vel	Gadag Vine	Folk
Vangueria spinosa	Pinditaka	Voa-Vanga	Ayurvedic
Vangueria spinosa	Snigdh-pinditaka	Voa-Vanga	Ayurvedic
Vangueria spinosa	Manakkarai	Voa-Vanga	Siddha/Tamil
Vangueria spinosa	Muyana	Voa-Vanga	Folk
Vangueria spinosa	Chiracholi	Voa-Vanga	Folk

Table Contd.

Botanical Name	Indian Name	English Name	Medicinal System
Vangueria spinosa	Alu	Voa-Vanga	Folk
Vateria indica	Sarja	White Damar, Indian Copal-Tree, Malabar Tallow Tree, Piney Varnish-Tree	Ayurvedic
Vateria indica	Sarjaka	White Damar, Indian Copal-Tree, Malabar Tallow Tree, Piney Varnish-Tree	Ayurvedic
Vateria indica	Karsya	White Damar, Indian Copal-Tree, Malabar Tallow Tree, Piney Varnish-Tree	Ayurvedic
Vateria indica	Sasyasumbara	White Damar, Indian Copal-Tree, Malabar Tallow Tree, Piney Varnish-Tree	Ayurvedic
Vateria indica	Devdhuupa	White Damar, Indian Copal-Tree, Malabar Tallow Tree, Piney Varnish-Tree	Ayurvedic
Vateria indica	Marich-patraka	White Damar, Indian Copal-Tree, Malabar Tallow Tree, Piney Varnish-Tree	Ayurvedic
Vateria indica	Chhaagakarna	White Damar, Indian Copal-Tree, Malabar Tallow Tree, Piney Varnish-Tree	Ayurvedic
Vateria indica	Raal	White Damar, Indian Copal-Tree, Malabar Tallow Tree, Piney Varnish-Tree	Unani
Vateria indica	Vellai kunthirikam	White Damar, Indian Copal-Tree, Malabar Tallow Tree, Piney Varnish-Tree	Siddha/Tamil
Vateria indica	Vellai Kundarakam	White Damar, Indian Copal-Tree, Malabar Tallow Tree, Piney Varnish-Tree	Siddha/Tamil
Ventilago denticulata	Raktavalli	Ventilago Black Vine	Ayurvedic
Ventilago denticulata	Pappili	Ventilago Black Vine	Folk
Ventilago denticulata	Raamadhaani	Ventilago Black Vine	Folk
Ventilago denticulata	Kevati (var.)	Ventilago Black Vine	Folk
Ventilago denticulata	Pitti	Ventilago Black Vine	Folk
Ventilago madraspatana	Taamravalli	Ventilago Vermilion Vine	Ayurvedic
Ventilago madraspatana	Kaivartikaa	Ventilago Vermilion Vine	Ayurvedic
Ventilago madraspatana	Vaamataruni	Ventilago Vermilion Vine	Ayurvedic
Ventilago madraspatana	Pappili-chaka	Ventilago Vermilion Vine	Siddha/Tamil

Table Contd.

Botanical Name	Indian Name	English Name	Medicinal System
Ventilago madraspatana	Lokhandi	Ventilago Vermilion Vine	Folk
Ventilago madraspatana	Kevati	Ventilago Vermilion Vine	Folk
Vepris bilocularis	Krishna-Agaru	Unarmed Black Deodar	Ayurvedic
Vepris bilocularis	Kaaragil	Unarmed Black Deodar	Siddha/Tamil
Veratrum viride	Hellebore	Indian Hellbore, False Hellebore, Indian Poke	Folk
Verbascum thapsus	Ban Tambaaku	Cow's Lungwort, Common Mullein	Ayurvedic
Verbascum thapsus	Gidar Tambaaku	Cow's Lungwort, Common Mullein	Ayurvedic
Verbascum thapsus	Phullaa	Cow's Lungwort, Common Mullein	Ayurvedic
Verbena officinalis	Saal-ul-hamaam	Vervain, Pigeon's Grass	Unani
Verbena officinalis	Faristariun	Vervain, Pigeon's Grass	Unani
Vernonia cinerea	Sahadevi	Ash Coloured Fleabane, Purple Fleabane	Ayurvedic
Vernonia cinerea	Uttamkanyaka	Ash Coloured Fleabane, Purple Fleabane	Ayurvedic
Vernonia cinerea	Dandotpalaa	Ash Coloured Fleabane, Purple Fleabane	Ayurvedic
Vernonia cinerea	Naichotte Poonde	Ash Coloured Fleabane, Purple Fleabane	Siddha/Tamil
Vernonia javanica	Shutthi	Java Fleabane	Siddha/Tamil
Vernonia roxburghii	Sahadevi	Himalayan Fleabane	Ayurvedic
Vernonia roxburghii	Doraa-baahaa	Himalayan Fleabane	Folk
Veronica beccabunga	Titalokiyaa	Brooklime	Folk
Veronica beccabunga	Tezhak	Brooklime	Folk
Vetiveria zizanioides	Ushira	Vetiver, Khas	Ayurvedic
Vetiveria zizanioides	Bahu-muulaka	Vetiver, Khas	Ayurvedic
Vetiveria zizanioides	Sugandhimuula	Vetiver, Khas	Ayurvedic
Vetiveria zizanioides	Jataamedaa	Vetiver, Khas	Ayurvedic
Vetiveria zizanioides	Indragupta	Vetiver, Khas	Ayurvedic
Vetiveria zizanioides	Nalada	Vetiver, Khas	Ayurvedic
Vetiveria zizanioides	Laamajjaka	Vetiver, Khas	Ayurvedic

Table Contd.

Botanical Name	Indian Name	English Name	Medicinal System
Viola tricolor	Banafashaa	Heartsease, Wild Pansy	Unani
Viscum album	Bandaaka	European Mistletoe	Ayurvedic
Viscum album	Suvarna-bandaaka	European Mistletoe	Ayurvedic
Viscum album	Vrikshaadani	European Mistletoe	Ayurvedic
Viscum album	Kishmish Kaabuli	European Mistletoe	Unani
Viscum articulatum	Bandaak	Napalese Mistletoe	Ayurvedic
Viscum articulatum	Jivantikaa	Napalese Mistletoe	Ayurvedic
Viscum articulatum	Kaamavriksha	Napalese Mistletoe	Ayurvedic
Viscum articulatum	Nilavalli	Napalese Mistletoe	Ayurvedic
Viscum articulatum	Panapuuduu	Napalese Mistletoe	Folk
Viscum articulatum	Bodobaando	Napalese Mistletoe	Folk
Viscum monoicum	Katukavalli	Himalayan Mistletoe	Ayurvedic
Viscum monoicum	Pashumo-hanikaa	Himalayan Mistletoe	Ayurvedic
Viscum monoicum	Kuchleikaa-malang	Himalayan Mistletoe	Folk
Viscum monoicum	Kuchlekaa-baandaa	Himalayan Mistletoe	Folk
Viscum monoicum	Pullurivi	Himalayan Mistletoe	Siddha/Tamil
Viscum monoicum	Pulluri	Himalayan Mistletoe	Folk/Tamil
Viscum orientale	Baandaa	Bengal Mistletoe	Folk
Vitex agnus-castus	Renukaa (seed)	Monk's Pepper-tree, Hemp Tree	Ayurvedic
Vitex agnus-castus	Sambhaalu	Monk's Pepper-tree, Hemp Tree	Unani
Vitex leucoxylon	Paaraavata-padi	Deccan Vitex	Ayurvedic
Vitex leucoxylon	Kaakajanghaa	Deccan Vitex	Ayurvedic
Vitex negundo	Nilanirgundi	Five-leaved Chaste Tree	Ayurvedic
Vitex negundo	Shephaalikaa	Five-leaved Chaste Tree	Ayurvedic
Vitex negundo	Sindhuka	Five-leaved Chaste Tree	Ayurvedic
Vitex negundo	Sindhuvaarak	Five-leaved Chaste Tree	Ayurvedic
Vitex negundo	Suvahaa	Five-leaved Chaste Tree	Ayurvedic
Vitex negundo	Sugandhikaa	Five-leaved Chaste Tree	Ayurvedic
Vitex negundo	Nila-sindhukaa	Five-leaved Chaste Tree	Ayurvedic

Table Contd.

Botanical Name	Indian Name	English Name	Medicinal System
Vitex negundo	Nilapushpaka	Five-leaved Chaste Tree	Ayurvedic
Vitex negundo	Bhuutakeshi	Five-leaved Chaste Tree	Ayurvedic
Vitex negundo	Sambhaalu	Five-leaved Chaste Tree	Unani
Vitex negundo	Fanjankisht	Five-leaved Chaste Tree	Unani
Vitex negundo	Dhanaka	Five-leaved Chaste Tree	Ayurvedic
Vitex negundo	Sheeta-bhiru	Five-leaved Chaste Tree	Ayurvedic
Vitex negundo	Nochchi	Five-leaved Chaste Tree	Siddha/Tamil
Vitex negundo	Nirkundi	Five-leaved Chaste Tree	Folk/Tamil
Vitex peduncularis	Kaakajanghaa	Assam Vitex	Ayurvedic
Vitex peduncularis	Chirai-godaa	Assam Vitex	Folk
Vitex peduncularis	Chirai-gorwaa	Assam Vitex	Folk
Vitex peduncularis	Naagpheni	Assam Vitex	Folk
Vitex trifolia	Sinduvaarak	Three-leaved Vitex	Ayurvedic
Vitex trifolia	Nirgundi (white var.)	Three-leaved Vitex	Ayurvedic
Vitex trifolia	Sveta-pushpaka	Three-leaved Vitex	Siddha/Tamil
Vitex trifolia	Sirunochi	Three-leaved Vitex	Siddha/Tamil
Vitex trifolia	Paani-Sambhaalu	Three-leaved Vitex	Folk
Vitis vinifera	Draakshaa	Wine Grape, European Grape	Ayurvedic
Vitis vinifera	Go-stani	Wine Grape, European Grape	Ayurvedic
Vitis vinifera	Mrdvikaa	Wine Grape, European Grape	Ayurvedic
Vitis vinifera	Daakh	Wine Grape, European Grape	Ayurvedic
Vitis vinifera	Munnakaa	Wine Grape, European Grape	Ayurvedic
Vitis vinifera	Kishmish	Wine Grape, European Grape	Ayurvedic
Vitis vinifera	Angoor	Wine Grape, European Grape	Unani
Vitis vinifera	Daakh	Wine Grape, European Grape	Unani
Vitis vinifera	Maweez	Wine Grape, European Grape	Unani
Vitis vinifera	Zabeeb	Wine Grape, European Grape	Unani
Vitis vinifera	Munaqqaa	Wine Grape, European Grape	Unani
Vitis vinifera	Kishmish	Wine Grape, European Grape	Unani
Vitis vinifera	Thiratchai, Draksha	Wine Grape, European Grape	Siddha/Tamil
Volutarella ramosa	Baadaavard	Volutarella	Unani

Table Contd.

Botanical Name	Indian Name	English Name	Medicinal System
Volutarella ramosa	Al-baavard	Volutarella	Unani
Volutarella ramosa	Shukaayi	Volutarella	Unani
Volutarella ramosa	Bhu-dandi	Volutarella	Folk
Volutarella ramosa	Sukaayi	Volutarella	Folk
Wagatea spicata	Okkadi-kodi	Western Ghat-Wakeri	Folk/Tamil
Wagatea spicata	Pulinak-kagondai	Western Ghat-Wakeri	Siddha/Tamil
Wagatea spicata	Vaakeri	Western Ghat-Wakeri	Folk
Wagatea spicata	Guchh-karanja	Western Ghat-Wakeri	Ayurvedic
Wahlenbergia marginata	Tosad kesari	Tenane (South Africa)	Folk
Wahlenbergia marginata	Dudma Saaga	Tenane (South Africa)	Folk
Walsura trifoliata	Cheddavokko	Walursi	Siddha/Tamil
Walsura trifoliata	Kanjiram	Walursi	Siddha/Tamil
Walsura trifoliata	Waalsuuraa	Walursi	Folk
Waltheria indica	Shembudu	Boater Bush, Buff Coat' Leather Coat, Sleepy Morning	Siddha/Tamil
Waltheria indica	Khar-Duudhi	Boater Bush, Buff Coat' Leather Coat, Sleepy Morning	Folk
Wedelia biflora	Bhringaraaja	Sea Coast Weldia	Ayurvedic
Wedelia calendulaceae	Bhringaraaja	Yellow-flowered Weldia	Ayurvedic
Wedelia calendulaceae	Pitabhringi	Yellow-flowered Weldia	Ayurvedic
Wedelia calendulaceae	Pitabhringa-raaja	Yellow-flowered Weldia	Ayurvedic
Wedelia calendulaceae	Avanti	Yellow-flowered Weldia	Ayurvedic
Wedelia calendulaceae	Kesharaaja	Yellow-flowered Weldia	Ayurvedic
Wedelia calendulaceae	Kesharaaga	Yellow-flowered Weldia	Ayurvedic
Wedelia calendulaceae	Manjal Karisaalai	Yellow-flowered Weldia	Siddha/Tamil
Wedelia calendulaceae	Potralai Kaiyan Tagarai	Yellow-flowered Weldia	Siddha/Tamil
Wedelia calendulaceae	Patalai Kaiantakerai	Yellow-flowered Weldia	Siddha/Tamil
Wendlandia exserta	Tilaka	Wendlandia	Ayurvedic
Wendlandia exserta	Tiliyaa	Wendlandia	Folk
Wendlandia exserta	Tilki	Wendlandia	Folk

Table Contd.

Botanical Name	Indian Name	English Name	Medicinal System
Wendlandia exserta	Mimri	Wendlandia	Folk
Wendlandia tinctoria	Tilak	Wendlandia	Ayurvedic
Wikstroemia indica	Salago	Small-Leaf Salago	Folk
Withania ashwagandha	Ashwagandhaa	Winter Cherry	Ayurvedic
Withania ashwagandha	Hayagandhaa	Winter Cherry	Ayurvedic
Withania ashwagandha	Ashwakanda	Winter Cherry	Ayurvedic
Withania ashwagandha	Gandharva-gandhaa	Winter Cherry	Ayurvedic
Withania ashwagandha	Turaga	Winter Cherry	Ayurvedic
Withania ashwagandha	Turaga-gandhaa	Winter Cherry	Ayurvedic
Withania ashwagandha	Turagaahvaa	Winter Cherry	Ayurvedic
Withania ashwagandha	Vaajigandhaa	Winter Cherry	Ayurvedic
Withania ashwagandha	Gokarnaa	Winter Cherry	Ayurvedic
Withania ashwagandha	Vrishaa	Winter Cherry	Ayurvedic
Withania ashwagandha	Varaahakarni	Winter Cherry	Ayurvedic
Withania ashwagandha	Varadaa	Winter Cherry	Ayurvedic
Withania ashwagandha	Balyaa	Winter Cherry	Ayurvedic
Withania ashwagandha	Vaajikari	Winter Cherry	Ayurvedic
Withania ashwagandha	Asgandh	Winter Cherry	Unani
Withania ashwagandha	Amukkuram-kishangu	Winter Cherry	Siddha/Tamil
Withania coagulans	Desi Asgandh	Vegetable Rennet, Indian Cheese-maker	Unani
Withania coagulans	Kaaknaj-e-Hindi	Vegetable Rennet, Indian Cheese-maker	Unani
Withania coagulans	Paneer	Vegetable Rennet, Indian Cheese-maker	Unani
Withania coagulans	Paneer-band	Vegetable Rennet, Indian Cheese-maker	Unani
Withania coagulans	Akri (fruit)	Vegetable Rennet, Indian Cheese-maker	Unani
Withania coagulans	Ammukkura	Vegetable Rennet, Indian Cheese-maker	Siddha/Tamil
Woodfordia fruticosa	Dhaataki	Fire-flame Bush, Shiranjitea	Ayurvedic
Woodfordia fruticosa	Dhaatri	Fire-flame Bush, Shiranjitea	Ayurvedic

Table Contd.

Botanical Name	Indian Name	English Name	Medicinal System
Woodfordia fruticosa	Kunjaraa	Fire-flame Bush, Shiranjitea	Ayurvedic
Woodfordia fruticosa	Taamrapushpi	Fire-flame Bush, Shiranjitea	Ayurvedic
Woodfordia fruticosa	Bahupushpi	Fire-flame Bush, Shiranjitea	Ayurvedic
Woodfordia fruticosa	Vahni-jwaalaa	Fire-flame Bush, Shiranjitea	Ayurvedic
Woodfordia fruticosa	Kaattaaththi-ppoo (Flower)	Fire-flame Bush, Shiranjitea	Siddha/Tamil
Wrightia tinctoria	Shveta Kutaja	Pala Indigo Plant	Ayurvedic
Wrightia tinctoria	Kutaja (Stree)	Pala Indigo Plant	Ayurvedic
Wrightia tinctoria	Indrayava (seeds)	Pala Indigo Plant	Ayurvedic
Wrightia tinctoria	Inderjao Shireen	Pala Indigo Plant	Unani
Wrightia tinctoria	Irum-paalai	Pala Indigo Plant	Siddha/Tamil
Wrightia tinctoria	Nila-paalai	Pala Indigo Plant	Siddha/Tamil
Wrightia tomentosa	Kutaja (Purush)	Red-flowered Wrightia	Ayurvedic
Wrightia tomentosa	Indrayava (seeds)	Red-flowered Wrightia	Ayurvedic
Wrightia tomentosa	Pala	Red-flowered Wrightia	Siddha/Tamil
Xanthium strumarium	Shankheshwara	Cocklebur, Burweed	Ayurvedic
Xanthium strumarium	Arishta	Cocklebur, Burweed	Ayurvedic
Xanthium strumarium	Aartagala	Cocklebur, Burweed	Ayurvedic
Xanthium strumarium	Maruloomatham	Cocklebur, Burweed	Siddha/Tamil
Xanthium strumarium	Adhasisi	Cocklebur, Burweed	Folk
Xanthium strumarium	Bana-okraa	Cocklebur, Burweed	Folk
Ximenia americana	Chiru-illantai	Tallow-Wood, False Sandal-Wood	Folk/Tamil
Ximenia americana	Kadaranji	Tallow-Wood, False Sandal-Wood	Folk/Tamil
Ximenia americana	Siruyilandai	Tallow-Wood, False Sandal-Wood	Folk/Tamil
Xylia xylocarpa	Irul	Irul Tree	Folk/Tamil
Xylia xylocarpa	Jambu	Irul Tree	Folk
Xylia xylocarpa	Suriaa	Irul Tree	Folk
Xylocarpus granatum	Somanthiri	The Puzzle Fruit Tree	Folk/Tamil
Xylocarpus granatum	Pussur	The Puzzle Fruit Tree	Folk
Xylocarpus granatum	Dhundul	The Puzzle Fruit Tree	Folk
Xylopia parviflora	Saanthu	Netawu, Atuketiya	Folk/Kerala

Table Contd.

Botanical Name	Indian Name	English Name	Medicinal System
Xylopia parviflora	Kalpottan	Netawu, Atuketiya	Folk/Kerala
Xylopia parviflora	Kalpootha	Netawu, Atuketiya	Folk/Tamil
Xylopia parviflora	Chiddavintai	Netawu, Atuketiya	Folk/Tamil
Xylopia parviflora	Ulli	Netawu, Atuketiya	Folk/Karnataka
Xylosma longifolium	Sallu	Dandal Tree, Kandhara Tree	Folk/Kumaun
Xylosma longifolium	Sailu	Dandal Tree, Kandhara Tree	Folk/Himachal
Xylosma longifolium	Dandal	Dandal Tree, Kandhara Tree	Folk
Xylosma longifolium	Katahaar	Dandal Tree, Kandhara Tree	Folk/Assam
Xyris commplanata	Kochelachi-pullu	Yellow-eyed Grass	Folk
Xyris indica	Daadmaari	Yellow-eyed Grass	Ayurvedic
Xyris indica	Dhobi Deeb	Yellow-eyed Grass	Ayurvedic
Xyris indica	Haabiduuba	Yellow-eyed Grass	Folk/Bengal
Yucca filamentosa	Yucca	Adam's Needle, Golden Sword	Folk
Yucca glorisa	Adamusi	Spanish Dagger-Plant, Adam's Needle	Folk
Zanonia indica	Chirpoti	Zanonia	Ayurvedic
Zanonia indica	Kuntali	Zanonia	Ayurvedic
Zanonia indica	Chirpotaa	Zanonia	Ayurvedic
Zanonia indica	Tiktaka	Zanonia	Ayurvedic
Zanonia indica	Penar-valli	Zanonia	Folk/Tamil
Zanonia indica	Parpoti	Zanonia	Folk
Zanthoxylum acanthopodium	Tumburu	Tumru Tree, Prickly Ash	Ayurvedic
Zanthoxylum acanthopodium	Nepaali Dhaniyaa	Tumru Tree, Prickly Ash	Folk
Zanthoxylum acanthopodium	Timur	Tumru Tree, Prickly Ash	Folk
Zanthoxylum americanum	Tumburu (Fruit)	Toothache Tree, Prickly Ash	Ayurvedic
Zanthoxylum armatum	Tumburu (Fruit)	Toothache Tree, Indian Prickly Ash	Ayurvedic
Zanthoxylum armatum	Tejabala	Toothache Tree, Indian Prickly Ash	Ayurvedic
Zanthoxylum armatum	Tejaswani	Toothache Tree, Indian Prickly Ash	Ayurvedic

Table Contd.

Botanical Name	Indian Name	English Name	Medicinal System
Zanthoxylum armatum	Tejohva	Toothache Tree, Indian Prickly Ash	Ayurvedic
Zanthoxylum armatum	Tejovati (stem bark)	Toothache Tree, Indian Prickly Ash	Ayurvedic
Zanthoxylum armatum	Faaghir	Toothache Tree, Indian Prickly Ash	Unani
Zanthoxylum armatum	Kabaab-e-Khandaan	Toothache Tree, Indian Prickly Ash	Unani
Zanthoxylum armatum	Tejyovathi	Toothache Tree, Indian Prickly Ash	Folk/South
Zanthoxylum armatum	Nepaali Dhaniyaa	Toothache Tree, Indian Prickly Ash	Folk
Zanthoxylum budrunga	Tumburu	Tumru Tree, Prickly Ash	Ayurvedic
Zanthoxylum budrunga	Ashvaghra	Tumru Tree, Prickly Ash	Ayurvedic
Zanthoxylum budrunga	Tejabala	Tumru Tree, Prickly Ash	Ayurvedic
Zanthoxylum budrunga	Iratechai	Tumru Tree, Prickly Ash	Siddha/Tamil
Zanthoxylum oxyphyllum	Mezenga	Tumru Tree, Prickly Ash	Folk
Zanthoxylum oxyphyllum	Timur	Tumru Tree, Prickly Ash	Folk
Zanthoxylum oxyphyllum	Bhansi	Tumru Tree, Prickly Ash	Folk
Zataria multiflora	Origanon	Wild Thyme	Unani
Zataria multiflora	Saatar Faarsi	Wild Thyme	Unani
Zataria multiflora	Al-Saatar	Wild Thyme	Unani
Zea mays	Mahaa-Kaaya	Maize, Corn, Indian Corn	Ayurvedic
Zea mays	Makkaa	Maize, Corn, Indian Corn	Unani
Zea mays	Zurraa Makkaa	Maize, Corn, Indian Corn	Unani
Zehneria umbellata	Pulivanji	Zehneria	Siddha/Tamil
Zehneria umbellata	Tarali	Zehneria	Folk
Zehneria umbellata	Gometi	Zehneria	Folk
Zehneria umbellata	Banakakaraa	Zehneria	Folk
Zehneria umbellata	Kudri	Zehneria	Folk
Zingiber cassumunar	Vanardraka	Cassumunar Ginger	Ayurvedic
Zingiber cassumunar	Peja	Cassumunar Ginger	Ayurvedic
Zingiber cassumunar	Peyu	Cassumunar Ginger	Ayurvedic
Zingiber cassumunar	Aardikaa	Cassumunar Ginger	Ayurvedic
Zingiber cassumunar	Shringaberikaa	Cassumunar Ginger	Ayurvedic

Table Contd.

Botanical Name	Indian Name	English Name	Medicinal System
Zingiber cassumunar	Adarakhi	Cassumunar Ginger	Folk
Zingiber cassumunar	Bana-adarakhi	Cassumunar Ginger	Folk
Zingiber officinale	Aadraka (Fresh rhizome)	Ginger	Ayurvedic
Zingiber officinale	Aadrikaa	Ginger	Ayurvedic
Zingiber officinale	Shrngibera	Ginger	Ayurvedic
Zingiber officinale	Shrngavera	Ginger	Ayurvedic
Zingiber officinale	Katubhadra	Ginger	Ayurvedic
Zingiber officinale	Shunthi (Dried rhizome)	Ginger	Ayurvedic
Zingiber officinale	Naagara	Ginger	Ayurvedic
Zingiber officinale	Naagaraa	Ginger	Ayurvedic
Zingiber officinale	Naagaraka	Ginger	Ayurvedic
Zingiber officinale	Aushadha	Ginger	Ayurvedic
Zingiber officinale	Mahaushadha	Ginger	Ayurvedic
Zingiber officinale	Vishvaa	Ginger	Ayurvedic
Zingiber officinale	Vishvabheshaja	Ginger	Ayurvedic
Zingiber officinale	Vishvaaushadha	Ginger	Ayurvedic
Zingiber officinale	Zanjabeel-e-Ratab (Fresh rhizome)	Ginger	Unani
Zingiber officinale	Al-Zanjabeel	Ginger	Unani
Zingiber officinale	Zanjabeel (Dried rhizome)	Ginger	Unani
Zingiber officinale	Zanjabeel-e-yaabis	Ginger	Unani
Zingiber officinale	Inji (Fresh rhizome)	Ginger	Siddha/Tamil
Zingiber officinale	Allam	Ginger	Siddha/Tamil
Zingiber officinale	Lokottai	Ginger	Siddha/Tamil
Zingiber officinale	Chukku (Dried rhizome)	Ginger	Siddha/Tamil
Zingiber officinale	Sunthi (Dried rhizome)	Ginger	Siddha/Tamil
Zingiber zerumbet	Mahaabhari-vachaa	Zerumbet Ginger	Ayurvedic
Zingiber zerumbet	Sthula-granthi	Zerumbet Ginger	Ayurvedic

Table Contd.

Botanical Name	Indian Name	English Name	Medicinal System
Zingiber zerumbet	Narkachoor	Zerumbet Ginger Curcuma caesia is also equated with Narkachoor	Unani
Zingiber zerumbet	Zarambaad	Zerumbet Ginger	Unani
Zingiber zerumbet	Karrallamu	Zerumbet Ginger	Folk
Ziziphus jujuba	Badar	Indian Jujube, Common Jujube	Ayurvedic
Ziziphus jujuba	Kola	Indian Jujube, Common Jujube	Ayurvedic
Ziziphus jujuba	Ber	Indian Jujube, Common Jujube	Unani
Ziziphus jujuba	Yelandai	Indian Jujube, Common Jujube	Siddha/Tamil
Ziziphus jujuba Mill.	Unnaab	Chinese Tsao	Unani
Ziziphus nummularia	Karkandhu	Wild Jujube	Ayurvedic
Ziziphus nummularia	Jharber	Wild Jujube	Unani
Ziziphus nummularia	Sadarber	Wild Jujube	Unani
Ziziphus oenoplia	Laghu-badara	Jackal Jujube	Ayurvedic
Ziziphus oenoplia	Shrgaala-badari	Jackal Jujube	Ayurvedic
Ziziphus oenoplia	Soorai	Jackal Jujube	Siddha/Tamil
Ziziphus rugosa	Charai Kattu Ilandai	White Jujube	Siddha/Tamil
Ziziphus rugosa	Kottaimaram	White Jujube	Siddha/Tamil
Ziziphus rugosa	Todari	White Jujube	Siddha/Tamil
Ziziphus rugosa	Churnaa	White Jujube	Folk
Ziziphus rugosa	Sekaraa	White Jujube	Folk
Ziziphus rugosa	Torana	White Jujube	Folk
Ziziphus trinervia	Karakattam	Jagged Jujube	Siddha/Tamil
Ziziphus xylopyra	Ghontaa	Lac-host Jujube	Ayurvedic
Ziziphus xylopyra	Ghonta-Phala	Lac-host Jujube Rangeeni lac is recovered from the tree.	Ayurvedic
Ziziphus xylopyra	Kottei	Lac-host Jujube	Siddha/Tamil
Ziziphus xylopyra	Kombarakku (Rangeeni Lac)	Lac-host Jujube	Siddha/Tamil
Zornia diphylla	Samraapani	Tasad Grass	Folk
Zornia diphylla	Dupatiyaa	Tasad Grass	Folk
Zygophyllum simplex	Alethi	Bean Caper	Folk
Zygophyllum simplex	Lunio	Bean Caper	Folk
Zygophyllum simplex	Lunwaa	Bean Caper	Folk

12

Synonyms by Indian Names

Indian Name	Botanical Name	English Name	Medicinal System
Aaabnuus	*Diospyros ebenum*	Ebony Persimmon, Malabar Ebony, Ceylon Ebony	Unani
Aaadaari	*Cassia auriculata*	Tanner's Cassia	Ayurvedic
Aaaduu	*Amygdalus persica*	Peach Tree	Unani
Aaakaasagarudan	*Corallocarpus epigaeus*	Indian Bryonia	Siddha/Tamil
Aaalamaram	*Ficus beng(h)alensis*	Banyan Tree	Siddha/Tamil
Aaamalaa	*Emblica officinalis*	Embic, Indian Gooseberry	Ayurvedic
Aaamalaka	*Emblica officinalis*	Embic, Indian Gooseberry	Ayurvedic
Aaamalaki	*Emblica officinalis*	Embic, Indian Gooseberry	Ayurvedic
Aaanaiittippili	*Rhaphidophora laciniata*	Pathos, Silver Vine	Folk
Aaavartaki	*Cassia auriculata*	Tanner's Cassia	Ayurvedic
Aabhaa	*Acacia arabica*	Babul, Black Babul, Indian Gum Arabic Tree	Ayurvedic
Aadaanpaaki	*Aerva lanata*	Mountain Knot Grass	Ayurvedic
Aadaari	*Acacia canescens*	Climbing Acacia	Ayurvedic
Aadaari	*Acacia pennata*	Feathery-shoot Acacia	Ayurvedic
Aadaari	*Acacia torta*	Twisted Acacia	Ayurvedic
Aadaathodai	*Adhatoda vasica*	Malabar Nut, Vasaca	Siddha/Tamil
Aadhaki	*Cajanus cajan*	Pigeon Pea, Red Gram	Ayurvedic
Aadhya	*Vetiveria zizanioides*	Vetiver, Khas	Ayurvedic
Aadityabhakta	*Cleome icosandra*	Wild Mustard	Ayurvedic
Aadraka (Fresh rhizome)	*Zingiber officinale*	Ginger	Ayurvedic
Aadrikaa	*Zingiber officinale*	Ginger	Ayurvedic

Table Contd.

Indian Name	Botanical Name	English Name	Medicinal System
Aadutheendaa-ppaalai	*Aristolochia bracteolata*	Bracteated Birthwort	Siddha/Tamil
Aaghaat	*Achyranthes aspera*	Prickly Chaff Flower	Ayurvedic
Aak	*Calotropis gigantea*	Swallow Wort	Unani
Aakaarakarabha	*Anacyclus pyrethrum*	Spanish, Pellitory, Pyrethrum Root	Ayurvedic
Aakaarakarabha	*Grangea maderaspatana*	Madras Carpet	Ayurvedic
Aakaarkarabha	*Spilanthes calva*	Para Cress	Ayurvedic
Aakaasha Neem	*Millingtonia hortensis*	Indian Cork Tree	Folk
Aakaashbel	*Cassytha filiformis*	Doddar-Laurel, Love-Vine	Ayurvedic
Aakaashvalli	*Cuscuta epithymum*	Lesser Doddar, Hellweed, Devil's Guts	Ayurvedic
Aakallaka	*Anacyclus pyrethrum*	Spanish, Pellitory, Pyrethrum Root	Ayurvedic
Aakh	*Calotropis procera*	Swallow-wort, Milk Weed, King's Crown	Unani
Aakharaa	*Tribulus alatus*	Winged Caltrops	Folk
Aakhukarni	*Evolvulus nummularius*	Round-leaf Bindweed	Ayurvedic
Aakhukarni	*Ipomoea eriocarpa*	Tiny Morning Glory, Wooly-Fruited Morning Glory	Ayurvedic
Aakhukarni	*Ipomoea reniformis*	Mouse-ear Shrub	Ayurvedic
Aakhukarni	*Salvinia cucullata*	Asian Watermoss	Ayurvedic
Aakhuparni	*Ipomoea reniformis*	Mouse-ear Shrub	Ayurvedic
Aakhuparnika	*Ipomoea reniformis*	Mouse-ear Shrub	Ayurvedic
Aakshiki	*Alangium begoniaefolium*	Sage-leaf Alangium	Ayurvedic
Aakshiki	*Euphoria longan*	Longan	Ayurvedic
Aakulakrit	*Anacyclus pyrethrum*	Spanish, Pellitory, Pyrethrum Root	Ayurvedic
Aalu-baalu	*Prunus cerasus*	Sour Cherry	Folk
Aaluka (var.)	*Dioscorea alata*	Wild Yam, Greater Yam, Asiatic Yam	Ayurvedic
Aaluka	*Prunus armeniaca*	Apricot	Ayurvedic
Aaluka	*Prunus persica*	Peach	Ayurvedic
Aaluka	*Solanum tuberosum*	Potato	Ayurvedic
Aalukas (yams)	*Dioscorea alata*	Wild Yam, Greater Yam, Asiatic Yam	Ayurvedic

Table Contd.

Indian Name	Botanical Name	English Name	Medicinal System
Aaluki	*Colocasia esculenta*	Taro, Edible Yam	Ayurvedic
Aaluu	*Solanum tuberosum*	Potato	Folk
Aaluubu-khaaraa	*Prunus domestica*	Prune	Ayurvedic
Aaluuchaa	*Prunus domestica*	Prune	Unani
Aam	*Mangifera indica*	Mango	Unani
Aamaabhaaji	*Acalypha indica*	Copperleaf Acalypha	Folk
Aamaashayaphala	*Artocarpus integrifolia*	Jackfruit, Jack Tree	Ayurvedic
Aamadaa	*Spondias pinnata*	Hog-Plum, Wild Mango	Ayurvedic
Aamalaa	*Emblica officinalis*	Embic, Indian Gooseberry	Unani
Aamaya	*Saussurea lappa*	Kuth, Costus	Ayurvedic
Aambaa Haldi	*Curcuma amada*	Mango-ginger, Wild Turmeric	Unani
Aambaalio Kanda	*Dioscorea oppositifolia*	Cylindrical Red Yam	Folk
Aamra	*Mangifera indica*	Mango	Ayurvedic
Aamra Haridraa	*Curcuma amada*	Mango-ginger, Wild Turmeric	Ayurvedic
Aamraata	*Spondias pinnata*	Hog-Plum, Wild Mango	Ayurvedic
Aamraataka	*Spondias pinnata*	Hog-Plum, Wild Mango	Ayurvedic
Aamragandha Karpuur	*Limnophila aromatica*	Turpentine Spinach	Folk
Aamragandhi Haridraa	*Curcuma amada*	Mango-ginger, Wild Turmeric	Ayurvedic
Aamrakeshi	*Mangifera indica*	Mango	Ayurvedic
Aanai nerunchil	*Pedalium murex*	Caltrops (bigger var.)	Siddha/Tamil
Aanaitippili	*Scindapsus officinalis*	Sal Forest Pepper	Siddha/Tamil
Aanaparuga	*Pothos scandens*	Money Plant	Siddha/Tamil
Aankha-phuutaa-mani	*Ctenolepis cerasiformis*	Ctenolepis	Folk
Aanthil	*Murraya exotica*	Chinese Boxwood, Andaman Satinwood	Folk
Aanvilam	*Tamarindus indica*	Tamarind Tree	Siddha/Tamil
Aapataa	*Bauhinia malabarica*	Malabar Mountain Ebony	Folk
Aapataa	*Bauhinia racemosa*	Kachnar Tree	Folk
Aaphuuka	*Papaver somniferum*	Opium Poppy	Ayurvedic
Aaqarqarhaa	*Anacyclus pyrethrum*	Spanish, Pellitory, Pyrethrum Root	Unani

Table Contd.

Indian Name	Botanical Name	English Name	Medicinal System
Aaragvadha	*Cassia fistula*	Indian Laburnum, Purging Cassia, Golden Shower	Ayurvedic
Aaramuri	*Indigofera articulata*	Egyptian Indigo, Arabian Indigo, Wild Indigo, Surat Indigo	Siddha/Tamil
Aarar	*Juniperus communis*	Common Juniper	Unani
Aardikaa	*Zingiber cassumunar*	Cassumunar Ginger	Ayurvedic
Aarevata	*Cassia fistula*	Indian Laburnum, Purging Cassia, Golden Shower	Ayurvedic
Aartagala	*Terminalia arjuna*	Arjun Terminalia	Ayurvedic
Aartagala	*Xanthium strumarium*	Cocklebur, Burweed	Ayurvedic
Aaruka	*Amygdalus persica*	Peach Tree	Ayurvedic
Aaruka	*Prunus domestica*	Prune	Ayurvedic
Aaruka	*Prunus persica*	Peach	Ayurvedic
Aaruka	*Solanum tuberosum*	Potato	Ayurvedic
Aarumathathandu	*Amaranthus blitum*	Trailing Amaranth, Wild Blite	Folk/Tamil
Aashaalim	*Lepidium sativum*	Gardencress, Tongue Grass	Ayurvedic
Aashaphala	*Euphoria longan*	Longan	Folk
Aasphota	*Calotropis procera*	Swallow-wort, Milk Weed, King's Crown	Ayurvedic
Aasphota	*Clitoria ternatea*	Butterfly Pea, Winged-leaved Clitoria, Mezereon	Ayurvedic
Aasphotaa	*Jasminum angustifolium*	Wild Jasmine	Ayurvedic
Aasphotaa	*Vallaris solanacea*	Bread Flower	Ayurvedic
Aasuri Raai	*Brassica juncea*	Chinese Mustard, Brown Mustard	Ayurvedic
Aataruushaka	*Adhatoda vasica*	Malabar Nut, Vasaca	Ayurvedic
Aathondan	*Capparis zeylanica*	Ceylon Caper	Siddha/Tamil
Aatmaguptaa	*Mucuna prurita*	Cowhage, Horse-eye Bean	Ayurvedic
Aatru Paalai	*Salix babylonica*	Weeping Willow	Siddha/Tamil
Aavaarai	*Cassia auriculata*	Tanner's Cassia	Siddha/Tamil
Aavartaki	*Helicteres isora*	East Indian Screw Tree	Ayurvedic
Aavartani	*Helicteres isora*	East Indian Screw Tree	Ayurvedic
Aavartphalaa	*Helicteres isora*	East Indian Screw Tree	Ayurvedic
Aazaad-Darakht-e-Hindi	*Azadirachta indica*	Neem Tree, Margosa Tree	Unani

Table Contd.

Indian Name	Botanical Name	English Name	Medicinal System
Abahal	*Juniperus communis*	Common Juniper	Unani
Abai	*Reinwardtia indica*	Winter-Flax, Yellow Flax	Folk
Abda	*Cyperus rotundus*	Nut Grass	Ayurvedic
Abhaya	*Vetiveria zizanioides*	Vetiver, Khas	Ayurvedic
Abhramaansi	*Valeriana dubia*	Common Valerian	Ayurvedic
Abhrangu	*Microcos paniculata*	Kadamb	Folk
Abhrapushpa	*Calamus rotang*	Rotang, Rattan, Chair Bottom Cane	Ayurvedic
Abini	*Papaver somniferum*	Opium	Siddha/Tamil
Abja	*Nelumbo nucifera*	East Indian Lotus, Sacred Lotus	Ayurvedic
Abu Khanjar	*Tropaeolum majus*	Garden Nasturtium, Indian Cress, Climbing-Nasturtium	Folk
Acca	*Feijoa sellowiana*	Feijoa, Pineapple Guava, New Zealand Banana	Folk (Nilgiri)
Acerola	*Malpighia glabra*	Barbados Cherry, Acerola	Folk
Acha-Thumbi	*Diospyros ebenum*	Ebony Persimmon, Malabar Ebony, Ceylon Ebony	Siddha/Tamil
Achhu	*Grewia populifolia*	Orange-red Phalsa, Tapadi	Siddha/Tamil
Adaasa	*Lens culinaris*	Lentil	Ayurvedic
Adagam	*Aristolochia indica*	Indian Birthwort	Siddha/Tamil
Adah-pushpi	*Trichodesma indicum*	Indian Borage	Ayurvedic
Adah-pushpi	*Trichodesma zeylanicum*	Ajovan	Ayurvedic
Adahshalya	*Achyranthes aspera*	Prickly Chaff Flower	Ayurvedic
Adalai	*Jatropha glandulifera*	Jatropha (South India)	Siddha/Tamil
Adambu	*Ipomoea pes-caprae*	Goat's Foot Creeper	Siddha/Tamil
Adamusi	*Yucca glorisa*	Spanish Dagger-Plant, Adam's Needle	Folk
Adarakhi	*Zingiber cassumunar*	Cassumunar Ginger	Folk
Addasarpa	*Alstonia venenata*	Devil's Tree, Dita Bark Tree	Folk/Kannada
Addula	*Ehretia laevis*	Datrang Tree	Siddha/Tamil
Adhasisi	*Xanthium strumarium*	Cocklebur, Burweed	Folk
Adhigandhaa	*Mucuna prurita*	Cowhage, Horse-eye Bean	Ayurvedic
Adhomukha	*Trichodesma indicum*	Indian Borage	Ayurvedic

Table Contd.

Indian Name	Botanical Name	English Name	Medicinal System
Aedagaja	*Cassia tora*	Sickle Senna, Ringworm Plant	Ayurvedic
Afarbiyuun	*Euphorbia resinifera*	Resin Spurge	Unani
Aflaatuun	*Balsamodendron mukul*	Indian Bdellium, Gum Guggul	Unani
Afsanteen-e-Hindi	*Artemisia vulgaris*	Indian Wormwood, Fleabane, Dungwort, Mugwort, Wild Wormwood	Unani
Afsanteen-ul-bahar	*Artemisia maritima*	Wormseed, Santonica	Unani
Aftimoon	*Cuscuta epithymum*	Lesser Doddar, Hellweed, Devil's Guts	Unani
Afyum	*Papaver somniferum*	Opium	Unani
Agachi	*Dillenia pentagyna*	Deer Apple	Folk
Agai	*Dillenia pentagyna*	Deer Apple	Folk
Agar-Agar	*Gelidium amansii*	Agar Agar, Japanese Isinglass	Folk
Agasatamarai	*Pistia stratiotes*	Water Lettuce, Tropical Duckweed	Ayurvedic
Agasti	*Sesbania grandiflora*	Agati Sesban, Swamp Pea	Ayurvedic
Agastya	*Sesbania grandiflora*	Agati Sesban, Swamp Pea	Ayurvedic
Agaththi	*Sesbania grandiflora*	Agati Sesban, Swamp Pea	Siddha/Tamil
Agethaa	*Premna integrifolia*	Headache Tree	Folk
Agethu (var.)	*Premna latifolia*	Dusky Fire Brand Bark	Folk
Aggali-chandanam	*Aquilaria agallocha*	Aloewood, Eaglewood, Agarwood	Folk/Tamil
Agil	*Excoecaria agallocha*	Blinding Tree	Siddha/Tamil
Agiyaa	*Striga asiatica*	Witchweed	Folk
Aglay	*Chukrasia tabularis*	Bastard Cedar, White Cedar, Indian Red Wood	Siddha/Tamil
Agmaki	*Melothria maderaspatana*	Rough Bryony	Folk
Agni	*Plumbago zeylanica*	Ceylon Leadwort	Ayurvedic
Agnik	*Semecarpus anacardium*	Marking-Nut	Ayurvedic
Agnimanth (var.)	*Premna tomentosa*	Bastard Teak	Ayurvedic
Agnimantha (var.)	*Premna latifolia*	Dusky Fire Brand Bark	Ayurvedic
Agnimantha	*Clerodendrum phlomidis*	Glory Bower	Ayurvedic
Agnimantha	*Premna integrifolia*	Headache Tree	Ayurvedic

Table Contd.

Indian Name	Botanical Name	English Name	Medicinal System
Agnimukha	*Semecarpus anacardium*	Marking-Nut	Ayurvedic
Agnipatri	*Ammannia baccifera*	Blistering Ammannia	Ayurvedic
Agnishikhaa	*Crocus sativus*	Saffron, Crocus	Ayurvedic
Agnishikhaa	*Gloriosa superba*	Glory Lily, Super Lily, Tiger's Claws	Ayurvedic
Agnivriksha	*Striga asiatica*	Witchweed	Ayurvedic
Agori	*Hugonia mystax*	Climbing Flax	Siddha/Tamil
Agragraahi	*Anacyclus pyrethrum*	Spanish, Pellitory, Pyrethrum Root	Ayurvedic
Agunivagil	*Dysoxylum binectariferum*	Termite-resistant Cedar	Siddha/Tamil
Aguru	*Aquilaria agallocha*	Aloewood, Eaglewood, Agarwood	Ayurvedic
Ahilekhana	*Melothria maderaspatana*	Rough Bryony	Ayurvedic
Ahimsra	*Capparis zeylanica*	Ceylon Caper	Ayurvedic
Ahiphala	*Trichosanthes anguina*	Snake-Gourd	Ayurvedic
Ahiphena	*Papaver somniferum*	Opium	Ayurvedic
Ahipushpa	*Mesua ferrea*	Iron-wood, Mesu	Ayurvedic
Aila	*Acacia pennata*	Feathery-shoot Acacia	Folk
Aila	*Acacia torta*	Twisted Acacia	Folk
Aindri	*Bacopa monnieri*	Thyme-leaved Gratiola	Ayurvedic
Aindri	*Citrullus colocynthis*	Colocynth Bitter Apple	Ayurvedic
Airaavata	*Citrus limon*	Lemon	Ayurvedic
Airaavati	*Bryophyllum pinnatum*	Air Plant, Mexican Love Plant	Ayurvedic
Airakaa	*Typha elephantina*	Elephant Grass, Indian Reed-Mace, Bulrush	Ayurvedic
Airakaa	*Typha laxmannii*	Scented Flag	Ayurvedic
Ajaaji	*Cuminum cyminum*	Cumin	Ayurvedic
Ajadaaa	*Mucuna prurita*	Cowhage, Horse-eye Bean	Ayurvedic
Ajadandi	*Lamprachaenium microcephalum*	Purple-flowered Brahmadandi	Folk
Ajagandhaa	*Elsholtzia cristata*	Himalayan Pseudo-Basil	Ayurvedic
Ajagandhaa	*Gynandropsis gynandra*	African Spider Plant	Ayurvedic
Ajagandhaa	*Thymus serphyllum*	Mother-of-thyme, Wild Thyme	Ayurvedic

Table Contd.

Indian Name	Botanical Name	English Name	Medicinal System
Ajakarna	*Dipterocarpus turbinatus*	Common Gurjun Tree, Wood Oil Tree	Ayurvedic
Ajamoda	*Trachyspermum roxburghianum*	Ajmud	Ayurvedic
Ajamodaa	*Trachyspermum roxburghianum*	Ajmud	Ayurvedic
Ajashringi	*Gymnema sylvestre*	Australian Cow Plant, Gymnema	Ayurvedic
Ajashringi	*Pistacia integerrima*	Horn-shaped Gall Tree, Kakra Gall Tree	Ayurvedic
Ajgandhikaa	*Ocimum basilicum*	Sweet Basil, Basil Herb	Ayurvedic
Ajmod	*Apium leptophyllum*	Celery	Unani
Ajmoda	*Apium graveolens*	Celery	Ayurvedic
Ajmodaa	*Apium graveolens*	Celery	Ayurvedic
Ajmodaa	*Apium leptophyllum*	Celery	Ayurvedic
Ajmodikaa	*Apium graveolens*	Celery	Ayurvedic
Ajmoja	*Trachyspermum roxburghianum*	Ajmud	Ayurvedic
Ajwaayin Khuraasaani	*Hyoscyamus muticus*	Egyptian Henbane	Unani
Akala Kohadi	*Tridax procumbens*	Mexican Daisy	Folk
Akal-ber	*Datisca cannabina*	False Hemp	Folk
Akarkaraa	*Tanacetum longifolium*	Long-leaved Tansy	Unani
Akarkaraa Sweet var.	*Tanacetum umbelliferum*	Sweet Pellitory	Unani
Akasa thammarai	*Eichhornia crassipes*	Water-Hyacinth, Bengal Terror, Blue Devil, The Million Dollar Weed	Siddha/Tamil
Akhaahi-lataa	*Trachelospermum fragrans*	Japanese Star-Jasmine	Folk
Akhani	*Alangium begoniaefolium*	Sage-leaf Alangium	Folk
Akhrot	*Juglans regia*	Walnut Tree	Unani
Akil kattai	*Aquilaria agallocha*	Aloewood, Eaglewood, Agarwood	Siddha/Tamil
Akkarakkaram	*Chrysanthemum indicum*	Chrysanthemum	Siddha/Tamil
Akkiraakaaram	*Anacyclus pyrethrum*	Spanish, Pellitory, Pyrethrum Root	Siddha/Tamil

Table Contd.

Indian Name	Botanical Name	English Name	Medicinal System
Aklaari	*Lodoicea maldivica*	Double Coconut Palm, Sea Coconut Palm	Siddha/Tamil
Akri (fruit)	*Withania coagulans*	Vegetable Rennet, Indian Cheese-maker	Unani
Akrottu	*Juglans regia*	Walnut Tree	Siddha/Tamil
Aksha	*Terminalia bellirica*	Belleric Myrobalan, Bastard Myrobalan	Ayurvedic
Akshaka	*Terminalia bellirica*	Belleric Myrobalan, Bastard Myrobalan	Ayurvedic
Akshi	*Morinda citrifolia*	Indian Mulberry	Ayurvedic
Akshiva	*Moringa pterygosperma*	Drumstick, Horse-Radish	Ayurvedic
Akshoda	*Juglans regia*	Walnut Tree	Ayurvedic
Akshodaka	*Juglans regia*	Walnut Tree	Ayurvedic
Akshota	*Aleurites moluccana*	Candlenut Tree	Ayurvedic
Akshota	*Juglans regia*	Walnut Tree	Ayurvedic
Alagai	*Agave americana*	Century Plant, American Aloe	Siddha/Tamil
Alambushaa	*Biophytum sensitivum*	Life Plant	Ayurvedic
Alambushaa	*Neptunia oleracea*	Sensitive Plant	Ayurvedic
Alambusta	*Sphaeranthus indicus*	East Indian Globe Thistle	Ayurvedic
Alarka	*Calotropis gigantea*	Swallow Wort	Ayurvedic
Alarka	*Calotropis procera*	Swallow-wort, Milk Weed, King's Crown	Ayurvedic
Alarka	*Solanum trilobatum*	Climbing Brinjal	Ayurvedic
Al-baavard	*Volutarella ramosa*	Volutarella	Unani
Alethi	*Zygophyllum simplex*	Bean Caper	Folk
Alfaajan	*Lavandula stoechas*	Arabian or French Lavender	Unani
Alfalfa	*Medicago sativa*	Alfalfa, Lucerne	Ayurvedic
Algerian Geranium	*Pelargonium graveolens*	Geranium	Folk
Aliar	*Dodonaea viscosa*	Jamacia Switch Sorrel	Folk
Alivirai	*Lepidium sativum*	Gardencress, Tongue Grass	Folk/Tamil
Ali-virail	*Linum usitatissimum*	Linseed, Flax	Siddha/Tamil
Al-kabar	*Capparis spinosa*	Caper Bush	Unani
Al-keenaa	*Cinchona officinalis*	Crown or Loxa Bark	Unani

Table Contd.

Indian Name	Botanical Name	English Name	Medicinal System
Allam	*Zingiber officinale*	Ginger	Siddha/Tamil
Alli	*Nymphaea alba*	European White Water-lily	Siddha/Tamil
Alli-tamarai	*Nymphaea rubra*	Indian Red Water-lily	Folk/Tamil
Al-murr	*Balsamodendron myrrha*	Myrrh, Herabol	Unani
Alpagada-pungam	*Prunus domestica*	Prune	Siddha/Tamil
Alpamaarish	*Amaranthus spinosus*	Spiny Amaranth, Thorny Amaranth, Spiny Pigweed	Ayurvedic
Alpamaarisha	*Amaranthus blitum*	Trailing Amaranth, Wild Blite	Ayurvedic
Alpikaa	*Phaseolus trilobus*	Wild Gram	Ayurvedic
Al-Saatar	*Zataria multiflora*	Wild Thyme	Unani
Alu	*Vangueria spinosa*	Voa-Vanga	Folk
Al-Zanjabeel	*Zingiber officinale*	Ginger	Unani
Amadok	*Laggera alata*	False Tobacco	Folk
Amalpori, Chivan amelpodi	*Rauvolfia serpentina*	Rauvolfia Root, Serpentina Root, Indian Snakeroot	Siddha/Tamil
Amaltaasa	*Cassia fistula*	Indian Laburnum, Purging Cassia, Golden Shower	Unani
Amam	*Glycosmis pentaphylla*	Orangeberry, Ginberry	Siddha/Tamil
Amaradaaru	*Cedrus deodara*	Himalayan Cedar, Deodar	Ayurvedic
Amarataru	*Cedrus deodara*	Himalayan Cedar, Deodar	Ayurvedic
Amarkanda	*Eulophia nuda*	Goruma Tuber, Riddhi	Ayurvedic
Amaruuda	*Psidium guajava*	Guava	Ayurvedic
Amarvalli	*Cassytha filiformis*	Doddar-Laurel, Love-Vine	Ayurvedic
Amarvalli	*Cuscuta epithymum*	Lesser Doddar, Hellweed, Devil's Guts	Ayurvedic
Amarvalli	*Cuscuta reflexa*	Doddar	Ayurvedic
Amarvel	*Pentatropis microphylla*	Ambervel, Beak-shaped Elliptic Flower	Folk
Amarvela	*Cuscuta epithymum*	Lesser Doddar, Hellweed, Devil's Guts	Ayurvedic
Ambaadi	*Hibiscus cannabinus*	Bimlipatam Jute, Kenaf, Mesta, Deccan Hemp	Folk
Ambah Shyaamaaka	*Echinochloa crus-galli*	Barnyard Millet	Ayurvedic

Table Contd.

Indian Name	Botanical Name	English Name	Medicinal System
Ambaj	*Mangifera indica*	Mango	Unani
Ambala-vriksham	*Excoecaria agallocha*	Blinding Tree	Siddha/Tamil
Ambar	*Pinus succinifera*	Baltic Amber, Succinite	Unani
Ambar Saayil	*Liquidambar orientalis*	Storax, Oriental Sweet Gum	Unani
Ambaratthi	*Trema orientalis*	Charcoal Tree, Indian Nettle Tree	Siddha/Tamil
Ambari	*Hibiscus cannabinus*	Bimlipatam Jute, Kenaf, Mesta, Deccan Hemp	Folk
Ambarkanda	*Eulophia nuda*	Goruma Tuber, Riddhi	Folk
Ambarvel	*Pentatropis spiralis*	Ambervel	Folk
Ambashthaa	*Chondrodendron tomentosum*	False Pareira Brava	Ayurvedic
Ambashthaa	*Cissampelos pareira*	Velvet-Leaf Pareira, Pareira Brava	Ayurvedic
Ambashtthaki	*Hibiscus sabdariffa*	Roselle, Jamaican Sorrel, Natal Sorrel, Red Sorrel	Ayurvedic
Ambel	*Nelumbo nucifera*	East Indian Lotus, Sacred Lotus	Siddha/Tamil
Ambgar	*Argyreia speciosa*	Elephant Creeper	Siddha/Tamil
Ambhas	*Coleus vettiveroides*	Coleus	Ayurvedic
Ambhoda	*Cyperus rotundus*	Nut Grass	Ayurvedic
Ambilonaa	*Oxalis corniculata*	Indian Sorrel	Folk
Ambodhara	*Cyperus rotundus*	Nut Grass	Ayurvedic
Ambu	*Coleus vettiveroides*	Coleus	Ayurvedic
Ambu	*Pavonia odorata*	Fragrant Sticky Mallow	Ayurvedic
Ambuda	*Cyperus rotundus*	Nut Grass	Ayurvedic
Ambuj	*Barringtonia acutangula*	Indian Oak	Ayurvedic
Ambuja	*Nelumbo nucifera*	East Indian Lotus, Sacred Lotus	Ayurvedic
Ambuli	*Limnophila aromatica*	Turpentine Spinach	Folk
Ambuli	*Limnophila indica*	Oil-of-lemons Spinach	Folk
Amburuha	*Ionidium suffruticosum*	Charati	Ayurvedic
Ambusaara	*Musa paradisiaca*	Banana, Plantain	Ayurvedic
Ambutaa Bhaaji	*Oxalis corniculata*	Indian Sorrel	Unani
Ambuvaasini	*Stereospermum personatum*	Trumpet Flower, Yellow Snake Tree	Ayurvedic

Table Contd.

Indian Name	Botanical Name	English Name	Medicinal System
Amla	*Emblica officinalis*	Embic, Indian Gooseberry	Ayurvedic
Amlaj	*Emblica officinalis*	Embic, Indian Gooseberry	Unani
Amlaparni	*Rheum emodi*	Indian Rhubarb, Himalayan Rhubarb	Ayurvedic
Amlapatrikaa	*Oxalis corniculata*	Indian Sorrel	Ayurvedic
Amlavetasa	*Garcinia pedunculata*	Bengal Brindleberry	Ayurvedic
Amlavrikshak	*Garcinia indica*	Kokam Butter Tree, Mangosteen Oil Tree	Ayurvedic
Amli	*Bauhinia malabarica*	Malabar Mountain Ebony	Folk
Amli	*Tamarindus indica*	Tamarind Tree	Ayurvedic
Amlikaa	*Oxalis corniculata*	Indian Sorrel	Ayurvedic
Amlikaa	*Tamarindus indica*	Tamarind Tree	Ayurvedic
Amlikaakanda (controversial)	*Dioscorea oppositifolia*	Cylindrical Yam	Ayurvedic
Amlora	*Rumex hastatus*	Toothed Dock	Folk
Amlosaa	*Bauhinia malabarica*	Malabar Mountain Ebony	Folk
Amlu	*Oxyria digyna*	Mountain Sorrel, Alpine Sorrel	Folk
Amman pachharisi	*Euphorbia hirta*	Euphorbia, Australian Asthma Weed, Pill-bearing Spurge	Siddha/Tamil
Ammanakku	*Ricinus communis*	Castor Seed	Siddha/Tamil
Ammukkura	*Withania coagulans*	Vegetable Rennet, Indian Cheese-maker	Siddha/Tamil
Amogha	*Embelia ribes*	Embelia	Ayurvedic
Amoghaa	*Emblica officinalis*	Embic, Indian Gooseberry	Ayurvedic
Amoghaa	*Stereospermum personatum*	Trumpet Flower, Yellow Snake Tree	Ayurvedic
Amrida-valli	*Tinospora cordifolia*	Heart-leaved Tinospora	Folk/Tamil
Amrita	*Aconitum ferox*	Indian Aconite, Wolfsbane, Monkshood	Ayurvedic
Amrita	*Eulophia campestris*	Salep Orchid	Ayurvedic
Amritaa	*Tinospora cordifolia*	Heart-leaved Tinospora	Ayurvedic
Amritalataa	*Tinospora cordifolia*	Heart-leaved Tinospora	Ayurvedic
Amritaphala	*Cydonia oblonga*	Quince Fruit	Ayurvedic
Amritaphala	*Emblica officinalis*	Embic, Indian Gooseberry	Ayurvedic
Amritaphala	*Trichosanthes cucumerina*	Coiled Snakegourd	Ayurvedic

Table Contd.

Indian Name	Botanical Name	English Name	Medicinal System
Amritavallari	*Tinospora cordifolia*	Heart-leaved Tinospora	Ayurvedic
Amritvallari	*Basella alba*	Indian Spinach	Ayurvedic
Amrul	*Oxalis acetosella*	Common Wood-Sorrel	Folk
Amsul	*Garcinia xanthochymus*	Egg Tree	Folk
Amsula	*Garcinia indica*	Kokam Butter Tree, Mangosteen Oil Tree	Ayurvedic
Amukkuram-kishangu	*Withania ashwagandha*	Winter Cherry	Siddha/Tamil
Amur	*Amoora cucullata*	Rohitak	Folk
Amutaa Saag	*Oxalis corniculata*	Indian Sorrel	Unani
Anaaghaalis	*Anagallis arvensis*	Bird's Eye, Bird's Tongue, Blue Pimpernel, Scarlet Pimpernel	Unani
Anaanaasa	*Ananas comosus*	Pineapple	Ayurvedic
Anaar	*Punica granatum*	Pomegranate	Unani
Anai-gundumani	*Adenanthera pavonina*	Coral Wood, Red Wood	Siddha/Tamil
Anaikkarai	*Lannea coromandelica*	Jhingan	Siddha/Tamil
Anaikkarai	*Typha elephantina*	Elephant Grass, Indian Reed-Mace, Bulrush	Siddha/Tamil
Anaittichal	*Tetracera laevis*	Sandpaper-Vine	Siddha/Tamil
Anakoranti	*Salacia macrosperma*	Saptrangi	Folk
Anannaas	*Ananas comosus*	Pineapple	Unani
Anantaa	*Cynodon dactylon*	Bermuda Grass, Bahama Grass, Couch Grass	Ayurvedic
Anantaa	*Fagonia cretica*	Thorny Fagonbush, Mantle of the Virgin	Ayurvedic
Anantaa	*Gloriosa superba*	Glory Lily, Super Lily, Tiger's Claws	Ayurvedic
Anantamuula	*Cryptolepis buchanani*	Indian Sarsaparilla	Folk
Anantmuula	*Hemidesmus indicus*	Indian Sarsaparilla	Ayurvedic
Anapendu	*Gnetum montanum*	Joint Fir	Siddha/Tamil
Anasippo	*Illicium verum*	Star Anise, Chinese Anise, Aniseed Stars	Siddha/Tamil
Anasphal	*Illicium verum*	Star Anise, Chinese Anise, Aniseed Stars	Folk
Anchhu	*Rubus ellipticus*	Gach Strawberry	Folk

Table Contd.

Indian Name	Botanical Name	English Name	Medicinal System
Arali	*Nerium indicum*	Indian Oleander, White Oleander	Siddha/Tamil
Aralu	*Ailanthus excelsa*	Tree of Heaven, Maharukh	Ayurvedic
Aralu	*Ailanthus glandulosa*	Ailanto	Ayurvedic
Aralu	*Oroxylum indicum*	Indian Trumpet Flower	Ayurvedic
Arand	*Ricinus communis*	Castor Seed	Unani
Arangaka	*Melia composita*	Hill Neem, Malabar Neem, Common Bead Tree	Ayurvedic
Aranthellia	*Antiaris toxicaria*	Sacking Tree, Upas Tree	Folk/Tamil
Aranya-Jiraka	*Centratherum anthelminticum*	Purple Flea-bane, Achenes	Ayurvedic
Aranya-kulathhikaa	*Cassia absus*	Four-leaved Cassia, Pig's Senna	Ayurvedic
Aranya-mudga	*Phaseolus adenanthus*	South American Snail Vine	Ayurvedic
Aranya-rajanikanda	*Curcuma aromatica*	Wild Turmeric, Yellow Zedoary	Ayurvedic
Aranyatikta	*Swertia chirayita*	Chiretta	Ayurvedic
Ararutgaddalu	*Curcuma angustifolia*	East Indian Arrowroot, Travancore Starch	Folk/Tamil
Arasam	*Ficus religiosa*	Peepal, Bot-tree	Siddha/Tamil
Aravinda	*Nelumbo nucifera*	East Indian Lotus, Sacred Lotus	Ayurvedic
Archa	*Rheum webbianum*	Himalayan Rhubarb	Folk
Arhar	*Cajanus cajan*	Pigeon Pea, Red Gram	Unani
Ari	*Acacia canescens*	Climbing Acacia	Folk
Ari	*Acacia pennata*	Feathery-shoot Acacia	Ayurvedic
Arimanja	*Acacia leucophloea*	White Babul	Ayurvedic
Arimeda	*Acacia farnesiana*	Cassie Flower, Cassie Absolute, Sweet Acacia	Ayurvedic
Arimeda	*Acacia leucophloea*	White Babul	Ayurvedic
Arimedaka	*Acacia leucophloea*	White Babul	Ayurvedic
Arishta	*Allium sativum*	Garlic	Ayurvedic
Arishta	*Azadirachta indica*	Neem Tree, Margosa Tree	Ayurvedic
Arishta	*Picrorhiza kurroa*	Picrorhiza	Ayurvedic
Arishta	*Xanthium strumarium*	Cocklebur, Burweed	Ayurvedic
Arishtaka	*Sapindus laurifolius*	Soapnut Tree of South India	Ayurvedic

Table Contd.

Indian Name	Botanical Name	English Name	Medicinal System
Arishtaka	*Sapindus mukorossi*	Chinese Soap Berry, Soap Nut Tree of North India	Ayurvedic
Arishtaphala	*Azadirachta indica*	Neem Tree, Margosa Tree	Ayurvedic
Arisi thippili	*Piper longum*	Indian Long Pepper, Joborandi	Siddha/Tamil
Arivalmanai-poondu	*Sida spinosa*	Prickly Mallow	Siddha/Tamil
Arjun	*Terminalia arjuna*	Arjun Terminalia	Unani
Arjuna	*Terminalia arjuna*	Arjun Terminalia	Ayurvedic
Arkamuula	*Aristolochia indica*	Indian Birthwort	Ayurvedic
Arkaparna	*Calotropis procera*	Swallow-wort, Milk Weed, King's Crown	Ayurvedic
Arkaparni	*Tylophora indica*	Emetic Swallow Wort, Indian or Country Ipecacuanha	Ayurvedic
Arkavallabha	*Pentapetes phoenicea*	Midday Flower, Copper Cup, Scarlet Mallow, Florimpia	Ayurvedic
Arkhar	*Rhus chinensis*	Chinese-Gall Rhus Tree	Folk
Arkkam	*Calotropis procera*	Swallow-wort, Milk Weed, King's Crown	Siddha/Tamil
Ark-pushpi	*Holostemma annularis*	Holostemma Creeper	Ayurvedic
Arshoghna	*Amorphophallus campanulatus*	Elephant's Foot Yam	Ayurvedic
Aru	*Prunus persica*	Peach	Ayurvedic
Arugampullu	*Cynodon dactylon*	Bermuda Grass, Bahama Grass, Couch Grass	Siddha/Tamil
Arulundi	*Azadirachta indica*	Neem Tree, Margosa Tree	Siddha/Tamil
Arunaa	*Aconitum heterophyllum*	Atis Root, Aconite	Ayurvedic
Arunaa	*Hibiscus rosa-sinensis*	Rose-of-China, Shoe-flower, Chinese Hibiscus	Ayurvedic
Arunaa	*Rubia cordifolia*	Indian Madder, Bengal Madder	Ayurvedic
Arunelli	*Garuga pinnata*	Grey Downy Balsam	Siddha/Tamil
Arunelli	*Phyllanthus distichus*	Country Gooseberry	Siddha/Tamil
Arusaa	*Adhatoda vasica*	Malabar Nut, Vasaca	Unani
Arushkara	*Semecarpus anacardium*	Marking-Nut	Ayurvedic
Aruvada	*Ruta chalepensis*	Fringed Rue	Siddha/Tamil
Aruvada	*Ruta graveolens*	Garden Rue	Siddha/Tamil

Table Contd.

Indian Name	Botanical Name	English Name	Medicinal System
Aruvadam-chedi	*Ruta chalepensis*	Fringed Rue	Siddha/Tamil
Arvi	*Colocasia esculenta*	Taro, Edible Yam	Folk
Arwan	*Lyonia ovalifolia*	Oval-leaved Staggerbush	Folk
Asaab-ul-Malik	*Melilotus officinalis*	Yellow Sweet Clover, Melilot	Unani
Asaanaa	*Bridelia montana*	Spinous Kino Tree	Folk
Asaaroon	*Asarum europaeum*	Asarbacca, Hazelwort, Wild Nard	Unani
Asaarun	*Valeriana hardwickii*	Himalayan Valerian	Folk
Asaarun	*Valeriana wallichii*	Indian Valerian	Folk
Asaarun	*Valeriana wallichii*	Indian Valerian	Unani
Asad	*Blepharis linariaefolia*	Acanthus	Unani
Asan	*Terminalia tomentosa*	Laurel (trade)	Folk/Bengal
Asana	*Bridelia retusa*	Spinous Kino Tree	Ayurvedic
Asana	*Pterocarpus marsupium*	Indian Kino Tree, Malabar Kino Tree	Ayurvedic
Asar	*Microcos paniculata*	Kadamb	Folk
Asbarg	*Delphinium zalil*	Zalil Larkspur	Unani
Asbarga	*Delphinium zalil*	Zalil Larkspur	Ayurvedic
Aselu	*Rubus ellipticus*	Gach Strawberry	Folk
Asgandh	*Withania ashwagandha*	Winter Cherry	Unani
Ashamtagam	*Trachyspermum roxburghianum*	Ajmud	Siddha/Tamil
Ashar	*Calotropis procera*	Swallow-wort, Milk Weed, King's Crown	Unani
Ashmagarbhaka	*Ougeinia dalbergioides*	Chariot Tree, Punjab Kino	Ayurvedic
Ashmantaka (var.)	*Ficus cordifolia*	Rumpf's Fig	Ayurvedic
Ashmantaka	*Bauhinia malabarica*	Malabar Mountain Ebony	Ayurvedic
Ashmantaka	*Bauhinia racemosa*	Kachnar Tree	Ayurvedic
Ashmantaka	*Bauhinia variegata*	Mountain Ebony, Buddhist Bauhinia	Ayurvedic
Ashmaribhadikaa	*Bergenia ligulata*	Elephant-Ear, Siberian Saxifrage	Ayurvedic
Ashmaribhit	*Bergenia ligulata*	Elephant-Ear, Siberian Saxifrage	Ayurvedic

Table Contd.

Indian Name	Botanical Name	English Name	Medicinal System
Ashmarighna	*Crataeva nurvala*	Steaved Tree, Sacred Barna	Ayurvedic
Ashmghna	*Bergenia ligulata*	Elephant-Ear, Siberian Saxifrage	Ayurvedic
Ashoka	*Saraca asoca*	Ashoka Tree	Ayurvedic
Ashoka	*Saraca asoca*	Ashoka Tree	Unani
Ashoka-rohini	*Erycibe paniculata*	Kari Climber (Assam)	Ayurvedic
Ashokarohinya	*Picrorhiza kurroa*	Picrorhiza	Ayurvedic
Ashoku	*Saraca asoca*	Ashoka Tree	Ayurvedic
Ashtaa	*Ficus cordifolia*	Rumpf's Fig	Folk
Ashvaghna	*Thevetia peruviana*	Yellow Oleander	Ayurvedic
Ashvaghra	*Zanthoxylum budrunga*	Tumru Tree, Prickly Ash	Ayurvedic
Ashvagola (var.)	*Plantago major*	Broadleaf Plantain	Ayurvedic
Ashvagola	*Plantago ovata*	Ispaghula, Spogel Seeds, Blond Psyllium	Ayurvedic
Ashvakatri	*Drynaria quercifolia*	Drynaria Fern	Ayurvedic
Ashvamaaraka	*Nerium indicum*	Indian Oleander, White Oleander	Ayurvedic
Ashvatham	*Ficus religiosa*	Peepal, Bot-tree	Siddha/Tamil
Ashvattha	*Ficus religiosa*	Peepal, Bot-tree	Ayurvedic
Ashwagandhaa	*Withania ashwagandha*	Winter Cherry	Ayurvedic
Ashwakanda	*Withania ashwagandha*	Winter Cherry	Ayurvedic
Ashwakarna	*Dipterocarpus alatus*	Gurjun	Ayurvedic
Ashwakarna	*Dipterocarpus turbinatus*	Common Gurjun Tree, Wood Oil Tree	Ayurvedic
Ashwakarna	*Plantago ovata*	Ispaghula, Spogel Seeds, Blond Psyllium	Ayurvedic
Ashwa-puchha	*Equisetum arvense*	Field Horsetail	Ayurvedic
Ashwa-shaakhota	*Glycosmis pentaphylla*	Orangeberry, Ginberry	Ayurvedic
Ashyuka	*Morinda citrifolia*	Indian Mulberry	Ayurvedic
Asipatra	*Saccharum officinarum*	Gannaa, Naishakar	Ayurvedic
Asita Jiraka	*Carum carvi*	Caraway	Ayurvedic
Asitaka	*Aquilaria agallocha*	Aloewood, Eaglewood, Agarwood	Ayurvedic
Asitkaaraka	*Diospyros embryopteris*	Gaub Persimmon, Riber Ebony	Ayurvedic
Asl-us-soos	*Glycyrrhiza glabra*	Licorice, Liquorice	Unani

Table Contd.

Indian Name	Botanical Name	English Name	Medicinal System
Asmaaniyaa	*Ephedra gerardiana*	Ephedra	Folk
Asmaaniyaabuuti	*Ephedra gerardiana*	Ephedra	Folk
Asokam	*Saraca asoca*	Ashoka Tree	Siddha/Tamil
Aspaghol	*Plantago amplexicaulis*	Brown Ispaghula	Unani
Aspaghol	*Plantago lanceolata*	Rib Grass, Ribwort Plantain, English Plantain, Buckhorn Plantain	Unani
Aspaghol	*Plantago ovata*	Ispaghula, Spogel Seeds, Blond Psyllium	Unani
Asperge	*Asparagus officinalis*	Asparagus, Sparrow Grass	Folk
Asphuka	*Vallaris solanacea*	Bread Flower	Ayurvedic
Asraash	*Asphodelus fistulosus*	Asphodel	Unani
Asthisamhaari	*Cissus quadrangula*	Square Stalked Vine, Adamant Creeper	Ayurvedic
Asthisamhrita	*Cissus quadrangula*	Square Stalked Vine, Adamant Creeper	Ayurvedic
Asthi-samyojaka	*Cissus quadrangula*	Square Stalked Vine, Adamant Creeper	Ayurvedic
Asthi-shrankhala	*Cissus quadrangula*	Square Stalked Vine, Adamant Creeper	Ayurvedic
Atangi	*Gordonia obtusa*	Loblolly Bay, Grey Laurel	Folk/South
Atari-lataa	*Reissantia indica*	Atari Vine	Folk
Atarunadaaru	*Argyreia speciosa*	Elephant Creeper	Ayurvedic
Atasi	*Linum usitatissimum*	Linseed, Flax	Ayurvedic
Atchy	*Morinda citrifolia*	Indian Mulberry	Ayurvedic
Athalaikai	*Momordica tuberosa*	Eight-ribbed Bitter Gourd	Siddha/Tamil
Athi Bala-chedi	*Sida rhombifolia*	Red-flowered Mallow	Siddha/Tamil
Athimathuram	*Glycyrrhiza glabra*	Licorice, Liquorice	Siddha/Tamil
Athividayam	*Aconitum heterophyllum*	Atis Root, Aconite	Siddha/Tamil
Aththi	*Ficus racemosa*	Cluster Fig, Country Fig	Siddha/Tamil
Atibalaa	*Abutilon indicum*	Country Mallow, Flowering Maples, Chinese Bell-flowers	Ayurvedic
Atimukta	*Hiptage benghalensis*	Hiptage	Ayurvedic
Atimuktaka	*Hiptage benghalensis*	Hiptage	Ayurvedic

Table Contd.

Indian Name	Botanical Name	English Name	Medicinal System
Atirasaa	*Asparagus racemosus*	Indian Asparagus, Wild Asparagus	Ayurvedic
Atirasaa	*Glycyrrhiza glabra*	Licorice, Liquorice	Ayurvedic
Atirasaa	*Marsdenia tenacissima*	White Turpeth	Ayurvedic
Atis	*Aconitum heterophyllum*	Atis Root, Aconite	Unani
Atisaurabha	*Mangifera indica*	Mango	Ayurvedic
Ativallabhaa	*Stereospermum personatum*	Trumpet Flower, Yellow Snake Tree	Ayurvedic
Ativisha	*Aconitum heterophyllum*	Atis Root, Aconite	Ayurvedic
Ativrihatphala	*Artocarpus integrifolia*	Jackfruit, Jack Tree	Ayurvedic
Atta	*Annona squamosa*	Custard Apple, Sugar Apple, Sweet-sop	Siddha/Tamil
Attalaree	*Polygonum glabrum*	Denseflower Knotweed	Siddha/Tamil
Attarasu	*Trewia nudiflora*	False White Teak, Gutel	Folk/Tamil
Attipurashadam	*Indigofera tinctoria*	Indigo	Folk/Tamil
Attukkal	*Ipomoea pes-caprae*	Goat's Foot Creeper	Folk/Tamil
Attupalai	*Salix tetrasperma*	Indian Willow	Siddha/Tamil
Aushadha	*Zingiber officinale*	Ginger	Ayurvedic
Ava-chiraayataa	*Exacum bicolor*	Pseudo-Chiretta	Ayurvedic
Avalguja	*Psoralea corylifolia*	Purple Fleabane	Ayurvedic
Avanti	*Wedelia calendulaceae*	Yellow-flowered Weldia	Ayurvedic
Avarin (Seed)	*Dolichos lablab*	Indian Butter Bean, Lablab Bean, Horsebean	Siddha/Tamil
Aviddhakarni	*Cissampelos pareira*	Velvet-Leaf Pareira, Pareira Brava	Ayurvedic
Avil thol	*Holoptelea integrifolia*	Indian Elm, Kanju Wood	Folk/Tamil
Avipriya	*Prangos pabularia*	Prangos, Yugan. Aju Chach	Ayurvedic
Avuri	*Indigofera tinctoria*	Indigo	Siddha/Tamil
Awaa	*Girardinia heterophylla*	Himalayan Nettle	Folk
Ayaapaana	*Eupatorium triplinerve*	Ayapana Tea	Ayurvedic
Ayamoda	*Trachyspermum roxburghianum*	Ajmud	Ayurvedic
Ayapanai	*Eupatorium triplinerve*	Ayapana Tea	Siddha/Tamil
Ayapani	*Eupatorium triplinerve*	Ayapana Tea	Folk
Ayil pattai (bark)	*Holoptelea integrifolia*	Indian Elm, Kanju Wood	Folk/Tamil

Table Contd.

Indian Name	Botanical Name	English Name	Medicinal System
Ayma	*Careya arborea*	Kumbi, Slow-Match Tree	Siddha/Tamil
Azaraaqi	*Strychnos nux-vomica*	Nux Vomica	Unani
Azhavanam	*Lawsonia inermis*	Henna	Siddha/Tamil
Azhinjil	*Alangium lamarckii*	Sage-leaf Alangium	Siddha/Tamil
Baabchi	*Psoralea corylifolia*	Purple Fleabane	Unani
Baabui Tulasi	*Ocimum basilicum*	Sweet Basil, Basil Herb	Ayurvedic
Baabunaa	*Matricaria chamomilla*	German Chamomile, Chamomile	Unani
Baadaam Shireen	*Prunus amygdalus*	Almond	Unani
Baadaavard	*Amberboa divaricata*	Volutarella	Unani
Baadaavard	*Volutarella ramosa*	Volutarella	Unani
Baadiyaan	*Foeniculum vulgare*	Fennel	Unani
Baadiyaan	*Illicium anisatum*	Star Anise	Unani
Baadiyaan-kohi	*Prangos pabularia*	Prangos, Yugan. Aju-Chach	Unani
Baadiyaanroomi	*Pimpinella anisum*	Anise, Aniseed	Unani
Baadranjboyaa	*Melissa officinalis*	Mountain Balm, Sweet or Lemon Balm	Unani
Baadranjbuuyaa	*Nepeta hindostana*	Catnip, Catnep, Catmint	Unani
Baadshaahi Saalab	*Allium macleanii*	Oriental Royal Salep	Unani
Baadyaan Khataai	*Illicium verum*	Star Anise, Chinese Anise, Aniseed Stars	Unani
Baahlika	*Ferula foetida*	Asafoetida	Ayurvedic
Baakuchi	*Psoralea corylifolia*	Purple Fleabane	Ayurvedic
Baala	*Coleus vettiveroides*	Coleus	Ayurvedic
Baala	*Pavonia odorata*	Fragrant Sticky Mallow	Ayurvedic
Baalaa	*Coleus vettiveroides*	Coleus	Ayurvedic
Baalaka	*Coleus vettiveroides*	Coleus	Ayurvedic
Baalaka	*Pavonia odorata*	Fragrant Sticky Mallow	Ayurvedic
Baalaka	*Valeriana leschenaultii*	Nilgiri Valerian	Folk
Baalaka	*Valeriana officinalis*	Valerian, Garden Heliotrope, Common Valerian	Ayurvedic
Baalaka	*Valeriana wallichii*	Indian Valerian	Folk
Baalakanda	*Eulophia nuda*	Goruma Tuber, Riddhi	Ayurvedic
Baalango	*Lallemantia royleana*	Balanga Seed	Unani

Table Contd.

Indian Name	Botanical Name	English Name	Medicinal System
Baalbach	*Iris ensata*	Japanese Iris	Ayurvedic
Baal-bach	*Iris germanica*	Orris, Iridis Rhizome, German Iris	Ayurvedic
Baal-bach	*Paris polyphylla*	Herb Paris, Tingling Rootstock Plant	Folk
Baalchhar	*Nardostachys jatamansi*	Spikenard, Musk-root	Unani
Baalu-ka-saag	*Gisekia pharnaceoides*	Jisucao (Chinese)	Folk
Baaman-haati	*Premna herbacea*	Bharangi Tree, Qian jie cao (Chinese)	Folk
Baamiyaa	*Abelmoschus esculentus*	Gumbo, Lady Finger, Okra	Unani
Baana	*Barleria prionitis*	Common Yellow Nail Dye Plant	Ayurvedic
Baandaa	*Dendrophthoe falcata*	Mango and Citrus Parasite	Folk
Baandaa	*Hedera nepalensis*	Nepal Ivy	Folk
Baandaa	*Loranthus falcatus*	Honeysuckle Mistletoe	Folk
Baandaa	*Loranthus pentandrus*	Mistletoe	Folk
Baandaa	*Vanda spathulata*	Plantain Tree, Tree-top Plantain	Ayurvedic
Baandaa	*Viscum orientale*	Bengal Mistletoe	Folk
Baandar-Baashing	*Drynaria quercifolia*	Drynaria Fern	Folk
Baaphali	*Corchorus fascicularis*	Chanchee Vegetable	Folk
Baaphali	*Peucedanum grande*	Wild Carrot	Folk
Baaqlaa	*Vicia faba*	Broad Bean, Windsor Bean	Unani
Baaraamaasi	*Rosa bourboniana*	Bourbon Rose	Ayurvedic
Baarak-kaant	*Pericampylus glaucus*	Broad-leaved Moonseed	Folk
Baartang	*Plantago lanceolata*	Rib Grass, Ribwort Plantain, English Plantain, Buckhorn Plantain	Unani
Baasanti	*Reinwardtia indica*	Winter-Flax, Yellow Flax	Ayurvedic
Baathu	*Chenopodium album*	Fat Hen, Lamb's Quarters, White Goosefoot, Wild Spinach, Pigweed	Unani
Baavari	*Acacia arabica*	Babul, Black Babul, Indian Gum Arabic Tree	Ayurvedic
Baayabirang	*Embelia robusta*	Broad-leaved Embelia	Folk
Babbu-goshaa	*Pyrus communis*	Common or European Pear	Folk
Babbuula	*Acacia arabica*	Babul, Black Babul, Indian Gum Arabic Tree	Ayurvedic

Table Contd.

Indian Name	Botanical Name	English Name	Medicinal System
Babbuuri	*Acacia arabica*	Babul, Black Babul, Indian Gum Arabic Tree	Ayurvedic
Babuul	*Acacia arabica*	Babul, Black Babul, Indian Gum Arabic Tree	Unani
Bacchanaag	*Aconitum ferox*	Indian Aconite, Wolfsbane, Monkshood	Folk
Bacho	*Rubia tinctorum*	Alizari, European Madder	Folk (Punjab)
Badaa Chaand	*Rauvolfia tetraphylla*	Wild Snakeroot	Folk
Badaam	*Amygdalus communis*	Almond	Unani
Badai	*Lilium wallichianum*	Trumpet-shaped Golden Lily	Folk
Badar	*Abies pindrow*	Pindrow-Fir, Silver-Fir, The West-Himalayan Low-Level Fir	Folk
Badar	*Abies webbiana*	Indian Silver Fir, The West-Himalayan High-Level Fir, The East-Himalayan Fir	Folk
Badar	*Ziziphus jujuba*	Indian Jujube, Common Jujube	Ayurvedic
Bael	*Aegle marmelos*	Bael Tree, Bengal Quince	Unani
Bagahul	*Osmanthus fragrans*	Sweet Olive Tree	Folk
Baghachuur	*Pisonia aculeata*	Devil's Claw	Folk
Bagharenda (var.)	*Jatropha curcas*	Physic Nut, Purging Nut	Folk
Bagharenda	*Jatropha glandulifera*	Jatropha (South India)	Folk
Bagu-goshaa	*Pyrus communis*	Common or European Pear	Folk
Baheraa	*Terminalia bellirica*	Belleric Myrobalan, Bastard Myrobalan	Unani
Bahir	*Imperata cylindrica*	Thatch Grass	Ayurvedic
Bahugranthikaa	*Tamarix indica*	Takut Galls	Ayurvedic
Bahukanda	*Cucumis melo*	Musk Melon, Sweet Melon	Ayurvedic
Bahulaa	*Amomum subulatum*	Greater or Nepal Cardamom	Ayurvedic
Bahulvalkala	*Betula utilis*	Himalayan Silver Birch, Indian Paper Tree	Ayurvedic
Bahulvalkala	*Buchanania lanzan*	Almondette Tree, Cheronjee, Buchanan's Mango	Ayurvedic
Bahumanjari	*Ocimum sanctum*	Holy Basil, Sacred Basil	Ayurvedic
Bahu-muulaka	*Vetiveria zizanioides*	Vetiver, Khas	Ayurvedic
Bahunetra	*Ananas comosus*	Pineapple	Ayurvedic

Table Contd.

Indian Name	Botanical Name	English Name	Medicinal System
Bahupaada	*Ficus beng(h)alensis*	Banyan Tree	Ayurvedic
Bahupatri	*Phyllanthus amarus*	Indian Chanca Piedra	Ayurvedic
Bahupatrikaa	*Trigonella foenum-graecum*	Fenugreek	Ayurvedic
Bahuphalaa	*Phyllanthus amarus*	Indian Chanca Piedra	Ayurvedic
Bahuprajaa	*Breynia retusa*	Cup Saucer Plant	Ayurvedic
Bahupushpi	*Woodfordia fruticosa*	Fire-flame Bush, Shiranjitea	Ayurvedic
Bahuputa	*Betula utilis*	Himalayan Silver Birch, Indian Paper Tree	Ayurvedic
Bahusutaa	*Asparagus racemosus*	Indian Asparagus, Wild Asparagus	Ayurvedic
Bahuvaara	*Cordia myxa*	Sabestan Plum	Ayurvedic
Bahuvaaraka	*Cordia wallichii*	Sebestan	Ayurvedic
Baibhita	*Terminalia bellirica*	Belleric Myrobalan, Bastard Myrobalan	Ayurvedic
Baikal	*Gymnosporia spinosa*	Celastrus Tree	Folk
Baingan	*Solanum melongena*	Eggplant, Brinjal	Folk
Baingan	*Solanum melongena*	Eggplant, Brinjal	Unani
Bairsinge	*Radermachera xylocarpa*	Padri Tree	Folk
Baishi	*Salix tetrasperma*	Indian Willow	Ayurvedic
Bajarbang	*Physochlaina praealta*	Hyoscyamine Plant	Folk
Bajradanti	*Potentilla arbuscula*	Shrubby Cinquefoil	Ayurvedic
Bajradanti	*Sibbaldia parviflora*	Sibbaldia	Ayurvedic
Bakaayan	*Melia azedarach*	Persian Lilac, Pride of India	Unani
Bakalpattaa	*Kalanchoe integra*	Never Die	Folk
Bakam	*Caesalpinia sappan*	Sappan	Unani
Bakam	*Haematoxylon campechianum*	Peachwood, Compeachy Tree	Ayurvedic
Bakam-Hindi	*Haematoxylon campechianum*	Logwood, Peachwood, Compeachy Tree	Unani
Bakli	*Lagerstroemia parviflora*	Lendi, Benteak	Folk
Bakuchi	*Psoralea corylifolia*	Purple Fleabane	Unani
Bakula	*Mimusops elengi*	Spanish-Cherry, West Indian Medlar, Bullet Wood	Ayurvedic
Bakula	*Osmanthus fragrans*	Sweet Olive Tree	Folk

Table Contd.

Indian Name	Botanical Name	English Name	Medicinal System
Balaa	*Sida acuta*	Hornbeam-Leaved Sida	Ayurvedic
Balaa	*Sida cordifolia*	Country Mallow	Ayurvedic
Balaadur	*Semecarpus anacardium*	Marking-Nut	Unani
Balaa-kantakini	*Sida spinosa*	Prickly Mallow	Ayurvedic
Balaamotaa	*Sesbania sesban*	Common Sesban	Ayurvedic
Balatang	*Plantago lanceolata*	Rib Grass, Ribwort Plantain, English Plantain, Buckhorn Plantain	Folk
Balbhra	*Gentiana kurroo*	Himalayan Gentian, Indian Gentian Root	Ayurvedic
Balelaa	*Terminalia bellirica*	Belleric Myrobalan, Bastard Myrobalan	Unani
Balini	*Sida cordifolia*	Country Mallow	Ayurvedic
Balkuwari	*Ginkgo biloba*	Maidenhair Tree	Folk
Balobalarao	*Ceriops candolleana*	Compound Cymed Mangrove	Folk (Trade)
Baloot	*Aesculus hippocastanum*	Horse Chestnut Tree	Unani
Baloot	*Quercus incana*	Grey Oak	Unani
Bal-raksha	*Gnaphalium luteo-album*	Jersey Cudweed, Cotton Weed, Cat's Foot, Everlasting Flower	Folk
Balsam	*Myroxylon balsamum*	Tolu Balsam Tree	Unani
Balsaan	*Balsamodendron opobalsamum*	Balsam Tree, Balsam of Mecca, Balsam of Gilead	Unani
Balsaan	*Hypericum perforatum*	Common St. John's Wort	Unani
Balu	*Rhododendron cinnabarinum*	Cinnamom-red flowered Azalea	Folk
Balvaja	*Eulaliopsis binata*	Baib Grass, Sabai Grass	Ayurvedic
Balyaa	*Withania ashwagandha*	Winter Cherry	Ayurvedic
Ban Kulathi	*Cassia absus*	Four-leaved Cassia, Pig's Senna	Folk
Ban Tambaaku	*Verbascum thapsus*	Cow's Lungwort, Common Mullein	Ayurvedic
Banaaalu	*Dioscorea bulbifera*	Patoto Yam, Bulb-bearing Yam, Air Potato, Dog Yam	Ayurvedic
Bana-adarakhi	*Zingiber cassumunar*	Cassumunar Ginger	Folk
Bana-bhantaa	*Solanum ferox*	Poison-Berry	Ayurvedic
Banachalit	*Leea crispa*	Grey-berry Holly	Folk

Table Contd.

Indian Name	Botanical Name	English Name	Medicinal System
Banachelt	*Leea crispa*	Grey-berry Holly	Folk
Banafashaa	*Viola biflora*	Yellow-flowered Violet	Unani
Banafashaa	*Viola cinerea*	White-flowered Violet	Unani
Banafashaa	*Viola odorata*	Sweet Violet	Unani
Banafashaa	*Viola patrinii*	Lilac-flowered Violet	Unani
Banafashaa	*Viola pilosa*	Banafshah-oil Violet	Unani
Banafashaa	*Viola sylvestris*	Pale Wood Violet, Wood Violet	Unani
Banafashaa	*Viola tricolor*	Heartsease, Wild Pansy	Unani
Banafsaj	*Viola odorata*	Sweet Violet	Unani
Banakakaraa	*Zehneria umbellata*	Zehneria	Folk
Bana-kakari	*Podophyllum hexandrum*	Indian Podophyllum	Folk
Banakalami	*Ipomoea sepiaria*	Big-flowered Morning Glory	Ayurvedic
Bana-Kapaasi	*Thespesia lampas*	Indian Hemp	Folk
Bana-laung	*Jussiaea suffruticosa*	Swamp Primrose	Ayurvedic
Bana-mallikaa	*Jasminum angustifolium*	Wild Jasmine	Ayurvedic
Bana-Nila	*Indigofera oblongifolia*	Wild Indigo, Mysore Panicled Indigo	Ayurvedic
Bana-Nimbu	*Glycosmis pentaphylla*	Orangeberry, Ginberry	Folk
Bana-okraa	*Xanthium strumarium*	Cocklebur, Burweed	Folk
Banarasi Raai	*Brassica nigra*	Black Mustard	Ayurvedic
Bana-Tulasi	*Ocimum basilicum*	Sweet Basil, Basil Herb	Folk
Bandaa	*Hedera nepalensis*	Nepal Ivy	Folk
Bandaak	*Viscum articulatum*	Napalese Mistletoe	Ayurvedic
Bandaaka (var.)	*Loranthus pentandrus*	Mistletoe	Ayurvedic
Bandaaka	*Dendrophthoe falcata*	Mango and Citrus Parasite	Ayurvedic
Bandaaka	*Loranthus falcatus*	Honeysuckle Mistletoe	Ayurvedic
Bandaaka	*Viscum album*	European Mistletoe	Ayurvedic
Bandaal	*Luffa echinata*	Bristly Luffa	Folk
Bandhujiva	*Pentapetes phoenicea*	Midday Flower, Copper Cup, Scarlet Mallow, Florimpia	Ayurvedic
Bandhuka	*Ixora coccinea*	Jungleflame Ixora	Ayurvedic
Bandhuuka	*Pentapetes phoenicea*	Midday Flower, Copper Cup, Scarlet Mallow, Florimpia	Ayurvedic
Ban-gulaab	*Rosa macrophylla*	Himalayan Rose	Folk

Table Contd.

Indian Name	Botanical Name	English Name	Medicinal System
Ban-haldi	*Hedychium spicatum*	Spiked Ginger Ivy	Folk
Banjhori	*Vicoa indica*	Banjauri	Folk
Ban-Jiraa	*Perilla frutescens*	Perilla, Wild Coleus	Folk
Ban-Karelaa	*Momordica dioica*	Small Bitter Gourd, burr Cucumber	Folk
Ban-Kevaraa	*Agave americana*	Century Plant, American Aloe	Folk
Bankharaa	*Dalbergia volubilis*	Cinnamom-scented Bark Tree	Folk
Bankhor	*Aesculus indica*	Indian Horse Chestnut, Himalayan Chestnut	Folk
Ban-mallikaa	*Jasminum sambac*	Arabian Jasmine, Tuscan Jasmine, Double Jasmine	Folk
Ban-Methi	*Melilotus indica*	Sweet Clover, Annual Yellow Sweet Clover, Small-flowered Melilot	Folk
Bannu	*Coffea arabica*	Arabian Coffee	Siddha/Tamil
Ban-pindaalu	*Gardenia latifolia*	Boxwood Gardenia	Folk
Ban-Reethaa	*Acacia concinna*	Soap-nut Acacia	Folk
Ban-Sangli	*Crataegeus oxyacantha*	English Hawthorn	Folk
Ban-Tulasi	*Elsholtzia cristata*	Himalayan Pseudo-Basil	Folk
Ban-tulasi	*Perilla frutescens*	Perilla, Wild Coleus	Folk
Banwaa	*Aconitum atrox*	Himalayan Napellus	Folk
Baobarang	*Embelia ribes*	Embelia	Unani
Baraahikand	*Dioscorea bulbifera*	Patoto Yam, Bulb-bearing Yam, Air Potato, Dog Yam	Unani
Baraas Kapoor	*Dryobalanops camphora*	Bornoe or Barus Camphor	Folk
Barachuli	*Limnanthemum indicum*	Aquatic Pseudo-Chiretta Plant	Folk
Barahantaa	*Solanum indicum*	Poison Berry	Folk
Baramdandi	*Lamprachaenium microcephalum*	Purple-flowered Brahmadandi	Unani
Baranaa	*Crataeva nurvala*	Steaved Tree, Sacred Barna	Unani
Barang Kaabuli	*Embelia ribes*	Embelia	Unani
Baranjaasif	*Leonurus cardiaca*	Common Motherwort	Unani
Baravat	*Rivea ornate*	Oliliuqui	Folk
Barbara	*Balsamodendron myrrha*	Myrrh, Herabol	Ayurvedic
Barbaraka	*Gynandropsis gynandra*	African Spider Plant	Ayurvedic

Table Contd.

Indian Name	Botanical Name	English Name	Medicinal System
Barbari	*Ocimum basilicum*	Sweet Basil, Basil Herb	Ayurvedic
Bargad	*Ficus beng(h)alensis*	Banyan Tree	Unani
Barhal	*Artocarpus lakoocha*	Monkey Jack	Folk
Barhishtha	*Pavonia odorata*	Fragrant Sticky Mallow	Ayurvedic
Barilla	*Salsola kali*	Glass-Wort, Russian Thistle, Prickly-Saltwort	Folk
Bariyaara	*Sida cordifolia*	Country Mallow	Unani
Bariyaara	*Sida rhombifolia*	Red-flowered Mallow	Unani
Barley	*Hordeum vulgare*	Barley	Unani
Barokalagoru	*Heterophragma roxburghii*	Karen Wood	Siddha/Tamil
Barphali	*Euonymus tingens*	Spindle Wood, Wahoo,	Folk
Barri	*Periploca aphylla*	Milk Broom	Folk
Barsanga	*Murraya koenigii*	Curry-Leaf Tree	Folk
Barsem	*Medicago sativa*	Alfalfa, Lucerne	Unani
Barunaa	*Crataeva nurvala*	Steaved Tree, Sacred Barna	Ayurvedic
Barz-ul-Banj	*Hyoscyamus niger*	Indian Henbane, Black Henbane	Unani
Basak	*Dichroa febrifuga*	Dichroa Quinine	Folk
Bashahr-Mohra	*Aconitum deinorrhizum*	Indian Aconite	Folk
Bassant	*Hypericum perforatum*	Common St. John's Wort	Unani
Bastaantri	*Argyreia speciosa*	Elephant Creeper	Ayurvedic
Basula	*Lippia geminata*	Melissa Lipia	Folk
Bathuaa	*Chenopodium album*	Fat Hen, Lamb's Quarters, White Goosefoot, Wild Spinach, Pigweed	Unani
Battal	*Sorbus aucuparia*	European Mountain Ash, Rowan Tree, Mountain Ash Berry	Folk
Batula	*Saussurea heteromalla*	Snow Lotus	Folk
Batvaasi	*Gouania leptostachya*	Soapy Chewing-stick Tree	Folk
Bazr-ul-khumkhum	*Lepidium iberis*	Peppercress	Unani
Bebina	*Mussaenda frondosa*	White Lady, White Rag Plant	Folk
Bebrang	*Myrsine africana*	Pseudo-Embelia	Folk
Bed	*Salix babylonica*	Weeping Willow	Folk

Table Contd.

Indian Name	Botanical Name	English Name	Medicinal System
Bed Mushk	*Salix caprea*	Sallow, Goat Willow, Common Willow	Unani
Bed Saadaa	*Salix alba*	White Willow, European Willow	Unani
Bedanjeer	*Ricinus communis*	Castor Seed	Unani
Bedina	*Mussaenda frondosa*	White Lady, White Rag Plant	Folk
Bed-Siyaah	*Salix nigra*	Black Willow	Unani
Beech	*Fagus sylvatica*	European Beech, Common Beech	Folk
Beedi-elai	*Diospyros melanoxylon*	Coromandel Ebony, Persimmon	Siddha/Tamil
Beejband (seeds)	*Rumex maritimus*	Golden Dock	Unani
Behman safed	*Centaurea behen*	White Rhapontic	Unani
Behman Surkh	*Salvia haematodes*	Blood-veined Sage	Unani
Behman-abyaz	*Centaurea behen*	White Rhapontic	Unani
Bekh-e-Baadiyaan	*Pimpinella saxifraga*	Burnet Saxifrage Root, Pimpinella Root	Folk
Belaa	*Jasminum sambac*	Arabian Jasmine, Tuscan Jasmine, Double Jasmine	Folk
Belambu	*Averrhoa bilimbi*	Bilimbi, Tree Sorrel	Unani
Beli	*Limonia crenulata*	Naringi, Beli	Folk
Belkangu	*Clematis gouriana*	Morvel, Virgin's Bower	Folk
Belu	*Agrimonia eupatoria*	Agrimony, Stickle Wort	Folk
Bendarali	*Lycopodium clavatum*	Common Club Moss	Folk
Ber	*Ziziphus jujuba*	Indian Jujube, Common Jujube	Unani
Berseem	*Trifolium pratense*	Red Clover	Unani
Berzad	*Pinus roxburghii*	Long-leaved Pine, Three-leaved Pine, Chir Pine	Unani
Bhaabar	*Eulaliopsis binata*	Baib Grass, Sabai Grass	Folk
Bhaandi	*Abelmoschus esculentus*	Gumbo, Lady Finger, Okra	Ayurvedic
Bhaandi	*Clerodendrum infortunatum*	Glory Bower	Ayurvedic
Bhaandira	*Clerodendrum infortunatum*	Glory Bower	Ayurvedic
Bhaang	*Cannabis sativa*	Hemp, Indian Hemp	Unani
Bhaanu	*Calotropis gigantea*	Swallow Wort	Ayurvedic

Table Contd.

Indian Name	Botanical Name	English Name	Medicinal System
Bhaaradwaaji	*Gossypium herbaceum*	Asiatic Cotton, Levant Cotton, Uppam Cotton	Ayurvedic
Bhaarangi	*Clerodendrum serratum*	Blue-flowered Glory Tree, Beetle Killer	Ayurvedic
Bhaarangi	*Pygmaeopremna herbacea*	Bharangi Tree, Qian jie cao (Chinese)	Ayurvedic
Bhaarati	*Bacopa monnieri*	Thyme-leaved Gratiola	Ayurvedic
Bhaargavi	*Cynodon dactylon*	Bermuda Grass, Bahama Grass, Couch Grass	Ayurvedic
Bhaargi	*Clerodendrum serratum*	Blue-flowered Glory Tree, Beetle Killer	Ayurvedic
Bhaasvanmuula	*Calotropis gigantea*	Swallow Wort	Ayurvedic
Bhadra	*Cyperus rotundus*	Nut Grass	Ayurvedic
Bhadra	*Gmelina arborea*	Candahar Tree, White Teak	Ayurvedic
Bhadraa	*Amomum subulatum*	Greater or Nepal Cardamom	Ayurvedic
Bhadraa	*Cyperus rotundus*	Nut Grass	Ayurvedic
Bhadraa	*Myrica nagi*	Box Myrtle	Ayurvedic
Bhadraaksh	*Guazuma ulmifolia*	Bastard Cedar	Ayurvedic
Bhadraaksha	*Scaevola frutescens*	Fan Flower, Malay Rice Paper Plant	Folk
Bhadrabalaa	*Convolvulus arvensis*	Deer's Foot, Devil's Garters	Ayurvedic
Bhadrabalaa	*Sida cordifolia*	Country Mallow	Ayurvedic
Bhadradaaru	*Cedrus deodara*	Himalayan Cedar, Deodar	Ayurvedic
Bhadrailaa	*Amomum subulatum*	Greater or Nepal Cardamom	Ayurvedic
Bhadraka	*Scaevola frutescens*	Fan Flower, Malay Rice Paper Plant	Folk
Bhadramuja	*Saccharum munja*	Munja Culms	Ayurvedic
Bhadramusta	*Cyperus rotundus*	Nut Grass	Ayurvedic
Bhadramustaa	*Cyperus rotundus*	Nut Grass	Ayurvedic
Bhadramustaka	*Cyperus rotundus*	Nut Grass	Ayurvedic
Bhadraparni	*Gmelina arborea*	Candahar Tree, White Teak	Ayurvedic
Bhadra-Shree	*Santalum album*	White Sandalwood	Ayurvedic
Bhadraudani	*Sida cordifolia*	Country Mallow	Ayurvedic
Bhadravalli	*Vallaris solanacea*	Bread Flower	Ayurvedic
Bhadravati	*Myrica nagi*	Box Myrtle	Ayurvedic

Table Contd.

Indian Name	Botanical Name	English Name	Medicinal System
Bhadrodumbara	*Ficus carica*	Common Fig	Ayurvedic
Bhakshantaka	*Pedalium murex*	Caltrops (bigger var.)	Ayurvedic
Bhakuraa	*Cucumis trigonus*	Wild Cucumber	Folk
Bhallaataka	*Semecarpus anacardium*	Marking-Nut	Ayurvedic
Bhallata	*Semecarpus anacardium*	Marking-Nut	Ayurvedic
Bhalluka	*Ailanthus excelsa*	Tree of Heaven, Maharukh	Ayurvedic
Bhalluka	*Oroxylum indicum*	Indian Trumpet Flower	Ayurvedic
Bhanda	*Geranium nepalense*	Nepal Geranium, Nepalese Crane's Bill	Ayurvedic
Bhandaa	*Geranium nepalense*	Nepal Geranium, Nepalese Crane's Bill	Ayurvedic
Bhandi	*Albizia lebbeck*	Siris Tree, East Indian Walnut	Ayurvedic
Bhandila	*Albizia lebbeck*	Siris Tree, East Indian Walnut	Ayurvedic
Bhangaa	*Cannabis sativa*	Hemp, Indian Hemp	Ayurvedic
Bhangaraa	*Eclipta alba*	Trailing Eclipta Plant	Folk
Bhangari	*Blepharis linariaefolia*	Acanthus	Folk/Rajasthan
Bhang-jala	*Datisca cannabina*	False Hemp	Folk
Bhanguraa	*Aconitum heterophyllum*	Atis Root, Aconite	Ayurvedic
Bhanjeer	*Perilla frutescens*	Perilla, Wild Coleus	Folk
Bhansi	*Zanthoxylum oxyphyllum*	Tumru Tree, Prickly Ash	Folk
Bhantaa	*Solanum melongena*	Eggplant, Brinjal	Ayurvedic
Bhantaa	*Solanum melongena*	Eggplant, Brinjal	Folk
Bhantaki	*Solanum melongena*	Eggplant, Brinjal	Ayurvedic
Bhanwar	*Ipomoea eriocarpa*	Tiny Morning Glory, Wooly-Fruited Morning Glory	Folk
Bhasindi	*Perilla frutescens*	Perilla, Wild Coleus	Folk
Bhat	*Glycine max*	Soybean, Soya	Folk
Bhatakataiyaa	*Solanum xanthocarpum*	Wild Eggplant, Yellow-Berried Nightshade	Ayurvedic
Bhatiaa	*Dalbergia volubilis*	Cinnamom-scented Bark Tree	Folk
Bhat-Karelaa	*Momordica cochinchinensis*	Chinese Cucumber, Mbiezi	Folk
Bhat-Karelaa	*Momordica dioica*	Small Bitter Gourd, burr Cucumber	Folk
Bhaulan	*Hymenodictyon excelsum*	Bridal Couch Tree	Folk

Table Contd.

Indian Name	Botanical Name	English Name	Medicinal System
Bhavya	*Dillenia indica*	Elephant Apple	Ayurvedic
Bhedas	*Syzygium zeylanicum*	Sumaich (Cambodia)	Folk
Bheet-chatti	*Lindenbergia indica*	Nettle-leaved Lindenbergia	Folk
Bhendaa	*Abelmoschus esculentus*	Gumbo, Lady Finger, Okra	Ayurvedic
Bheria	*Chloroxylon swietenia*	Indian Satinwood Tree	Folk
Bherul	*Chloroxylon swietenia*	Indian Satinwood Tree	Folk
Bhikshu	*Asteracantha longifolia*	Hygrophilla	Ayurvedic
Bhilaavaan	*Semecarpus anacardium*	Marking-Nut	Folk
Bhilaavaan	*Semecarpus anacardium*	Marking-Nut	Unani
Bhilaayan	*Semecarpus anacardium*	Marking-Nut	Unani
Bhillotaka	*Euonymus tingens*	Spindle Wood, Wahoo,	Ayurvedic
Bhimseni Kapoor	*Dryobalanops camphora*	Bornoe or Barus Camphor	Ayurvedic
Bhindaka	*Abelmoschus esculentus*	Gumbo, Lady Finger, Okra	Ayurvedic
Bhindi	*Abelmoschus esculentus*	Gumbo, Lady Finger, Okra	Folk
Bhinjir	*Turnera ulmifolia*	West Indian Holly, Sagerose	Folk/ Maharashtra
Bhiru	*Asparagus racemosus*	Indian Asparagus, Wild Asparagus	Ayurvedic
Bhojapatra	*Betula alnoides*	Indian Birch, Naga Birch	Ayurvedic
Bhootakeshi	*Corydalis govaniana*	Dutchman's Breeches	Ayurvedic
Bhotiaa Badaam	*Corylus colurna*	Turkish Hazel	Folk
Bhotia-baadaam	*Dicentra canadensis*	Squirrel Corn	Folk
Bhragubhavaa	*Clerodendrum serratum*	Blue-flowered Glory Tree, Beetle Killer	Ayurvedic
Bhramarchhali	*Hymenodictyon excelsum*	Bridal Couch Tree	Folk
Bhramar-chhalikaa	*Hymenodictyon excelsum*	Bridal Couch Tree	Ayurvedic
Bhringaahva	*Eclipta alba*	Trailing Eclipta Plant	Ayurvedic
Bhringaja	*Eclipta alba*	Trailing Eclipta Plant	Ayurvedic
Bhringaraaja	*Eclipta alba*	Trailing Eclipta Plant	Ayurvedic
Bhringaraaja	*Wedelia biflora*	Sea Coast Weldia	Ayurvedic
Bhringaraaja	*Wedelia calendulaceae*	Yellow-flowered Weldia	Ayurvedic
Bhringa-vriksha	*Hymenodictyon excelsum*	Bridal Couch Tree	Ayurvedic

Table Contd.

Indian Name	Botanical Name	English Name	Medicinal System
Bhringaraaja	*Eclipta alba*	Trailing Eclipta Plant	Ayurvedic
Bhrngaparnikaa	*Elettaria cardamomum*	Lesser Cardamom	Ayurvedic
Bhubhaazi	*Malva sylvestris*	Common Mallow, Blue Mallow, High Mallow	Unani
Bhu-dandi	*Volutarella ramosa*	Volutarella	Folk
Bhui Aaamalaa	*Phyllanthus amarus*	Indian Chanca Piedra	Unani
Bhui-champaa	*Kaempferia rotunda*	Rounded Galanga	Folk
Bhui-erendi	*Sebastiana chamaelea*	Snake's Tongue	Folk
Bhui-kumhraa	*Trichosanthes cordata*	Snake-Gourd	Folk
Bhui-lukham	*Osbeckia chinensis*	Chinese Osbeckia	Folk
Bhuin Kakhaaru	*Ipomoea digitata*	Milky Yam	Folk
Bhui-nila	*Indigofera enneaphylla*	Trailing Indigo	Folk
Bhujangalataa	*Piper betle*	Betel Pepper	Ayurvedic
Bhumi Jambu	*Syzygium cerasoideum*	Piaman Tree	Ayurvedic
Bhumibalaa	*Sida veronicaefolia*	Prostrate Mallow	Ayurvedic
Bhumichakkarai	*Maerua arenaria*	Desert Maerua, Hemkand	Siddha/Tamil
Bhumi-jambu	*Pygmaeopremna herbacea*	Bharangi Tree, Qian jie cao (Chinese)	Ayurvedic
Bhumi-Naagaranga	*Naregamia alata*	Goanese Ipecacuanha	Folk
Bhumyaamalaki (var.)	*Phyllanthus simplex*	Wild Chanca Piedra	Ayurvedic
Bhunsari	*Hyptis suaveolens*	American Mint, American Patchouli	Folk
Bhurangi	*Picrasma quassioides*	Quassia	Ayurvedic
Bhuri-chharilla	*Parmelia perlata*	Parmelia Lichen	Ayurvedic
Bhutakesha	*Mussaenda frondosa*	White Lady, White Rag Plant	Folk
Bhutali	*Elaeocarpus tuberculatus*	Western Ghat Olive-Nut Tree	Folk
Bhutvrkshaka	*Cordia myxa*	Sabestan Plum	Ayurvedic
Bhuu-champaka	*Kaempferia rotunda*	Rounded Galanga	Ayurvedic
Bhuudhaatri	*Phyllanthus amarus*	Indian Chanca Piedra	Ayurvedic
Bhuukadamba	*Sphaeranthus indicus*	East Indian Globe Thistle	Ayurvedic
Bhuu-lavanga	*Jussiaea suffruticosa*	Swamp Primrose	Ayurvedic
Bhuumi-champaka	*Kaempferia rotunda*	Rounded Galanga	Ayurvedic

Table Contd.

Indian Name	Botanical Name	English Name	Medicinal System
Bhuumichhatra	*Agaricus campestris*	Field Mushroom, Edible Mushroom	Ayurvedic
Bhuumi-kushmaanda	*Pueraria tuberosa*	Indian Kudze	Ayurvedic
Bhuumi-kushmaanda	*Trichosanthes cordata*	Snake-Gourd	Ayurvedic
Bhuumikuush-maanda	*Ipomoea digitata*	Milky Yam	Ayurvedic
Bhuumimudga	*Arachis hypogaea*	Groundnut, Peanut, Monkeynut	Ayurvedic
Bhuuminimbaka	*Andrographis paniculata*	Creat	Ayurvedic
Bhuumisaha	*Tectona grandis*	Teak Tree	Ayurvedic
Bhuumitaala	*Curculigo orchioides*	Black Musali	Ayurvedic
Bhuumyaamalaki (var.)	*Phyllanthus urinaria*	Cultivated Field Chanca Piedra	Ayurvedic
Bhuumyaamalaki	*Phyllanthus amarus*	Indian Chanca Piedra	Ayurvedic
Bhuumyaamalaki	*Phyllanthus niruri*	Chanca Piedra	Ayurvedic
Bhuunimba	*Andrographis paniculata*	Creat	Ayurvedic
Bhuunimba	*Swertia chirayita*	Chiretta	Ayurvedic
Bhuurirasa	*Saccharum officinarum*	Gannaa, Naishakar	Ayurvedic
Bhuurja	*Betula utilis*	Himalayan Silver Birch, Indian Paper Tree	Ayurvedic
Bhuurkunda	*Hymenodictyon excelsum*	Bridal Couch Tree	Folk
Bhuuta-bhairavi	*Lygodium flexuosum*	Wolfberry, Scrambling Fern	Folk
Bhuutaghna	*Eruca sativa*	Rocket-Salad	Ayurvedic
Bhuutaghni	*Ocimum sanctum*	Holy Basil, Sacred Basil	Ayurvedic
Bhuutajataa	*Nardostachys jatamansi*	Spikenard, Musk-root	Ayurvedic
Bhuutakeshi	*Selinum tenuifolium*	Cow Parsley	Folk
Bhuutakeshi	*Seseli sibiricum*	Himalayan Seseli	Ayurvedic
Bhuutakeshi	*Vitex negundo*	Five-leaved Chaste Tree	Ayurvedic
Bhuuta-raaj	*Lygodium flexuosum*	Wolfberry, Scrambling Fern	Folk
Bhuutavaasa	*Streblus asper*	Siamese Rough Brush	Ayurvedic
Bhuutika	*Cymbopogon citratus*	Lemongrass	Ayurvedic
Bhuutikaa	*Cymbopogon citratus*	Lemongrass	Ayurvedic
Bhuu-Tulasi	*Salvia plebeia*	Common Sage	Folk
Bhuu-tumbi	*Ceropegia bulbosa*	Candlestick Ceropegia	Folk

Table Contd.

Indian Name	Botanical Name	English Name	Medicinal System
Bibhita	*Terminalia bellirica*	Belleric Myrobalan, Bastard Myrobalan	Ayurvedic
Bibhitaka	*Terminalia bellirica*	Belleric Myrobalan, Bastard Myrobalan	Ayurvedic
Bibhitaki	*Terminalia bellirica*	Belleric Myrobalan, Bastard Myrobalan	Ayurvedic
Bicchuu-buuti	*Urtica dioica*	Stinging Nettle	Folk
Bichhuu	*Martynia annua*	Devil's Claw, Tiger Claw	Folk
Bichhuu-booti	*Girardinia heterophylla*	Himalayan Nettle	Folk
Bichhuu-buuti	*Portulaca tuberosa*	Loniya Weed	Ayurvedic
Bidhaaraa	*Argyreia speciosa*	Elephant Creeper	Folk
Bidhaaraa	*Ipomoea petaloidea*	False Jalap, Hawaii Morning Glory	Folk
Bihi	*Cydonia oblonga*	Quince Fruit	Unani
Bihidaanaa	*Cydonia oblonga*	Quince Fruit	Unani
Bijaahva	*Citrus medica*	Citron	Ayurvedic
Bijagarbha	*Trichosanthes dioica*	Patol, Pointed Gourd	Ayurvedic
Bijaka	*Pterocarpus marsupium*	Indian Kino Tree, Malabar Kino Tree	Ayurvedic
Bijaysaar	*Pterocarpus marsupium*	Indian Kino Tree, Malabar Kino Tree	Unani
Bijoraa	*Citrus medica*	Citron	Folk
Bijpuura	*Citrus medica*	Citron	Ayurvedic
Bikh	*Aconitum falconeri*	Indian Aconite	Folk
Bikhamaa	*Aconitum palmatum*	Himalayan Aconite	Folk
Bikshu	*Hygrophila auriculata*	Indian Swampweed	Ayurvedic
Bilaaikanda	*Ipomoea digitata*	Milky Yam	Folk
Billilotan	*Melissa axillaris*	Lemon Balm	Unani
Billilotan	*Melissa officinalis*	Mountain Balm, Sweet or Lemon Balm	Unani
Billilotan	*Nepeta hindostana*	Catnip, Catnep, Catmint	Unani
Billori	*Polygonum viviparum*	Viviparous Bistort	Folk
Bilpat	*Melochia corchorifolia*	Chocolate-Weed	Folk
Bilva	*Aegle marmelos*	Bael Tree, Bengal Quince	Ayurvedic
Bilvaparni	*Limonia crenulata*	Naringi, Beli	Ayurvedic

Table Contd.

Indian Name	Botanical Name	English Name	Medicinal System
Bimbi	*Coccinia indica*	Ivy-Gourd	Ayurvedic
Binthaa	*Limonia crenulata*	Naringi, Beli	Folk
Binyi	*Larix griffithiana*	Himalayan Larch, Sikkim Larch	Folk
Biranj Saathi	*Oryza sativa*	Rice	Unani
Biranjaasif	*Achillea millefolium*	Milfoil, Yarrow, Thousand Leaf	Unani
Biriyaaraa	*Triumfetta rhomboidea*	Burbush, Burweed	Folk
Birmi	*Taxus baccata*	European Yew	Folk
Birm-kanwal	*Saussurea obvallata*	Sah du goh ghoo (Chinese)	Folk
Bisakhaparaa	*Trianthema decandra*	Horse Purslane	Folk
Bisbaasaa (Mace)	*Myristica fragrans*	Nutmeg	Unani
Bisfaayaj	*Polypodium vulgare*	Polypody Fern	Unani
Bish	*Aconitum falconeri*	Indian Aconite	Folk
Bish	*Aconitum ferox*	Indian Aconite, Wolfsbane, Monkshood	Folk
Bish	*Aconitum ferox*	Indian Aconite, Wolfsbane, Monkshood	Unani
Bishkhaparaa	*Boerhavia diffusa*	Red-flowered Hogweed	Unani
Bishnaag	*Aconitum ferox*	Indian Aconite, Wolfsbane, Monkshood	Unani
Biskandri	*Chlorophytum arundinaceum*	White Musali	Unani
Biskhaparaa	*Trianthema portulacastrum*	Horse Purslane	Unani
Bithuaa	*Dalbergia lanceolaria*	Takoliwood	Folk
Bitkil-chaand	*Gouania leptostachya*	Soapy Chewing-stick Tree	Folk
Black Locust	*Robinia pseudoacacia*	Locust Tree, Robinia, False Acacia, Black Locust	Folk
Boargasella	*Larix griffithiana*	Himalayan Larch, Sikkim Larch	Folk
Bodhaini	*Trigonella foenum-graecum*	Fenugreek	Ayurvedic
Bodhidru	*Ficus religiosa*	Peepal, Bot-tree	Ayurvedic
Bodhivrkisha	*Ficus religiosa*	Peepal, Bot-tree	Ayurvedic
Bodobaando	*Viscum articulatum*	Napalese Mistletoe	Folk

Table Contd.

Indian Name	Botanical Name	English Name	Medicinal System
Bokat	*Asphodelus fistulosus*	Asphodel	Folk
Bol	*Kleinhovia hospita*	Crowned Bol Tree	Folk
Bola	*Balsamodendron myrrha*	Myrrh, Herabol	Ayurvedic
Bond Vel	*Lettsomia elliptica*	Silverweed	Folk
Boogri	*Pittosporum dasycaulon*	Pittosporum Cheesewood	Folk
Boorjapattirum (Leaves)	*Betula utilis*	Himalayan Silver Birch, Indian Paper Tree	Siddha/Tamil
Bovai	*Elsholtzia cristata*	Himalayan Pseudo-Basil	Folk
Braahmany-ashtikaa	*Clerodendrum serratum*	Blue-flowered Glory Tree, Beetle Killer	Ayurvedic
Braahmi	*Bacopa monnieri*	Thyme-leaved Gratiola	Ayurvedic
Brahmadandi	*Amberboa divaricata*	Volutarella	Ayurvedic
Brahmadandi	*Echinops echinatus*	Globe-Thistle, Camel's Thistle	Ayurvedic
Brahmadandi	*Tricholepis angustifolia*	Camel's Thistle	Ayurvedic
Brahmadandi	*Tricholepis glaberrima*	Smooth Tricholepis	Ayurvedic
Brahma-Dhaniyaa	*Eryngium foetidum*	Sea Holly	Folk
Brahma-kamal	*Saussurea obvallata*	Sah du goh ghoo (Chinese)	Folk
Brahmamanduuki	*Centella asiatica*	Asiatic Pennywort, Indian Pennywort	Ayurvedic
Brahmamanduuki	*Hydrocotyle javanica*	Java Pennywort	Folk
Brahma-suvarchalaa	*Drosera peltata*	Sundew	Ayurvedic
Brahmavriksha	*Butea monosperma*	Flame of the Forest, Butea Gum, Bengal Kino	Ayurvedic
Brahmdandi	*Lamprachaenium microcephalum*	Purple-flowered Brahmadandi	Folk
Brahmi	*Bacopa monnieri*	Thyme-leaved Gratiola	Unani
Brahmi-vazhukkai	*Bacopa monnieri*	Thyme-leaved Gratiola	Siddha/Tamil
Brihat Lonikaa	*Portulaca oleracea*	Common Purslane	Ayurvedic
Brihat-Danti	*Jatropha multifida*	Coral Plant, Physic Nut	Ayurvedic
Brihatgokshura	*Pedalium murex*	Caltrops (bigger var.)	Ayurvedic
Brihati	*Solanum Aculeatissimum*	Cockroach Berry, Indian Love Apple, Devil's Apple	Ayurvedic
Brihati	*Solanum albicaule*	Narkanta Prikly Shrub	Ayurvedic

Table Contd.

Indian Name	Botanical Name	English Name	Medicinal System
Brihati	*Solanum ferox*	Poison-Berry	Ayurvedic
Brihati	*Solanum indicum*	Poison Berry	Ayurvedic
Brihati	*Solanum torvum*	West Indian Turkey Berry	Ayurvedic
Brihatikaa	*Solanum ferox*	Poison-Berry	Ayurvedic
Brihat-patra Kamal	*Victoria regia*	Royal Waterlily, Water Maize (seeds)	Ayurvedic
Broom	*Cytisus scoparius*	Broom, Scotch Broom, Yellow Broom	Folk/South
Buchbuchaa	*Stellaria media*	Common Chickweed	Folk
Buckbean	*Menyanthes trifoliata*	Bogbean, Buckbean, Goat's Bean, Marsh Trefoil	Folk
Buckthorn	*Rhamnus procumbens*	Buckthorn	Folk
Buckthorn	*Rhamnus purshiana*	Buckthorn, Cascara Sagrada, Sacred Bark	Folk
Budeolaa	*Stellaria aquatica*	Chickweed, Water Starwort	Folk
Bu-e-Jahudaan	*Balsamodendron mukul*	Indian Bdellium, Gum Guggul	Unani
Bui	*Aerva lanata*	Mountain Knot Grass	Folk
Bui-chholi	*Kochia indica*	Kochia Weed	Folk
Buin	*Platanus orientalis*	Oriental Plane, Oriental Sycamore, European Plane Tree	Folk
Bukham	*Caesalpinia sappan*	Sappan	Folk
Bukkum Booti	*Lippia nodiflora*	Wild Sage	Unani
Bundaar	*Eupatorium cannabinum*	Hemp Agrimony, Water Hemp, Hemp Eupatorium	Folk
Bunduq	*Corylus avellana*	European Hazel, Filbert	Unani
Buqqam	*Haematoxylon campechianum*	Logwood, Peachwood, Compeachy Tree	Unani
Burans	*Rhododendron arboreum*	Tree-Rhododendron, Rose-Tree	Folk
Bustaani Kaasani	*Cichorium endivia*	Succory, Endive	Unani
Butcher's Broom	*Ruscus aculeatus*	Butcher's Broom, Jew's Myrtle	Folk
Buujidaan	*Tanacetum umbelliferum*	Sweet Pellitory	Unani
Buuk	*Osmanthus fragrans*	Sweet Olive Tree	Folk
Canary Tree	*Liriodendron tulipifera*	Tulip Tree	Folk
Candy-tuft	*Iberis amara*	Rocket Candy-tuft, Clown's Mustard	Folk

Table Contd.

Indian Name	Botanical Name	English Name	Medicinal System
Carnation	*Dianthus caryophyllus*	Carnation, Clove Pink	Folk
Celery-keerai	*Apium graveolens*	Celery	Siddha/Tamil
Cembil	*Dysoxylum binectariferum*	Termite-resistant Cedar	Siddha/Tamil
Chaah	*Camellia sinensis*	Tea Plant	Unani
Chaai	*Camellia sinensis*	Tea Plant	Unani
Chaaksu	*Cassia absus*	Four-leaved Cassia, Pig's Senna	Unani
Chaalmogra	*Taraktogenos kurzii*	Kalawa Tree	Folk
Chaalmograa	*Gynocardia odorata*	Oleum Gynocardiae	Ayurvedic
Chaalmograa	*Hydnocarpus kurzii*	Chalmogra	Unani
Chaalmograa	*Hydnocarpus laurifolia*	Soorty Oil Tree	Ayurvedic
Chaalmograa	*Hydnocarpus laurifolia*	Soorty Oil Tree	Unani
Chaaltaa	*Dillenia indica*	Elephant Apple	Folk
Chaampeya	*Mesua ferrea*	Iron-wood, Mesu	Ayurvedic
Chaampeya	*Michelia champaca*	Champak, Golden Champa	Ayurvedic
Chaandani	*Ipomoea bona-nox*	Moon Flower	Folk
Chaandani	*Tabernaemontana coronaria*	East Indian Rosebay	Folk
Chaandri	*Psoralea corylifolia*	Purple Fleabane	Ayurvedic
Chaangeri	*Oxalis acetosella*	Common Wood-Sorrel	Ayurvedic
Chaangeri	*Oxalis corniculata*	Indian Sorrel	Ayurvedic
Chaarapaatu	*Ruellia suffruticosa*	Petunia	Folk
Chaaraparaad	*Ruellia suffruticosa*	Petunia	Folk
Chaaru Vaalhika	*Crocus sativus*	Saffron, Crocus	Ayurvedic
Chaarukesharaa	*Rosa centifolia*	Cabbage Rose, Provence Rose, Hundred-leaved Rose	Ayurvedic
Chaaval-mungari	*Gynocardia odorata*	Oleum Gynocardiae	Folk
Chadolaa	*Rhamnus virgata*	Indian Buckthorn	Folk
Chaembu	*Colocasia esculenta*	Taro, Edible Yam	Siddha/Tamil
Chainhari	*Trigonella incisa*	Winter burr Clover	Folk
Chakavad	*Cassia tora*	Sickle Senna, Ringworm Plant	Folk
Chakondaa	*Cassia obtusifolia*	Arsenic Weed, Sicklepod	Folk
Chakotra	*Citrus maxima*	Pummelo, Shaddock	Unani
Chakotraa	*Citrus paradisi*	Grapefruit, 'Marsh' Grapefruit	Folk

Table Contd.

Indian Name	Botanical Name	English Name	Medicinal System
Chakraangi	*Crinum latifolium*	Wide-leaved Crinum	Ayurvedic
Chakraangi	*Picrorhiza kurroa*	Picrorhiza	Ayurvedic
Chakramarda	*Cassia obtusifolia*	Arsenic Weed, Sicklepod	Ayurvedic
Chakramarda	*Cassia tora*	Sickle Senna, Ringworm Plant	Ayurvedic
Chakravarti	*Rumex vesicarius*	Bladder-Dock, Country Sorrel	Ayurvedic
Chakri	*Cassia tora*	Sickle Senna, Ringworm Plant	Ayurvedic
Chakshushya	*Strychnos potatorum*	Clearing Nut Tree	Ayurvedic
Chakshushyaa	*Cassia absus*	Four-leaved Cassia, Pig's Senna	Ayurvedic
Chakuliya	*Hemionitis arifolia*	Male Fern	Folk
Chakwar	*Cassia obtusifolia*	Arsenic Weed, Sicklepod	Folk
Chalangada	*Pterocarpus dalbergioides*	Andaman Paduak, Andaman Redwood	Folk
Chalapatra	*Ficus religiosa*	Peepal, Bot-tree	Ayurvedic
Chalnundar	*Iris nepalensis*	Nepal Iris	Folk
Chamariyaa	*Artemisia vestita*	Russian Wormwood	Folk
Chambul	*Ranunculus arvensis*	Corn Buttercup	Folk
Chameli (var.)	*Jasminum arborescens*	Tree Jasmine	Folk
Chameli (var.)	*Jasminum flexile*	Jasmine, Juhi	Folk
Chameli	*Jasminum officinale*	Spanish Jasmine	Ayurvedic
Champa Methi	*Trigonella corniculata*	Kasuri Fenugreek	Folk
Champaka	*Artabotrys hexapetalus*	Yling-Yling Vine	Ayurvedic
Champaka	*Michelia champaca*	Champak, Golden Champa	Ayurvedic
Chamror	*Ehretia laevis*	Datrang Tree	Folk
Chanaka	*Cicer arietinum*	Bengal Gram, Chick Pea	Ayurvedic
Chanakaa	*Cicer arietinum*	Bengal Gram, Chick Pea	Ayurvedic
Chanchu	*Corchorus aestuans*	White Jute	Ayurvedic
Chanchu	*Corchorus fascicularis*	Chanchee Vegetable	Ayurvedic
Chanchu	*Ricinus communis*	Castor Seed	Ayurvedic
Chanchu Shaaka	*Corchorus fascicularis*	Chanchee Vegetable	Folk
Chanchuka	*Corchorus fascicularis*	Chanchee Vegetable	Ayurvedic
Chandaa	*Angelica archangelica*	Angelica	Ayurvedic
Chandaamshuka	*Angelica archangelica*	Angelica	Ayurvedic

Table Contd.

Indian Name	Botanical Name	English Name	Medicinal System
Chandan Betu	*Chenopodium album*	Fat Hen, Lamb's Quarters, White Goosefoot, Wild Spinach, Pigweed	Folk/Bengal
Chandana	*Santalum album*	White Sandalwood	Ayurvedic
Chandanam	*Santalum album*	White Sandalwood	Siddha/Tamil
Chandikaa	*Tamarindus indica*	Tamarind Tree	Ayurvedic
Chandmalla	*Limnanthemum cristatum*	Aquatic Pseudo-Chiretta Plant	Folk
Chandra	*Cinnamomum camphora*	Camphor Tree	Ayurvedic
Chandra	*Mallotus philippensis*	Kamala Tree, Monkey Face Tree	Ayurvedic
Chandra Prabhaa	*Cinnamomum camphora*	Camphor Tree	Ayurvedic
Chandrakaanti	*Ipomoea bona-nox*	Moon Flower	Ayurvedic
Chandramuula	*Kaempferia galanga*	Maraba	Ayurvedic
Chandramulika	*Kaempferia galanga*	Maraba	Ayurvedic
Chandrashuura	*Lepidium sativum*	Gardencress, Tongue Grass	Ayurvedic
Chandrikaa	*Lepidium sativum*	Gardencress, Tongue Grass	Ayurvedic
Chapalaa	*Piper longum*	Indian Long Pepper, Joborandi	Ayurvedic
Charai Kattu Ilandai	*Ziziphus rugosa*	White Jujube	Siddha/Tamil
Charas	*Cannabis sativa*	Hemp, Indian Hemp	Unani
Charchari	*Tetrastigma serrulatum*	Lizard Plant	Folk/Nepal
Charmakashaa	*Euphorbia dracunculoides*	Dragon Spurge	Ayurvedic
Charmarangaa	*Cassia auriculata*	Tanner's Cassia	Ayurvedic
Charmasaahvaa	*Euphorbia dracunculoides*	Dragon Spurge	Ayurvedic
Charmi	*Betula utilis*	Himalayan Silver Birch, Indian Paper Tree	Ayurvedic
Charmi-vrksha	*Ehretia laevis*	Datrang Tree	Ayurvedic
Chathurakkali	*Euphorbia antiquorum*	Triangular Spurge	Siddha/Tamil
Chathuramulla	*Myxopyrum serratulum*	Yellow-flowered Myxopyrum	Folk
Chathuravalli	*Myxopyrum serratulum*	Yellow-flowered Myxopyrum	Folk
Chatrod	*Berberis vulgaris*	Common Barberry, True Barberry	Folk

Table Contd.

Indian Name	Botanical Name	English Name	Medicinal System
Chaturaangi	*Lantana camara*	Lantana, Wild Sage, Surinam Tea Plant	Ayurvedic
Chaturangula	*Cassia fistula*	Indian Laburnum, Purging Cassia, Golden Shower	Ayurvedic
Chaturdhaaraa	*Cissus quadrangula*	Square Stalked Vine, Adamant Creeper	Ayurvedic
Chatushpatri	*Blepharis edulis*	Acanthus	Ayurvedic
Chatushpatri	*Marsilea minuta*	Dwarf Waterclover, Pepperwort	Ayurvedic
Chauhaara	*Artemisia maritima*	Wormseed, Santonica	Ayurvedic
Chaupaitra	*Marsilea minuta*	Dwarf Waterclover, Pepperwort	Ayurvedic
Chavika	*Piper chaba*	Java Long Pepper	Ayurvedic
Chavya	*Balanophora involucrata*	Knotted-Cup Vine	Ayurvedic
Chavya	*Piper chaba*	Java Long Pepper	Ayurvedic
Chebisa	*Peristrophe bicalyculata*	Panicled Peristrophe	Siddha/Tamil
Cheddavokko	*Walsura trifoliata*	Walursi	Siddha/Tamil
Cheeku	*Achras zapota*	Sapota, Sapodilla Plum, Chicle	Unani
Cheemaat	*Scutia myrtina*	Chimat Fruit	Folk
Cheenaa	*Panicum miliaceum*	Common Millet, Proso Millet, Hog Millet	Ayurvedic
Cheenia-Gulaab	*Rosa bourboniana*	Bourbon Rose	Ayurvedic
Cheenitroghaans	*Geranium nepalense*	Nepal Geranium, Nepalese Crane's Bill	Folk/Nepalese
Cheerakam	*Cuminum cyminum*	Cumin	Siddha/Tamil
Chemmulli	*Barleria prionitis*	Common Yellow Nail Dye Plant	Siddha/Tamil
Chenaa	*Panicum miliaceum*	Common Millet, Proso Millet, Hog Millet	Folk
Chenaikkizhangu	*Amorphophallus campanulatus*	Elephant's Foot Yam	Siddha/Tamil
Chench Shaaka	*Corchorus aestuans*	White Jute	Folk
Chendurakam	*Carthamus tinctorius*	Safflower	Siddha/Tamil
Cheppu-nerinjal	*Rotula aquatica*	Aquatic Rotula	Siddha/Tamil
Cheppunerinjil	*Indigofera enneaphylla*	Trailing Indigo	Siddha/Tamil
Cherailu	*Rhododendron campanulatum*	Paper-bark Azalea	Folk

Table Contd.

Indian Name	Botanical Name	English Name	Medicinal System
Cherutekku	*Clerodendrum serratum*	Blue-flowered Glory Tree, Beetle Killer	Siddha/Tamil
Chetikaa	*Jasminum officinale*	Spanish Jasmine	Ayurvedic
Chhaagakarna	*Dipterocarpus turbinatus*	Common Gurjun Tree, Wood Oil Tree	Ayurvedic
Chhaagakarna	*Vateria indica*	White Damar, Indian Copal-Tree, Malabar Tallow Tree, Piney Varnish-Tree	Ayurvedic
Chhaagalaantri	*Ipomoea petaloidea*	False Jalap, Hawaii Morning Glory	Ayurvedic
Chhaagalshrngi	*Gymnema sylvestre*	Australian Cow Plant, Gymnema	Ayurvedic
Chhaalia	*Areca catechu*	Areca Nut, Betel Nut	Unani
Chhaatim	*Alstonia scholaris*	Devil's Tree, Dita Bark Tree	Unani
Chhaduaa	*Rhamnus virgata*	Indian Buckthorn	Folk
Chhagalaantri	*Ipomoea pes-caprae*	Goat's Foot Creeper	Ayurvedic
Chhagul-bati	*Naravelia zeylanica*	Naravelia Climber	Ayurvedic
Chhail	*Capparis sepiaria*	Indian Caper	Folk
Chhardana	*Randia dumetorum*	Common Emetic Nut	Ayurvedic
Chharela	*Cetraria islandica*	Cetraria, Iceland Lichen, Liceland Moss	Folk
Chharelaa	*Parmelia perlata*	Parmelia Lichen	Unani
Chhatraa	*Coriandrum sativum*	Coriander	Ayurvedic
Chhatraamlikaa	*Oxalis corniculata*	Indian Sorrel	Ayurvedic
Chhatrakam	*Agaricus campestris*	Field Mushroom, Edible Mushroom	Ayurvedic
Chhatri	*Leea indica*	Purple-berry Holly	Ayurvedic
Chhatri	*Mahonia nepaulensis*	Holly Leaved Berberry	Folk
Chhengam	*Capparis aphylla*	Caper Berry	Siddha/Tamil
Chhikkikaa	*Centipeda orbicularis*	Sneezewort	Ayurvedic
Chhikkini	*Centipeda orbicularis*	Sneezewort	Ayurvedic
Chhilihinta	*Cocculus hirsutus*	Broom-Creeper, Ink-Berry	Ayurvedic
Chhinipatra	*Evolvulus nummularius*	Round-leaf Bindweed	Folk
Chhitavan	*Alstonia scholaris*	Devil's Tree, Dita Bark Tree	Folk
Chhochhidan	*Momordica balsamina*	Balsam Apple	Folk

Table Contd.

Indian Name	Botanical Name	English Name	Medicinal System
Chhotaa Chand	*Rauvolfia serpentina*	Rauvolfia Root, Serpentina Root, Indian Snakeroot	Folk
Chhotaa Chirayataa	*Enicostemma littorale*	Indian Gentian	Folk
Chhotaa Kuuta	*Sagittaria trifolia*	Old World Arrowhead	Folk
Chhuhaaraa (dry date)	*Phoenix dactylifera*	Date Palm	Ayurvedic
Chhuharaa	*Phoenix dactylifera*	Date Palm	Unani
Chhuimui	*Mimosa pudica*	Sensitive-plant, Humble-Plant	Unani
Chichidaa	*Achyranthes aspera*	Prickly Chaff Flower	Folk
Chichinda	*Trichosanthes anguina*	Snake-Gourd	Ayurvedic
Chichoda	*Cyperus esculentus*	Earth Almond, Chufa, Rush Nut, Tiger Nut	Ayurvedic
Chichodaa	*Cyperus esculentus*	Earth Almond, Chufa, Rush Nut, Tiger Nut	Folk
Chichodaa	*Scirpus articulatus*	Paddyfield Club-Rush	Folk
Chiddavintai	*Xylopia parviflora*	Netawu, Atuketiya	Folk/Tamil
Chikesoppu	*Tetragonia expansa*	New Zealand Spinach	Folk/Karnataka
Chikondaa	*Trichosanthes anguina*	Snake-Gourd	Folk
Chikrassy	*Chukrasia tabularis*	Bastard Cedar, White Cedar, Indian Red Wood	Folk/Bengal
Chikri	*Buxus wallichiana*	Himalayan Boxwood Tree	Folk
Chikri	*Girardinia heterophylla*	Himalayan Nettle	Folk
Chikti	*Triumfetta rhomboidea*	Burbush, Burweed	Folk
Chilanti	*Ochna jabotapita*	Bird's Eye Bush	Folk/Tamil
Chilar	*Acacia torta*	Twisted Acacia	Folk
Chilauni	*Schima wallichii*	Chilauni Needle Wood	Folk
Chilgozaa	*Pinus gerardiana*	Neosia Pine, Edible Pine, Chilgoza Pine	Unani
Chilhaka	*Casearia tomentosa*	Fish-Poison Wood	Ayurvedic
Chillaa	*Casearia tomentosa*	Fish-Poison Wood	Folk
Chillaa	*Pinus excelsa*	Indian Blue Pine, Bhutan Pine, Five-leaved Pine	Folk
Chillika	*Chenopodium album*	Fat Hen, Lamb's Quarters, White Goosefoot, Wild Spinach, Pigweed	Ayurvedic

Table Contd.

Indian Name	Botanical Name	English Name	Medicinal System
Chiru Thekku	*Premna herbacea*	Bharangi Tree, Qian jie cao (Chinese)	Siddha/Tamil
Chiru-illantai	*Ximenia americana*	Tallow-Wood, False Sandal-Wood	Folk/Tamil
Chirukila chiru	*Carissa opaca*	Karaunda	Siddha/Tamil
Chitra	*Citrullus colocynthis*	Colocynth Bitter Apple	Ayurvedic
Chitraa	*Ricinus communis*	Castor Seed	Ayurvedic
Chitrabija	*Ricinus communis*	Castor Seed	Ayurvedic
Chitraka	*Plumbago zeylanica*	Ceylon Leadwort	Ayurvedic
Chitrakrt	*Ougeinia dalbergioides*	Chariot Tree, Punjab Kino	Ayurvedic
Chitraparni	*Uraria picta*	Trailing Uraria	Ayurvedic
Chitrapatra	*Betula utilis*	Himalayan Silver Birch, Indian Paper Tree	Ayurvedic
Chitraphalaa	*Bryonopsis laciniosa*	Bryony	Ayurvedic
Chitraphalaa	*Citrullus colocynthis*	Colocynth Bitter Apple	Ayurvedic
Chitraraththai	*Alpinia officinarum*	Lesser Galangal, Alpinia, Catarrh Root, Chinese Ginger	Siddha/Tamil
Chitraraththai	*Alpinia speciosa*	Light Galangal	Siddha/Tamil
Chitratandula	*Embelia ribes*	Embelia	Ayurvedic
Chitrmutti	*Sida rhombifolia*	Red-flowered Mallow	Siddha/Tamil
Chittavarai	*Rhynchosia minima*	Rhynchosia	Folk
Chitti-ita	*Phoenix pusilla*	Wild Coromandel Palm	Folk/Telugu
Chittramoolam	*Plumbago zeylanica*	Ceylon Leadwort	Siddha/Tamil
Chivuka	*Pterospermum acerifolium*	Hathipaila	Ayurvedic
Chobachini (bigger var.)	*Smilax glabra*	Bulbous China Root	Ayurvedic
Chobachini	*Smilax china*	China Root	Ayurvedic
Chobchini	*Smilax china*	China Root	Unani
Chob-hayaat	*Guaiacum officinale*	Lignum Vitae, Tree-of-life, Pockwood Tree	Unani
Chochaa	*Cinnamomum zeylanicum*	Cinnamon, Ceylon Cinnamon	Ayurvedic
Choh-hanka	*Oxyria digyna*	Mountain Sorrel, Alpine Sorrel	Siddha/Tamil
Chokkala	*Callicarpa macrophylla*	Perfumed Cherry	Siddha/Tamil
Chona Atthi	*Ficus hispida*	Devil's Fig, Rough-leaved Fig	Siddha/Tamil

Table Contd.

Indian Name	Botanical Name	English Name	Medicinal System
Choncha	*Cinnamomum zeylanicum*	Cinnamon, Ceylon Cinnamon	Ayurvedic
Chopachini	*Smilax china*	China Root	Ayurvedic
Chopra	*Euonymus tingens*	Spindle Wood, Wahoo	Folk
Choraka	*Angelica glauca*	Angelica	Ayurvedic
Chorakaa	*Angelica glauca*	Angelica	Ayurvedic
Chorakaakhya	*Angelica glauca*	Angelica	Ayurvedic
Chorakapatra (var.)	*Ficus altissima*	Council Tree, Lofty Fig Tree	Ayurvedic
Choraka-patra	*Ficus cunia*	Indian Fig	Ayurvedic
Chorpaat	*Laportea crenulata*	Devil Nettle, Fever Nettle	Folk
Chowri	*Ceriops candolleana*	Compound Cymed Mangrove	Folk/Kannada
Chuglam	*Terminalia bialata*	Andamans Ash, Silver Grey Wood	Folk
Chuhaari Ajawaayin	*Artemisia maritima*	Wormseed, Santonica	Ayurvedic
Chuhai	*Phlogacanthus thyrsiflorus*	Nongmangkha, Banheka	Folk
Chukandar	*Beta vulgaris*	Beet Root, Garden Beet, Chard	Folk
Chukku (Dried rhizome)	*Zingiber officinale*	Ginger	Siddha/Tamil
Chuko	*Amaranthus caudatus*	Love-Lies-Bleeding, Tassel Flower	Folk
Chuko	*Rumex acetosella*	Sheep Sorrel	Ayurvedic
Chuko	*Rumex vesicarius*	Bladder Dock, Country Sorrel	Ayurvedic
Chukra	*Garcinia indica*	Kokam Butter Tree, Mangosteen Oil Tree	Ayurvedic
Chukra	*Rumex crispus*	Yellow Dock, Curled Dock	Ayurvedic
Chukra	*Rumex vesicarius*	Bladder-Dock, Country Sorrel	Ayurvedic
Chukraa	*Oxalis corniculata*	Indian Sorrel	Ayurvedic
Chukraa	*Tamarindus indica*	Tamarind Tree	Ayurvedic
Chukram	*Rumex acetosa*	Garden Sorrel, Sorrel Dock	Ayurvedic
Chukrikaa	*Oxalis corniculata*	Indian Sorrel	Ayurvedic
Chukrikaa	*Rumex acetosella*	Sheep Sorrel	Ayurvedic
Chukrikaa	*Rumex crispus*	Yellow Dock, Curled Dock	Ayurvedic
Chukrikaa	*Tamarindus indica*	Tamarind Tree	Ayurvedic

Table Contd.

Indian Name	Botanical Name	English Name	Medicinal System
Chumaa	*Hippophae rhamnoides*	Seabuckthorn, Sand Thorn	Folk
Chumlora	*Rumex hastatus*	Toothed Dock	Folk
Chunch	*Melochia corchorifolia*	Chocolate-Weed	Folk
Chunchu	*Corchorus aestuans*	White Jute	Ayurvedic
Chunda kadalai	*Cicer arietinum*	Bengal Gram, Chick Pea	Siddha/Tamil
Chundai	*Solanum erianthum*	Mullen Nightshade	Folk
Chundai	*Solanum torvum*	West Indian Turkey Berry	Siddha/Tamil
Chundan	*Salacia oblonga*	Saptrangi	Folk
Chungi	*Lagerstroemia parviflora*	Lendi, Benteak	Folk
Churnaa	*Ziziphus rugosa*	White Jujube	Folk
Chuta	*Mangifera indica*	Mango	Ayurvedic
Chuttakulaatigaa	*Aspidopterys indica*	Bokadvel	Folk/Telugu
Chuukaa	*Rumex acetosa*	Garden Sorrel, Sorrel Dock	Ayurvedic
Chuukaa	*Rumex scutatus*	French-Sorrel	Folk
Ciminukku	*Swietenia mahagoni*	West Indian Mahogany	Siddha/Tamil
Cleaver	*Galium aparine*	Goosegrass, Cleavers	Folk
Cleaver	*Galium verum*	Lady's Bedstraw, Cheese Rennet	Folk
Clover	*Trifolium pratense*	Red Clover	Unani
Cocoa	*Theobroma cacao*	Cocoa, Theobroma, Chocolate Tree	Folk
Cohosh	*Cimicifuga racemosa*	Black Cohosh Root, Black Snake Root	Folk
Cranberry Bark	*Viburnum opulus*	Cranberry Bush, Crampbark, Guelder Rose	Folk
Cress, Indian Posey	*Barbarea vulgaris*	Bitter Cress, Hedge Mustard, Yellow Rocket, Winter Cress	Folk
Cuscus	*Vetiveria zizanioides*	Vetiver, Khas	Unani
Cylon-keerai	*Talinum triangulare*	Ceylon Spinach, Surinam Purslane, Flame Flower, Sweet Heart, Water Leaf, Ceylon Spinach	Folk/Tamil
Daabh	*Imperata cylindrica*	Thatch Grass	Folk
Daadamaari	*Cassia tora*	Sickle Senna, Ringworm Plant	Folk

Table Contd.

Indian Name	Botanical Name	English Name	Medicinal System
Daadari	*Acalypha ciliata*	Smaller var. Acalypha	Folk
Daadima	*Punica granatum*	Pomegranate	Ayurvedic
Daadimachhada	*Aphanamixis polystachya*	Amoora	Ayurvedic
Daadimapushpaka	*Aphanamixis polystachya*	Amoora	Ayurvedic
Daadimba	*Punica granatum*	Pomegranate	Ayurvedic
Daadimchhada	*Tecomella undulata*	Rohida Tree	Ayurvedic
Daadim-pushpaka	*Tecomella undulata*	Rohida Tree	Ayurvedic
Daadmaari	*Ammannia baccifera*	Blistering Ammannia	Folk
Daadmaari	*Cassia alata*	Ringworm Cassia	Folk
Daadmaari	*Xyris indica*	Yellow-eyed Grass	Ayurvedic
Daakh	*Vitis vinifera*	Wine Grape, European Grape	Ayurvedic
Daakh	*Vitis vinifera*	Wine Grape, European Grape	Unani
Daalchini	*Cinnamomum cassia*	Chinese Cinnamon, Cassia bark	Ayurvedic
Daantiraa	*Ficus heterophylla*	Oak-Leaf Fig	Folk
Daarchini	*Cinnamomum zeylanicum*	Cinnamon, Ceylon Cinnamon	Unani
Daarchob	*Curcuma amada*	Mango-ginger, Wild Turmeric	Unani
Daarchob	*Curcuma aromatica*	Wild Turmeric, Yellow Zedoary	Unani
Daarfilfil	*Piper longum*	Indian Long Pepper, Joborandi	Unani
Daarhald	*Berberis aristata*	Indian Barberry	Unani
Daaru	*Berberis aristata*	Indian Barberry	Ayurvedic
Daaru	*Cedrus deodara*	Himalayan Cedar, Deodar	Ayurvedic
Daaruchini	*Cinnamomum zeylanicum*	Cinnamon, Ceylon Cinnamon	Ayurvedic
Daaruharidraa	*Berberis aristata*	Indian Barberry	Ayurvedic
Daaruharidraa	*Berberis chitria*	Barberry	Ayurvedic
Daaruka	*Cedrus deodara*	Himalayan Cedar, Deodar	Ayurvedic
Daarunaj Aqrabi	*Doronicum hookeri*	Leopard's Bane	Unani
Daarunaj Aqrabi	*Doronicum pardalianches*	Leopard's Bane	Unani
Daarunaj Aqrabi Hindi	*Doronicum roylei*	Leopard's Bane	Unani

Table Contd.

Indian Name	Botanical Name	English Name	Medicinal System
Daarunishaa	*Berberis aristata*	Indian Barberry	Ayurvedic
Daarurajani	*Berberis aristata*	Indian Barberry	Ayurvedic
Daarusitaa	*Cinnamomum zeylanicum*	Cinnamon, Ceylon Cinnamon	Ayurvedic
Daarvi	*Berberis aristata*	Indian Barberry	Ayurvedic
Dabi	*Cadaba fruticosa*	Indian Cadaba	Folk
Dadap	*Erythrina indica*	Indian Coral Tree	Ayurvedic
Dadhiphala	*Feronia limonia*	Wood Apple	Ayurvedic
Dadhipushpi	*Trichosanthes anguina*	Snake-Gourd	Ayurvedic
Dadhittha	*Feronia limonia*	Wood Apple	Ayurvedic
Dadrughna	*Cassia alata*	Ringworm Cassia	Ayurvedic
Dadrughna	*Cassia tora*	Sickle Senna, Ringworm Plant	Ayurvedic
Dadrumardana	*Cassia alata*	Ringworm Cassia	Ayurvedic
Dahana	*Paullinia asiatica*	Lopez Root Tree, Wild Orange Tree, Forest Pepper	Ayurvedic
Dahana	*Plumbago zeylanica*	Ceylon Leadwort	Ayurvedic
Daitya	*Selinum tenuifolium*	Cow Parsley	Ayurvedic
Dakhini Babool	*Pithecellobium dulce*	Minila Tamarind, Madras Thorn, Quamachil	Folk
Daleek (Fruit)	*Rosa damascena*	Damask Rose	Unani
Dalme	*Securinega suffruticosa*	Securinega	Folk
Dalmi	*Osyris wightiana*	African Sandalwood, Zanzibar Lawa Wood	Folk
Dalmia	*Osyris wightiana*	African Sandalwood, Zanzibar Lawa Wood	Folk
Damanaa	*Artemisia vulgaris*	Indian Wormwood, Fleabane, Dungwort, Mugwort, Wild Wormwood	Folk
Damanaka	*Artemisia vulgaris*	Indian Wormwood, Fleabane, Dungwort, Mugwort, Wild Wormwood	Ayurvedic
Dambu	*Phragmites communis*	Common Reed	Folk/Punjab
Damm-ul-Akhwain	*Daemonorops draco*	East Indian Dragon's Blood	Unani

Table Contd.

Indian Name	Botanical Name	English Name	Medicinal System
Dammul-Akhwain	*Dracaena cinnabari*	Dragon's Blood	Unani
Dandal	*Xylosma longifolium*	Dandal Tree, Kandhara Tree	Folk
Dandotpalaa	*Vernonia cinerea*	Ash Coloured Fleabane, Purple Fleabane	Ayurvedic
Dankuni	*Canscora decussata*	Conch-flowered Bindweed	Ayurvedic
Danshir	*Reissantia grahamii*	Pristimera Root	Folk
Dantabijaa	*Punica granatum*	Pomegranate	Ayurvedic
Dantashatha	*Citrus limon*	Lemon	Ayurvedi
Dantchhadaa	*Coccinia indica*	Ivy-Gourd	Ayurvedic
Dantdhaavan	*Acacia catechu*	Cutch tree, Catechu	Ayurvedic
Danti	*Baliospermum montanum*	False Croton	Ayurvedic
Danti	*Gymnosporia spinosa*	Celastrus Tree	Folk/Telugu
Danti	*Jatropha multifida*	Coral Plant, Physic Nut	Folk
Dantibija	*Croton tiglium*	Purging Croton	Ayurvedic
Dantshatha	*Feronia limonia*	Wood Apple	Ayurvedic
Daphni	*Laurus nobilis*	Laurel, Sweet Bay	Unani
Daradharsha	*Eruca sativa*	Rocket-Salad	Ayurvedic
Darakht e Reesh	*Ficus beng(h)alensis*	Banyan Tree	Unani
Darbha	*Imperata cylindrica*	Thatch Grass	Ayurvedic
Darduradalaa	*Bacopa monnieri*	Thyme-leaved Gratiola	Ayurvedic
Dariyaayee Naariyal	*Lodoicea maldivica*	Double Coconut Palm, Sea Coconut Palm	Ayurvedic
Darkht-e-Shaan	*Abutilon indicum*	Country Mallow, Flowering Maples, Chinese Bell-flowers	Unani
Daruharidraa	*Berberis vulgaris*	Common Barberry, True Barberry	Ayurvedic
Darvipatraa	*Onosma bracteatum*	Borage	Ayurvedic
Dasbaha	*Belamcanda chinensis*	Leopard Lily	Folk/Bengal
Dasbichandi	*Belamcanda chinensis*	Leopard Lily	Folk/Bengal
Dasmori	*Elytraria crenata*	Dasmori	Folk
Datarangi	*Ehretia laevis*	Datrang Tree	Folk
Datura (American)	*Brugmansia suaveolens*	Angel's Trumpet, Angel's Tears	Folk

Table Contd.

Indian Name	Botanical Name	English Name	Medicinal System
Daturaa	*Physochlaina praealta*	Hyoscyamine Plant	Folk
Daunaa	*Artemisia vulgaris*	Indian Wormwood, Fleabane, Dungwort, Mugwort, Wild Wormwood	Folk
Daushir	*Reissantia grahamii*	Pristimera Root	Folk
Davaa-e-junoon	*Rauvolfia serpentina*	Rauvolfia Root, Serpentina Root, Indian Snakeroot	Unani
Dayaa-kunji	*Hyssopus officinalis*	Hyssop	Ayurvedic
Deepamaal	*Leonotis nepetaefolia*	Christmas Candlestick, Jonny Collins, Lion's Ear, Lion's Tail	Folk
Deodaar	*Cedrus deodara*	Himalayan Cedar, Deodar	Unani
Desi Ajawaayin	*Trachyspermum ammi*	Ammi, Lovage, Carum, Ajowan	Unani
Desi Akarkaraa	*Spilanthes calva*	Para Cress	Folk
Desi Akarkaraa	*Spilanthes oleracea*	Brazilian Cress, Para Cress	Ayurvedic
Desi Asgandh	*Withania coagulans*	Vegetable Rennet, Indian Cheese-maker	Unani
Desi Baadaam	*Terminalia catappa*	Indian Almond, Tropical Almond	Folk
Desi Gokharu	*Tribulus alatus*	Winged Caltrops	Folk
Desi Gulab	*Rosa bourboniana*	Bourbon Rose	Folk
Desi Ushbaa	*Decalepis hamiltonii*	Sweet Sarsaparilla	Unani
Devaahvaa	*Cedrus deodara*	Himalayan Cedar, Deodar	Ayurvedic
Devadaali	*Luffa echinata*	Bristly Luffa	Ayurvedic
Devadaari	*Polyalthia longifolia*	Mast Tree, Fake Asoka Tree, False Devadaru, Cemetry Tree	Ayurvedic
Devadaaru	*Cedrus deodara*	Himalayan Cedar, Deodar	Ayurvedic
Devadaram	*Erythroxylum monogynum*	Bastard Sandal, Red Cedar	Siddha/Tamil
Devadhoop	*Balsamodendron mukul*	Indian Bdellium, Gum Guggul	Ayurvedic
Devadruma	*Cedrus deodara*	Himalayan Cedar, Deodar	Ayurvedic
Deva-dundhubhi	*Ocimum sanctum*	Holy Basil, Sacred Basil	Ayurvedic
Devakaashtha	*Cedrus deodara*	Himalayan Cedar, Deodar	Ayurvedic
Devakusum	*Syzygium aromaticum*	Clove	Ayurvedic
Devanala (var.)	*Lobelia leschenaultiana*	Poisonous Pukeweed	Folk

Table Contd.

Indian Name	Botanical Name	English Name	Medicinal System
Devanala	*Lobelia inflata*	Indian Tabacco, Pukeweed	Ayurvedic
Devanala	*Lobelia nicotianaefolia*	Wild Tobacco	Ayurvedic
Devapushpa	*Syzygium aromaticum*	Clove	Ayurvedic
Devarigaanl	*Polygonatum cirrhifolium*	Solomon's Seal	Folk
Devataadaka	*Luffa echinata*	Bristly Luffa	Ayurvedic
Devataruni	*Rosa centifolia*	Cabbage Rose, Provence Rose, Hundred-leaved Rose	Ayurvedic
Devdhuupa	*Vateria indica*	White Damar, Indian Copal-Tree, Malabar Tallow Tree, Piney Varnish-Tree	Ayurvedic
Devi	*Marsdenia tenacissima*	White Turpeth	Ayurvedic
Dhaak	*Butea monosperma*	Flame of the Forest, Butea Gum, Bengal Kino	Unani
Dhaamaargava	*Luffa cylindrica*	Smooth Luffa, Sponge-gourd, Sponge Cucumber	Ayurvedic
Dhaaman	*Grewia tiliaefolia*	Dhaman	Folk
Dhaamin	*Grewia tiliaefolia*	Dhaman	Folk
Dhaanaa	*Coriandrum sativum*	Coriander	Ayurvedic
Dhaanya	*Coriandrum sativum*	Coriander	Ayurvedic
Dhaanyaka	*Coriandrum sativum*	Coriander	Ayurvedic
Dhaanya-ruk	*Claviceps purpurea*	Ergot of Rye, Fungus of Rye	Ayurvedic
Dhaanyeyaka	*Coriandrum sativum*	Coriander	Ayurvedic
Dhaaraa-kadamba	*Adina cordifolia*	Yellow Teak, Saffron Teak	Ayurvedic
Dhaaru	*Brunella vulgaris*	Self-heal	Folk
Dhaaru	*Lavandula stoechas*	Arabian or French Lavender	Folk
Dhaataki	*Woodfordia fruticosa*	Fire-flame Bush, Shiranjitea	Ayurvedic
Dhaatri	*Emblica officinalis*	Embic, Indian Gooseberry	Ayurvedic
Dhaatri	*Woodfordia fruticosa*	Fire-flame Bush, Shiranjitea	Ayurvedic
Dhaatriparni	*Abies webbiana*	Indian Silver Fir, The West-Himalayan High-Level Fir, The East-Himalayan Fir	Ayurvedic

Table Contd.

Indian Name	Botanical Name	English Name	Medicinal System
Dhaatripatra	*Abies webbiana*	Indian Silver Fir, The West-Himalayan High-Level Fir, The East-Himalayan Fir	Ayurvedic
Dhaatri-patra	*Taxus baccata*	European Yew	Ayurvedic
Dhaatriphala	*Emblica officinalis*	Embic, Indian Gooseberry	Ayurvedic
Dhaavaa	*Anogeissus latifolia*	Axle-wood, Button Tree, Ghatti Tree	Unani
Dhaavani	*Solanum xanthocarpum*	Wild Eggplant, Yellow-Berried Nightshade	Ayurvedic
Dhaavani	*Uraria picta*	Trailing Uraria	Ayurvedic
Dhabbar	*Anagallis arvensis*	Bird's Eye, Bird's Tongue, Blue Pimpernel, Scarlet Pimpernel	Folk (Punjab)
Dhamaasaa	*Fagonia cretica*	Thorny Fagonbush, Mantle of the Virgin	Unani
Dhamana	*Arundo donax*	Great Reed, Spanish-Bamboo-Reed, Giant-Bamboo-Reed	Ayurvedic
Dhanaka	*Vitex negundo*	Five-leaved Chaste Tree	Ayurvedic
Dhananjaya	*Terminalia arjuna*	Arjun Terminalia	Ayurvedic
Dhanavalli	*Naravelia zeylanica*	Naravelia Climber	Ayurvedic
Dhanhar	*Angelica glauca*	Angelica	Ayurvedic
Dhanika	*Coriandrum sativum*	Coriander	Ayurvedic
Dhanikaa	*Coriandrum sativum*	Coriander	Ayurvedic
Dhaniyaa	*Coriandrum sativum*	Coriander	Ayurvedic
Dhanur-vriksha	*Grewia tiliaefolia*	Dhaman	Ayurvedic
Dhanvana	*Grewia sclerophylla*	Bhokota	Ayurvedic
Dhanvana	*Grewia tiliaefolia*	Dhaman	Ayurvedic
Dhanvayaasa	*Fagonia cretica*	Thorny Fagonbush, Mantle of the Virgin	Ayurvedic
Dhanvayaasaka	*Fagonia cretica*	Thorny Fagonbush, Mantle of the Virgin	Ayurvedic
Dhanvayavaasa	*Fagonia cretica*	Thorny Fagonbush, Mantle of the Virgin	Ayurvedic
Dhanvi	*Mimusops elengi*	Spanish-Cherry, West Indian Medlar, Bullet Wood	Ayurvedic

Table Contd.

Indian Name	Botanical Name	English Name	Medicinal System
Dharba	*Imperata cylindrica*	Thatch Grass	Siddha/Tamil
Dhar-Karelaa	*Momordica dioica*	Small Bitter Gourd, burr Cucumber	Folk
Dhastura	*Datura metel*	Thornapple, Downy Datura	Ayurvedic
Dhattuura	*Datura alba*	Thornapple	Ayurvedic
Dhattuura	*Datura innoxia*	Angel's Trumpet, Sacred Datura	Ayurvedic
Dhattuura	*Datura metel*	Thornapple, Downy Datura	Ayurvedic
Dhaturaa	*Datura alba*	Thornapple	Unani
Dhaturaa	*Datura innoxia*	Angel's Trumpet, Sacred Datura	Unani
Dhaturaa	*Datura metel*	Thornapple, Downy Datura	Unani
Dhaturaa	*Datura stramonium*	Thornapple, Jimsonweed, Stramonium	Unani
Dhaulaa-findauri	*Nothosaerva brachiata*	Grains of Selim	Folk
Dhauli Musali	*Chlorophytum tuberosum*	White Musali	Folk
Dhauraa	*Lagerstroemia parviflora*	Lendi, Benteak	Folk
Dhava	*Anogeissus latifolia*	Axle-wood, Button Tree, Ghatti Tree	Ayurvedic
Dhaval-baruaa	*Rauvolfia serpentina*	Rauvolfia Root, Serpentina Root, Indian Snakeroot	Folk
Dheniaani	*Olax scandens*	Olax	Ayurvedic
Dhira	*Microstylis wallichii*	Rshabhaka	Ayurvedic
Dhobi Deeb	*Xyris indica*	Yellow-eyed Grass	Ayurvedic
Dhohan	*Grewia villosa*	Tamthar	Folk
Dhol	*Lindenbergia indica*	Nettle-leaved Lindenbergia	Folk
Dholphuli	*Aerva javanica*	Javanese Wool Plant	Folk
Dholsamudra	*Leea macrophylla*	Tuberous Holly	Folk
Dhruv	*Ficus beng(h)alensis*	Banyan Tree	Ayurvedic
Dhumrapatra	*Aristolochia bracteolata*	Bracteated Birthwort	Ayurvedic
Dhundul	*Xylocarpus granatum*	The Puzzle Fruit Tree	Folk
Dhurandhara	*Anogeissus latifolia*	Axle-wood, Button Tree, Ghatti Tree	Ayurvedic

Table Contd.

Indian Name	Botanical Name	English Name	Medicinal System
Dhurchuk	*Hippophae rhamnoides*	Seabuckthorn, Sand Thorn	Folk
Dhurpi Saaga	*Leucas cephalotes*	Dhurpi Vegetable	Folk
Dhustuura	*Datura metel*	Thornapple, Downy Datura	Ayurvedic
Dhustuuraka	*Datura metel*	Thornapple, Downy Datura	Ayurvedic
Dhuumrapatraa	*Nicotiana tabacum*	Tobacco	Ayurvedic
Dhuup	*Jurinea macrocephala*	Temple Incense Root	Folk
Dhuupavriksha	*Pinus roxburghii*	Long-leaved Pine, Three-leaved Pine, Chir Pine	Ayurvedic
Dhuupa-vriksha	*Shorea robusta*	Sal Tree	Ayurvedic
Dhuurta	*Datura metel*	Thornapple, Downy Datura	Ayurvedic
Dhuurta	*Datura stramonium*	Thornapple, Jimsonweed, Stramonium	Ayurvedic
Dhvankshamaachi	*Solanum nigrum*	Black Nightshade	Ayurvedic
Dhyaamaka	*Cymbopogon martinii*	Rosha Grass, Palmarosa	Ayurvedic
Dhyaamaka	*Valeriana pyrolaefolia*	Smaller-rhizome Jatamansi	Ayurvedic
Didhi	*Sonchus asper*	Spinyleaved Sow Thistle	Folk
Dieng-soh kajut	*Phlogacanthus thyrsiflorus*	Nongmangkha, Banheka	Folk
Diflaa	*Nerium indicum*	Indian Oleander, White Oleander	Unani
Digsaa	*Pinus khasya*	Khasi Pine	Folk
Dikaamaali	*Gardenia gummifera*	Gummy Cape Jasmine	Unani
Dikaamaali	*Gardenia resinifera*	Brilliant Gardenia, Cambi Resin Tree	Unani
Dikamalli	*Gardenia gummifera*	Gummy Cape Jasmine	Siddha/Tamil
Dikkamalli	*Gardenia resinifera*	Brilliant Gardenia, Cambi Resin Tree	Siddha/Tamil
Dil	*Phragmites communis*	Common Reed	Folk/Punjab
Dill	*Indigofera oblongifolia*	Wild Indigo, Mysore Panicled Indigo	Ayurvedic
Dimok	*Mycrotomia benthami*	Pseudo-Ratanjot	Folk
Dinesh	*Calotropis gigantea*	Swallow Wort	Ayurvedic
Dineshavalli	*Alkanna tinctoria*	Alkanet, Dyers' or Spanish Bugloss	Siddha/Tamil
Dipani	*Trigonella foenum-graecum*	Fenugreek	Ayurvedic

Table Contd.

Indian Name	Botanical Name	English Name	Medicinal System
Dipyaka	*Apium graveolens*	Celery	Ayurvedic
Dipyaka	*Apium leptophyllum*	Celery	Ayurvedic
Dipyaka	*Trachyspermum ammi*	Ammi, Lovage, Carum, Ajowan	Ayurvedic
Dipyaka	*Trachyspermum roxburghianum*	Ajmud	Ayurvedic
Dirgha-chhada	*Saccharum officinarum*	Gannaa, Naishakar	Ayurvedic
Dirghakeelaka	*Alangium lamarckii*	Sage-leaf Alangium	Ayurvedic
Dirghapatrakaa	*Diospyros melanoxylon*	Coromandel Ebony, Persimmon	Ayurvedic
Dirghavalli	*Cocculus hirsutus*	Broom-Creeper, Ink-Berry	Ayurvedic
Dirghavranta	*Ailanthus excelsa*	Tree of Heaven, Maharukh	Ayurvedic
Dirghkantaka	*Balanites aegyptiaca*	Desert Date	Ayurvedic
Dirmanah	*Artemisia maritima*	Wormseed, Santonica	Unani
Dittany	*Dictamnus albus*	Gas Plant, Dittany, Burning Bush	Folk
Divi-divi	*Caesalpinia coriaria*	American Sumac, Divi-divi Plant	Folk
Divyapushpa	*Nerium indicum*	Indian Oleander, White Oleander	Ayurvedic
Divyapushpa	*Thevetia peruviana*	Yellow Oleander	Ayurvedic
Diyaanku	*Hyssopus officinalis*	Hyssop	Folk
Dochunty	*Ageratum conyzoides*	Goat Weed, White Weed	Ayurvedic
Dodaka	*Sonchus oleraceus*	Milk Thistle	Folk
Dodishaak	*Leptadenia reticulata*	Dodi Vegetable	Folk
Doraa-baahaa	*Vernonia roxburghii*	Himalayan Fleabane	Folk
Draakshaa	*Vitis vinifera*	Wine Grape, European Grape	Ayurvedic
Draavida	*Curcuma zedoaria*	Zedoary, Zerumbet	Ayurvedic
Draavidi	*Elettaria cardamomum*	Lesser Cardamom	Ayurvedic
Dravanti	*Croton tiglium*	Purging Croton	Ayurvedic
Dreka	*Melia azedarach*	Persian Lilac, Pride of India	Ayurvedic
Drekaa	*Thlaspi arvense*	Pennycress, Fanweed	Folk
Droma	*Potentilla anserina*	Silverweed, Goose Grass	Folk/Tibet
Dronpushpi	*Leucas aspera*	White Dead Nettle	Ayurvedic
Dronpushpi	*Leucas cephalotes*	Dhurpi Vegetable	Ayurvedic
Dronpushpi	*Leucas lavandulaefolia*	Sacred Flower-Weed	Ayurvedic

Table Contd.

Indian Name	Botanical Name	English Name	Medicinal System
Feranjmushk	*Dracocephalum moldavica*	Dragon's Head	Unani
Filfil Daraaz	*Piper longum*	Indian Long Pepper, Joborandi	Unani
Filfil Safed	*Piper nigrum*	White Pepper	Unani
Filfil Siyaah	*Piper nigrum*	Black Pepper	Unani
Filfil-e-Ahmar	*Capsicum annuum*	Chilli, Red Pepper	Unani
Filfil-e-Surkh	*Capsicum annuum*	Chilli, Red Pepper	Unani
Findora	*Lilium wallichianum*	Trumpet-shaped Golden Lily	Folk
Fitraasaaliyum	*Petroselinum crispum*	Parsley	Unani
Fitraasaaliyun	*Prangos pabularia*	Prangos, Yugan. Aju-Chach	Unani
Frashbean	*Phaseolus vulgaris*	Kidney Bean, French Bean, Haricot Bean	Unani
Fritillary	*Fritillaria imperialis*	Crown Imperial, Imperial Fritillary	Folk
Fufal	*Areca catechu*	Areca Nut, Betel Nut	Unani
Funduq	*Corylus avellana*	European Hazel, Filbert	Unani
Gaajar	*Daucus carota*	Carrot, Cultivated Carrot, Wild Carrot	Unani
Gaajara	*Daucus carota*	Carrot, Cultivated Carrot, Wild Carrot	Ayurvedic
Gaandhaari	*Fagonia cretica*	Thorny Fagonbush, Mantle of the Virgin	Ayurvedic
Gaangeru (ki)	*Grewia populifolia*	Orange-red Phalsa, Tapadi	Ayurvedic
Gaanjaa	*Cannabis sativa*	Hemp, Indian Hemp	Ayurvedic
Gaayatri	*Acacia catechu*	Cutch tree, Catechu	Ayurvedic
Gaayotraa	*Lilium giganteum*	Giant Lily	Folk
Gada	*Saussurea lappa*	Kuth, Costus	Ayurvedic
Gadaga-vel	*Vandellia pedunculata*	Gadag Vine	Folk
Gadaha-purnaa	*Boerhavia diffusa*	Red-flowered Hogweed	Folk
Gadera	*Ceriops candolleana*	Compound Cymed Mangrove	Folk/Telugu
Gadgubar	*Ficus altissima*	Council Tree, Lofty Fig Tree	Folk
Gager-kanda	*Ranunculus arvensis*	Corn Buttercup	Folk
Gagger vurmi	*Rhododendron campanulatum*	Paper-bark Azalea	Folk
Gaidar	*Notonia grandiflora*	Common Fleshy Rag-weed	Folk

Table Contd.

Indian Name	Botanical Name	English Name	Medicinal System
Gajabhaksha	*Ficus religiosa*	Peepal, Bot-tree	Ayurvedic
Gajabhakshyaa	*Boswellia serrata*	Indian Frankincense, Indian Olibanum	Ayurvedic
Gajakrishna	*Scindapsus officinalis*	Sal Forest Pepper	Ayurvedic
Gajanaa	*Ficus cordifolia*	Rumpf's Fig	Folk
Gajapaadapa	*Ficus arnottiana*	Indian Rock Fig	Ayurvedic
Gajapippali	*Piper chaba*	Java Long Pepper	Ayurvedic
Gajapippali	*Scindapsus officinalis*	Sal Forest Pepper	Ayurvedic
Gajavaajipriyaa	*Ipomoea digitata*	Milky Yam	Ayurvedic
Gajavaajipriyaa	*Pueraria tuberosa*	Indian Kudze	Ayurvedic
Galgal	*Citrus limon*	Lemon	Folk
Galls—Chhoti-Maayin	*Tamarix aphylla*	Athel, Tamarisk	Folk
Galls-Maayin	*Tamarix dioica*	Tamarisk	Folk
Galot	*Ceropegia bulbosa*	Candlestick Ceropegia	Folk
Gambhaari	*Gmelina arborea*	Candahar Tree, White Teak	Ayurvedic
Gambhaari	*Gmelina asiatica*	Small Cashmere Tree	Ayurvedic
Gambhaari	*Trewia nudiflora*	False White Teak, Gutel	Ayurvedic
Ganda-Duurvaa	*Cyperus rotundus*	Nut Grass	Ayurvedic
Gandagaatra	*Annona squamosa*	Custard Apple, Sugar Apple, Sweet-sop	Ayurvedic
Gandam-gundu	*Lycopus europaeus*	Gipsywort, Bugleweed	Folk
Gandana	*Achillea millefolium*	Milfoil, Yarrow, Thousand Leaf	Folk
Gandanaa	*Allium ascalonicum*	Shellot	Unani
Gandbabuul	*Acacia farnesiana*	Cassie Flower, Sweet Acacia	Unani
Gandhaaddhyaa	*Rosa centifolia*	Cabbage Rose, Provence Rose, Hundred-leaved Rose	Ayurvedic
Gandhaari	*Bauhinia variegata*	Mountain Ebony, Buddhist Bauhinia	Ayurvedic
Gandhaarikaa	*Hedychium spicatum*	Spiked Ginger Ivy	Ayurvedic
Gandhabhaaduli	*Paederia foetida*	Skunk Vine	Folk
Gandha-daaru	*Lindera neesiana*	Spicebush, Benjamin Bush	Folk
Gandhadravya	*Cinnamomum camphora*	Camphor Tree	Ayurvedic
Gandhakuti	*Selinum tenuifolium*	Cow Parsley	Ayurvedic

Table Contd.

Indian Name	Botanical Name	English Name	Medicinal System
Gandhalataa	*Saccolabium papillosum*	Small Warty Acampe	Folk
Gandhali	*Paederia foetida*	Skunk Vine	Folk
Gandhamuulikaa	*Hedychium spicatum*	Spiked Ginger Ivy	Ayurvedic
Gandha-Palaasa	*Miliusa velutina*	Sal-Forest Miliusa	Folk
Gandhapalaashi	*Hedychium spicatum*	Spiked Ginger Ivy	Ayurvedic
Gandhaphala	*Trigonella foenum-graecum*	Fenugreek	Ayurvedic
Gandha-prasaarini	*Paederia foetida*	Skunk Vine	Ayurvedic
Gandha-priyangu	*Prunus mahaleb*	Mahaleb Cherry	Ayurvedic
Gandhapushpa	*Saraca asoca*	Ashoka Tree	Ayurvedic
Gandha-pushpika	*Trichodesma indicum*	Indian Borage	Ayurvedic
Gandhapuura	*Gaultheria fragrantissima*	Fragrant Wintergreen, Indian Wintergreen	Ayurvedic
Gandhapuurna	*Gaultheria fragrantissima*	Fragrant Wintergreen, Indian Wintergreen	Ayurvedic
Gandharaaja	*Gardenia jasminoides*	Cape Jasmine	Ayurvedic
Gandharasa	*Balsamodendron myrrha*	Myrrh, Herabol	Ayurvedic
Gandharva-gandhaa	*Withania ashwagandha*	Winter Cherry	Ayurvedic
Gandharvahastaa	*Ricinus communis*	Castor Seed	Ayurvedic
Gandhashathi	*Hedychium spicatum*	Spiked Ginger Ivy	Ayurvedic
Gandhavadhuu	*Hedychium spicatum*	Spiked Ginger Ivy	Ayurvedic
Gandhavati	*Selinum tenuifolium*	Cow Parsley	Ayurvedic
Gandh-Bihrojaa (Oleo-resin)	*Pinus roxburghii*	Long-leaved Pine, Three-leaved Pine, Chir Pine	Unani
Gandhela	*Murraya koenigii*	Curry-Leaf Tree	Folk
Gandh-giri	*Erythroxylum monogynum*	Bastard Sandal, Red Cedar	Folk
Gandhi-buuti	*Glinus lotoides*	Lotus Sweetjuice, Damascisa	Folk
Gandhini Revatikaa	*Rheum emodi*	Indian Rhubarb, Himalayan Rhubarb	Ayurvedic
Gandhmuulaka	*Curcuma zedoaria*	Zedoary, Zerumbet	Ayurvedic
Gandhnaakuli	*Aristolochia indica*	Indian Birthwort	Ayurvedic
Gandhotkata	*Artemisia vulgaris*	Indian Wormwood, Fleabane, Dungwort, Mugwort, Wild Wormwood	Ayurvedic

Table Contd.

Indian Name	Botanical Name	English Name	Medicinal System
Gandhphali	*Callicarpa macrophylla*	Perfumed Cherry	Ayurvedic
Gandhpriyangu	*Callicarpa macrophylla*	Perfumed Cherry	Ayurvedic
Gandhraayana	*Heracleum candicans*	Cowparsnip	Folk
Gandhsaara	*Santalum album*	White Sandalwood	Ayurvedic
Gandira	*Cayratia carnosa*	Cayratia	Ayurvedic
Gandira	*Coleus barbatus*	Coleus	Ayurvedic
Gandira	*Rubia cordifolia*	Indian Madder, Bengal Madder	Ayurvedic
Ganerukaa	*Pterospermum acerifolium*	Hathipaila	Ayurvedic
Ganesh-kand	*Rhaphidophora laciniata*	Pathos, Silver Vine	Folk
Gangaa Tulasi	*Artemisia vestita*	Russian Wormwood	Ayurvedic
Gangaa Tulasi	*Hyptis suaveolens*	American Mint American Patchouli	Folk
Gangaapatri	*Blumea balsamifera*	Nagai Camphor	Ayurvedic
Gangaati	*Sida spinosa*	Prickly Mallow	Ayurvedic
Ganga-muula	*Saussurea affinis*	East Asian Saw-wort	Folk
Gangawaa	*Excoecaria agallocha*	Blinding Tree	Folk
Gangeran	*Grewia populifolia*	Orange-red Phalsa, Tapadi	Folk
Gangeruki	*Canthium parviflorum*	Wild Jasmine	Ayurvedic
Gangeti	*Sida spinosa*	Prickly Mallow	Folk
Ganikaarikaa	*Clerodendrum phlomidis*	Glory Bower	Ayurvedic
Ganikaarikaa	*Premna integrifolia*	Headache Tree	Ayurvedic
Ganiyaari	*Premna integrifolia*	Headache Tree	Folk
Ganjamkorai	*Ocimum canum*	Hoary Basil	Folk/Tamil
Ganjikaa	*Cannabis sativa*	Hemp, Indian Hemp	Folk
Gannaa	*Saccharum officinarum*	Gannaa, Naishakar	Unani
Ganther	*Neuracanthus sphaerostachyus*	Pin Cushion Plant	Folk
Gaosheer	*Ferula galbaniflua*	Galbanum	Unani
Gaozabaan	*Anchusa italica*	Cow's Tongue Plant	Unani
Gaozabaan	*Borago officinalis*	Borage, Cow's Tongue Plant	Unani
Gaozabaan	*Caccinia crassifolia*	False Gaozaban	Unani
Gaozabaan	*Onosma bracteatum*	Borage	Unani
Gapasundi	*Pittosporum dasycaulon*	Pittosporum Cheesewood	Folk

Table Contd.

Indian Name	Botanical Name	English Name	Medicinal System
Garaagari	*Luffa echinata*	Bristly Luffa	Ayurvedic
Garaheduaa	*Coix lacryma-jobi*	Job's Tears	Folk
Garala	*Aconitum ferox*	Indian Aconite, Wolfsbane, Monkshood	Ayurvedic
Garbhanut	*Gloriosa superba*	Glory Lily, Super Lily, Tiger's Claws	Ayurvedic
Garbhapaatana	*Sapindus laurifolius*	Soapnut Tree of South India	Ayurvedic
Garbhapaatani	*Gloriosa superba*	Glory Lily, Super Lily, Tiger's Claws	Ayurvedic
Garbha-phool	*Anastatica hierochuntica*	Jericho Rose	Folk
Garbhda	*Putranjiva roxburghii*	Child-life Tree, Indian Amulet Plant, Spurious Wild Olive	Ayurvedic
Gardabhaanda	*Thespesia populnea*	Portia Tree, Tulip Tree, Umbrella Tree, False Rosewood	Ayurvedic
Gardel	*Entada scandens*	Garbee Bean, Mackay Bean, Elephant Creeper	Folk
Gargari	*Coix lacryma-jobi*	Job's Tears	Folk
Gariki	*Scutia myrtina*	Chimat Fruit	Folk
Garjan	*Dipterocarpus alatus*	Gurjun	Ayurvedic
Garjara	*Daucus carota*	Carrot, Cultivated Carrot, Wild Carrot	Ayurvedic
Garmar	*Coleus barbatus*	Coleus	Folk
Garnaa	*Carissa opaca*	Karaunda	Folk
Gartkalambukaa	*Alternanthera sessilis*	Sessile Joyweed	Ayurvedic
Garudaphala	*Hydnocarpus laurifolia*	Soorty Oil Tree	Ayurvedic
Gatbhanjan	*Borreria articularis*	Shaggy Button Weed	Folk
Gathivan	*Leonotis nepetaefolia*	Christmas Candlestick, Jonny Collins, Lion's Ear, Lion's Tail	Folk
Gauri	*Curcuma longa*	Turmeric	Ayurvedic
Gauripushpa	*Nerium indicum*	Indian Oleander, White Oleander	Ayurvedic
Gaur-kadamba	*Adina cordifolia*	Yellow Teak, Saffron Teak	Ayurvedic
Gavaakshi	*Citrullus colocynthis*	Colocynth Bitter Apple	Ayurvedic
Gavedhukaa	*Coix lacryma-jobi*	Job's Tears	Ayurvedic

Table Contd.

Indian Name	Botanical Name	English Name	Medicinal System
Gehun	*Triticum aestivum*	Wheat	Folk
Gendaa	*Tagetes erecta*	Big Marigold, Aztec or African Marigold	Ayurvedic
Genneru	*Nerium indicum*	Indian Oleander, White Oleander	Folk/Telugu
Germander	*Teucrium scordium*	Water-Germander	Folk/Kashmir
Geru	*Sarcococca saligna*	Christmas Box	Folk
Gethiaa	*Premna herbacea*	Bharangi Tree, Qian jie cao (Chinese)	Folk
Gevaa	*Excoecaria agallocha*	Blinding Tree	Folk
Ghaafis	*Agrimonia eupatoria*	Agrimony, Stickle Wort	Unani
Ghaafis	*Gentiana kurroo*	Himalayan Gentian, Indian Gentian Root	Unani
Ghaajuraan	*Salsola kali*	Glass-Wort, Russian Thistle, Prickly-Saltwort	Unani
Ghaaneri	*Lantana camara*	Lantana, Wild Sage, Surinam Tea Plant	Folk
Ghaariqoon	*Polyporus officinalis*	White Agaric	Unani
Ghaati-Parpata	*Justicia procumbens*	Fumitary (Western Ghats)	Ayurvedic
Ghainchu	*Limnanthemum cristatum*	Aquatic Pseudo-Chiretta Plant	Folk
Ghamchi	*Abrus precatorius*	Indian Wild Liquorice, Jequirity, Crab's Eye, Precatory Bean	Unani
Ghana	*Cyperus rotundus*	Nut Grass	Ayurvedic
Ghanasaara	*Cinnamomum camphora*	Camphor Tree	Ayurvedic
Ghanaskandha	*Schleichera oleosa*	Lac Tree, Macassar Oil Tree, Honey Tree, Ceylon Oak	Ayurvedic
Ghandh-Birojaa	*Pinus roxburghii*	Long-leaved Pine, Three-leaved Pine, Chir Pine	Ayurvedic
Ghanti-chi-bhaaji	*Borreria articularis*	Shaggy Button Weed	Folk
Ghantu Bhaarangi	*Premna herbacea*	Bharangi Tree, Qian jie cao (Chinese)	Folk
Gharaiqoon	*Agaricus albus*	Purging Agaric	Unani
Ghatti (Gum)	*Anogeissus latifolia*	Axle-wood, Button Tree, Ghatti Tree	Folk
Ghaulaa	*Prunus mahaleb*	Mahaleb Cherry	Folk

Table Contd.

Indian Name	Botanical Name	English Name	Medicinal System
Gheekuwaar	*Aloe barbadensis*	Curacao Aloe, Barbados Aloe, Indian Aloe, Jaffarabad Aloe	Unani
Ghenu	*Viburnum cotinifolium*	Wooly-leaved Guelder Rose	Folk
Ghima	*Polycarpon prostratum*	Four-leaved Allseed	Folk
Ghingaaru	*Crataegus crenulata*	Himalayan Hawthorn	Folk
Ghinwaa	*Viburnum cotinifolium*	Wooly-leaved Guelder Rose	Folk
Ghodaa-tulasi	*Scoparia dulcis*	Sweet Broomweed	Folk
Ghoddhika	*Portulaca oleracea*	Common Purslane	Ayurvedic
Ghogar	*Garuga pinnata*	Grey Downy Balsam	Folk
Ghontaa	*Areca catechu*	Areca Nut, Betel Nut	Ayurvedic
Ghontaa	*Ziziphus xylopyra*	Lac-host Jujube	Ayurvedic
Ghonta-Phala	*Ziziphus xylopyra*	Lac-host Jujube Rangeeni lac is recovered from the tree	Ayurvedic
Ghorant	*Areca catechu*	Areca Nut, Betel Nut	Ayurvedic
Ghorbach	*Acorus calamus*	Sweet Flag, Calamus	Ayurvedic
Ghosa-vel	*Neuracanthus sphaerostachyus*	Pin Cushion Plant	Folk
Ghotikaa	*Portulaca oleracea*	Common Purslane	Ayurvedic
Ghot-vel	*Smilax ovalifolia*	Wild China Root	Folk
Ghritkumaarika	*Aloe barbadensis*	Curacao Aloe, Barbados Aloe, Indian Aloe, Jaffarabad Aloe	Ayurvedic
Ghritpuur	*Derris indica*	Indian Beech, Pongamia Oil Tree	Ayurvedic
Ghrusrrn	*Crocus sativus*	Saffron, Crocus	Ayurvedic
Ghuggi	*Saussurea gossypiphora*	Himalayan Saw-wort	Folk/Garhwal
Ghuggi	*Saussurea sacra*	Yogiraj Plant, Sacred Saussurea	Folk/Garhwal
Ghuiyaa	*Colocasia esculenta*	Taro, Edible Yam	Folk
Ghumchi	*Adenanthera pavonina*	Coral Wood, Red Wood	Folk
Ghunapriyaa	*Aconitum heterophyllum*	Atis Root, Aconite	Ayurvedic
Ghunavallabhaa	*Aconitum heterophyllum*	Atis Root, Aconite	Ayurvedic
Ghunghchi	*Abrus precatorius*	Indian Wild Liquorice, Jequirity, Crab's Eye, Precatory Bean	Unani
Gidaangu	*Stephania glabra*	Indian Tape Vine	Folk
Gidar Tambaaku	*Verbascum thapsus*	Cow's Lungwort, Common Mullein	Ayurvedic

Table Contd.

Indian Name	Botanical Name	English Name	Medicinal System
Gilaas	*Prunus avium*	Sweet Cherry	Folk
Gilaas	*Prunus cerasus*	Sour Cherry	Folk
Gil-gaachh	*Entada scandens*	Garbee Bean, Mackay Bean, Elephant Creeper	Folk
Gilo	*Tinospora cordifolia*	Heart-leaved Tinospora	Unani
Gilodya	*Ceropegia bulbosa*	Candlestick Ceropegia	Folk
Gilothi	*Ceropegia bulbosa*	Candlestick Ceropegia	Folk
Giloya	*Tinospora cordifolia*	Heart-leaved Tinospora	Folk
Gineri (var.)	*Premna tomentosa*	Bastard Teak	Folk
Gio	*Trema orientalis*	Charcoal Tree, Indian Nettle Tree	Folk
Gippit	*Triumfetta rhomboidea*	Burbush, Burweed	Ayurvedic
Girijaa	*Gentiana kurroo*	Himalayan Gentian, Indian Gentian Root	Ayurvedic
Girikadamba	*Adina cordifolia*	Yellow Teak, Saffron Teak	Ayurvedic
Giri-kadamba	*Mitragyna parvifolia*	Kaim Kadamb	Ayurvedic
Girikanyaa	*Clitoria ternatea*	Butterfly Pea, Winged-leaved Clitoria, Mezereon	Ayurvedic
Girikarnikaa	*Clitoria ternatea*	Butterfly Pea, Winged-leaved Clitoria, Mezereon	Ayurvedic
Girimallikaa	*Clitoria ternatea*	Butterfly Pea, Winged-leaved Clitoria, Mezereon	Ayurvedic
Girimallikaa	*Holarrhena antidysenterica*	Easter Tree, Ivory Tree, Tellicherry Bark	Ayurvedic
Giriparpata	*Podophyllum hexandrum*	Indian Podophyllum	Ayurvedic
Girishaanujaa	*Gentiana kurroo*	Himalayan Gentian, Indian Gentian Root	Ayurvedic
Giur	*Salix babylonica*	Weeping Willow	Folk
Gnaazhal	*Aglaia roxburghiana*	Priyangu Mahogany	Siddha/Tamil
Gnazhal	*Callicarpa macrophylla*	Perfumed Cherry	Siddha/Tamil
Godaar	*Millettia auriculata*	Evergreen Wisteria	Folk
Godaar	*Millettia racemosa*	Evergreen Wisteria	Folk
Godhaapadi	*Cayratia pedata*	Cayratia	Ayurvedic
Godhaa-skandha	*Acacia leucophloea*	White Babul	Ayurvedic

Table Contd.

Indian Name	Botanical Name	English Name	Medicinal System
Godhuuma	*Triticum aestivum*	Wheat	Ayurvedic
Gogji-mul	*Geum urbanum*	Avens Root, Herb Bennet, Wood Avens	Folk/Kashmir
Gojihvaa	*Elephantopus scaber*	Prickly-leaved Elephant's Foot	Ayurvedic
Gojihvaa	*Launaea pinnatifida*	Bhonpatri	Ayurvedic
Gojihvaa	*Onosma bracteatum*	Borage	Ayurvedic
Gojihvikaa	*Anchusa italica*	Cow's Tongue Plant	Ayurvedic
Gokantaka	*Pedalium murex*	Caltrops (bigger var.)	Ayurvedic
Gokarnaa	*Withania ashwagandha*	Winter Cherry	Ayurvedic
Gokarni	*Marsdenia tenacissima*	White Turpeth	Ayurvedic
Gokharu Kalaan	*Pedalium murex*	Caltrops (bigger var.)	Unani
Gokharu-kalaan	*Tribulus alatus*	Winged Caltrops	Unani
Gokshura	*Tribulus alatus*	Winged Caltrops	Ayurvedic
Gokshura	*Tribulus terrestris*	Land-Caltrops, Puncture Vine	Ayurvedic
Gokshuraka	*Tribulus terrestris*	Land-Caltrops, Puncture Vine	Ayurvedic
Golaalu	*Solanum tuberosum*	Potato	Ayurvedic
Golden-rod	*Solidago virgaurea*	European Goldenrod, Woundwort	Folk
Golomi	*Acorus calamus*	Sweet Flag, Calamus	Ayurvedic
Golomi	*Cynodon dactylon*	Bermuda Grass, Bahama Grass, Couch Grass	Ayurvedic
Golomikaa	*Launaea pinnatifida*	Bhonpatri	Ayurvedic
Gometi	*Zehneria umbellata*	Zehneria	Folk
Gond Kateeraa	*Sterculia urens*	Bissy Nuts, Karaya Gum	Unani
Gondani	*Bridelia retusa*	Spinous Kino Tree	Folk
Gondapateraa	*Typha australis*	Lesser Indian Reed-Mace	Folk
Gondapateraa	*Typha elephantina*	Elephant Grass, Indian Reed-Mace, Bulrush	Folk
Gondi	*Cordia rothii*	Sebestan	Folk
Gondi	*Cordia wallichii*	Sebestan	Folk
Gondni	*Bridelia montana*	Spinous Kino Tree	Folk
Gondui	*Bridelia retusa*	Spinous Kino Tree	Folk
Gonyuch	*Lepidium latifolium*	Peppercress	Folk
Gopaa	*Hemidesmus indicus*	Indian Sarsaparilla	Ayurvedic

Table Contd.

Indian Name	Botanical Name	English Name	Medicinal System
Gopabhadra	*Gmelina asiatica*	Small Cashmere Tree	Ayurvedic
Gopakantaa	*Flacourtia indica*	Ramontchi, Madagascar Plum, Mauritius Plum, Governor's Plum	Ayurvedic
Gopakanyaa	*Hemidesmus indicus*	Indian Sarsaparilla	Ayurvedic
Gopasutaa	*Hemidesmus indicus*	Indian Sarsaparilla	Ayurvedic
Gopavadhu	*Cryptolepis buchanani*	Indian Sarsaparilla	Ayurvedic
Gopavalli	*Hemidesmus indicus*	Indian Sarsaparilla	Ayurvedic
Gopavalli	*Ichnocarpus frutescens*	Black Creeper	Ayurvedic
Gopi	*Cryptolepis buchanani*	Indian Sarsaparilla	Ayurvedic
Gopi	*Hemidesmus indicus*	Indian Sarsaparilla	Ayurvedic
Gorakh	*Dalbergia lanceolaria*	Takoliwood	Folk
Gorakh amli	*Adansonia digitata*	Baobab, Monkey Bread Tree, African Calabash	Unani
Gorakh Chinchaa	*Adansonia digitata*	Baobab, Monkey Bread Tree, African Calabash	Folk
Gorakh Imli	*Adansonia digitata*	Baobab, Monkey Bread Tree, African Calabash	Folk
Gorakhi	*Dalbergia volubilis*	Cinnamom-scented Bark Tree	Ayurvedic
Gorakh-mundi	*Sphaeranthus indicus*	East Indian Globe Thistle	Folk
Goraksha	*Dalbergia latifolia*	East Indian Rosewood, Bombay Blackwood	Ayurvedic
Gorakshaganjaa	*Aerva lanata*	Mountain Knot Grass	Ayurvedic
Goraksha-phalini	*Cyamopsis tetragonoloba*	Cluster Bean, Guar	Ayurvedic
Gorakshi	*Adansonia digitata*	Baobab, Monkey Bread Tree, African Calabash	Ayurvedic
Goriaa-loti	*Pericampylus glaucus*	Broad-leaved Moonseed	Folk
Goshtha-vaartaaku	*Solanum torvum*	West Indian Turkey Berry	Ayurvedic
Go-stani	*Vitis vinifera*	Wine Grape, European Grape	Ayurvedic
Goth-begun	*Solanum torvum*	West Indian Turkey Berry	Folk
Gouri-phal	*Rubus ellipticus*	Gach Strawberry	Folk
Graamya	*Ocimum sanctum*	Holy Basil, Sacred Basil	Ayurvedic
Gramyaa	*Indigofera tinctoria*	Indigo	Ayurvedic

Table Contd.

Indian Name	Botanical Name	English Name	Medicinal System
Hansapadi	*Adiantum lunulatum*	Walking Maidenhair Fern, Black Maidenhair	Ayurvedic
Hansaraaja	*Adiantum capillus-veneris*	American Maidenhair Fern, Venus Hair, Rock Fern	Ayurvedic
Hansaraaja	*Adiantum lunulatum*	Walking Maidenhair Fern, Black Maidenhair	Ayurvedic
Hanumaan-buuti	*Indigofera enneaphylla*	Trailing Indigo	Folk
Hanumaan-Vel	*Ipomoea sepiaria*	Big-flowered Morning Glory	Ayurvedic
Hanzal	*Citrullus colocynthis*	Colocynth Bitter Apple	Unani
Hapushaa	*Juniperus communis*	Common Juniper	Ayurvedic
Hara Champaa	*Artabotrys hexapetalus*	Yling-Yling Vine	Ayurvedic
Harad	*Terminalia chebula*	Chebulic Myrobalan, Black Myrobalan	Unani
Haraduaa-kadamba	*Adina cordifolia*	Yellow Teak, Saffron Teak	Ayurvedic
Harakuch	*Enhydra fluctuans*	Marsh Herb, Water Cress	Folk
Haramal	*Peganum harmala*	Wild Rue, Foreign Henna, Syrian Rue	Ayurvedic
Haranpagaa	*Convolvulus arvensis*	Deer's Foot, Devil's Garters	Ayurvedic
Harapriya	*Datura metel*	Thornapple, Downy Datura	Ayurvedic
Harasingaar	*Nyctanthes arbor-tristis*	Tree of Sorrow, Night Jasmine, Coral Jasmine	Unani
Hargozaa	*Acanthus ilicifolius*	Sea Holly	Folk
Hariaa	*Smilax lanceifolia*	Himalayan China Root	Folk
Harichandana	*Coscinium fenestratum*	False Calumba	Ayurvedic
Haridraa	*Curcuma longa*	Turmeric	Ayurvedic
Haridru	*Adina cordifolia*	Yellow Teak, Saffron Teak	Ayurvedic
Haridruma	*Curcuma longa*	Turmeric	Ayurvedic
Harimantha	*Cicer arietinum*	Bengal Gram, Chick Pea	Ayurvedic
Haritaki	*Terminalia chebula*	Chebulic Myrobalan, Black Myrobalan	Ayurvedic
Haritaki	*Terminalia citrina*	Bengal Myrobalan	Folk/Bengal
Haritamanjari	*Acalypha indica*	Copperleaf Acalypha	Ayurvedic
Haritaparna	*Eucalyptus globulus*	Blue-gum Tree, Australian Gum Tree	Ayurvedic
Haritashaaka	*Moringa pterygosperma*	Drumstick, Horse-Radish	Ayurvedic

Table Contd.

Indian Name	Botanical Name	English Name	Medicinal System
Harivaaluka	*Prunus avium*	Sweet Cherry	Ayurvedic
Harshaf	*Cynara scolymus*	Globe Artichoke	Unani
Hasaka	*Tribulus alatus*	Winged Caltrops	Folk
Hashish-ut-Dinaar	*Humulus lupulus*	Hops	Unani
Hastikanda	*Leea macrophylla*	Tuberous Holly	Ayurvedic
Hasti-karna Palaasha	*Leea macrophylla*	Tuberous Holly	Ayurvedic
Hastikarni	*Alocasia indica*	Giant Taro	Ayurvedic
Hastipippali	*Scindapsus officinalis*	Sal Forest Pepper	Ayurvedic
Hastishundi	*Heliotropium indicum*	Scorpion Tail	Ayurvedic
Hastyaaluka	*Dioscorea daemona*	Asiatic Bitter Yam	Ayurvedic
Hatermuula	*Senecio jacquemontianus*	Jacquemont's Senecio	Folk
Hathajori	*Martynia annua*	Devil's Claw, Tiger Claw	Folk
Hathokane	*Kalanchoe integra*	Never Die	Folk
Hatkan	*Leea macrophylla*	Tuberous Holly	Folk
Hattavilaasini	*Curcuma longa*	Turmeric	Ayurvedic
Hattha	*Emblica officinalis*	Embic, Indian Gooseberry	Ayurvedic
Hatthaa jodi	*Selaginella involvens*	Spike Moss	Folk
Hatthaajodi	*Selaginella rupestris*	Little Clubmoss, Rock Spike-Moss	Folk
Havushaa	*Juniperus communis*	Common Juniper	Ayurvedic
Hayagandhaa	*Withania ashwagandha*	Winter Cherry	Ayurvedic
Hayamaaraka	*Nerium indicum*	Indian Oleander, White Oleander	Ayurvedic
Hayapriya	*Hordeum vulgare*	Barley	Ayurvedic
Hayeshtha	*Hordeum vulgare*	Barley	Ayurvedic
Hazaar-mani	*Phyllanthus urinaria*	Cultivated Field Chanca Piedra	Folk
Heel Habshi	*Aframomum melegueta*	Grains of Paradise, Alligator Pepper, Meleguetta Pepper	Unani
Heel Kalaan	*Amomum subulatum*	Greater or Nepal Cardamom	Unani
Heel Khurd	*Elettaria cardamomum*	Lesser Cardamom	Unani
Heeng	*Ferula foetida*	Asafoetida	Unani
Heeng	*Ferula narthex*	Narthex Asafoetida	Unani

Table Contd.

Indian Name	Botanical Name	English Name	Medicinal System
Heens	*Capparis sepiaria*	Indian Caper	Folk
Heeraadokhi	*Daemonorops draco*	East Indian Dragon's Blood	Ayurvedic
Heeraadokhi	*Dracaena cinnabari*	Dragon's Blood	Ayurvedic
Hellebore	*Veratrum viride*	Indian Hellbore, False Hellebore, Indian Poke	Folk
Hema	*Datura metel*	Thornapple, Downy Datura	Ayurvedic
Hemaahvaa	*Argemone mexicana*	Prickly Poppy, Mexican Poppy	Ayurvedic
Hema-daudhaka	*Ficus racemosa*	Cluster Fig, Country Fig	Ayurvedic
Hemajivanti	*Dregea volubilis*	Wattakaka	Ayurvedic
Hemapushpa	*Michelia champaca*	Champak, Golden Champa	Ayurvedic
Hemapushpikaa	*Jasminum humile*	Yellow Jasmine, Nepal Jasmine, Italian Jasmine	Ayurvedic
Hemar	*Ulmus wallichiana*	Himalayan Elm	Folk
Hemavati	*Argemone mexicana*	Prickly Poppy, Mexican Poppy	Ayurvedic
Hemavati	*Leptadenia reticulata*	Dodi Vegetable	Ayurvedic
Hem-maalati	*Myxopyrum serratulum*	Yellow-flowered Myxopyrum	Folk
Hempushpa	*Saraca asoca*	Ashoka Tree	Ayurvedic
Hemsaagar	*Kalanchoe laciniata*	Christmastree Plant	Folk
Hemsaagar	*Kalanchoe pinnata*	Christmastree Plant	Ayurvedic
Herb Robert	*Geranium robertianum*	Herb-Robert Geranium	Folk
Herniary	*Herniaria glabra*	Smooth Rupture-Wort	Folk
Hetenuriyaa	*Trichodesma zeylanicum*	Ajovan	Folk
Heufaariqoon	*Hypericum perforatum*	Common St. John's Wort	Unani
Hijjala	*Barringtonia acutangula*	Indian Oak	Ayurvedic
Hillua	*Asparagus officinalis*	Asparagus, Sparrow Grass	Folk
Hil-mochikaa	*Enhydra fluctuans*	Marsh Herb, Water Cress	Ayurvedic
Hilteet	*Ferula foetida*	Asafoetida	Unani
Hilteet	*Ferula narthex*	Narthex Asafoetida	Unani
Hima	*Santalum album*	White Sandalwood	Ayurvedic
Himaavati	*Argemone mexicana*	Prickly Poppy, Mexican Poppy	Ayurvedic
Himakara	*Cinnamomum camphora*	Camphor Tree	Ayurvedic
Hima-valukaa	*Cinnamomum camphora*	Camphor Tree	Ayurvedic

Table Contd.

Indian Name	Botanical Name	English Name	Medicinal System
Him-Champaa	*Magnolia grandiflora*	Bull Bay, Great Laurel Magnolia, Southern Magnolia	Ayurvedic
Himopala	*Cinnamomum camphora*	Camphor Tree	Ayurvedic
Him-Paadapa	*Monotropa uniflora*	Indian Pipe, Ice Plant	Folk
Himsraa	*Capparis sepiaria*	Indian Caper	Ayurvedic
Himsraa	*Capparis spinosa*	Caper Bush	Ayurvedic
Hinaa	*Lawsonia inermis*	Henna	Unani
Hind-baa-al-Barri	*Taraxacum officinale*	Common Dandelion	Unani
Hindi Chobachini	*Smilax lanceifolia*	Himalayan China Root	Ayurvedic
Hindubaa	*Cichorium intybus*	Chicory, Indian Endive	Unani
Hingan	*Balanites aegyptiaca*	Desert Date	Unani
Hingol	*Balanites aegyptiaca*	Desert Date	Folk
Hingota	*Balanites aegyptiaca*	Desert Date	Folk
Hingothaa	*Balanites aegyptiaca*	Desert Date	Folk
Hingu (var.)	*Ferula narthex*	Narthex Asafoetida	Ayurvedic
Hingu	*Ferula foetida*	Asafoetida	Ayurvedic
Hinguka	*Ferula foetida*	Asafoetida	Ayurvedic
Hinguli	*Solanum ferox*	Poison-Berry	Ayurvedic
Hingupatri	*Ferula jaeschkeana*	Kashmiri Ferula	Ayurvedic
Hingupatri	*Gardenia gummifera*	Gummy Cape Jasmine	Ayurvedic
Hingupatrikaa	*Gardenia gummifera*	Gummy Cape Jasmine	Ayurvedic
Hingushivaatikaa	*Gardenia gummifera*	Gummy Cape Jasmine	Ayurvedic
Hinsaalu	*Rubus ellipticus*	Gach Strawberry	Folk
Hintala	*Phoenix paludosa*	Bengal Palm	Ayurvedic
Hintalamu	*Phoenix paludosa*	Bengal Palm	Folk
Hiraa	*Gmelina arborea*	Candahar Tree, White Teak	Ayurvedic
Hiraabola	*Balsamodendron myrrha*	Myrrh, Herabol	Ayurvedic
Hiran-chaaro	*Lepidagathis cristata*	Spotted White-flowered Pluchea	Folk
Hirankhuri	*Convolvulus arvensis*	Deer's Foot, Devil's Garters	Ayurvedic
Hirankhuri	*Emilia sonchifolia*	Emilia Salad	Unani
Hiranpadi	*Convolvulus arvensis*	Deer's Foot, Devil's Garters	Ayurvedic
Hiran-vel	*Paederia foetida*	Skunk Vine	Folk

Table Contd.

Indian Name	Botanical Name	English Name	Medicinal System
Hiranyatuttha	*Colchicum luteum*	Hermodactyls, Colchicum, Meadow Saffron, Golden Collyrium	Ayurvedic
Hiravi	*Euphorbia thomsoniana*	Hirvi Spurge	Folk
Hiruberaka	*Coleus vettiveroides*	Coleus	Ayurvedic
Hirva Champaa	*Artabotrys hexapetalus*	Yling-Yling Vine	Folk
Hital	*Phoenix paludosa*	Bengal Palm	Folk
Hiyaavali	*Euphorbia thomsoniana*	Hirvi Spurge	Ayurvedic
Holly	*Ilex aquifolium*	English Holly, Common Holly	Folk
Hooirjo	*Begonia laciniata*	Beefsteak Geraniums, Elephant's Ear	Folk/Bengal
Horse-radish	*Armoracia lapathifolia*	Red Cole, Pepperrot, Great Raifort	Folk
Horseradish	*Cochlearia armoracia*	Red Cole	Folk
Houseleek	*Sempervivum tectorum*	Houseleek	Folk
Hriddgandhaa	*Jasminum officinale*	Spanish Jasmine	Ayurvedic
Hriddhaatri	*Smilax china*	China Root	Ayurvedic
Hriswaanga	*Microstylis musifera*	Jivaka	Ayurvedic
Hritpatri	*Digitalis lanata*	Grecian Foxglove	Ayurvedic
Hritpatri	*Digitalis purpurea*	Digitalis, Foxglove	Ayurvedic
Hrivera	*Coleus vettiveroides*	Coleus	Ayurvedic
Hrivera	*Pavonia odorata*	Fragrant Sticky Mallow	Ayurvedic
Hubb-ul-arar	*Juniperus communis*	Common Juniper	Unani
Hubb-ul-Malook	*Croton tiglium*	Purging Croton	Unani
Hulbaa	*Trigonella foenum-graecum*	Fenugreek	Unani
Hum	*Fraxinus hookery*	European Ash, Weeping Ash	Folk
Huraa	*Excoecaria agallocha*	Blinding Tree	Folk
Hurhur	*Cleome icosandra*	Wild Mustard	Ayurvedic
Hurnaa	*Sapium indicum*	Tallow Tree	Folk
Hutaasha	*Plumbago zeylanica*	Ceylon Leadwort	Ayurvedic
Huttian	*Ceiba pentandra*	White Silk Cotton Tree	Folk
Ibha-muulaka	*Fimbristylis ovata*	Fringe-Rush	Ayurvedic
Ichchi	*Ficus lacor*	White Fig	Siddha/Tamil

Table Contd.

Indian Name	Botanical Name	English Name	Medicinal System
Ielaikkali	*Euphorbia neriifolia*	Holy Milk Hedge, Dog's Tongue	Siddha/Tamil
Ielavampisin (gum)	*Salmalia malabarica*	Silk Cotton Tree, Semul Tree	Siddha/Tamil
Ielavum	*Ceiba pentandra*	White Silk Cotton Tree	Siddha/Tamil
Ieluppai	*Madhuca indica*	Mahua Tree, Moha	Siddha/Tamil
Ijjala	*Barringtonia acutangula*	Indian Oak	Ayurvedic
Ikil-ul-Malik	*Astragalus hamosus*	Tonkin Bean, Melilot, King's Crown, King's Clover	Unani
Iklil-ul-Malik	*Melilotus officinalis*	Yellow Sweet Clover, Melilot	Unani
Iklil-ul-Malik	*Trigonella uncata*	Tonkin Bean, Melilot, King's Crown	Unani
Ikshavaaku	*Lagenaria siceraria*	Bitter Bottle-Gourd	Ayurvedic
Ikshu	*Saccharum officinarum*	Gannaa, Naishakar	Ayurvedic
Ikshugandhaa	*Pueraria tuberosa*	Indian Kudze	Ayurvedic
Ikshukandaa	*Ipomoea digitata*	Milky Yam	Ayurvedic
Ikshura	*Asteracantha longifolia*	Hygrophilla	Ayurvedic
Ikshura	*Hygrophila auriculata*	Indian Swampweed	Ayurvedic
Ikshuraka	*Asteracantha longifolia*	Hygrophilla	Ayurvedic
Ikshuraka	*Hygrophila auriculata*	Indian Swampweed	Ayurvedic
Ilaayachi	*Elettaria cardamomum*	Lesser Cardamom	Folk
Ilakotta	*Eriobotrya japonica*	Loquat, Japanese Medlar	Siddha/Tamil
Ilangu	*Artocarpus lakoocha*	Monkey Jack	Folk/Tamil
Ilkil-ul-Malik	*Melilotus alba*	White Sweet Clover	Unani
Ilkil-ul-Malik	*Melilotus indica*	Sweet Clover, Annual Yellow Sweet Clover, Small-flowered Melilot	Unani
Ilk-ul-Ambaat (resin)	*Pistacia vera*	Pistachio, Green Almond	Unani
Illupei	*Madhuca longifolia*	South Indian Mahua	Siddha/Tamil
Iluppei	*Bassia longifolia*	Mowra Butter Tree, South Indian Mahua	Folk/Tamil
Inbooral	*Oldenlandia umbellata*	Indian Madder, Chay-Root	Siddha/Tamil
Inbud-dub	*Arctostaphylos uva-ursi*	Bearberry	Unani
Indan	*Acacia pennata*	Feathery-shoot Acacia	Siddha/Tamil
Inderjao Shireen	*Wrightia tinctoria*	Pala Indigo Plant	Unani

Table Contd.

Indian Name	Botanical Name	English Name	Medicinal System
Iruvi	*Dryopteris filix-mas*	Male Fern, Aspidium	Siddha/Tamil
Isabgol	*Plantago major*	Broadleaf Plantain	Folk
Isabgol	*Plantago ovata*	Ispaghula, Spogel Seeds, Blond Psyllium	Folk
Isapppa	*Plantago ovata*	Ispaghula, Spogel Seeds, Blond Psyllium	Siddha/Tamil
Isarmuula	*Aristolochia indica*	Indian Birthwort	Folk
Isband	*Peganum harmala*	Wild Rue, Foreign Henna, Syrian Rue	Ayurvedic
Isband-laahauri	*Peganum harmala*	Wild Rue, Foreign Henna, Syrian Rue	Folk
Isfahaan Marv	*Phyllanthus maderaspatensis*	Kanocha Seed	Unani
Isferaaz	*Asparagus officinalis*	Asparagus, Sparrow Grass	Unani
Ishalingi	*Bryonopsis laciniosa*	Bryony	Ayurvedic
Ishvari	*Aristolochia indica*	Indian Birthwort	Ayurvedic
Ishwara	*Ixora parviflora*	Torchwood Tree	Ayurvedic
Ishwar-jataa	*Pogostemon benghalensis*	Bengal Pogostemon	Folk
Ispast	*Trifolium pratense*	Red Clover	Unani
Isqueel-e-Hindi	*Urginea indica*	Indian Squill, Sea Onion (red and white varieties)	Unani
Isrola	*Aristolochia indica*	Indian Birthwort	Folk
Ita	*Phoenix dactylifera*	Date Palm	Siddha/Tamil
Itarilaal	*Ammi majus*	Bishop's Weed-Amee, Greater Ammi	Unani
Ithi	*Phoenix pusilla*	Wild Coromandel Palm	Folk/Tamil
Itkata (var.)	*Sesbania bispinosa*	Prickly Sesban, Dhaincha	Ayurvedic
Itsit	*Boerhavia diffusa*	Red-flowered Hogweed	Unani
Itthi	*Ficus talboti*	Pakar Tree	Siddha/Tamil
Itti	*Ficus microcarpa*	Indian Laurel Fig	Folk
Izkhar	*Cymbopogon jwarancusa*	Vetiver-scented Grass	Unani
Izkhar	*Cymbopogon schoenanthus*	Camel-Hay	Unani
Jaadippatiri (Mace)	*Myristica fragrans*	Nutmeg	Siddha/Tamil

Table Contd.

Indian Name	Botanical Name	English Name	Medicinal System
Jaamphal	*Citrus limon*	Lemon	Ayurvedic
Jaamun	*Syzygium cuminii*	Java Plum, Jambolan, Black Plum	Unani
Jaarul	*Lagerstroemia flos-reginae*	Pride of India, Queen's Flowers, Queen Crape Myrtle	Folk
Jaathikkai	*Myristica fragrans*	Nutmeg	Siddha/Tamil
Jaati	*Jasminum officinale*	Spanish Jasmine	Ayurvedic
Jaatikaa	*Jasminum officinale*	Spanish Jasmine	Ayurvedic
Jaatikosha (Mace)	*Myristica fragrans*	Nutmeg	Ayurvedic
Jaatimalli	*Jasminum officinale*	Spanish Jasmine	Ayurvedic
Jaatipatra	*Myristica fragrans*	Nutmeg	Ayurvedic
Jaatipatraka	*Myristica fragrans*	Nutmeg	Ayurvedic
Jaatipatri	*Myristica fragrans*	Nutmeg	Ayurvedic
Jaatiphala	*Myristica fragrans*	Nutmeg	Ayurvedic
Jaatishasya	*Myristica fragrans*	Nutmeg	Ayurvedic
Jaatukanda	*Jurinea macrocephala*	Temple Incense Root	Ayurvedic
Jabara	*Bixa orellana*	Annatto	Siddha/Tamil
Jaborandi	*Pilocarpus microphyllus*	Jaborandi	Folk
Jadwaar Khataai	*Delphinium denudatum*	Larkspur	Unani
Jai	*Clerodendrum phlomidis*	Glory Bower	Ayurvedic
Jainta	*Sesbania sesban*	Common Sesban	Folk
Jala	*Coleus vettiveroides*	Coleus	Ayurvedic
Jala	*Pavonia odorata*	Fragrant Sticky Mallow	Ayurvedic
Jalaapaa	*Exogonium purga*	Jalap	Unani
Jalaapaa	*Ipomoea purga*	Jalap	Folk
Jalada	*Cyperus rotundus*	Nut Grass	Ayurvedic
Jaladudhi	*Oxystelma secamone*	Dudhni, Chamuuk plaa lot (Thai)	Folk
Jalaja	*Ceratophyllum demersum*	Coontail, Hornwort	Ayurvedic
Jalaja	*Nelumbo nucifera*	East Indian Lotus, Sacred Lotus	Ayurvedic
Jalajali	*Stachytarpheta jamaicensis*	Brazilian Tea, Bastard Vervain, Aaron's Rod	Folk
Jalajamani	*Cocculus hirsutus*	Broom-Creeper, Ink-Berry	Ayurvedic

Table Contd.

Indian Name	Botanical Name	English Name	Medicinal System
Jalakarnaa	*Lippia nodiflora*	Wild Sage	Ayurvedic
Jalakumbhi	*Eichhornia crassipes*	Water-Hyacinth, Bengal Terror, Blue Devil, The Million Dollar Weed	Ayurvedic
Jalakumbhi	*Pistia stratiotes*	Water Lettuce, Tropical Duckweed	Ayurvedic
Jala-lavanga (var.)	*Jussiaea tenella*	Swamp Primrose	Ayurvedic
Jala-lavanga	*Jussiaea suffruticosa*	Swamp Primrose	Ayurvedic
Jala-Madhuuka	*Madhuca longifolia*	South Indian Mahua	Folk
Jala-Mahuaa	*Madhuca longifolia*	South Indian Mahua	Folk
Jalaneem	*Bacopa monnieri*	Thyme-leaved Gratiola	Folk
Jala-papr	*Mollugo spergula*	Falsely-whorled Carpetweed	Folk
Jalaphala	*Trapa bispinosa*	Water Chestnut	Ayurvedic
Jalapippali	*Lippia nodiflora*	Wild Sage	Ayurvedic
Jalapippali	*Phyla nodiflora*	Fogfruit, Sawtooth Fogfruit	Ayurvedic
Jalasirasa	*Trichodesma zeylanicum*	Ajovan	Folk
Jalavaasa	*Vetiveria zizanioides*	Vetiver, Khas	Ayurvedic
Jala-vetasa	*Salix acmophylla*	Wild Weeping Willow	Ayurvedic
Jalavetasa	*Salix alba*	White Willow, European Willow	Ayurvedic
Jalavetasa	*Salix tetrasperma*	Indian Willow	Ayurvedic
Jal-dhaniyaa	*Ranunculus sceleratus*	Blister Buttercup, Celery-leaved Crowfoot	Folk
Jaldhara	*Cyperus rotundus*	Nut Grass	Ayurvedic
Jalidar	*Grewia villosa*	Tamthar	Folk
Jalkanda	*Trapa bispinosa*	Water Chestnut	Ayurvedic
Jallil	*Vallisneria spiralis*	Eel-Grass, Tape Grass, Wild Celery	Ayurvedic
Jalneem	*Lycopus europaeus*	Gipsywort, Bugleweed	Folk
Jalnili	*Ceratophyllum demersum*	Coontail, Hornwort	Ayurvedic
Jamaalgotaa	*Croton tiglium*	Purging Croton	Unani
Jambaka	*Citrus limon*	Lemon	Ayurvedic
Jambir Nimbu	*Citrus limon*	Lemon	Ayurvedic
Jambira	*Citrus limon*	Lemon	Ayurvedic

Table Contd.

Indian Name	Botanical Name	English Name	Medicinal System
Jambir-trn	*Cymbopogon nardus*	Ceylon Citronella Grass	Ayurvedic
Jambu	*Syzygium cuminii*	Java Plum, Jambolan, Black Plum	Ayurvedic
Jambu	*Xylia xylocarpa*	Irul Tree	Folk
Jambuka	*Pandanus fascicularis*	Screw Pine	Ayurvedic
Jambupatraa Saarivaa	*Cryptolepis buchanani*	Indian Sarsaparilla	Ayurvedic
Jamiri Nimbu	*Citrus limon*	Lemon	Ayurvedic
Jamrasi (gum)	*Elaeodendron glaucum*	Jamrasi Gum Tree	Folk
Jangaddi	*Chenopodium botrys*	Feather Geramium, Jerusalem-Oak	Folk
Jangali Kaalimirchi	*Paullinia asiatica*	Lopez Root Tree, Wild Orange Tree, Forest Pepper	Folk
Jangali Kaali-mirch	*Toddalia asiatica*	Wild Orange Tree, Forest Pepper	Folk
Jangali Aam	*Spondias pinnata*	Hog-Plum, Wild Mango	Folk
Jangali Akharot	*Aleurites moluccana*	Candlenut Tree	Ayurvedic
Jangali Baadaam	*Canarium commune*	Jave Almond, Kenari Nut	Folk
Jangali Baadaam	*Sterculia foetida*	Kola Seeds, Gurru Nuts	Folk
Jangali Baadaam	*Terminalia catappa*	Indian Almond, Tropical Almond	Folk
Jangali Fraas	*Populus alba*	White Poplar	Folk
Jangali Gaajar *(var.)*	*Eryngium foetidum*	Sea Holly	Folk
Jangali Gaajar	*Portulaca tuberosa*	Loniya Weed	Folk
Jangali Gulaab	*Rosa sericea*	Mountain Rose	Folk
Jangali Karelaa	*Momordica balsamina*	Balsam Apple	Ayurvedic
Jangali Karelaa	*Momordica dioica*	Small Bitter Gourd, burr Cucumber	Folk
Jangali Karondaa	*Carissa opaca*	Karaunda	Folk
Jangali Maruaa	*Origanum majorana*	Sweet Marjoram	Folk
Jangali Methi	*Desmodium triflorum*	Matty Trefoil	Folk
Jangali Methi	*Sida acuta*	Hornbeam-Leaved Sida	Folk
Jangali Moong	*Phaseolus trilobus*	Wild Gram	Folk
Jangali Paalak	*Rumex acetosella*	Sheep Sorrel	Unani

Table Contd.

Indian Name	Botanical Name	English Name	Medicinal System
Jangali Paalak	*Rumex dentatus*	Toothed Dock	Folk
Jangali Paalak	*Rumex maritimus*	Golden Dock	Unani
Jangali Paan	*Piper hamiltonii*	Wild Pepper	Folk
Jangali Paan	*Piper thomsoni*	Sikkim Betel	Folk
Jangali Phaalsaa	*Grewia sclerophylla*	Bhokota	Folk
Jangali Piyaaz	*Urginea indica*	Indian Squill, Sea Onion (red and white varieties)	Unani
Jangali Pudinaa	*Mentha longifolia*	English Horsemint	Unani
Jangali Pudinaa	*Thymus serphyllum*	Mother-of-thyme, Wild Thyme	Unani
Jangali sawuk	*Echinochloa colonum*	Shama Millet	Folk
Jangali Sudaab	*Ruta chalepensis*	Fringed Rue	Unani
Jangali Suuran	*Dracontium polyphyllum*	Stunk Weed, Poleca Weed	Folk
Jangali Ushbaa	*Smilax zeylanica*	Indian China Root	Unani
Jangali-erandi	*Jatropha glandulifera*	Jatropha (South India)	Folk
Jangali-methi	*Sida spinosa*	Prickly Mallow	Folk
Jangli Jamaalgotaa	*Baliospermum montanum*	False Croton	Folk
Jangli Piyaz	*Scilla indica*	South Indian Squill	Unani
Jangli Tur	*Atylosia scarabaeoides*	Peanut Grass	Folk
Jantughna	*Embelia ribes*	Embelia	Ayurvedic
Jantuka	*Gardenia resinifera*	Brilliant Gardenia, Cambi Resin Tree	Ayurvedic
Jantunaashana	*Embelia ribes*	Embelia	Ayurvedic
Jantuphala	*Ficus racemosa*	Cluster Fig, Country Fig	Ayurvedic
Jao Birahnaa	*Avena sativa*	Oat, Common Oat	Unani
Jao Gandum	*Avena sativa*	Oat, Common Oat	Unani
Jao Shaeer	*Hordeum vulgare*	Barley	Unani
Japaa	*Hibiscus rosa-sinensis*	Rose-of-China, Shoe-flower, Chinese Hibiscus	Ayurvedic
Jaraayupriya	*Erigeron canadensis*	Canadian Fleabane	Ayurvedic
Jarandruma	*Dipterocarpus alatus*	Gurjun	Ayurvedic
Jastimadhu	*Scoparia dulcis*	Sweet Broomweed	Folk
Jataadhaari	*Celosia cristata*	Cock's Comb	Ayurvedic
Jataamaansi	*Nardostachys jatamansi*	Spikenard, Musk-root	Ayurvedic

Table Contd.

Indian Name	Botanical Name	English Name	Medicinal System
Jataamedaa	*Vetiveria zizanioides*	Vetiver, Khas	Ayurvedic
Jateraa	*Oenanthe javanica*	Water Dropwort	Folk
Jatilaa	*Nardostachys jatamansi*	Spikenard, Musk-root	Ayurvedic
Jatuka	*Ferula foetida*	Asafoetida	Ayurvedic
Jauzbuwaa (Seed)	*Myristica fragrans*	Nutmeg	Unani
Jauz-ul-Qai	*Randia dumetorum*	Common Emetic Nut	Unani
Javaa	*Hibiscus rosa-sinensis*	Rose-of-China, Shoe-flower, Chinese Hibiscus	Ayurvedic
Jawaasaa	*Alhagi pseudalhagi*	Camel Thorn, Persian Manna Plant	Unani
Jawaasheer	*Ferula galbaniflua*	Galbanum	Unani
Jayaa	*Clerodendrum phlomidis*	Glory Bower	Ayurvedic
Jayaa	*Sesbania sesban*	Common Sesban	Ayurvedic
Jayanti (var.)	*Sesbania bispinosa*	Prickly Sesban, Dhaincha	Ayurvedic
Jayanti	*Clerodendrum phlomidis*	Glory Bower	Ayurvedic
Jayanti	*Sesbania sesban*	Common Sesban	Ayurvedic
Jayanti	*Tridax procumbens*	Mexican Daisy	Ayurvedic
Jayantikaa	*Sesbania sesban*	Common Sesban	Ayurvedic
Jayapaala	*Croton tiglium*	Purging Croton	Ayurvedic
Jayee	*Premna integrifolia*	Headache Tree	Ayurvedic
Jeem Shaak	*Mollugo cerviana*	Carpetweed	Folk
Jeem Shaak	*Mollugo spergula*	Falsely-whorled Carpetweed	Folk
Jenghani	*Anagallis arvensis*	Bird's Eye, Bird's Tongue, Blue Pimpernel, Scarlet Pimpernel	Folk
Jethi-madh	*Taverniera cuneifolia*	East Indian Moneywort	Folk
Jhaar Phaanuus	*Kigelia pinnata*	Common Sausage Tree	Folk
Jhaaramaaricha	*Ipomoea nil*	Pharbitis Seeds	Ayurvedic
Jhaau	*Casuarina equisetifolia*	Casuarina, She-Oak, Australian or Whistling Pine, Beefwood	Ayurvedic
Jhaau	*Tamarix dioica*	Tamarisk	Folk
Jhaau	*Tamarix ericoides*	Tamarisk Mucronta	Folk
Jhaau	*Tamarix indica*	Takut Galls	Folk
Jhaavuka	*Tamarix indica*	Takut Galls	Ayurvedic

Table Contd.

Indian Name	Botanical Name	English Name	Medicinal System
Jhalai	*Biophytum sensitivum*	Life Plant	Folk
Jhandu	*Tagetes erecta*	Big Marigold, Aztec or African Marigold	Ayurvedic
Jhangi (smaller var.)	*Utricularia bifida*	Bladder Wort	Folk
Jhanjhaniaa	*Crotalaria juncea*	Sun Hemp	Folk
Jhanjhaniaa	*Crotalaria verrucosa*	Sun Hemp	Folk
Jharber	*Ziziphus nummularia*	Wild Jujube	Unani
Jharihaldi	*Coscinium fenestratum*	False Calumba	Folk
Jhill	*Indigofera oblongifolia*	Wild Indigo, Mysore Panicled Indigo	Ayurvedic
Jhingan	*Lannea coromandelica*	Jhingan	Ayurvedic
Jhingi	*Trichodesma zeylanicum*	Ajovan	Ayurvedic
Jhinjhireetaa	*Triumfetta rhomboidea*	Burbush, Burweed	Ayurvedic
Jhinki	*Rhynchosia minima*	Rhynchosia	Folk
Jhinti	*Barleria buxifolia*	Box-leaved Barleria	Folk
Jhinti	*Barleria prionitis*	Common Yellow Nail Dye Plant	Folk
Jhuri	*Osyris wightiana*	African Sandalwood, Zanzibar Lawa Wood	Folk
Jighanaa	*Anagallis arvensis*	Bird's Eye, Bird's Tongue, Blue Pimpernel, Scarlet Pimpernel	Folk
Jimikipoo	*Vicoa indica*	Banjauri	Siddha/Tamil
Jimuuta	*Luffa echinata*	Bristly Luffa	Ayurvedic
Jinghini	*Trichodesma zeylanicum*	Ajovan	Folk
Jingi	*Rubia cordifolia*	Indian Madder, Bengal Madder	Ayurvedic
Jingini	*Lannea coromandelica*	Jhingan	Ayurvedic
Jinko-banafashaa	*Viola cinerea*	White-flowered Violet	Folk
Jipachi	*Laminum amplexicaule*	Henbit Dead Nettle	Folk
Jiraa	*Carum carvi*	Caraway	Ayurvedic
Jiraa Siyaah	*Carum bulbocastanum*	Black Caraway	Unani
Jiraka	*Cuminum cyminum*	Cumin	Ayurvedic
Jirjeer	*Eruca sativa*	Rocket-Salad	Unani
Jirki	*Ipomoea hederacea*	Ivy-leaved Morning Glory	Folk

Table Contd.

Indian Name	Botanical Name	English Name	Medicinal System
Jiuenti	*Cimicifuga racemosa*	Black Cohosh Root, Black Snake Root	Folk
Jivadaaru	*Guaiacum officinale*	Lignum Vitae, Tree-of-life, Pockwood Tree	Ayurvedic
Jivaka	*Microstylis musifera*	Jivaka	Ayurvedic
Jivaka-Rshabhaka	*Lipasis rostrata*	Jivak Orchid	Ayurvedic
Jivan	*Cicer arietinum*	Bengal Gram, Chick Pea	Ayurvedic
Jivana	*Leptadenia reticulata*	Dodi Vegetable	Ayurvedic
Jivaniya	*Leptadenia reticulata*	Dodi Vegetable	Ayurvedic
Jivanti	*Dendrobium ovatum*	Pigeon Orchid, Cooktown Orchid	Ayurvedic
Jivanti	*Leptadenia reticulata*	Dodi Vegetable	Ayurvedic
Jivanti	*Pholidota articulata*	Coelogyne Orchid	Ayurvedic
Jivanti	*Tinospora cordifolia*	Heart-leaved Tinospora	Ayurvedic
Jivanti	*Trema orientalis*	Charcoal Tree, Indian Nettle Tree	Ayurvedic
Jivantikaa	*Viscum articulatum*	Napalese Mistletoe	Ayurvedic
Jivapushpa	*Leptadenia reticulata*	Dodi Vegetable	Ayurvedic
Jiyaapotaa	*Putranjiva roxburghii*	Child-life Tree, Indian Amulet Plant, Spurious Wild Olive	Folk
Jogi Paashaah	*Saussurea gossypiphora*	Himalayan Saw-wort	Folk/Kashmir
Jogi-paadshaah	*Saussurea sacra*	Yogiraj Plant, Sacred Saussurea	Folk/Kashmir
Jongaka	*Aquilaria agallocha*	Aloewood, Eaglewood, Agarwood	Ayurvedic
Jonkmaari	*Anagallis arvensis*	Bird's Eye, Bird's Tongue, Blue Pimpernel, Scarlet Pimpernel	Folk
Jowaar	*Sorghum vulgare*	Sorghum, Broomcorn	Folk
Joz Maasil	*Datura innoxia*	Angel's Trumpet, Sacred Datura	Unani
Jui lataa	*Pogostemon benghalensis*	Bengal Pogostemon	Folk
Junaar	*Thysanolaena agrostis*	Bouquet-Grass, Broom-Grass, Tiger-Grass, Amliso	Folk
Jungli Nimbu	*Atalantia monophylla*	Wild Lime	Folk

Table Contd.

Indian Name	Botanical Name	English Name	Medicinal System
Juuhi (yellow var.)	*Jasminum heterophyllum*	Yellow Jasmine	Folk
Juuhi (yellow var.)	*Jasminum humile*	Yellow Jasmine, Nepal Jasmine, Italian Jasmine	Folk
Juuhi	*Jasminum auriculatum*	Cultivated Jasmine	Folk
Juurnaa	*Thysanolaena agrostis*	Bouquet-Grass, Broom-Grass, Tiger-Grass, Amliso	Ayurvedic
Juurnaahv	*Thysanolaena agrostis*	Bouquet-Grass, Broom-Grass, Tiger-Grass, Amliso	Ayurvedic
Jvalanaakhya	*Plumbago zeylanica*	Ceylon Leadwort	Ayurvedic
Jwaalaamukhi	*Sesbania sesban*	Common Sesban	Ayurvedic
Jyotishmati	*Celastrus paniculatus*	Staff Tree, Intellect Tree	Ayurvedic
Kaabuli Kikar	*Prosopis chilensis*	Mestique Gum Tree	Folk
Kaafoor	*Cinnamomum camphora*	Camphor Tree	Unani
Kaagadolia	*Mucuna monosperma*	Negro Bean	Folk
Kaagazi Nimbu	*Citrus aurantifolia*	Acid or Sour Lime, Country Lime	Folk
Kaahuu Barri (var.)	*Lactuca virosa*	Bitter Lettuce, Wild Lettuce	Unani
Kaahuu Barri	*Lactuca serriola*	Wild Lettuce, Prickly Lettuce	Unani
Kaahuu Bustaani	*Lactuca sativa*	Garden Lettuce	Unani
Kaahuu Sahrai (var.)	*Lactuca virosa*	Bitter Lettuce, Wild Lettuce	Unani
Kaahuu Sahrai	*Lactuca serriola*	Wild Lettuce, Prickly Lettuce	Unani
Kaajar-vel	*Strychnos colubrina*	Trumpet Wood	Folk
Kaaju	*Anacardium occidentale*	Cashew Nut Tree	Unani
Kaakaadani	*Anamirta cocculus*	Levant Berry, Fish Berry, Poison Berry, Crow Killer	Ayurvedic
Kaakaadani	*Cardiospermum halicacabum*	Balloon Vine, Winter Pea, Heartseed	Ayurvedic
Kaakaahya	*Solanum nigrum*	Black Nightshade	Ayurvedic
Kaakaandaki	*Celastrus paniculatus*	Staff Tree, Intellect Tree	Ayurvedic
Kaakaandolaa	*Mucuna monosperma*	Negro Bean	Ayurvedic
Kaakaangi	*Martynia annua*	Devil's Claw, Tiger Claw	Ayurvedic
Kaakaangi	*Pentatropis microphylla*	Ambervel, Beak-shaped Elliptic Flower	Ayurvedic

Table Contd.

Indian Name	Botanical Name	English Name	Medicinal System
Kaakajanghaa	*Leea aequata*	Black-berry Holly	Ayurvedic
Kaakajanghaa	*Peristrophe bicalyculata*	Panicled Peristrophe	Ayurvedic
Kaakajanghaa	*Vitex leucoxylon*	Deccan Vitex	Ayurvedic
Kaakajanghaa	*Vitex peduncularis*	Assam Vitex	Ayurvedic
Kaakamaachi	*Solanum nigrum*	Black Nightshade	Ayurvedic
Kaakamaachi-vishesha	*Solanum dulcamara*	Woody Night Shade, Bittersweet, Bitter Nightshade, Felonwort	Ayurvedic
Kaakamaari	*Anamirta cocculus*	Levant Berry, Fish Berry, Poison Berry, Crow Killer	Ayurvedic
Kaakamaataa	*Solanum nigrum*	Black Nightshade	Ayurvedic
Kaakamudraa	*Phaseolus trilobus*	Wild Gram	Ayurvedic
Kaakanaasaa	*Pentatropis microphylla*	Ambervel, Beak-shaped Elliptic Flower	Ayurvedic
Kaakanaasaa	*Pentatropis spiralis*	Ambervel	Ayurvedic
Kaakanaasikaa	*Asclepias curassavica*	Curassavian Swallow-Wort, West Indian Ipecacuanha, Blood-Flower	Ayurvedic
Kaakanaasikaa	*Martynia annua*	Devil's Claw, Tiger Claw	Ayurvedic
Kaakanaasikaa	*Pentatropis microphylla*	Ambervel, Beak-shaped Elliptic Flower	Ayurvedic
Kaakananti	*Abrus precatorius*	Indian Wild Liquorice, Jequirity, Crab's Eye, Precatory Bean	Ayurvedic
Kaakaparni	*Phaseolus trilobus*	Wild Gram	Ayurvedic
Kaakapiluka	*Strychnos nux-vomica*	Nux Vomica	Ayurvedic
Kaakapuchha	*Leonotis nepetaefolia*	Christmas Candlestick, Jonny Collins, Lion's Ear, Lion's Tail	Ayurvedic
Kaakatikta	*Peristrophe bicalyculata*	Panicled Peristrophe	Ayurvedic
Kaakatiktaa	*Cardiospermum halicacabum*	Balloon Vine, Winter Pea, Heartseed	Ayurvedic
Kaaka-tinduka	*Diospyros montana*	Mountain Persimmon	Ayurvedic
Kaakatinduka	*Strychnos nux-vomica*	Nux Vomica	Ayurvedic
Kaakchinchi	*Abrus precatorius*	Indian Wild Liquorice, Jequirity, Crab's Eye, Precatory Bean	Ayurvedic
Kaakdaani	*Capparis sepiaria*	Indian Caper	Ayurvedic

Table Contd.

Indian Name	Botanical Name	English Name	Medicinal System
Kaakdaani	*Capparis spinosa*	Caper Bush	Ayurvedic
Kaakekshu	*Asteracantha longifolia*	Hygrophilla	Ayurvedic
Kaakekshu	*Hygrophila auriculata*	Indian Swampweed	Ayurvedic
Kaakendu	*Strychnos nux-vomica*	Nux Vomica	Ayurvedic
Kaakibeeraa	*Hugonia mystax*	Climbing Flax	Folk
Kaakkaik-kollividai	*Anamirta cocculus*	Levant Berry, Fish Berry, Poison Berry, Crow Killer	Siddha/Tamil
Kaakkanam	*Clitoria ternatea*	Butterfly Pea, Winged-leaved Clitoria, Mezereon	Siddha/Tamil
Kaakkattan	*Ipomoea nil*	Pharbitis Seeds	Folk/Tamil
Kaaknaj	*Physalis alkekengi*	Strawberry Tomato, Winter Cherry	Unani
Kaaknaj-e-Hindi	*Withania coagulans*	Vegetable Rennet, Indian Cheese-maker	Unani
Kaakodumbara	*Ficus hispida*	Devil's Fig, Rough-leaved Fig	Ayurvedic
Kaakoli	*Lilium polyphyllum*	Kakoli Tuber Lily	Ayurvedic
Kaakoli	*Roscoea procera*	Kaakoli	Ayurvedic
Kaakraasingi	*Pistacia integerrima*	Horn-shaped Gall Tree, Kakra Gall Tree	Unani
Kaakraasingi	*Rhus succedanea*	Japanese Wax Tree, Wild Varnish Tree	Unani
Kaaktundphalaa	*Pentatropis microphylla*	Ambervel, Beak-shaped Elliptic Flower	Ayurvedic
Kaakubha	*Terminalia arjuna*	Arjun Terminalia	Ayurvedic
Kaala Shaaka	*Corchorus capsularis*	White Jute	Ayurvedic
Kaala Titmuliyaa	*Viburnum coriaceum*	Guelder Rose, Snowball Tree	Folk
Kaalaa Til	*Guizotia abyssinica*	Nigerseed	Folk
Kaalaa-aduusaa	*Graptophyllum picum*	Caricature Plant, Jamaican Cotton	Folk
Kaalaadaanaa	*Ipomoea hederacea*	Ivy-leaved Morning Glory	Folk
Kaalaadaanaa	*Ipomoea nil*	Pharbitis Seeds	Ayurvedic
Kaalaadaanaa	*Ipomoea nil*	Pharbitis Seeds	Unani
Kaalaajaaji	*Nigella sativa*	Black Cumin, Small Fennel	Ayurvedic
Kaalaa-Kirayaat	*Haplanthus verticillatus*	Black Creat, Kiryaat	Folk

Table Contd.

Indian Name	Botanical Name	English Name	Medicinal System
Kaalaanjani	*Ipomoea nil*	Pharbitis Seeds	Ayurvedic
Kaalaanusaari	*Valeriana wallichii*	Indian Valerian	Ayurvedic
Kaalaanu-saarikaa	*Valeriana wallichii*	Indian Valerian	Ayurvedic
Kaalaanu-saarthaka	*Parmelia perlata*	Parmelia Lichen	Ayurvedic
Kaalakushtha	*Garcinia hanburyi*	Siam Gamboge	Ayurvedic
Kaalaloha	*Aquilaria agallocha*	Aloewood, Eaglewood, Agarwood	Ayurvedic
Kaalameshi	*Operculina turpethum*	Indian Jalap, Turpeth	Ayurvedic
Kaalameshika	*Rubia cordifolia*	Indian Madder, Bengal Madder	Ayurvedic
Kaala-mokhaa	*Elaeodendron glaucum*	Jamrasi Gum Tree	Folk
Kaalaskandha	*Diospyros embryopteris*	Gaub Persimmon, Riber Ebony	Ayurvedic
Kaala-umar	*Ficus asperrima*	Brahma's Banyan, Sandpaper Fig	Folk
Kaalghatika	*Cryptolepis buchanani*	Indian Sarsaparilla	Ayurvedic
Kaali Haldi	*Curcuma caesia*	Black Zedorary	Ayurvedic
Kaali Kamboi	*Breynia retusa*	Cup Saucer Plant	Folk
Kaali Sarson	*Brassica napus*	Mustard, Indian Rape	Unani
Kaali Tulasi	*Ocimum canum*	Hoary Basil	Ayurvedic
Kaali-jarri	*Salvia moorcroftiana*	Wild Sage	Folk
Kaalijiri	*Centratherum anthelminticum*	Purple Flea-bane, Achenes	Ayurvedic
Kaalikaa	*Indigofera tinctoria*	Indigo	Ayurvedic
Kaalinda	*Citrullus vulgaris*	Watermelon	Ayurvedic
Kaalinga	*Holarrhena antidysenterica*	Easter Tree, Ivory Tree, Tellicherry Bark	Ayurvedic
Kaalisar	*Ichnocarpus frutescens*	Black Creeper	Folk
Kaaliyaka	*Coscinium fenestratum*	False Calumba	Ayurvedic
Kaaliziri (Seed)	*Saussurea heteromalla*	Snow Lotus	Folk
Kaalmegha	*Andrographis paniculata*	Creat	Ayurvedic
Kaama-duuti	*Stereospermum personatum*	Trumpet Flower, Yellow Snake Tree	Ayurvedic
Kaamaghna	*Terminalia bellirica*	Belleric Myrobalan, Bastard Myrobalan	Ayurvedic
Kaamalataa	*Ipomoea quamoclit*	Cypress Vine, Indian Pink	Ayurvedic

Table Contd.

Indian Name	Botanical Name	English Name	Medicinal System
Kaamavridhi	*Blepharis edulis*	Acanthus	Ayurvedic
Kaamavriksha	*Viscum articulatum*	Napalese Mistletoe	Ayurvedic
Kaamboja	*Teramnus labialis*	Blue Wiss	Ayurvedic
Kaamboji	*Breynia retusa*	Cup Saucer Plant	Ayurvedic
Kaamboji	*Kirganelia reticulata*	Black-berried Featherfoil	Ayurvedic
Kaamini	*Murraya exotica*	Chinese Boxwood, Andaman Satinwood	Folk
Kaamuka	*Hiptage benghalensis*	Hiptage	Ayurvedic
Kaan	*Leea macrophylla*	Tuberous Holly	Folk
Kaanam	*Dolichos biflorus*	Horsegram	Siddha/Tamil
Kaanan-eranda	*Jatropha curcas*	Physic Nut, Purging Nut	Ayurvedic
Kaanan-mallikaa	*Jasminum angustifolium*	Wild Jasmine	Ayurvedic
Kaanchana	*Bauhinia variegata*	Mountain Ebony, Buddhist Bauhinia	Ayurvedic
Kaanchana	*Paullinia asiatica*	Lopez Root Tree, Wild Orange Tree, Forest Pepper	Ayurvedic
Kaanchanaara (Rakta)	*Bauhinia purpurea*	Camel's Foot Tree, Pink Bauhinia, Butterfly Tree, Geramium Tree, Orchid Tree	Ayurvedic
Kaanchanaara	*Bauhinia malabarica*	Malabar Mountain Ebony	Ayurvedic
Kaanchanaara	*Bauhinia variegata*	Mountain Ebony, Buddhist Bauhinia	Ayurvedic
Kaanchanaaraka	*Bauhinia variegata*	Mountain Ebony, Buddhist Bauhinia	Ayurvedic
Kaanchani	*Curcuma longa*	Turmeric	Ayurvedic
Kaanchankshiri	*Argemone mexicana*	Prickly Poppy, Mexican Poppy	Ayurvedic
Kaanchnaara	*Bauhinia acuminata*	Dwarf White Bauhinia	Ayurvedic
Kaandakatuka	*Ranunculus sceleratus*	Blister Buttercup, Celery-leaved Crowfoot	Ayurvedic
Kaandaruhaa	*Picrorhiza kurroa*	Picrorhiza	Ayurvedic
Kaandira (var.)	*Ranunculus trichophyllus*	Water Crowfoot, Water Fennel	Ayurvedic
Kaandira	*Ranunculus sceleratus*	Blister Buttercup, Celery-leaved Crowfoot	Ayurvedic
Kaanful	*Taraxacum officinale*	Common Dandelion	Unani
Kaantaa	*Callicarpa macrophylla*	Perfumed Cherry	Ayurvedic

Table Contd.

Indian Name	Botanical Name	English Name	Medicinal System
Kaantaa	*Solanum ferox*	Poison-Berry	Ayurvedic
Kaantaa-Gulaab	*Rosa chinensis*	Bengal Rose, Monthly Rose	Folk
Kaantaahvaa	*Callicarpa macrophylla*	Perfumed Cherry	Ayurvedic
Kaantaalu	*Dioscorea pentaphylla*	Cylindrical Brown Yam	Folk
Kaantaasaru	*Lasia spinosa*	Prickly Lasia	Folk
Kaantala	*Agave americana*	Century Plant, American Aloe	Ayurvedic
Kaapi	*Coffea arabica*	Arabian Coffee	Siddha/Tamil
Kaaragil	*Vepris bilocularis*	Unarmed Black Deodar	Siddha/Tamil
Kaarali-Kanda	*Momordica tuberosa*	Eight-ribbed Bitter Gourd	Ayurvedic
Kaaravella	*Momordica charantia*	Bitter Gourd, Balsam Pear, Carilla	Ayurvedic
Kaaravellajalaja	*Momordica cochinchinensis*	Chinese Cucumber, Mbiezi	Ayurvedic
Kaaravellaka	*Momordica charantia*	Bitter Gourd, Balsam Pear, Carilla	Ayurvedic
Kaaravi	*Carum carvi*	Caraway	Ayurvedic
Kaaravi	*Cuminum cyminum*	Cumin	Ayurvedic
Kaari	*Clerodendrum infortunatum*	Glory Bower	Ayurvedic
Kaari	*Miliusa velutina*	Sal-Forest Miliusa	Folk
Kaarpaasa	*Gossypium barbadense*	Egyptian Cotton, Sea-Island Cotton	Ayurvedic
Kaarpaasa	*Gossypium herbaceum*	Asiatic Cotton, Levant Cotton, Uppam Cotton	Ayurvedic
Kaarpaasaka	*Gossypium herbaceum*	Asiatic Cotton, Levant Cotton, Uppam Cotton	Ayurvedic
Kaarpaasi	*Gossypium arboreum*	Tree Cotton, Desi Cotton	Ayurvedic
Kaarpaasi	*Gossypium herbaceum*	Asiatic Cotton, Levant Cotton, Uppam Cotton	Ayurvedic
Kaarvi	*Strobilanthes callosus*	Carvia Callosa	Folk
Kaasaalu	*Dioscorea anguina*	Foetid Yam	Ayurvedic
Kaasaari	*Cassia occidentalis*	Coffee Senna, Foetid Cassia, Negro Coffee	Ayurvedic
Kaasamarda	*Cassia occidentalis*	Coffee Senna, Foetid Cassia, Negro Coffee	Ayurvedic
Kaasamarda	*Cassia sophera*	Sophera Senna	Ayurvedic

Table Contd.

Indian Name	Botanical Name	English Name	Medicinal System
Kaasani	*Cichorium endivia*	Succory, Endive	Ayurvedic
Kaasani Dashti	*Cichorium intybus*	Chicory, Indian Endive	Unani
Kaasani Dashti	*Taraxacum officinale*	Common Dandelion	Unani
Kaasani Sahraayi	*Taraxacum officinale*	Common Dandelion	Unani
Kaasha	*Saccharum spontaneum*	Thatch Grass, Wild Sugarcane	Ayurvedic
Kaashmari	*Gmelina arborea*	Candahar Tree, White Teak	Ayurvedic
Kaashmarya	*Gmelina arborea*	Candahar Tree, White Teak	Ayurvedic
Kaashmira	*Crocus sativus*	Saffron, Crocus	Ayurvedic
Kaashmira	*Inula racemosa*	Elecampane	Ayurvedic
Kaashmira	*Saussurea lappa*	Kuth, Costus	Ayurvedic
Kaashmiraa	*Aconitum heterophyllum*	Atis Root, Aconite	Ayurvedic
Kaashmirajiraka	*Carum bulbocastanum*	Black Caraway	Ayurvedic
Kaashmirajiraka	*Carum carvi*	Caraway	Ayurvedic
Kaashmiraka	*Crocus sativus*	Saffron, Crocus	Ayurvedic
Kaashthaaluka	*Dioscorea alata*	Wild Yam, Greater Yam, Asiatic Yam	Ayurvedic
Kaashtodumbara	*Ficus hispida*	Devil's Fig, Rough-leaved Fig	Ayurvedic
Kaasim	*Alstonia scholaris*	Devil's Tree, Dita Bark Tree	Unani
Kaasukkatti (Heartwood extract)	*Acacia catechu*	Cutch tree, Catechu	Siddha/Tamil
Kaat	*Acacia catechu*	Cutch tree, Catechu	Unani
Kaathilla	*Momordica charantia*	Bitter Gourd, Balsam Pear, Carilla	Ayurvedic
Kaathukarunai	*Amorphophallus campanulatus*	Elephant's Foot Yam	Siddha/Tamil
Kaattaaththippoo (Flower)	*Woodfordia fruticosa*	Fire-flame Bush, Shiranjitea	Siddha/Tamil
Kaattu-milagu	*Piper wallichii*	Nepal Pepper	Siddha/Tamil
Kaattupaagala	*Momordica dioica*	Small Bitter Gourd, burr Cucumber	Siddha/Tamil
Kaatu Kunthumani	*Coix lacryma-jobi*	Job's Tears	Siddha/Tamil
Kaatu Mullangi	*Blumea lacera*	Nagai Camphor	Siddha/Tamil
Kaatu Seerakam	*Centratherum anthelminticum*	Purple Flea-bane, Achenes	Siddha/Tamil

Table Contd.

Indian Name	Botanical Name	English Name	Medicinal System
Kaatukollu	*Cassia absus*	Four-leaved Cassia, Pig's Senna	Siddha/Tamil
Kaatumalli	*Jasminum angustifolium*	Wild Jasmine	Siddha/Tamil
Kaatumurungai	*Moringa concanensis*	Drumstick, Horse-Radish	Siddha/Tamil
Kaatupayaru	*Phaseolus trilobus*	Wild Gram	Siddha/Tamil
Kaayaaputi	*Melaleuca leucadendron*	Cajeput Tree, Swamp Tea Tree, White Tea Tree	Folk
Kaayaphal	*Myrica nagi*	Box Myrtle	Unani
Kaayasthaa	*Emblica officinalis*	Embic, Indian Gooseberry	Ayurvedic
Kaayasthaa	*Terminalia chebula*	Chebulic Myrobalan, Black Myrobalan	Ayurvedic
Kaayasthikaa	*Fritillaria roylei*	Pei-mu (China), Kakoli	Ayurvedic
Kabaabchini	*Piper cubeba*	Cubeb, Tailed Pepper	Unani
Kabaab-e-Khandaan	*Zanthoxylum armatum*	Toothache Tree, Indian Prickly Ash	Unani
Kabar	*Capparis aphylla*	Caper Berry	Unani
Kabara	*Capparis sepiaria*	Indian Caper	Ayurvedic
Kabara	*Capparis spinosa*	Caper Bush	Ayurvedic
Kabar-e-Hindi	*Capparis aphylla*	Caper Berry	Unani
Kabar-ul-Hind	*Capparis aphylla*	Caper Berry	Unani
Kabjaka	*Abrus precatorius*	Indian Wild Liquorice, Jequirity, Crab's Eye, Precatory Bean	Ayurvedic
Kacchuraa	*Mucuna prurita*	Cowhage, Horse-eye Bean	Ayurvedic
Kachhuraa	*Fagonia cretica*	Thorny Fagonbush, Mantle of the Virgin	Ayurvedic
Kachloraa	*Pithecellobium monadelphum*	Grasshopper Tree	Folk
Kachnaal	*Bauhinia acuminata*	Dwarf White Bauhinia	Unani
Kachnaala	*Bauhinia racemosa*	Kachnar Tree	Folk
Kachnaar	*Bauhinia racemosa*	Kachnar Tree	Unani
Kachnaar	*Bauhinia tomentosa*	Yellow Bauhinia, St. Thomas Tree, Bell Bauhinia	Folk
Kacholaki-zhangu	*Kaempferia galanga*	Maraba	Siddha/Tamil

Table Contd.

Indian Name	Botanical Name	English Name	Medicinal System
Kadalai	*Lagerstroemia flos-reginae*	Pride of India, Queen's Flowers, Queen Crape Myrtle	Folk/Tamil
Kadali	*Musa paradisiaca*	Banana, Plantain	Ayurvedic
Kadalranchi	*Olax scandens*	Olax	Folk/Tamil
Kadalthengai	*Lodoicea maldivica*	Double Coconut Palm, Sea Coconut Palm	Siddha/Tamil
Kadam Karai	*Canthium parviflorum*	Wild Jasmine	Siddha/Tamil
Kadamba (var.)	*Mitragyna parvifolia*	Kaim Kadamb	Ayurvedic
Kadamba	*Anthocephalus cadamba*	Wild Cinchona	Ayurvedic
Kadambaka	*Adina cordifolia*	Yellow Teak, Saffron Teak	Ayurvedic
Kadambu	*Microcos paniculata*	Kadamb	Folk/Tamil
Kadambu	*Siegesbeckia orientalis*	The Holy Herb, Sieges-beckia	Siddha/Tamil
Kadappai	*Barringtonia acutangula*	Indian Oak	Siddha/Tamil
Kadara	*Acacia catechu*	Cutch tree, Catechu	Ayurvedic
Kadara	*Acacia suma*	White Babul	Ayurvedic
Kadaranarathai	*Citrus medica*	Citron	Siddha/Tamil
Kadaranji	*Ximenia americana*	Tallow-Wood, False Sandal-Wood	Folk/Tamil
Kadashing	*Radermachera xylocarpa*	Padri Tree	Folk
Kaddalattai	*Dolichandrone falcate*	Corky-winged-seed Tree	Siddha/Tamil
Kaddu-e-Roomi	*Benincasa hispida*	Ash Gourd, White Gourd, Wax Gourd, White Pumpkin	Unani
Kaddu-e-Sheerin	*Cucurbita maxima*	Red Gourd, Red Pumpkin	Unani
Kaddu-e-talkh	*Lagenaria siceraria*	Bitter Bottle-Gourd	Unani
Kadichai	*Casearia tomentosa*	Fish-Poison Wood	Siddha/Tamil
Kadir Pachai	*Pogostemon patchouli*	Patchouli	Siddha/Tamil
Kadiram	*Acacia catechu*	Cutch tree, Catechu	Siddha/Tamil
Kadugu	*Brassica campestris*	Field Mustard, Turnip Rape	Siddha/Tamil
Kadugu	*Brassica juncea*	Chinese Mustard, Brown Mustard	Siddha/Tamil
Kadugu	*Brassica nigra*	Black Mustard	Siddha/Tamil
Kaduguragini	*Picrorhiza kurroa*	Picrorhiza	Siddha/Tamil
Kaduka poo (Gall)	*Pistacia integerrima*	Horn-shaped Gall Tree, Kakra Gall Tree	Siddha/Tamil

Table Contd.

Indian Name	Botanical Name	English Name	Medicinal System
Kadukanni	*Panicum miliaceum*	Common Millet, Proso Millet, Hog Millet	Folk/Tamil
Kadukapoo (galls)	*Rhus succedanea*	Japanese Wax Tree, Wild Varnish Tree	Siddha/Tamil
Kadukkaai	*Terminalia chebula*	Chebulic Myrobalan, Black Myrobalan	Siddha/Tamil
Kadusinde	*Solanum erianthum*	Mullen Nightshade	Folk
Kafe-aaishaa	*Anastatica hierochuntica*	Jericho Rose	Unani
Kafemariyam	*Anastatica hierochuntica*	Jericho Rose	Unani
Kagdown	*Asparagus officinalis*	Asparagus, Sparrow Grass	Folk
Kagoti	*Ficus arnottiana*	Indian Rock Fig	Siddha/Tamil
Kahruubaa	*Pinus succinifera*	Baltic Amber, Succinite	Unani
Kahvaa	*Coffea arabica*	Arabian Coffee	Unani
Kailaashi	*Oxyria digyna*	Mountain Sorrel, Alpine Sorrel	Folk
Kaindal	*Heracleum candicans*	Cowparsnip	Folk
Kairaata	*Swertia chirayita*	Chiretta	Ayurvedic
Kaith	*Feronia limonia*	Wood Apple	Folk
Kaitrya	*Careya arborea*	Kumbi, Slow-Match Tree	Ayurvedic
Kaivartikaa	*Ventilago madraspatana*	Ventilago Vermilion Vine	Ayurvedic
Kakahi	*Abutilon indicum*	Country Mallow, Flowering Maples, Chinese Bell-flowers	Folk
Kakahiyaa	*Abutilon indicum*	Country Mallow, Flowering Maples, Chinese Bell-flowers	Folk
Kakaiyaa	*Flacourita indica*	Ramontchi, Madagascar Plum, Mauritius Plum, Governor's Plum	Folk
Kakanti	*Abrus precatorius*	Indian Wild Liquorice, Jequirity, Crab's Eye, Precatory Bean	Ayurvedic
Kakapu	*Torenia travancorica*	Wishbone Flower	Folk
Kakar	*Pistacia integerrima*	Horn-shaped Gall Tree, Kakra Gall Tree	Unani
Kakari	*Cucumis melo*	Musk Melon, Sweet Melon	Unani

Table Contd.

Indian Name	Botanical Name	English Name	Medicinal System
Kakaronda	*Blumea eriantha*	Nagai Camphor	Unani
Kakarondaa	*Blumea balsamifera*	Nagai Camphor	Unani
Kakarondaa	*Blumea fastulosa*	Nagai Camphor	Unani
Kakarondaa	*Blumea lacera*	Nagai Camphor	Unani
Kakatundi	*Asclepias curassavica*	Curassavian Swallow-Wort, West Indian Ipecacuanha, Blood-Flower	Folk
Kakatundi	*Martynia annua*	Devil's Claw, Tiger Claw	Siddha/Tamil
Kakhum	*Myrsine africana*	Pseudo-Embelia	Folk
Kakkaippilai	*Casearia esculenta*	Boxwood	Siddha/Tamil
Kakkarikkay	*Cucumis melo*	Musk Melon, Sweet Melon	Folk/Tamil
Kakkattan	*Ipomoea hederacea*	Ivy-leaved Morning Glory	Folk
Kakkola	*Piper cubeba*	Cubeb, Tailed Pepper	Ayurvedic
Kakolaa	*Amomum subulatum*	Greater or Nepal Cardamom	Folk
Kakosh	*Viola odorata*	Sweet Violet	Unani
Kakranda	*Blumea lacera*	Nagai Camphor	Folk
Kakrol	*Momordica cochinchinensis*	Chinese Cucumber, Mbiezi	Folk
Kakrol	*Momordica tuberosa*	Eight-ribbed Bitter Gourd	Folk
Kakubha	*Terminalia arjuna*	Arjun Terminalia	Ayurvedic
Kakubha	*Terminalia myriocarpa*	Hollock	Ayurvedic
Kal Aal	*Ficus dalhousiae*	Carica Fig	Siddha/Tamil
Kal Ichi	*Ficus microcarpa*	Indian Laurel Fig	Siddha/Tamil
Kal Itthi	*Ficus talboti*	Pakar Tree	Siddha/Tamil
Kalaaya	*Lathyrus sativus*	Chickling Vetch, Grass Pea	Folk
Kalakke	*Carissa carandas*	Christ's Thorn, Bengal Currant	Siddha/Tamil
Kalambaka	*Coscinium fenestratum*	False Calumba	Ayurvedic
Kalambaka	*Jateorhiza palmata*	Calumba, Colombo	Ayurvedic
Kalambi	*Ipomoea aquatica*	Swamp Cabbage	Ayurvedic
Kalangu	*Phoenix pusilla*	Wild Coromandel Palm	Siddha/Tamil
Kalappanki-zhangu	*Gloriosa superba*	Glory Lily, Super Lily, Tiger's Claws	Siddha/Tamil
Kal-arasu	*Ficus asperrima*	Brahma's Banyan, Sandpaper Fig	Siddha/Tamil

Table Contd.

Indian Name	Botanical Name	English Name	Medicinal System
Kalasan	*Lannea coromandelica*	Jhingan	Siddha/Tamil
Kalashi	*Uraria picta*	Trailing Uraria	Ayurvedic
Kalawa	*Salvadora oleoides*	Mustard Tree, Salt Bush Tree, Tooth Brush Tree	Siddha/Tamil
Kalhudaitumbai	*Trichodesma indicum*	Indian Borage	Siddha/Tamil
Kaliaar	*Bauhinia purpurea*	Camel's Foot Tree, Pink Bauhinia, Butterfly Tree, Geramium Tree, Orchid Tree	Folk
Kalidrum	*Terminalia bellirica*	Belleric Myrobalan, Bastard Myrobalan	Ayurvedic
Kalihaari	*Gloriosa superba*	Glory Lily, Super Lily, Tiger's Claws	Ayurvedic
Kalihaari	*Meconopsis aculeata*	Blue Poppy	Folk
Kalikaa	*Nigella sativa*	Black Cumin, Small Fennel	Ayurvedic
Kalikaari	*Gloriosa superba*	Glory Lily, Super Lily, Tiger's Claws	Ayurvedic
Kalingaka	*Holarrhena antidysenterica*	Easter Tree, Ivory Tree, Tellicherry Bark	Ayurvedic
Kalisam	*Prosopis spicigera*	Mestique Gum Tree	Siddha/Tamil
Kaliyana-murukkan	*Erythrina indica*	Indian Coral Tree	Siddha/Tamil
Kalkashunda	*Cassia occidentalis*	Coffee Senna, Foetid Cassia, Negro Coffee	Folk/Bengal
Kallalnaram	*Ficus lacor*	White Fig	Siddha/Tamil
Kalli	*Euphorbia nivulia*	Corky-barked Spurge	Siddha/Tamil
Kalmi-lataa	*Rivea hypocrateriformis*	Midnapore Creeper	Folk
Kalo Bikhmo	*Aconitum laciniatum*	Himalayan Aconite	Folk
Kalonji	*Nigella sativa*	Black Cumin, Small Fennel	Unani
Kalpakku	*Pithecellobium monadelphum*	Grasshopper Tree	Siddha/Tamil
Kalpanaatha	*Andrographis paniculata*	Creat	Ayurvedic
Kal-passi	*Parmelia perlata*	Parmelia Lichen	Siddha/Tamil
Kalpootha	*Xylopia parviflora*	Netawu, Atuketiya	Folk/Tamil
Kalpottan	*Xylopia parviflora*	Netawu, Atuketiya	Folk/Kerala
Kalupatti	*Mallotus philippensis*	Kamala Tree, Monkey Face Tree	Siddha/Tamil

Table Contd.

Indian Name	Botanical Name	English Name	Medicinal System
Kanyaa	*Aloe barbadensis*	Curacao Aloe, Barbados Aloe, Indian Aloe, Jaffarabad Aloe	Ayurvedic
Kanyaasaara (Dried leaf juice)	*Aloe barbadensis*	Curacao Aloe, Barbados Aloe, Indian Aloe, Jaffarabad Aloe	Ayurvedic
Kanyong	*Dipterocarpus turbinatus*	Common Gurjun Tree, Wood Oil Tree	Folk/ Meghalaya
Kaoashund	*Geranium wallichianum*	Wallich Crane's Bill	Folk
Kapaasa	*Gossypium arboreum*	Tree Cotton, Desi Cotton	Folk
Kapaasa	*Gossypium barbadense*	Egyptian Cotton, Sea-Island Cotton	Folk
Kapaasi	*Corylus colurna*	Turkish Hazel	Folk
Kapavila	*Vinca pusilla*	Bengal Periwinkle	Folk
Kaphal	*Garcinia cowa*	Indo-Malayan Brindleberry	Folk
Kapikacchuu	*Mucuna prurita*	Cowhage, Horse-eye Bean	Ayurvedic
Kapilaa	*Dalbergia latifolia*	East Indian Rosewood, Bombay Blackwood	Ayurvedic
Kapilu	*Strychnos nux-vomica*	Nux Vomica	Ayurvedic
Kapipriya	*Feronia limonia*	Wood Apple	Ayurvedic
Kapitaila	*Liquidambar orientalis*	Storax, Oriental Sweet Gum	Ayurvedic
Kapitaila	*Styrax officinale*	The True Storax Tree	Ayurvedic
Kapitana	*Albizia lebbeck*	Siris Tree, East Indian Walnut	Ayurvedic
Kapitana	*Spondias pinnata*	Hog-Plum, Wild Mango	Ayurvedic
Kapitana	*Thespesia populnea*	Portia Tree, Tulip Tree, Umbrella Tree, False Rosewood	Ayurvedic
Kapittha	*Feronia limonia*	Wood Apple	Ayurvedic
Kaplila	*Mallotus philippensis*	Kamala Tree, Monkey Face Tree	Siddha/Tamil
Kapoor Ghass	*Themeda arundinacea*	Ulla Grass	Folk
Kapotavankaa	*Bacopa monnieri*	Thyme-leaved Gratiola	Ayurvedic
Kapurijadi	*Aerva lanata*	Mountain Knot Grass	Folk
Kapuur-Bhendi	*Turraea villosa*	Wild Honeysuckle	Folk
Kapuuri	*Hemidesmus indicus*	Indian Sarsaparilla	Ayurvedic
Kapuurkachari	*Hedychium spicatum*	Spiked Ginger Ivy	Ayurvedic
Kapuurkachari	*Hedychium spicatum*	Spiked Ginger Ivy	Unani
Kapuurkachari	*Kaempferia galanga*	Marba	Folk

Table Contd.

Indian Name	Botanical Name	English Name	Medicinal System
Karachunai	*Tacca pinnatifida*	Fiji Arrowroot, Tahiti Arrowroot	Siddha/Tamil
Karafs	*Apium graveolens*	Celery	Unani
Karafs-e-Hindi	*Apium leptophyllum*	Celery	Unani
Karafs-e-Hindi	*Trachyspermum roxburghianum*	Ajmud	Unani
Karafs-e-Kohi	*Petroselinum crispum*	Parsley	Unani
Karafs-e-kohi	*Prangos pabularia*	Prangos, Yugan. Aju-Chach	Unani
Karahaata	*Gardenia turgida*	Bharangi Bark Tree	Ayurvedic
Karai	*Sterculia urens*	Bissy Nuts, Karaya Gum	Folk
Kara-jodi-kanda	*Selaginella involvens*	Spike Moss	Ayurvedic
Kara-jodi-kanda	*Selaginella rupestris*	Little Clubmoss, Rock Spike-Moss	Ayurvedic
Karakatiyaa (Seeds)	*Ipomoea purpurea*	Tall Morning-Glory	Folk
Karakattam	*Ziziphus trinervia*	Jagged Jujube	Siddha/Tamil
Karalli	*Carallia brachiata*	Freshwater Mangrove	Folk
Karamarda	*Carissa carandas*	Christ's Thorn, Bengal Currant	Ayurvedic
Karamardikaa	*Carissa opaca*	Karaunda	Ayurvedic
Karangalli	*Acacia catechu*	Cutch tree, Catechu	Siddha/Tamil
Karanja	*Derris indica*	Indian Beech, Pongamia Oil Tree	Ayurvedic
Karanja	*Pongamia pinnata*	Pongam Oil Tree, Indian Beech	Ayurvedic
Karanjin	*Caesalpinia bonduc*	Fever Nut, Bonduc Nut, Nikkar Nut	Ayurvedic
Karanjuaa	*Caesalpinia bonduc*	Fever Nut, Bonduc Nut, Nikkar Nut	Unani
Karanoi	*Roylea cinerea*	Roylea Mint	Folk
Karantaa	*Cryptolepis buchanani*	Indian Sarsaparilla	Ayurvedic
Karantaa	*Cryptolepis buchanani*	Indian Sarsaparilla	Folk
Karantaa	*Ichnocarpus frutescens*	Black Creeper	Folk
Karapilly	*Pithecellobium dulce*	Minila Tamarind, Madras Thorn, Quamachil	Siddha/Tamil
Karaveera	*Nerium indicum*	Indian Oleander, White Oleander	Ayurvedic

Table Contd.

Indian Name	Botanical Name	English Name	Medicinal System
Karaveeraka	*Nerium oleander*	Indian Oleander, White Oleander	Siddha/Tamil
Karaviram	*Nerium indicum*	Indian Oleander, White Oleander	Siddha/Tamil
Karbudaar	*Olax scandens*	Olax	Ayurvedic
Karchuura	*Curcuma zedoaria*	Zedoary, Zerumbet	Ayurvedic
Karelaa	*Momordica charantia*	Bitter Gourd, Balsam Pear, Carilla	Unani
Kareruaa	*Capparis zeylanica*	Ceylon Caper	Folk
Karila	*Capparis aphylla*	Caper Berry	Ayurvedic
Karimulli	*Solanum ferox*	Poison-Berry	Siddha/Tamil
Karindu	*Pisonia aculeata*	Devil's Claw	Siddha/Tamil
Karinga	*Gardenia jasminoides*	Cape Jasmine	Siddha/Tamil
Karinjottei	*Quassia indica*	Niepa Bark Tree	Folk/Tamil
Karinkaara	*Carissa carandas*	Christ's Thorn, Bengal Currant	Ayurvedic
Karintakaali	*Geophila repens*	Corrida, Yerba de guava (US)	Folk
Karipattaa	*Murraya koenigii*	Curry-Leaf Tree	Unani
Karir	*Capparis aphylla*	Caper Berry	Folk
Karirak	*Capparis aphylla*	Caper Berry	Ayurvedic
Karisalaan-kanni	*Eclipta alba*	Trailing Eclipta Plant	Siddha/Tamil
Karivempu	*Murraya koenigii*	Curry-Leaf Tree	Siddha/Tamil
Kariyartharani	*Stachytarpheta jamaicensis*	Brazilian Tea, Bastard Vervain, Aaron's Rod	Ayurvedic
Kariyundu	*Acacia torta*	Twisted Acacia	Siddha/Tamil
Karjiri	*Centratherum anthelminticum*	Purple Flea-bane, Achenes	Ayurvedic
Karkaaruka	*Cucurbita maxima*	Red Gourd, Red Pumpkin	Ayurvedic
Karkandhu	*Ziziphus nummularia*	Wild Jujube	Ayurvedic
Karkani	*Leea indica*	Purple-berry Holly	Folk
Karkar	*Iris kumaonensis*	Kumaon Iris	Folk
Karkash	*Mallotus philippensis*	Kamala Tree, Monkey Face Tree	Ayurvedic
Karkasha	*Trichosanthes dioica*	Patol, Pointed Gourd	Ayurvedic
Karkashchhada	*Trichosanthes dioica*	Patol, Pointed Gourd	Ayurvedic

Table Contd.

Indian Name	Botanical Name	English Name	Medicinal System
Karkata	*Pistacia integerrima*	Horn-shaped Gall Tree, Kakra Gall Tree	Ayurvedic
Karkataakhya	*Pistacia integerrima*	Horn-shaped Gall Tree, Kakra Gall Tree	Ayurvedic
Karkatajihvaa	*Leea indica*	Purple-berry Holly	Ayurvedic
Karkataka	*Momordica cochinchinensis*	Chinese Cucumber, Mbiezi	Ayurvedic
Karkata-kasringi	*Rhus succedanea*	Japanese Wax Tree, Wild Varnish Tree	Siddha/Tamil
Karkatashringee	*Rhus succedanea*	Japanese Wax Tree, Wild Varnish Tree	Ayurvedic
Karkatashringi	*Pistacia integerrima*	Horn-shaped Gall Tree, Kakra Gall Tree	Ayurvedic
Karkatashringikaa	*Pistacia integerrima*	Horn-shaped Gall Tree, Kakra Gall Tree	Ayurvedic
Karkati	*Cucumis melo*	Musk Melon, Sweet Melon	Ayurvedic
Karkota	*Momordica dioica*	Small Bitter Gourd, burr Cucumber	Ayurvedic
Karkotaka	*Momordica dioica*	Small Bitter Gourd, burr Cucumber	Ayurvedic
Karkotikaa	*Momordica dioica*	Small Bitter Gourd, burr Cucumber	Ayurvedic
Karkotikaa-vandhyaa	*Momordica dioica*	Small Bitter Gourd, burr Cucumber	Ayurvedic
Karmal	*Averrhoa carambola*	Carambola, Star Fruit, Chinese Gooseberry	Unani
Karmaranga	*Averrhoa carambola*	Carambola, Star Fruit, Chinese Gooseberry	Ayurvedic
Karna-kusha	*Cymbopogon jwarancusa*	Vetiver-scented Grass	Folk/Bengal
Karnamorata	*Commelina benghalensis*	Tropical Spiderwort	Ayurvedic
Karnasphota	*Commelina benghalensis*	Tropical Spiderwort	Ayurvedic
Karnikaa	*Lilium polyphyllum*	Kakoli Tuber Lily	Ayurvedic
Karnikaa	*Rosa centifolia*	Cabbage Rose, Provence Rose, Hundred-leaved Rose	Ayurvedic
Karnikaara	*Cassia fistula*	Indian Laburnum, Purging Cassia, Golden Shower	Ayurvedic

Table Contd.

Indian Name	Botanical Name	English Name	Medicinal System
Karnikaara	*Pterospermum acerifolium*	Hathipaila	Ayurvedic
Karnsphotaa	*Cardiospermum halicacabum*	Balloon Vine, Winter Pea, Heartseed	Ayurvedic
Karondaa	*Carissa carandas*	Christ's Thorn, Bengal Currant	Unani
Karparaal	*Juglans regia*	Walnut Tree	Ayurvedic
Karpari	*Ficus lacor*	White Fig	Ayurvedic
Karpookarisi	*Psoralea corylifolia*	Purple Fleabane	Siddha/Tamil
Karpooramaram	*Eucalyptus globulus*	Blue-gum Tree, Australian Gum Tree	Siddha/Tamil
Karpoorvalli	*Coleus amboinicus*	Indian Borage	Siddha/Tamil
Karpura	*Cinnamomum camphora*	Camphor Tree	Ayurvedic
Karpura Tulasi	*Ocimum kilimandscharicum*	Camphor Basil	Ayurvedic
Karpuraa	*Curcuma amada*	Mango-ginger, Wild Turmeric	Ayurvedic
Karpuraa	*Curcuma aromatica*	Wild Turmeric, Yellow Zedoary	Ayurvedic
Karpuravalli	*Anisochilus carnosus*	Wild Violet	Folk (South)
Karpuur	*Limnophila aromatica*	Turpentine Spinach	Folk
Karpuur	*Limnophila indica*	Oil-of-lemons Spinach	Folk
Karrallamu	*Zingiber zerumbet*	Zerumbet Ginger	Folk
Karramarda	*Terminalia tomentosa*	Laurel (trade)	Folk/Tamil
Karre Vembu	*Garuga pinnata*	Grey Downy Balsam	Siddha/Tamil
Karshaphala	*Terminalia bellirica*	Belleric Myrobalan, Bastard Myrobalan	Ayurvedic
Karsya	*Vateria indica*	White Damar, Indian Copal-Tree, Malabar Tallow Tree, Piney Varnish-Tree	Ayurvedic
Karu Karunai Kizhangu	*Typhonium trilobatum*	Bengal Arum	Folk/Tamil
Karui	*Roylea cinerea*	Roylea Mint	Folk
Karui Buuti	*Ainsliaea aptera*	Bitter Ainsli	Folk
Karukandu	*Dioscorea daemona*	Asiatic Bitter Yam	Folk
Karukanni	*Clerodendrum infortunatum*	Glory Bower	Siddha/Tamil
Karum Dumbi	*Diospyros melanoxylon*	Coromandel Ebony, Persimmon	Siddha/Tamil

Table Contd.

Indian Name	Botanical Name	English Name	Medicinal System
Karumboraju	*Chloroxylon swietenia*	Indian Satinwood Tree	Siddha/Tamil
Karumbu	*Saccharum officinarum*	Gannaa, Naishakar	Siddha/Tamil
Karumcheerakam	*Nigella damascena*	Love-in-a-mist	Siddha/Tamil
Karumpul	*Echinochloa colonum*	Shama Millet	Siddha/Tamil
Karum-sumbai (leaf)	*Sesbania sesban*	Common Sesban	Siddha/Tamil
Karunaabhi	*Aconitum ferox*	Indian Aconite, Wolfsbane, Monkshood	Siddha/Tamil
Karunannari	*Ichnocarpus frutescens*	Black Creeper	Siddha/Tamil
Karuncheerakam Seeragm	*Nigella sativa*	Black Cumin, Small Fennel	Siddha/Tamil
Karunchivadai	*Operculina turpethum*	Indian Jalap, Turpeth	Siddha/Tamil
Karundan	*Scirpus kysoor*	Kaseru Tuber	Siddha/Tamil
Karundoroiral	*Dalbergia latifolia*	East Indian Rosewood, Bombay Blackwood	Siddha/Tamil
Karunjurai	*Capparis sepiaria*	Indian Caper	Siddha/Tamil
Karunkaali (Bark)	*Acacia catechu*	Cutch tree, Catechu	Siddha/Tamil
Karunkungiliyam	*Canarium strictum*	Black Dammar	Siddha/Tamil
Karunkuvalai	*Kaempferia rotunda*	Rounded Galanga	Siddha/Tamil
Karunochhi	*Justicia gendarussa*	Blue-flowered Vasaka, Chinese Justicia	Siddha/Tamil
Karupalai	*Putranjiva roxburghii*	Child-life Tree, Indian Amulet Plant, Spurious Wild Olive	Siddha/Tamil
Karupali	*Drypetes roxburghii*	Putrajiva	Siddha/Tamil
Karupporam	*Cinnamomum camphora*	Camphor Tree	Siddha/Tamil
Karu-velamaram	*Acacia arabica*	Babul, Black Babul, Indian Gum Arabic Tree	Siddha/Tamil
Karuvelei	*Acacia arabica*	Babul, Black Babul, Indian Gum Arabic Tree	Siddha/Tamil
Karuveppilai	*Murraya koenigii*	Curry-Leaf Tree	Siddha/Tamil
Karuvoomatthai	*Datura metel*	Thornapple, Downy Datura	Siddha/Tamil
Karwaa	*Viburnum coriaceum*	Guelder Rose, Snowball Tree	Folk
Kasaalu	*Alocasia indica*	Giant Taro	Ayurvedic
Kasaalu	*Dioscorea anguina*	Foetid Yam	Ayurvedic
Kasai	*Memecylon edule*	Iron Wood	Siddha/Tamil

Table Contd.

Indian Name	Botanical Name	English Name	Medicinal System
Kasakasa (Seeds)	*Papaver somniferum*	Opium Poppy	Siddha/Tamil
Kasakasa	*Papaver rhoeas*	Corn Poppy, Red Poppy	Siddha/Tamil
Kaseru (Punjab)	*Cyperus esculentus*	Earth Almond, Chufa, Rush Nut, Tiger Nut	Folk
Kaseru	*Scirpus kysoor*	Kaseru Tuber	Folk
Kasheru	*Scirpus kysoor*	Kaseru Tuber	Ayurvedic
Kasheruka	*Eleocharis dulcis*	Chinese Water Chestnut	Ayurvedic
Kasheruka	*Scirpus kysoor*	Kaseru Tuber	Ayurvedic
Kashmal	*Berberis vulgaris*	Common Barberry, True Barberry	Folk
Kashmiri Gaozabaan	*Arnebia benthamii*	Himalayan Arnebia	Folk
Kashmiri Kahzabaan	*Arnebia benthamii*	Himalayan Arnebia	Folk
Kashphala	*Piper cubeba*	Cubeb, Tailed Pepper	Ayurvedic
Kasini	*Hibiscus cannabinus*	Bimlipatam Jute, Kenaf, Mesta, Deccan Hemp	Folk/Tamil
Kasinikkeerai	*Cichorium intybus*	Chicory, Indian Endive	Siddha/Tamil
Kasittumbai	*Impatiens balsamina*	Garden Balsam	Siddha/Tamil
Kasondi	*Cassia occidentalis*	Coffee Senna, Foetid Cassia, Negro Coffee	Unani
Kasondi	*Cassia sophera*	Sophera Senna	Unani
Kasoos	*Cuscuta reflexa*	Doddar	Unani
Kastoori Manjal	*Curcuma aromatica*	Wild Turmeric, Yellow Zedoary	Siddha/Tamil
Kastoori Vendai	*Pavonia odorata*	Fragrant Sticky Mallow	Siddha/Tamil
Kasturi Mogaraa	*Jasminum multiflorum*	Downy Jasmine	Ayurvedic
Kasturi Mogaraa	*Jasminum multiflorum*	Downy Jasmine	Folk
Kasturi-vendai	*Hibiscus abelmoschus*	Musk Seed, Ambette Seed, Muskmallow	Siddha/Tamil
Kastuurivelam	*Acacia farnesiana*	Cassie Flower, Sweet Acacia	Siddha/Tamil
Kasuri Methi	*Trigonella corniculata*	Kasuri Fenugreek	Folk
Kata Champaa	*Artabotrys hexapetalus*	Yling-Yling Vine	Folk
Kataad	*Astragalus gummifer*	Tragacanth Gum	Unani
Kataai Kalaan	*Solanum indicum*	Poison Berry	Unani
Kataai Khurd	*Solanum xanthocarpum*	Wild Eggplant, Yellow-Berried Nightshade	Unani

Table Contd.

Indian Name	Botanical Name	English Name	Medicinal System
Kataaya	*Flacourtia indica*	Ramontchi, Madagascar Plum, Mauritius Plum, Governor's Plum	Folk
Katabhi	*Careya arborea*	Kumbi, Slow-Match Tree	Ayurvedic
Katahaar	*Xylosma longifolium*	Dandal Tree, Kandhara Tree	Folk/Assam
Katahal	*Artocarpus integrifolia*	Jackfruit, Jack Tree	Folk
Katai Kalaan	*Solanum ferox*	Poison-Berry	Unani
Kataka	*Cassia absus*	Four-leaved Cassia, Pig's Senna	Ayurvedic
Kataka	*Strychnos potatorum*	Clearing Nut Tree	Ayurvedic
Katakaphala	*Strychnos potatorum*	Clearing Nut Tree	Ayurvedic
Katambal	*Rumex hastatus*	Toothed Dock	Folk
Katampam	*Siegesbeckia orientalis*	The Holy Herb, Sieges-beckia	Siddha/Tamil
Kateri (bigger var.)	*Solanum ferox*	Poison-Berry	Ayurvedic
Kateri (bigger var.)	*Solanum indicum*	Poison Berry	Ayurvedic
Kateri Indryaayana	*Ecballium elaterium*	Squirting Cucumber	Folk
Kath Safed	*Acacia leucophloea*	White Babul	Unani
Kathaalu	*Dioscorea alata*	Wild Yam, Greater Yam, Asiatic Yam	Folk
Kathachampaa	*Pavetta indica*	White-Pavetta	Ayurvedic
Kathachoraa	*Angelica archangelica*	Angelica	Ayurvedic
Kathapahaariaa	*Reissantia indica*	Atari Vine	Folk
Kathela	*Picea smithiana*	West Himalayan Spruce	Folk
Kathirikai	*Solanum melongena*	Eggplant, Brinjal	Siddha/Tamil
Kathmahuli	*Bauhinia retusa*	Semla Gum Tree	Folk
Kathneem	*Murraya koenigii*	Curry-Leaf Tree	Folk
Kaththakkaambu	*Uncaria gambier*	Pale Catechu, Gambier	Siddha/Tamil
Katili-chaulai	*Amaranthus spinosus*	Spiny Amaranth, Thorny Amaranth, Spiny Pigweed	Folk
Katiraa	*Astragalus gummifer*	Tragacanth Gum	Unani
Katol	*Salsola kali*	Glass-Wort, Russian Thistle, Prickly-Saltwort	Ayurvedic

Table Contd.

Indian Name	Botanical Name	English Name	Medicinal System
Katphala	*Myrica nagi*	Box Myrtle	Ayurvedic
Katplaaster	*Anaphalis neelgerriana*	Katplaster	Folk
Katsaraiyaa	*Barleria cristata*	Crested Philippine Violet	Folk
Katsaraiyaa	*Barleria prionitis*	Common Yellow Nail Dye Plant	Folk
Kattagatti	*Cadaba fruticosa*	Indian Cadaba	Siddha/Tamil
Kattaka	*Brassica napus*	Mustard, Indian Rape	Ayurvedic
Kattalari-palai	*Tabernaemontana dichotoma*	Eve's Apple, Forbidden Fruit	Siddha/Tamil
Kattan	*Linum usitatissimum*	Linseed, Flax	Unani
Kattanam	*Gmelina arborea*	Candahar Tree, White Teak	Siddha/Tamil
Kattaphala	*Hibiscus abelmoschus*	Musk Seed, Ambette Seed, Muskmallow	Ayurvedic
Kattarohini	*Picrorhiza kurroa*	Picrorhiza	Ayurvedic
Kattasambadam	*Chenopodium ambrosioides*	Indian Wormseed, Sweet Pigweed, Mexican Tea	Siddha/Tamil
Kattatti	*Diospyros embryopteris*	Gaub Persimmon, Riber Ebony	Siddha/Tamil
Kattavuri	*Indigofera articulata*	Egyptian Indigo, Arabian Indigo, Wild Indigo, Surat Indigo	Siddha/Tamil
Katthaa (Heartwood extract)	*Acacia catechu*	Cutch tree, Catechu	Unani
Katthakkaambu (Heartwood extract)	*Acacia chundra*	Red Cutch	Siddha/Tamil
Katthilla	*Boerhavia diffusa*	Red-flowered Hogweed	Ayurvedic
Katthinjara	*Digera muricata*	Gitana Weed	Ayurvedic
Kattraazhai	*Aloe barbadensis*	Curacao Aloe, Barbados Aloe, Indian Aloe, Jaffarabad Aloe	Siddha/Tamil
Kattu alari	*Homonoia riparia*	Willow-leaved Water Croton	Siddha/Tamil
Kattu Amanaku	*Jatropha curcas*	Physic Nut, Purging Nut	Siddha/Tamil
Kattu elam	*Amomum subulatum*	Greater or Nepal Cardamom	Folk/Tamil
Kattu elumicchai	*Atalantia monophylla*	Wild Lime	Siddha/Tamil
Kattu Jhadi	*Myristica malabarica*	Malabar Nutmeg, False Nutmeg, Bombay Nutmeg, Bombay Mace	Siddha/Tamil

Table Contd.

Indian Name	Botanical Name	English Name	Medicinal System
Kattu Kadali	*Grewia sclerophylla*	Bhokota	Siddha/Tamil
Kattu Karun-ayikkilangu	*Dracontium polyphyllum*	Stunk Weed, Poleca Weed	Siddha/Tamil
Kattu Milagu	*Toddalia asiatica*	Wild Orange Tree, Forest Pepper	Siddha/Tamil
Kattu Narangam	*Atalantia monophylla*	Wild Lime	Siddha/Tamil
Kattu Pey Pudal	*Trichosanthes cucumerina*	Coiled Snakegourd	Siddha/Tamil
Kattu Sampangi	*Pittosporum floribundum*	Ginger-bark Pittosporum	Siddha/Tamil
Kattu talai	*Ipomoea muricata*	Traveller's Midnight Lilies	Folk/Tamil
Kattu velvengayam	*Scilla indica*	South Indian Squill	Siddha/Tamil
Kattuchandanam	*Erythroxylum monogynum*	Bastard Sandal, Red Cedar	Ayurvedic
Kattu-kadugu	*Rorippa dufia*	Field Cress	Siddha/Tamil
Kattukkar-chammathi	*Indigofera oblongifolia*	Wild Indigo, Mysore Panicled Indigo	Siddha/Tamil
Kattukodi	*Cocculus hirsutus*	Broom-Creeper, Ink-Berry	Siddha/Tamil
Kattuma	*Spondias pinnata*	Hog-Plum, Wild Mango	Siddha/Tamil
Kattumalligei	*Jasminum rottlerianum*	Wild jasmine (Western Ghats)	Siddha/Tamil
Kattumilaaku	*Piper attenuatum*	Oval-leaved Pepper Plant	Siddha/Tamil
Kattumilagu	*Paullinia asiatica*	Lopez Root Tree, Wild Orange Tree, Forest Pepper	Siddha/Tamil
Kattupala	*Cryptolepis buchanani*	Indian Sarsaparilla	Folk/Tamil
Kattupayaru	*Phaseolus adenanthus*	South American Snail Vine	Siddha/Tamil
Kattuppirandai	*Cayratia pedata*	Cayratia	Siddha/Tamil
Kattuppugaiyilai	*Lobelia nicotianaefolia*	Wild Tobacco	Siddha/Tamil
Kattusuragam	*Aristolochia bracteolata*	Bracteated Birthwort	Siddha/Tamil
Kattu-thrithava	*Orthosiphon tomentosus*	Cat's Whiskers	Folk
Kattutumatti	*Cucumis trigonus*	Wild Cucumber	Folk/Tamil
Kattuulandu	*Teramnus labialis*	Blue Wiss	Siddha/Tamil
Kattuveppilai	*Murraya koenigii*	Curry-Leaf Tree	Siddha/Tamil
Kattuvettilai	*Ehretia buxifolia*	Carmonia Shrub	Siddha/Tamil
Katubhadra	*Zingiber officinale*	Ginger	Ayurvedic

Table Contd.

Indian Name	Botanical Name	English Name	Medicinal System
Katudugu	*Hardwickia binata*	Copaiba-grade Balsam	Siddha/Tamil
Katuka	*Hibiscus abelmoschus*	Musk Seed, Ambette Seed, Muskmallow	Ayurvedic
Katukaa	*Picrorhiza kurroa*	Picrorhiza	Ayurvedic
Katukala	*Flacourtia indica*	Ramontchi, Madagascar Plum, Mauritius Plum, Governor's Plum	Siddha/Tamil
Katu-Kapittha	*Hydnocarpus laurifolia*	Soorty Oil Tree	Ayurvedic
Katukavalli	*Viscum monoicum*	Himalayan Mistletoe	Ayurvedic
Katuki	*Picrorhiza kurroa*	Picrorhiza	Ayurvedic
Katukikaa	*Picrorhiza kurroa*	Picrorhiza	Ayurvedic
Katukoshataki	*Luffa acutangula*	Ribbed or Ridged Gourd (bitter var.)	Ayurvedic
Katumbaa	*Leucas cephalotes*	Dhurpi Vegetable	Ayurvedic
Katunaahi	*Corallocarpus epigaeus*	Indian Bryonia	Ayurvedic
Katuparni	*Argemone mexicana*	Prickly Poppy, Mexican Poppy	Ayurvedic
Katuparni	*Euphorbia thomsoniana*	Hirvi Spurge	Ayurvedic
Katurohini	*Picrorhiza kurroa*	Picrorhiza	Ayurvedic
Katusneha	*Brassica napus*	Mustard, Indian Rape	Ayurvedic
Katutikta	*Swertia chirayita*	Chiretta	Ayurvedic
Katu-tumbi	*Lagenaria siceraria*	Bitter Bottle-Gourd	Ayurvedic
Katuveekaa	*Celastrus paniculatus*	Staff Tree, Intellect Tree	Ayurvedic
Katuviraa	*Capsicum annuum*	Chilli, Red Pepper	Ayurvedic
Katuviraa	*Capsicum frutescens*	Bird Chilli	Ayurvedic
Katvanga	*Ailanthus excelsa*	Tree of Heaven, Maharukh	Ayurvedic
Kaur	*Amphicome emodi*	False Chirayita	Folk (Kashmir)
Kaur	*Roylea cinerea*	Roylea Mint	Folk
Kauraro	*Kochia indica*	Kochia Weed	Folk
Kauri	*Roylea cinerea*	Roylea Mint	Folk
Kaushika	*Balsamodendron mukul*	Indian Bdellium, Gum Guggul	Ayurvedic
Kavacha	*Fumaria parviflora*	Fumitory	Ayurvedic
Kavalai	*Clerodendrum indicum*	Turk's Turban, Tube-Flower	Siddha/Tamil
Kavala-kodi	*Dioscorea oppositifolia*	Cylindrical Red Yam	Siddha/Tamil
Kavalam	*Sterculia urens*	Bissy Nuts, Karaya Gum	Siddha/Tamil

Table Contd.

Indian Name	Botanical Name	English Name	Medicinal System
Kavathampillu	*Cymbopogon martinii*	Rosha Grass, Palmarosa	Folk/Tamil
Kayappankottai	*Strychnos ignatii*	Ignatus Beans	Siddha/Tamil
Kazharchikkaai	*Caesalpinia bonduc*	Fever Nut, Bonduc Nut, Nikkar Nut	Siddha/Tamil
Kazurati	*Reissantia indica*	Atari Vine	Folk
Kebu	*Costus speciosus*	Canereed, Wild Ginger	Folk
Kebuka	*Costus speciosus*	Canereed, Wild Ginger	Ayurvedic
Keechey	*Primula denticulata*	Himalayan Primrose	Folk
Keerippaalai	*Leptadenia reticulata*	Dodi Vegetable	Siddha/Tamil
Keerippundu	*Ophiorrhiza mungos*	Mongoose Plant	Folk/Tamil
Keezh Kai Nelli	*Phyllanthus amarus*	Indian Chanca Piedra	Siddha/Tamil
Kekidandaa	*Leea macrophylla*	Tuberous Holly	Ayurvedic
Kelaa	*Musa paradisiaca*	Banana, Plantain	Unani
Kelp	*Fucus vesiculosus*	Bladderwrack	Folk
Kembuka	*Costus speciosus*	Canereed, Wild Ginger	Ayurvedic
Kembumalligai	*Ipomoea quamoclit*	Cypress Vine, Indian Pink	Siddha/Tamil
Kenaa	*Commelina benghalensis*	Tropical Spiderwort	Folk
Kenaa	*Commelina nudiflora*	Day Flower, Kenna vegetable	Folk
Keoraa	*Pandanus fascicularis*	Screw Pine	Unani
Keraari	*Ceriops candolleana*	Compound Cymed Mangrove	Folk/Kannada
Keshahantri	*Prosopis spicigera*	Mestique Gum Tree	Ayurvedic
Keshara	*Crocus sativus*	Saffron, Crocus	Ayurvedic
Keshara	*Mimusops elengi*	Spanish-Cherry, West Indian Medlar, Bullet Wood	Ayurvedic
Kesharaaga	*Wedelia calendulaceae*	Yellow-flowered Weldia	Ayurvedic
Kesharaaja	*Eclipta alba*	Trailing Eclipta Plant	Ayurvedic
Kesharaaja	*Wedelia calendulaceae*	Yellow-flowered Weldia	Ayurvedic
Kesharanjan	*Eclipta alba*	Trailing Eclipta Plant	Ayurvedic
Keshruuhaa	*Sesbania sesban*	Common Sesban	Ayurvedic
Kesri	*Polygonum aviculare*	Knotgrass, Knotweed, Mexican Sanguinaria	Folk
Ketaka	*Pandanus fascicularis*	Screw Pine	Ayurvedic
Ketakark	*Pandanus fascicularis*	Screw Pine	Ayurvedic

Table Contd.

Indian Name	Botanical Name	English Name	Medicinal System
Ketaki	*Pandanus fascicularis*	Screw Pine	Ayurvedic
Ketaki	*Pandanus utilis*	Stilt-rooted Screw Pine	Ayurvedic
Keteri (smaller var.)	*Solanum xanthocarpum*	Wild Eggplant, Yellow-Berried Nightshade	Ayurvedic
Kevaanch	*Mucuna prurita*	Cowhage, Horse-eye Bean	Ayurvedic
Kevati (var.)	*Ventilago denticulata*	Ventilago Black Vine	Folk
Kevati	*Ventilago madraspatana*	Ventilago Vermilion Vine	Folk
Kezhvaregu	*Eleusine coracana*	Finger Millet, African Millet, Ragi	Siddha/Tamil
Khaajaa	*Bridelia retusa*	Spinous Kino Tree	Folk
Khaakasi	*Descurainia sophia*	Flix Weed, Flax Weed	Unani
Khaaksi	*Sisymbrium irio*	London Rocket	Ayurvedic
Khaarchu	*Marsdenia roylei*	Marua Vine	Folk
Khaar-e-khasak Kalaan	*Pedalium murex*	Caltrops (bigger var.)	Unani
Khaar-e-shutur	*Alhagi pseudalhagi*	Camel Thorn, Persian Manna Plant	Unani
Khadira	*Acacia catechu*	Cutch tree, Catechu	Ayurvedic
Khadira	*Acacia chundra*	Red Cutch	Ayurvedic
Khadira	*Uncaria gambier*	Pale Catechu, Gambier	Ayurvedic
Khadirkaa	*Mimosa pudica*	Sensitive-plant, Humble-Plant	Ayurvedic
Khair	*Acacia catechu*	Cutch tree, Catechu	Unani
Khairi	*Dichrostachys cinerea*	Chinese Lantern, Kalihari Christmastree	Folk
Khairposh	*Limnanthemum nymphaeoides*	Fringed Water-Lily	Folk
Khairwaal	*Bauhinia purpurea*	Camel's Foot Tree, Pink Bauhinia, Butterfly Tree, Geramium Tree, Orchid Tree	Folk
Khajuur	*Phoenix dactylifera*	Date Palm	Unani
Khajuur Desi	*Phoenix sylvestris*	Wild Date Palm	Folk
Khalah	*Ammi majus*	Bishop's Weed-Amee, Greater Ammi	Unani
Khalva	*Dolichos biflorus*	Horsegram	Ayurvedic
Khamaan	*Sambucus ebulus*	Dwarf Elder	Unani

Table Contd.

Indian Name	Botanical Name	English Name	Medicinal System
Khamaan Kabir	*Sambucus nigra*	European Elder, Black Elder	Unani
Khamaan Saghir	*Sambucus ebulus*	Dwarf Elder	Unani
Khamaan-ul-Arzaa	*Sambucus ebulus*	Dwarf Elder	Unani
Khamman	*Sambucus ebulus*	Dwarf Elder	Siddha/Tamil
Khamraq	*Averrhoa carambola*	Carambola, Star Fruit, Chinese Gooseberry	Unani
Khappar-kaddu	*Ceropegia bulbosa*	Candlestick Ceropegia	Folk
Kharachada	*Tectona grandis*	Teak Tree	Ayurvedic
Kharachhada	*Streblus asper*	Siamese Rough Brush	Ayurvedic
Kharahaara	*Gardenia turgida*	Bharangi Bark Tree	Ayurvedic
Kharamanjari	*Achyranthes aspera*	Prickly Chaff Flower	Ayurvedic
Kharamati	*Grewia villosa*	Tamthar	Folk
Kharaoli	*Streblus asper*	Siamese Rough Brush	Folk
Kharapatra	*Ficus asperrima*	Brahma's Banyan, Sandpaper Fig	Ayurvedic
Kharapushpaa	*Achyranthes aspera*	Prickly Chaff Flower	Ayurvedic
Khara-yashtikaa	*Sida cordifolia*	Country Mallow	Ayurvedic
Kharbaq Siyah	*Helleborus niger*	Black Hellebore, Christmas Rose	Unani
Kharbaq-e-Hindi	*Picrorhiza kurroa*	Picrorhiza	Unani
Khardal Safed	*Brassica alba*	White Mustard	Unani
Khardal Siyah	*Brassica nigra*	Black Mustard	Unani
Khardi	*Cressa cretica*	Mediterranean Bindweed	Folk
Khar-Duudhi	*Waltheria indica*	Boater Bush, Buff Coat' Leather Coat, Sleepy Morning	Folk
Khar-e-Khasak Khurd	*Tribulus terrestris*	Land-Caltrops, Puncture Vine	Unani
Kharhar	*Plesmonium margaritiferum*	Kharhar Tuber	Folk
Khar-indraayana	*Cucumis prophetarum*	Wild Cucumber	Folk
Kharjuura	*Phoenix dactylifera*	Date Palm	Ayurvedic
Kharjuuraka	*Phoenix dactylifera*	Date Palm	Ayurvedic
Kharjuuri	*Phoenix sylvestris*	Wild Date Palm	Ayurvedic
Kharjuurikaa	*Phoenix dactylifera*	Date Palm	Ayurvedic

Table Contd.

Indian Name	Botanical Name	English Name	Medicinal System
Kharmor	*Rungia repens*	Creeping Rungia	Folk
Kharnuub Shaami	*Ceratonia siliqua*	Locust Bean, St. John's Bread, Carob Tree	Unani
Kharpata	*Garuga pinnata*	Grey Downy Balsam	Ayurvedic
Kharpatraa	*Onosma bracteatum*	Borage	Ayurvedic
Kharpushpa	*Ocimum basilicum*	Sweet Basil, Basil Herb	Ayurvedic
Kharshaak	*Clerodendrum serratum*	Blue-flowered Glory Tree, Beetle Killer	Ayurvedic
Kharsing	*Radermachera xylocarpa*	Padri Tree	Folk
Kharskandha	*Buchanania lanzan*	Almondette Tree, Cheronjee, Buchanan's Mango	Ayurvedic
Kharunb Nabti	*Acacia concinna*	Soap-nut Acacia	Unani
Khar-zaharah	*Nerium indicum*	Indian Oleander, White Oleander	Unani
Khas	*Andropogon muricatus*	Vetiver, Cuscus	Unani
Khas	*Vetiveria zizanioides*	Vetiver, Khas	Unani
Khashbulhayyh	*Asparagus officinalis*	Asparagus, Sparrow Grass	Unani
Khatmi	*Althaea officinalis*	Marshmallow, Hollyhock	Unani
Khatraq	*Artemisia absinthium*	Wormwood, Madderwood	Unani
Khattaa	*Citrus aurantium*	Citrus Dulcis, Sour Orange, Sweet Orange	Folk
Khattimal	*Rumex hastatus*	Toothed Dock	Folk
Khatuaa	*Chenopodium ambrosioides*	Indian Wormseed, Sweet Pigweed, Mexican Tea	Folk
Khedari	*Lettsomia elliptica*	Silverweed	Folk
Kheechar Chirchataa	*Lycium barbarum*	Boxthorn, Matrimony Vine	Folk
Kheep	*Leptadenia spartium*	Khimp Leptadenia	Folk
Khejaraa (var.)	*Prosopis stephaniana*	Syrian Mestique Gum Tree	Folk
Khejaraa	*Prosopis chilensis*	Mestique Gum Tree	Folk
Khesaari	*Lathyrus sativus*	Chickling Vetch, Grass Pea	Folk
Kheta Kadam	*Adina cordifolia*	Yellow Teak, Saffron Teak	Folk
Khet-chiraayataa	*Erythraea roxburghii*	Pseudo-Chiretta	Folk
Khimor	*Viburnum cotinifolium*	Wooly-leaved Guelder Rose	Folk
Khimp	*Leptadenia spartium*	Khimp Leptadenia	Folk

Table Contd.

Indian Name	Botanical Name	English Name	Medicinal System
Khiraa	*Cucumis sativus*	Cucumber	Folk
Khiraa	*Cucumis sativus*	Cucumber	Unani
Khireti	*Sida cordifolia*	Country Mallow	Unani
Khirhati	*Sida cordifolia*	Country Mallow	Unani
Khirni	*Manilkara kauki*	Kauki	Ayurvedic
Khiyaar	*Cucumis sativus*	Cucumber	Unani
Khodiki Raasanaa	*Tylophora tenuis*	Backwater Swallow-wort	Folk/ Maharashtra
Khokh	*Amygdalus persica*	Peach Tree	Unani
Khokli	*Acalypha indica*	Copperleaf Acalypha	Folk
Khoobkalaan	*Rorippa dufia*	Field Cress	Unani
Khoon-kharaabaa	*Daemonorops draco*	East Indian Dragon's Blood	Ayurvedic
Khoonkharaabaa	*Dracaena cinnabari*	Dragon's Blood	Ayurvedic
Khor	*Acacia suma*	White Babul	Unani
Khubb	*Descurainia sophia*	Flix Weed, Flax Weed	Unani
Khubbaazi	*Malva sylvestris*	Common Mallow, Blue Mallow, High Mallow	Unani
Khubhaazi	*Malva rotundifolia*	Round-leaved Mallow, Drawf Mallow, Cheese Cake Flower	Unani
Khukhudi	*Polygonum affine*	Hogweed, Knotweed	Folk
Khul	*Aerva javanica*	Javanese Wool Plant	Folk
Khulanjaan	*Alpinia galanga*	Greater Galangal	Unani
Khulanjaan	*Alpinia officinarum*	Lesser Galangal, Alpinia, Catarrh Root, Chinese Ginger	Unani
Khumaa	*Strobilanthes flaccidifolius*	Assam Indigo	Folk
Khumani	*Sophora mollis*	Himalayan Laburnum, Low Mountain Laurel	Folk/Kumaun
Khumbi	*Agaricus campestris*	Field Mushroom, Edible Mushroom	Folk
Khunsaa	*Asphodelus fistulosus*	Asphodel	Unani
Khuraasaani Kutaki	*Helleborus niger*	Black Hellebore, Christmas Rose	Ayurvedic
Khuraasaani Ajwaayin	*Hyoscyamus niger*	Indian Henbane, Black Henbane	Ayurvedic

Table Contd.

Indian Name	Botanical Name	English Name	Medicinal System
Khuraasaani Ajwaayin	*Hyoscyamus niger*	Indian Henbane, Black Henbane	Unani
Khuraasaani Kutaki	*Helleborus niger*	Black Hellebore, Christmas Rose	Unani
Khuraashaanikaa	*Hyoscyamus niger*	Indian Henbane, Black Henbane	Ayurvedic
Khurasani Omam	*Hyoscyamus niger*	Indian Henbane, Black Henbane	Siddha/Tamil
Khurbanti	*Ajuga bracteosa*	Bugle	Folk
Khurfaa	*Portulaca oleracea*	Common Purslane	Unani
Khurmaa	*Phoenix dactylifera*	Date Palm	Unani
Khursaa	*Portulaca oleracea*	Common Purslane	Ayurvedic
Khusyaat-us-Saalab	*Orchis latifolia*	Orchis, Salep	Unani
Khuubaani	*Prunus armeniaca*	Apricot	Unani
Khuubkalaan	*Descurainia sophia*	Flix Weed, Flax Weed	Unani
Khuubkalaan	*Sisymbrium irio*	London Rocket	Unani
Khyaarshambar	*Cassia fistula*	Indian Laburnum, Purging Cassia, Golden Shower	Unani
Kichaka	*Bambusa bambos*	Spiny or Thorny Bamboo	Ayurvedic
Kichhilik-kizhangu	*Curcuma zedoaria*	Zedoary, Zerumbet	Siddha/Tamil
Kichilikizangu	*Hedychium spicatum*	Spiked Ginger Ivy	Siddha/Tamil
Kierpa	*Carallia brachiata*	Freshwater Mangrove	Folk
Kikar	*Acacia arabica*	Babul, Black Babul, Indian Gum Arabic Tree	Unani
Kilapalam	*Vaccinium symplocifolium*	Indian Bilberry, Blueberry	Folk
Kilar	*Casearia esculenta*	Boxwood	Siddha/Tamil
Kimshuka	*Butea monosperma*	Flame of the Forest, Butea Gum, Bengal Kino	Ayurvedic
Kindal (trade)	*Terminalia paniculata*	Flowering Murdah	Folk
Kinjal	*Terminalia paniculata*	Flowering Murdah	Folk
Kinkini	*Flacourtia sepiaria*	Governor's Plum	Ayurvedic
Kinkiraata	*Acacia arabica*	Babul, Black Babul, Indian Gum Arabic Tree	Ayurvedic

Table Contd.

Indian Name	Botanical Name	English Name	Medicinal System
Kintodaa	*Berberis chitria*	Barberry	Folk
Kiraamaar	*Aristolochia bracteolata*	Bracteated Birthwort	Unani
Kiraambu	*Syzygium aromaticum*	Clove	Siddha/Tamil
Kiraata (sweet var.)	*Swertia angustifolia*	Hill Chiretta	Ayurvedic
Kiraata	*Swertia chirayita*	Chiretta	Ayurvedic
Kiraataka	*Swertia chirayita*	Chiretta	Ayurvedic
Kiraata-tikta	*Andrographis paniculata*	Creat	Ayurvedic
Kiraatatikta	*Swertia affinis*	Hill Chiretta	Ayurvedic
Kiraatatikta	*Swertia chirayita*	Chiretta	Ayurvedic
Kiraatatikta	*Swertia ciliata*	Black Chiretta	Ayurvedic
Kiraatatikta	*Swertia densifolia*	Dense-leaved Chiretta	Ayurvedic
Kiraatatikta	*Swertia lawii*	Western Ghat Chiretta	Ayurvedic
Kiraatatiktaka	*Swertia chirayita*	Chiretta	Ayurvedic
Kiraat-tikta	*Erythraea roxburghii*	Pseudo-Chiretta	Ayurvedic
Kiraitandu	*Amaranthus blitum*	Trailing Amaranth, Wild Blite	Folk/Tamil
Kirantitakkaaram	*Ruellia strepens*	Wild Petunia	Folk
Kirmalaa	*Artemisia maritima*	Wormseed, Santonica	Unani
Kirmani Ajawaayin	*Artemisia maritima*	Wormseed, Santonica	Folk
Kirmani Yavaani	*Artemisia maritima*	Wormseed, Santonica	Ayurvedic
Kirmani-ajmo	*Artemisia maritima*	Wormseed, Santonica	Folk
Kirmani-owaa	*Artemisia maritima*	Wormseed, Santonica	Folk
Kirni	*Canthium parviflorum*	Wild Jasmine	Folk
Kiryaat	*Andrographis paniculata*	Creat	Unani
Kishli-keerai	*Hibiscus surattensis*	Wild Sour, Bush Sorrel	Siddha/Tamil
Kishmish	*Vitis vinifera*	Wine Grape, European Grape	Ayurvedic
Kishmish	*Vitis vinifera*	Wine Grape, European Grape	Unani
Kishmish Kaabuli	*Viscum album*	European Mistletoe	Unani
Kishneez	*Coriandrum sativum*	Coriander	Unani
Kitamaara	*Ulmus wallichiana*	Himalayan Elm	Folk
Kitamaari	*Aristolochia bracteolata*	Bracteated Birthwort	Ayurvedic
Kitamaataa	*Adiantum lunulatum*	Walking Maidenhair Fern, Black Maidenhair	Ayurvedic

Table Contd.

Indian Name	Botanical Name	English Name	Medicinal System
Kitani	*Derris uliginosa*	Tuba Root	Folk
Kitav	*Datura stramonium*	Thornapple, Jimsonweed, Stramonium	Ayurvedic
Kithi	*Dioscorea deltoidea*	Lice-killer Yam	Folk
Kitran	*Ecballium elaterium*	Squirting Cucumber	Folk
Klitaka	*Glycyrrhiza glabra*	Licorice, Liquorice	Ayurvedic
Kochelachipullu	*Xyris commplanata*	Yellow-eyed Grass	Folk
Kodaga-saleh	*Rungia repens*	Creeping Rungia	Siddha/Tamil
Kodaittani	*Gironniera reticulata*	Diancaoxieshu (Chinese)	Siddha/Tamil
Kodakkapuli	*Garcinia cambogia*	Gamboge Tree	Siddha/Tamil
Kodapalai	*Hardwickia binata*	Copaiba-grade Balsam	Siddha/Tamil
Kodapalai	*Kingiodendron pinnatum*	Piney	Siddha/Tamil
Kodaparuavalli	*Tiliacora acuminata*	Bega Climber	Siddha/Tamil
Kodarsi	*Securinega suffruticosa*	Securinega	Folk
Kodhab	*Cadaba fruticosa*	Indian Cadaba	Folk
Kodi Athi	*Ficus heterophylla*	Oak-Leaf Fig	Siddha/Tamil
Kodi-kilangu	*Dioscorea bulbifera*	Patoto Yam, Bulb-bearing Yam, Air Potato, Dog Yam	Siddha/Tamil
Kodippalai	*Dregea volubilis*	Wattakaka	Siddha/Tamil
Kodivelam	*Caesalpinia coriaria*	American Sumac, Divi-divi Plant	Siddha/Tamil
Kodo	*Paspalum scrobiculatum*	Kodo Millet	Folk
Kodrava	*Paspalum scrobiculatum*	Kodo Millet	Ayurvedic
Kodukkaa Puli	*Pithecellobium dulce*	Minila Tamarind, Madras Thorn, Quamachil	Siddha/Tamil
Kohal Kirmaani	*Astragalus sarcocolla*	Sarcocola	Unani
Kohlu	*Salicornia brachiata*	Glasswort, Pickleweed, Marsh Samphire	Folk
Koilaara	*Bauhinia purpurea*	Camel's Foot Tree, Pink Bauhinia, Butterfly Tree, Geramium Tree, Orchid Tree	Folk
Koilangu	*Ipomoea aquatica*	Swamp Cabbage	Siddha/Tamil
Koilekhaa	*Barleria strigosa*	Blue-flowered Barleria	Folk
Kokam (var.)	*Garcinia cambogia*	Gamboge Tree	Ayurvedic

Table Contd.

Indian Name	Botanical Name	English Name	Medicinal System
Kokam	*Garcinia indica*	Kokam Butter Tree, Mangosteen Oil Tree	Ayurvedic
Kokam	*Garcinia indica*	Kokam Butter Tree, Mangosteen Oil Tree	Folk
Kokilaa	*Clitoria ternatea*	Butterfly Pea, Winged-leaved Clitoria, Mezereon	Ayurvedic
Kokilaa	*Luvunga eleutherandra*	Woody Clove Vine	Folk
Kokilaaksha	*Asteracantha longifolia*	Hygrophilla	Ayurvedic
Kokilaaksha	*Hygrophila auriculata*	Indian Swampweed	Ayurvedic
Kokilaakshi	*Asteracantha longifolia*	Hygrophilla	Ayurvedic
Kokilaakshi	*Hygrophila auriculata*	Indian Swampweed	Ayurvedic
Kokkumandarai	*Bauhinia racemosa*	Kachnar Tree	Siddha/Tamil
Kokkumandarai	*Bauhinia tomentosa*	Yellow Bauhinia, St. Thomas Tree, Bell Bauhinia	Siddha/Tamil
Kokoon	*Stellaria media*	Common Chickweed	Folk
Kola	*Ziziphus jujuba*	Indian Jujube, Common Jujube	Ayurvedic
Kolaa	*Piper longum*	Indian Long Pepper, Joborandi	Ayurvedic
Kolaka	*Piper cubeba*	Cubeb, Tailed Pepper	Ayurvedic
Kolakanda	*Urginea indica*	Indian Squill, Sea Onion (red and white varieties)	Ayurvedic
Kolakkaai	*Gaultheria fragrantissima*	Fragrant Wintergreen, Indian Wintergreen	Siddha/Tamil
Kolakottathekku pinari	*Premna tomentosa*	Bastard Teak	Siddha/Tamil
Kolaoyila	*Anthocephalus cadamba*	Wild Cinchona	Folk/Tamil
Kollankovai	*Corallocarpus epigaeus*	Indian Bryonia	Siddha/Tamil
Kollimulli	*Acanthus ilicifolius*	Sea Holly	Siddha/Tamil
Kollu	*Dolichos biflorus*	Horsegram	Siddha/Tamil
Kollukkaivelai	*Tephrosia purpurea*	Purple Tephrosia, Wild Indigo	Folk/Tamil
Kollukkayvelai	*Tephrosia purpurea*	Purple Tephrosia, Wild Indigo	Siddha/Tamil
Kolo	*Dioscorea daemona*	Asiatic Bitter Yam	Folk
Kolumbu	*Jateorhiza palmata*	Calumba, Colombo	Siddha/Tamil
Kolunchi	*Tephrosia purpurea*	Purple Tephrosia, Wild Indigo	Folk/Tamil

Table Contd.

Indian Name	Botanical Name	English Name	Medicinal System
Komal	*Prangos pabularia*	Prangos, Yugan. Aju-Chach	Folk
Kombarakku (Rangeeni Lac)	*Ziziphus xylopyra*	Lac-host Jujube	Siddha/Tamil
Kombe	*Strophanthus kombe*	Kombe Arrow Poison, Large-leaved Poison Rope	Folk
Kombu Pudalai	*Trichosanthes nervifolia*	Bitter Chinese Cucumber	Siddha/Tamil
Kon, jib (Baluchistan)	*Astragalus strobiliferus*	Milk vetch	Unani
Konatekkali	*Symphorema involucratum*	Bhingri	Folk
Konchh	*Mucuna prurita*	Cowhage, Horse-eye Bean	Unani
Konda Potari	*Kydia calycina*	Pula Tree	Folk
Kondachinta	*Peltophorum pterocarpum*	Copper Pod, Rusty Shield-Bearer	Folk/Telugu
Konda-gengura	*Hibiscus cannabinus*	Bimlipatam Jute, Kenaf, Mesta, Deccan Hemp	Folk/Telugu
Kondai	*Flacourtia sepiaria*	Governor's Plum	Folk
Kondal	*Trichosanthes bracteata*	Redball Snakegourd	Folk
Kondari	*Flacourtia sepiaria*	Governor's Plum	Folk
Kongilavu	*Cochlospermum gossypium*	Golden Silk Tree, White Silk Cotton Tree	Siddha/Tamil
Konji	*Glycosmis pentaphylla*	Orangeberry, Ginberry	Siddha/Tamil
Konji	*Murraya exotica*	Chinese Boxwood, Andaman Satinwood	Siddha/Tamil
Konkanada (red)	*Nelumbo nucifera*	East Indian Lotus, Sacred Lotus	Ayurvedic
Kookaineer	*Maranta arundinacea*	Arrowroot	Siddha/Tamil
Koovaikizhangu	*Maranta arundinacea*	Arrowroot	Siddha/Tamil
Koovilam	*Aegle marmelos*	Bael Tree, Bengal Quince	Siddha/Tamil
Kopanaa	*Angelica glauca*	Angelica	Ayurvedic
Kopparai	*Cocos nucifera*	Coconut Palm	Siddha/Tamil
Koraikkilangu	*Cyperus scariosus*	Nut Grass	Siddha/Tamil
Koraikkizhangu	*Cyperus rotundus*	Nut Grass	Siddha/Tamil
Koraka	*Piper cubeba*	Cubeb, Tailed Pepper	Ayurvedic
Korakizhangu	*Cyperus scariosus*	Nut Grass	Folk/Malayalam
Koranda	*Barleria prionitis*	Common Yellow Nail Dye Plant	Ayurvedic

Table Contd.

Indian Name	Botanical Name	English Name	Medicinal System
Korandaka	*Barleria prionitis*	Common Yellow Nail Dye Plant	Ayurvedic
Koranti	*Salacia reticulata*	Saptrangi	Folk/South
Korattai	*Trichosanthes bracteata*	Redball Snakegourd	Siddha/Tamil
Korduusha	*Paspalum scrobiculatum*	Kodo Millet	Ayurvedic
Korikanda	*Scilla indica*	South Indian Squill	Ayurvedic
Korivi	*Ixora parviflora*	Torchwood Tree	Folk/Tamil
Korukkai	*Arundo donax*	Great Reed, Spanish-Bamboo-Reed, Giant-Bamboo-Reed	Siddha/Tamil
Koshaamra	*Schleichera oleosa*	Lac Tree, Macassar Oil Tree, Honey Tree, Ceylon Oak	Ayurvedic
Koshakanda	*Dioscorea anguina*	Foetid Yam	Folk
Koshapushpi	*Murdannia nudiflora*	Nakedstem Dewflower	Ayurvedic
Kostum	*Saussurea lappa*	Kuth, Costus	Siddha/Tamil
Kothaphala	*Luffa echinata*	Bristly Luffa	Ayurvedic
Kothaveray	*Cyamopsis tetragonoloba*	Cluster Bean, Guar	Folk/Tamil
Koththamalli	*Coriandrum sativum*	Coriander	Siddha/Tamil
Kottai Paakku	*Areca catechu*	Areca Nut, Betel Nut	Siddha/Tamil
Kottaikarandai	*Sphaeranthus indicus*	East Indian Globe Thistle	Siddha/Tamil
Kottaimaram	*Ziziphus rugosa*	White Jujube	Siddha/Tamil
Kottam	*Costus speciosus*	Canereed, Wild Ginger	Siddha/Tamil
Kottam	*Saussurea lappa*	Kuth, Costus	Siddha/Tamil
Kottargovai	*Casearia esculenta*	Boxwood	Siddha/Tamil
Kottavan	*Cardiospermum halicacabum*	Balloon Vine, Winter Pea, Heartseed	Siddha/Tamil
Kottei	*Microcos paniculata*	Kadamb	Folk/Tamil
Kottei	*Ziziphus xylopyra*	Lac-host Jujube	Siddha/Tamil
Kotu	*Fagopyrum esculentum*	Buckwheat	Ayurvedic
Kousso	*Brayera anthelmintica*	Cusso, Brayera	Folk
Kovidaara	*Bauhinia acuminata*	Dwarf White Bauhinia	Ayurvedic
Kovidaara	*Bauhinia purpurea*	Camel's Foot Tree, Pink Bauhinia, Butterfly Tree, Geramium Tree, Orchid Tree	Ayurvedic
Kovvai	*Coccinia indica*	Ivy-Gourd	Siddha/Tamil

Table Contd.

Indian Name	Botanical Name	English Name	Medicinal System
Kshdra	*Trianthema portulacastrum*	Horse Purslane	Ayurvedic
Kshemaka	*Angelica glauca*	Angelica	Ayurvedic
Kshetrabalaa	*Sida rhombifolia*	Red-flowered Mallow	Ayurvedic
Kshetraparpata	*Hedyotis corymbosa*	Old World Diamond Flower	Ayurvedic
Kshetra-vaastuuka	*Chenopodium ambrosioides*	Indian Wormseed, Sweet Pigweed, Mexican Tea	Ayurvedic
Kshira	*Lilium polyphyllum*	Kakoli Tuber Lily	Ayurvedic
Kshira Champaa	*Plumeria acuminata*	Pagoda Tree	Ayurvedic
Kshira Champaka	*Plumeria alba*	White Champaka	Ayurvedic
Kshira Champaka	*Plumeria rubra*	Red Jasmine	Ayurvedic
Kshiradruma	*Ficus religiosa*	Peepal, Bot-tree	Ayurvedic
Kshira-Kaakoli	*Fritillaria roylei*	Pei-mu (China), Kakoli	Ayurvedic
Kshira-Kaakoli	*Roscoea procera*	Kaakoli	Ayurvedic
Kshirapushpi	*Convolvulus pluricaulis*	Conch-flowered Bindweed, White-flowered Shankhpushpi	Ayurvedic
Kshira-vidaari	*Ipomoea digitata*	Milky Yam	Ayurvedic
Kshirparna	*Calotropis procera*	Swallow-wort, Milk Weed, King's Crown	Ayurvedic
Kshirphena	*Carissa carandas*	Christ's Thorn, Bengal Currant	Ayurvedic
Kshirvalli	*Ipomoea digitata*	Milky Yam	Ayurvedic
Kshouraka	*Pedalium murex*	Caltrops (bigger var.)	Ayurvedic
Kshudra Gokharu	*Tribulus terrestris*	Land-Caltrops, Puncture Vine	Ayurvedic
Kshudra Paashaana-bheda	*Homonoia riparia*	Willow-leaved Water Croton	Ayurvedic
Kshudra Panas	*Artocarpus lakoocha*	Monkey Jack	Ayurvedic
Kshudra Shimbi	*Cyamopsis tetragonoloba*	Cluster Bean, Guar	Ayurvedic
Kshudraa	*Solanum xanthocarpum*	Wild Eggplant, Yellow-Berried Nightshade	Ayurvedic
Kshudra-aamra	*Persea macrantha*	Machilus	Folk
Kshudraamra	*Schleichera oleosa*	Lac Tree, Macassar Oil Tree, Honey Tree, Ceylon Oak	Ayurvedic
Kshudra-bhantaaki	*Solanum indicum*	Poison Berry	Ayurvedic
Kshudra-bhantaki	*Solanum ferox*	Poison-Berry	Ayurvedic

Table Contd.

Indian Name	Botanical Name	English Name	Medicinal System
Kshudrailaa	*Elettaria cardamomum*	Lesser Cardamom	Ayurvedic
Kshudra-Paa-shaanabheda	*Didymocarpus pedicellata*	Rock Flower, Stone-Breaker	Ayurvedic
Kshudra-patra	*Acorus calamus*	Sweet Flag, Calamus	Ayurvedic
Kshumaa	*Linum usitatissimum*	Linseed, Flax	Ayurvedic
Kshurak	*Asteracantha longifolia*	Hygrophilla	Ayurvedic
Kshuraka	*Hygrophila auriculata*	Indian Swampweed	Ayurvedic
Kshurapatra	*Desmostachya bipinnata*	Sacrificial Grass	Ayurvedic
Ksuchalaa	*Strychnos nux-vomica*	Nux Vomica	Ayurvedic
Kubajaka	*Rosa bourboniana*	Bourbon Rose	Ayurvedic
Kuberaakshi	*Caesalpinia bonduc*	Fever Nut, Bonduc Nut, Nikkar Nut	Ayurvedic
Kuberaakshi	*Stereospermum personatum*	Trumpet Flower, Yellow Snake Tree	Ayurvedic
Kubjaka	*Rosa moschata*	Himalayan Musk Rose	Ayurvedic
Kuchandan	*Juniperus virginiana*	Pencil Cedar, Red Cedar	Folk
Kuchandana	*Caesalpinia sappan*	Sappan	Ayurvedic
Kuchilaa	*Strychnos nux-vomica*	Nux Vomica	Ayurvedic
Kuchilaa-lataa	*Strychnos colubrina*	Trumpet Wood	Ayurvedic
Kuchlaa	*Strychnos nux-vomica*	Nux Vomica	Unani
Kuchleikaa-malang	*Viscum monoicum*	Himalayan Mistletoe	Folk
Kuchlekaa-baandaa	*Viscum monoicum*	Himalayan Mistletoe	Folk
Kudasappaalai-pattai (Bark)	*Holarrhena antidysenterica*	Easter Tree, Ivory Tree, Tellicherry	Siddha/Tamil
Kudasappaalai-vidai (Seed)	*Holarrhena antidysenterica*	Easter Tree, Ivory Tree, Tellicherry	Siddha/Tamil
Kudavuboraju	*Chloroxylon swietenia*	Indian Satinwood Tree	Siddha/Tamil
Kudirai Pidukku	*Sterculia foetida*	Kola Seeds, Gurru Nuts	Siddha/Tamil
Kudiram	*Canthium parviflorum*	Wild Jasmine	Siddha/Tamil
Kudiyotti	*Argemone mexicana*	Prickly Poppy, Mexican Poppy	Siddha/Tamil
Kudri	*Zehneria umbellata*	Zehneria	Folk
Kudrraivali pillu	*Echinochloa frumentacea*	Japanese Barnyard Millet	Siddha/Tamil

Table Contd.

Indian Name	Botanical Name	English Name	Medicinal System
Kudu-hunchi	*Momordica tuberosa*	Eight-ribbed Bitter Gourd	Ayurvedic
Ku-Jaavitri	*Myristica malabarica*	Malabar Nutmeg, False Nutmeg, Bombay Nutmeg, Bombay Mace	Ayurvedic
Kujai	*Rosa moschata*	Himalayan Musk Rose	Folk
Kujithekera	*Garcinia cowa*	Indo-Malayan Brindleberry	Folk
Kukarondh	*Pluchea indica*	Indian Fleabane	Folk
Kukkur-kaashtha	*Piscidia piscipula*	Jamaica Dogwood	Folk
Kukumadona	*Kedrostis foetidissima*	Lobed-leaf Foetid Plant	Folk
Kukundara	*Blumea balsamifera*	Nagai Camphor	Ayurvedic
Kukundara	*Blumea densiflora*	Nagai Camphor	Ayurvedic
Kukundara	*Blumea eriantha*	Nagai Camphor	Ayurvedic
Kukundara	*Blumea fastulosa*	Nagai Camphor	Ayurvedic
Kukundara	*Blumea lacera*	Nagai Camphor	Ayurvedic
Kukuradru	*Blumea lacera*	Nagai Camphor	Ayurvedic
Kukurjihvaa	*Leea indica*	Purple-berry Holly	Ayurvedic
Kulaka	*Trichosanthes dioica*	Patol, Pointed Gourd	Ayurvedic
Kulanjan	*Alpinia officinarum*	Lesser Galangal, Alpinia, Catarrh Root, Chinese Ginger	Ayurvedic
Kulanjana	*Alpinia galanga*	Greater Galangal	Ayurvedic
Kula-pannai	*Glycosmis pentaphylla*	Orangeberry, Ginberry	Siddha/Tamil
Kulattha	*Dolichos biflorus*	Horsegram	Ayurvedic
Kulatthikaa	*Dolichos falcatus*	Kapik	Ayurvedic
Kulavi	*Garcinia xanthochymus*	Egg Tree	Siddha/Tamil
Kulfaa	*Portulaca oleracea*	Common Purslane	Unani
Kulinaval	*Myrtus communis*	Myrtle, Clove Myrtle, Spanish Myrtle	Folk
Kulirashringaaya	*Pistacia integerrima*	Horn-shaped Gall Tree, Kakra Gall Tree	Ayurvedic
Kuliravishaanikaa	*Pistacia integerrima*	Horn-shaped Gall Tree, Kakra Gall Tree	Ayurvedic
Kulittha	*Dolichos biflorus*	Horsegram	Ayurvedic
Kullai	*Grewia villosa*	Tamthar	Siddha/Tamil
Kullai	*Ixora coccinea*	Jungleflame Ixora	Folk/Tamil

Table Contd.

Indian Name	Botanical Name	English Name	Medicinal System
Kulli	*Rumex nepalensis*	Nepal Dock	Folk
Kulthi	*Atylosia scarabaeoides*	Peanut Grass	Folk
Kulthi	*Dolichos biflorus*	Horsegram	Unani
Kulu Naaspaati	*Persea americana*	Avacado, Alligator Pear	Folk
Kum	*Fraxinus hookery*	European Ash, Weeping Ash	Folk
Kumaarak	*Crataeva nurvala*	Steaved Tree, Sacred Barna	Ayurvedic
Kumaari	*Aloe barbadensis*	Curacao Aloe, Barbados Aloe, Indian Aloe, Jaffarabad Aloe	Ayurvedic
Kumaari	*Aloe barbadensis*	Curacao Aloe, Barbados Aloe, Indian Aloe, Jaffarabad Aloe	Siddha/Tamil
Kumaarikaa	*Aloe barbadensis*	Curacao Aloe, Barbados Aloe, Indian Aloe, Jaffarabad Aloe	Ayurvedic
Kumal	*Abroma augusta*	Perennial Indian Hemp, Devil's Cotton	Folk
Kumbay	*Gardenia latifolia*	Boxwood Gardenia	Siddha/Tamil
Kumbha	*Balsamodendron mukul*	Indian Bdellium, Gum Guggul	Ayurvedic
Kumbha	*Operculina turpethum*	Indian Jalap, Turpeth	Ayurvedic
Kumbha	*Sesbania grandiflora*	Agati Sesban, Swamp Pea	Ayurvedic
Kumbhi	*Careya arborea*	Kumbi, Slow-Match Tree	Ayurvedic
Kumbhika	*Careya arborea*	Kumbi, Slow-Match Tree	Ayurvedic
Kumbhipushpi	*Stereospermum personatum*	Trumpet Flower, Yellow Snake Tree	Ayurvedic
Kumbi	*Careya arborea*	Kumbi, Slow-Match Tree	Siddha/Tamil
Kumbi	*Cochlospermum gossypium*	Golden Silk Tree, White Silk Cotton Tree	Folk
Kumgumappoo	*Crocus sativus*	Saffron, Crocus	Siddha/Tamil
Kumhraa	*Cucurbita pepo*	Pumpin, Marrow	Unani
Kumizham	*Gmelina arborea*	Candahar Tree, White Teak	Siddha/Tamil
Kumizham	*Gmelina asiatica*	Small Cashmere Tree	Siddha/Tamil
Kumkuma	*Crocus sativus*	Saffron, Crocus	Ayurvedic
Kumshmaanda	*Cucurbita moschata*	Squash	Ayurvedic
Kumuda	*Nymphaea alba*	European White Water-lily	Ayurvedic
Kumuda	*Nymphaea rubra*	Indian Red Water-lily	Ayurvedic
Kumudini	*Limnanthemum cristatum*	Aquatic Pseudo-Chiretta Plant	Folk

Table Contd.

Indian Name	Botanical Name	English Name	Medicinal System
Kunaashak	*Alhagi pseudalhagi*	Camel Thorn, Persian Manna Plant	Ayurvedic
Kunanjara	*Digera muricata*	Gitana Weed	Ayurvedic
Kunanjara	*Rumex maritimus*	Golden Dock	Ayurvedic
Kunati	*Coriandrum sativum*	Coriander	Ayurvedic
Kunayi	*Sida cordifolia*	Country Mallow	Unani
Kunda	*Jasminum multiflorum*	Downy Jasmine	Ayurvedic
Kunda	*Meconopsis aculeata*	Blue Poppy	Folk
Kundali	*Azima tetracantha*	Mistletoe Berrythorn	Folk
Kundali	*Clerodendrum inerme*	Smooth Volkameria	Ayurvedic
Kundalini	*Spondias pinnata*	Hog-Plum, Wild Mango	Ayurvedic
Kundalini	*Tinospora cordifolia*	Heart-leaved Tinospora	Ayurvedic
Kundiyaa	*Artemisia vestita*	Russian Wormwood	Folk
Kundur (Gum)	*Boswellia serrata*	Indian Frankincense, Indian Olibanum	Unani
Kunduru (Gum)	*Boswellia serrata*	Indian Frankincense, Indian Olibanum	Ayurvedic
Kunduru	*Coccinia indica*	Ivy-Gourd	Ayurvedic
Kungiliyam	*Shorea robusta*	Sal Tree	Siddha/Tamil
Kungli	*Boswellia serrata*	Indian Frankincense, Indian Olibanum	Siddha/Tamil
Kuniyun	*Conium maculatum*	Spotted Hemlock, Poison Hemlock	Unani
Kunjad	*Sesamum indicum*	Sesame, Gingelly	Unani
Kunjaraa	*Woodfordia fruticosa*	Fire-flame Bush, Shiranjitea	Ayurvedic
Kunjuyaa	*Urena lobata*	Pink Chinese Burr, Burr Mallow	Folk
Kunku	*Euonymus tingens*	Spindle Wood, Wahoo	Folk
Kunri	*Abrus precatorius*	Indian Wild Liquorice, Jequirity, Crab's Eye, Precatory Bean	Siddha/Tamil
Kuntali	*Zanonia indica*	Zanonia	Ayurvedic
Kupilu-lataa	*Strychnos colubrina*	Trumpet Wood	Ayurvedic
Kuppaimeni	*Acalypha fruticosa*	Birch-leaved Acalypha	Siddha/Tamil
Kuppaimeni	*Acalypha indica*	Copperleaf Acalypha	Siddha/Tamil

Table Contd.

Indian Name	Botanical Name	English Name	Medicinal System
Kuppi (Smaller variety)	*Acalypha ciliata*	Smaller var. Acalypha	Ayurvedic
Kuppi	*Acalypha indica*	Copperleaf Acalypha	Ayurvedic
Kuppi	*Acalypha indica*	Copperleaf Acalypha	Folk
Kuptaa	*Ehretia laevis*	Datrang Tree	Folk
Kuraa	*Tarenna asiatica*	Komi Tree	Folk
Kuranta	*Barleria prionitis*	Common Yellow Nail Dye Plant	Ayurvedic
Kurantaka	*Barleria prionitis*	Common Yellow Nail Dye Plant	Ayurvedic
Kuranti	*Striga asiatica*	Witchweed	Ayurvedic
Kurbak	*Rhododendron arboreum*	Tree-Rhododendron, Rose-Tree	Folk
Kurbak	*Rhododendron barbatum*	Giantblood Rhododendron	Folk
Kurcha	*Microstylis musifera*	Jivaka	Ayurvedic
Kurchi (Bark)	*Holarrhena antidysenterica*	Easter Tree, Ivory Tree, Tellicherry	Ayurvedic
Kureli	*Murdannia scapiflora*	Few-flowered Dewflower	Folk
Kuri	*Bidens pilosa*	Beggar's Tick, Devil's Needle	Folk
Kurinji	*Nilgirianthus ciliatus*	Kurunji	Siddha/Tamil
Kurinji	*Perilepta auriculata*	Pandai	Siddha/Tamil
Kuru	*Limnanthemum nymphaeoides*	Fringed Water-Lily	Folk
Kurugu	*Ficus lacor*	White Fig	Siddha/Tamil
Kurunthotti	*Sida cordifolia*	Country Mallow	Siddha/Tamil
Kuruver	*Coleus vettiveroides*	Coleus	Siddha/Tamil
Kuruvingi	*Ehretia buxifolia*	Carmonia Shrub	Siddha/Tamil
Kusha	*Desmostachya bipinnata*	Sacrificial Grass	Ayurvedic
Kushbhikaa	*Myrica nagi*	Box Myrtle	Ayurvedic
Kushimshapaa	*Dalbergia sissoides*	Malabar Blackwood	Ayurvedic
Kusht	*Saussurea lappa*	Kuth, Costus	Ayurvedic
Kushtavairi	*Hydnocarpus laurifolia*	Soorty Oil Tree	Ayurvedic
Kushtha	*Saussurea hypoleuca*	Himalayan Saw-wort	Ayurvedic
Kushtha	*Saussurea lappa*	Kuth, Costus	Ayurvedic
Kushtha-bheda	*Inula racemosa*	Elecampane	Ayurvedic
Kustumburu	*Coriandrum sativum*	Coriander	Ayurvedic
Kusum	*Carthamus tinctorius*	Safflower	Ayurvedic

Table Contd.

Indian Name	Botanical Name	English Name	Medicinal System
Kusumbha	*Carthamus tinctorius*	Safflower	Ayurvedic
Kutaja (Purush)	*Wrightia tomentosa*	Red-flowered Wrightia	Ayurvedic
Kutaja (Stree)	*Wrightia tinctoria*	Pala Indigo Plant	Ayurvedic
Kutaja	*Holarrhena antidysenterica*	Easter Tree, Ivory Tree, Tellicherry Bark	Ayurvedic
Kutambaka	*Leucas aspera*	White Dead Nettle	Ayurvedic
Kutannata	*Oroxylum indicum*	Indian Trumpet Flower	Ayurvedic
Kutilal	*Daphne oleoides*	Mezereon	Folk
Kutki	*Picrorhiza kurroa*	Picrorhiza	Unani
Kutri	*Solanum erianthum*	Mullen Nightshade	Folk
Kuttra	*Limnophila aromatica*	Turpentine Spinach	Folk
Kuttra	*Limnophila indica*	Oil-of-lemons Spinach	Folk
Kutu (var.)	*Fagopyrum tataricum*	Tatary Duckwheat	Folk
Kutu	*Fagopyrum esculentum*	Buckwheat	Folk
Kuujaa	*Rosa moschata*	Himalayan Musk Rose	Folk
Kuurchshirshaka	*Cocos nucifera*	Coconut Palm	Ayurvedic
Kuushmaanda	*Benincasa hispida*	Ash Gourd, White Gourd, Wax Gourd, White Pumpkin	Ayurvedic
Kuushmaandaka	*Benincasa hispida*	Ash Gourd, White Gourd, Wax Gourd, White Pumpkin	Ayurvedic
Kuushmaandaka	*Cucurbita maxima*	Red Gourd, Red Pumpkin	Ayurvedic
Kuushmaandi	*Benincasa hispida*	Ash Gourd, White Gourd, Wax Gourd, White Pumpkin	Ayurvedic
Kuusmaandi	*Cucurbita maxima*	Red Gourd, Red Pumpkin	Ayurvedic
Kuuthan-Kali	*Salvia lanata*	Scarlet Sage	Folk
Kuvet	*Feronia limonia*	Wood Apple	Unani
Laajavanti	*Mimosa pudica*	Sensitive-plant, Humble-Plant	Ayurvedic
Laajwanti	*Mimosa pudica*	Sensitive-plant, Humble-Plant	Unani
Laakheri	*Melastoma malabathricum*	Indian Rhododendron	Folk
Laakshaa	*Rosa centifolia*	Cabbage Rose, Provence Rose, Hundred-leaved Rose	Ayurvedic
Laakshaa-vriksha	*Ficus cunia*	Indian Fig	Ayurvedic
Laal Bagharenda	*Jatropha gossypifolia*	Physic Nut, Purging Nut	Folk
Laal Indraayana	*Trichosanthes bracteata*	Redball Snakegourd	Folk

Table Contd.

Indian Name	Botanical Name	English Name	Medicinal System
Laal Jadi	*Geranium wallichianum*	Wallich Crane's Bill	Folk
Laal Jahri	*Geranium wallichianum*	Wallich Crane's Bill	Folk
Laal Jhaau	*Tamarix aphylla*	Athel, Tamarisk	Folk
Laal Kaskas	*Papaver rhoeas*	Corn Poppy, Red Poppy	Folk
Laal Khair	*Acacia chundra*	Red Cutch	Folk
Laal Marashaa	*Amaranthus tricolor*	Chinese Spinach, Garden Amaranth, Fountain Plant	Folk
Laal Posta	*Papaver rhoeas*	Corn Poppy, Red Poppy	Folk
Laal Shaak	*Amaranthus tricolor*	Chinese Spinach, Garden Amaranth, Fountain Plant	Folk
Laal-Aghaadaa	*Plectranthus mollis*	Country Borage	Folk
Laal-ambaari	*Hibiscus sabdariffa*	Roselle, Jamaican Sorrel, Natal Sorrel, Red Sorrel	Folk
Laal-bhui-aamlaa	*Phyllanthus urinaria*	Cultivated Field Chanca Piedra	Folk
Laal-chameli	*Quisqualis indica*	Rangoon Creeper	Folk
Laal-chandan	*Pterocarpus santalinus*	Red Sandalwood, Red Sanders	Folk
Laal-giyaa	*Striga gesneroides*	Cowpea Witchweed	Folk
Laal-Naagakeshar	*Ochrocarpus longifolius*	Red-dye-flowerbud, Pseudo-Mesua ferra	Folk
Laamaajja	*Cymbopogon jwarancusa*	Vetiver-scented Grass	Ayurvedic
Laamajjaka	*Cymbopogon jwarancusa*	Vetiver-scented Grass	Ayurvedic
Laamajjaka	*Vetiveria zizanioides*	Vetiver, Khas	Ayurvedic
Laanaa-buuti	*Salsola kali*	Glass-Wort, Russian Thistle, Prickly-Saltwort	Ayurvedic
Laangalaki	*Gloriosa superba*	Glory Lily, Super Lily, Tiger's Claws	Ayurvedic
Laangali (Kerala)	*Hydrolea zeylanica*	Ceylon Hydrolea	Ayurvedic
Laangali	*Cocos nucifera*	Coconut Palm	Ayurvedic
Laangali	*Gloriosa superba*	Glory Lily, Super Lily, Tiger's Claws	Ayurvedic
Laangali	*Lippia nodiflora*	Wild Sage	Ayurvedic
Laangali	*Phyla nodiflora*	Fogfruit, Sawtooth Fogfruit	Ayurvedic

Table Contd.

Indian Name	Botanical Name	English Name	Medicinal System
Laangaliki	*Gloriosa superba*	Glory Lily, Super Lily, Tiger's Claws	Ayurvedic
Laanglaahva	*Gloriosa superba*	Glory Lily, Super Lily, Tiger's Claws	Ayurvedic
Laangtaan	*Physochlaina praealta*	Hyoscyamine Plant	Folk
Laanguli	*Mucuna prurita*	Cowhage, Horse-eye Bean	Ayurvedic
Lab Laab	*Dolichos lablab*	Indian Butter Bean, Lablab Bean, Horsebean	Unani
Lablaab	*Convolvulus arvensis*	Deer's Foot, Devil's Garters	Ayurvedic
Lablab	*Hedera nepalensis*	Nepal Ivy	Folk
Laddaakhi-Sevati	*Rosa webbiana*	Webb's Rose	Ayurvedic
Laderi	*Parthenocissus himalayana*	Kandur Tree	Folk
Laghu Arni	*Clerodendrum phlomidis*	Glory Bower	Folk
Laghu Kasheruka	*Scirpus articulatus*	Paddyfield Club-Rush	Ayurvedic
Laghu-badara	*Ziziphus oenoplia*	Jackal Jujube	Ayurvedic
Laghu-lonikaa	*Portulaca quadrifida*	Chicken Weed	Ayurvedic
Laghu-muulaka	*Raphanus sativus*	Radish	Ayurvedic
Laghu-shleshmaataka	*Cordia rothii*	Sebestan	Ayurvedic
Laghu-udumbara	*Ficus cunia*	Indian Fig	Ayurvedic
Lahsun	*Allium sativum*	Garlic	Unani
Lahsuvaa	*Digera muricata*	Gitana Weed	Folk
Lajjaalu (var.)	*Neptunia oleracea*	Sensitive Plant	Ayurvedic
Lajjaalu	*Biophytum sensitivum*	Life Plant	Ayurvedic
Lajjaalu	*Mimosa pudica*	Sensitive-plant, Humble-Plant	Ayurvedic
Lajoni	*Biophytum sensitivum*	Life Plant	Folk
Lakajana	*Biophytum sensitivum*	Life Plant	Folk
Lakshaa vrksha	*Schleichera oleosa*	Lac Tree, Macassar Oil Tree, Honey Tree, Ceylon Oak	Ayurvedic
Lakshmanaa	*Ipomoea marginata*	Purple Heart Morning Glory	Ayurvedic
Lakshmanaa	*Mandragora autumnalis*	Mandrake	Ayurvedic
Lakuch	*Artocarpus lakoocha*	Monkey Jack	Ayurvedic
Lal Murga	*Celosia cristata*	Cock's Comb	Folk

Table Contd.

Indian Name	Botanical Name	English Name	Medicinal System
Lamia	*Lamium album*	White Dead Nettle, Archangel	Folk
Lanjai	*Clerodendrum inerme*	Smooth Volkameria	Folk
Lankaa	*Capsicum annuum*	Chilli, Red Pepper	Ayurvedic
Larkspur	*Delphinium consolida*	Forking Larkspur, Larkspur, Lark's Claw, Knight's Spur	Folk
Larkspur Tagara	*Delphinium cashmirianum*	Kashmir Larkspur	Ayurvedic
Lashuna	*Allium sativum*	Garlic	Ayurvedic
Lasobaval	*Leucaena glauca*	White Popinac, Lead Tree	Folk
Lasodaa	*Cordia myxa*	Sabestan Plum	Unani
Lassuni	*Dysoxylum binectariferum*	Termite-resistant Cedar	Folk
Lasunghaas	*Medicago sativa*	Alfalfa, Lucerne	Ayurvedic
Lataa Khadira	*Acacia torta*	Twisted Acacia	Ayurvedic
Lataa-karanja	*Caesalpinia bonduc*	Fever Nut, Bonduc Nut, Nikkar Nut	Ayurvedic
Lataakasturi	*Hibiscus abelmoschus*	Musk Seed, Ambette Seed, Muskmallow	Ayurvedic
Lataakasturikaa	*Hibiscus abelmoschus*	Musk Seed, Ambette Seed, Muskmallow	Ayurvedic
Lataakhadira	*Acacia pennata*	Feathery-shoot Acacia	Ayurvedic
Lataa-Palaash	*Butea superba*	Flame of the Forest	Ayurvedic
Lataaphatakari	*Cardiospermum halicacabum*	Balloon Vine, Winter Pea, Heartseed	Folk
Latari	*Lathyrus sativus*	Chickling Vetch, Grass Pea	Folk
Latjeeraa	*Achyranthes aspera*	Prickly Chaff Flower	Folk
Lat-latiaa	*Siegesbeckia orientalis*	The Holy Herb, Sieges-beckia	Folk
Lat-mahuriaa	*Digera muricata*	Gitana Weed	Folk
Latmi	*Amoora cucullata*	Rohitak	Folk
Latputiyaa	*Nasturtium officinale*	Watercress	Folk
Laung	*Syzygium aromaticum*	Clove	Unani
Lavali-phala	*Phyllanthus distichus*	Country Gooseberry	Ayurvedic
Lavanga	*Syzygium aromaticum*	Clove	Ayurvedic
Lavanga-lataa (var.)	*Luvunga eleutherandra*	Woody Clove Vine	Ayurvedic
Lavanga-lataa	*Luvunga scandens*	Woody Clove Vine	Ayurvedic

Table Contd.

Indian Name	Botanical Name	English Name	Medicinal System
Lavangam	*Syzygium aromaticum*	Clove	Siddha/Tamil
Lavender	*Lavandula angustifolia*	Lavender	Unani
Leechai kottai keerai	*Pisonia grandis*	Grand Devil's Claws	Siddha/Tamil
Leemu	*Citrus limon*	Lemon	Unani
Leemu-e-khaarki	*Citrus limon*	Lemon	Unani
Leihruisen (Lushai)	*Lonicera japonica*	Japanese Honeysuckle	Folk
Lekhyapatra	*Borassus flabellifer*	Palmyra Palm, Brab Tree	Ayurvedic
Lekhyapatraka	*Betula utilis*	Himalayan Silver Birch, Indian Paper Tree	Ayurvedic
"Lemon Queen"	*Santolina chamaecyparissus*	Lavender Cotton	Folk
Lendaphala	*Salacia macrosperma*	Saptrangi	Folk
Lendira (trade)	*Lagerstroemia parviflora*	Lendi, Benteak	Folk
Libi-dibi	*Caesalpinia coriaria*	American Sumac, Divi-divi Plant	Folk
Lichi	*Litchi chinensis*	Litchi, Lychee	Folk
Lichkuraa	*Siegesbeckia orientalis*	The Holy Herb, Sieges-beckia	Folk
Lilac	*Syringa vulgaris*	Common Lilac	Folk
Lilakaathi	*Polygala crotalarioides*	Himalayan Milkwort	Folk
Lilakanthi	*Polygala crotalarioides*	Himalayan Milkwort	Folk
Limri	*Paullinia asiatica*	Lopez Root Tree, Wild Orange Tree, Forest Pepper	Folk
Limu Kaghzi	*Citrus aurantifolia*	Acid or Sour Lime, Country Lime	Unani
Lingadonda	*Bryonopsis laciniosa*	Bryony	Folk/Telugu
Lingikaa	*Bryonopsis laciniosa*	Bryony	Ayurvedic
Lingini	*Bryonopsis laciniosa*	Bryony	Ayurvedic
Lisodaa	*Cordia myxa*	Sabestan Plum	Ayurvedic
Lisodaa	*Cordia rothii*	Sebestan	Ayurvedic
Lobaan	*Styrax benzoin*	True Gum Benzoin, Sumatra Benzoin or Gum Benjamin	Unani
Lobia	*Phaseolus vulgaris*	Kidney Bean	Unani

Table Contd.

Indian Name	Botanical Name	English Name	Medicinal System
Lobiyaa	*Phaseolus lunatus*	Double Bean, Lima Bean, Burma Bean	Unani
Lodh Pathaani	*Symplocos paniculata*	Sapphire Berry	Unani
Lodh Pathaani	*Symplocos racemosa*	Lodh Tree, Sapphire Berry	Unani
Lodhra	*Symplocos racemosa*	Lodh Tree, Sapphire Berry	Ayurvedic
Lodhra-Pattikaa	*Symplocos paniculata*	Sapphire Berry	Ayurvedic
Loha	*Aquilaria agallocha*	Aloewood, Eaglewood, Agarwood	Ayurvedic
Loha-Kaashtha	*Guaiacum officinale*	Lignum Vitae, Tree-of-life, Pockwood Tree	Ayurvedic
Loha-lakkar	*Guaiacum officinale*	Lignum Vitae, Tree-of-life, Pockwood Tree	Folk
Lohitpushpaka	*Punica granatum*	Pomegranate	Ayurvedic
Lokaat	*Eriobotrya japonica*	Loquat, Japanese Medlar	Unani
Lokhandi	*Memecylon edule*	Iron Wood	Folk
Lokhandi	*Quassia indica*	Niepa Bark Tree	Folk
Lokhandi	*Reissantia grahamii*	Pristimera Root	Folk
Lokhandi	*Reissantia indica*	Atari Vine	Folk
Lokhandi	*Ventilago madraspatana*	Ventilago Vermilion Vine	Folk
Lokottai	*Zingiber officinale*	Ginger	Siddha/Tamil
Lomash-parni	*Teramnus labialis*	Blue Wiss	Ayurvedic
Lombardy	*Populus nigra*	River Birch	Folk
Lonaa	*Portulaca oleracea*	Common Purslane	Ayurvedic
Loni	*Portulaca oleracea*	Common Purslane	Ayurvedic
Lot-loti	*Urena lobata*	Pink Chinese Burr, Burr Mallow	Folk
Lottaaka	*Eriobotrya japonica*	Loquat, Japanese Medlar	Ayurvedic
Lowani Hariphala	*Phyllanthus distichus*	Country Gooseberry	Ayurvedic
Loz	*Amygdalus communis*	Almond	Unani
Loz	*Prunus amygdalus*	Almond	Unani
Lubis firmun	*Lithospermum officinale*	Corn Gromwell	Folk
Luffaah	*Atropa acuminata*	Indian Belladonna, Indian Atropa	Unani
Luffaah-Barri	*Atropa acuminata*	Indian Belladonna, Indian Atropa	Unani

Table Contd.

Indian Name	Botanical Name	English Name	Medicinal System
Lugro-maarpro	*Pedicularis pectinata*	Lousewort	Folk/Kashmir
Lunga	*Citrus medica*	Citron	Ayurvedic
Lunio	*Zygophyllum simplex*	Bean Caper	Folk
Lunwaa	*Zygophyllum simplex*	Bean Caper	Folk
Lusan	*Medicago sativa*	Alfalfa, Lucerne	Ayurvedic
Luutaari	*Taraxacum officinale*	Common Dandelion	Ayurvedic
Luvuni	*Annona reticulata*	Bull's Heart, Common Custard Apple	Folk
Maa	*Mangifera indica*	Mango	Folk/Tamil
Maacheeka	*Tamarix aphylla*	Athel, Tamarisk	Ayurvedic
Maachika	*Tamarix ericoides*	Tamarisk Mucronta	Ayurvedic
Maachikaa	*Tamarix aphylla*	Athel, Tamarisk	Ayurvedic
Maachikaa	*Tamarix dioica*	Tamarisk	Ayurvedic
Maachipatri	*Grangea maderaspatana*	Madras Carpet	Folk
Maadani	*Cannabis sativa*	Hemp, Indian Hemp	Ayurvedic
Maadhavi	*Hiptage benghalensis*	Hiptage	Ayurvedic
Maadhavi	*Hiptage benghalensis*	Hiptage	Siddha/Tamil
Maagadha	*Piper longum*	Indian Long Pepper, Joborandi	Ayurvedic
Maagadhaa	*Piper longum*	Indian Long Pepper, Joborandi	Ayurvedic
Maagadhi	*Piper longum*	Indian Long Pepper, Joborandi	Ayurvedic
Maagadhikaa	*Piper longum*	Indian Long Pepper, Joborandi	Ayurvedic
Maajuphalaka	*Quercus infectoria*	Oak Galls, Aleppo Galls, Mecca Galls	Ayurvedic
Maakaal	*Trichosanthes bracteata*	Redball Snakegourd	Folk
Maakhaniaa Mahuaa	*Madhuca butyracea*	Phulwara, Indian Butter Tree	Folk
Maalaakanda	*Eulophia nuda*	Goruma Tuber, Riddhi	Ayurvedic
Maalati (var.)	*Jasminum arborescens*	Tree Jasmine	Folk
Maalati (var.)	*Jasminum flexile*	Jasmine, Juhi	Ayurvedic
Maalati	*Jasminum officinale*	Spanish Jasmine	Ayurvedic
Maalatiphala	*Myristica fragrans*	Nutmeg	Ayurvedic
Maaliyaka	*Aquilaria agallocha*	Aloewood, Eaglewood, Agarwood	Ayurvedic
Maalkaanguni	*Celastrus paniculatus*	Staff Tree, Intellect Tree	Ayurvedic

Table Contd.

Indian Name	Botanical Name	English Name	Medicinal System
Maalkangani	*Celastrus paniculatus*	Staff Tree, Intellect Tree	Unani
Maaluura	*Aegle marmelos*	Bael Tree, Bengal Quince	Ayurvedic
Maalvaa	*Basella alba*	Indian Spinach	Ayurvedic
Maamajjaka	*Enicostemma littorale*	Indian Gentian	Ayurvedic
Maamekh	*Polygonum viviparum*	Viviparous Bistort	Folk
Maamiraa	*Coptis teeta*	Gold Thread	Ayurvedic
Maamisaa	*Coptis teeta*	Gold Thread	Ayurvedic
Maana	*Alocasia indica*	Giant Taro	Ayurvedic
Maanaka	*Alocasia indica*	Giant Taro	Ayurvedic
Maanakand	*Remusatia vivipara*	Hitch-hiker Elephant Ear	Folk
Maanduuki	*Centella asiatica*	Asiatic Pennywort, Indian Pennywort	Ayurvedic
Maangalya	*Leptadenia reticulata*	Dodi Vegetable	Ayurvedic
Maangalya Kusuma	*Convolvulus pluricaulis*	Conch-flowered Bindweed, White-flowered Shankhpushpi	Ayurvedic
Maangalyaa	*Acorus calamus*	Sweet Flag, Calamus	Ayurvedic
Maankanda	*Alocasia indica*	Giant Taro	Ayurvedic
Maansi	*Nardostachys jatamansi*	Spikenard, Musk-root	Ayurvedic
Maansrohini	*Soymida febrifuga*	Indian Red-Wood, Bastard Cedar	Ayurvedic
Maaphal	*Quercus infectoria*	Oak Galls, Aleppo Galls, Mecca Galls	Unani
Maaraajuti	*Elephantopus scaber*	Prickly-leaved Elephant's Foot	Folk
Maarchob	*Asparagus officinalis*	Asparagus, Sparrow Grass	Unani
Maargiyaah	*Asparagus officinalis*	Asparagus, Sparrow Grass	Unani
Maarisha-rakta	*Amaranthus tricolor*	Chinese Spinach, Garden Amaranth, Fountain Plant	Ayurvedic
Maarjaar-gandhikaa	*Phaseolus trilobus*	Wild Gram	Ayurvedic
Maarka	*Eclipta alba*	Trailing Eclipta Plant	Ayurvedic
Maarkandi	*Cassia angustifolia*	Indian senna, Tinnevelly senna	Ayurvedic
Maarkandikaa	*Cassia angustifolia*	Indian senna, Tinnevelly senna	Ayurvedic
Maarkandikaa	*Cassia obovata*	Spanish, Sudan Senna	Ayurvedic
Maarkava	*Eclipta alba*	Trailing Eclipta Plant	Ayurvedic

Table Contd.

Indian Name	Botanical Name	English Name	Medicinal System
Maarwaari Methi	*Trigonella corniculata*	Kasuri Fenugreek	Folk
Maasha	*Phaseolus mungo*	Kidney Bean, Black Gram	Ayurvedic
Maashaparni	*Atylosia goensis*	Maashparni	Ayurvedic
Maashaparni	*Teramnus labialis*	Blue Wiss	Ayurvedic
Maasikkaai	*Quercus infectoria*	Oak Galls, Aleppo Galls, Mecca Galls	Siddha/Tamil
Maasipathri	*Grangea maderaspatana*	Madras Carpet	Siddha/Tamil
Maasipattiri	*Artemisia vulgaris*	Indian Wormwood, Fleabane, Dungwort, Mugwort, Wild Wormwood	Siddha/Tamil
Maathulai	*Punica granatum*	Pomegranate	Siddha/Tamil
Maatiryaaq	*Delphinium denudatum*	Larkspur	Unani
Maattan-kodi	*Cryptolepis buchanani*	Indian Sarsaparilla	Folk/Tamil
Maatul	*Datura stramonium*	Thornapple, Jimsonweed, Stramonium	Ayurvedic
Maatula	*Datura metel*	Thornapple, Downy Datura	Ayurvedic
Maatulaani	*Cannabis sativa*	Hemp, Indian Hemp	Ayurvedic
Maatulaka	*Citrus medica*	Citron	Ayurvedic
Maatulunga	*Citrus medica*	Citron	Ayurvedic
Maavilingam	*Crataeva nurvala*	Steaved Tree, Sacred Barna	Siddha/Tamil
Maayaaphala (var.)	*Quercus ilex*	Holly or Holm Oak	Ayurvedic
Maayaaphala	*Quercus infectoria*	Oak Galls, Aleppo Galls, Mecca Galls	Ayurvedic
Maayakku	*Quercus infectoria*	Oak Galls, Aleppo Galls, Mecca Galls	Ayurvedic
Maayeen Kalaan	*Tamarix indica*	Takut Galls	Unani
Maayeen Khurd	*Tamarix indica*	Takut Galls	Unani
Maayin Khurd	*Tamarix aphylla*	Athel, Tamarisk	Unani
Maazu	*Quercus infectoria*	Oak Galls, Aleppo Galls, Mecca Galls	Unani
Machhechhi	*Alternanthera sessilis*	Sessile Joyweed	Unani
Machhipatri	*Parthenium hysterophorus*	Congress Grass	Folk
Machipatri	*Artemisia absinthium*	Wormwood, Madderwood	Siddha/Tamil

Table Contd.

Indian Name	Botanical Name	English Name	Medicinal System
Machoti	*Polygonum aviculare*	Knotgrass, Knotweed, Mexican Sanguinaria	Folk
Machuttai	*Rivea ornate*	Oliliuqui	Siddha/Tamil
Madaar	*Calotropis gigantea*	Swallow Wort	Unani
Madaar	*Calotropis procera*	Swallow-wort, Milk Weed, King's Crown	Unani
Madan	*Datura stramonium*	Thornapple, Jimsonweed, Stramonium	Ayurvedic
Madana	*Randia dumetorum*	Common Emetic Nut	Ayurvedic
Madana Ghanti	*Spermacoce hispida*	Saggy Buttonweed	Ayurvedic
Madana-ghanti	*Borreria articularis*	Shaggy Button Weed	Ayurvedic
Madayansambrani	*Kingiodendron pinnatum*	Piney	Siddha/Tamil
Madayanti	*Jasminum sambac*	Arabian Jasmine, Tuscan Jasmine, Double Jasmine	Ayurvedic
Madayanti	*Lawsonia inermis*	Henna	Ayurvedic
Madayantikaa	*Lawsonia inermis*	Henna	Ayurvedic
Madhu Shigru	*Moringa pterygosperma*	Drumstick, Horse-Radish	Ayurvedic
Madhuchhadaa	*Actiniopteris dichotoma*	Peacock's Tail	Ayurvedic
Madhudoot	*Mangifera indica*	Mango	Ayurvedic
Madhu-duuti	*Stereospermum personatum*	Trumpet Flower, Yellow Snake Tree	Ayurvedic
Madhugandha	*Mimusops elengi*	Spanish-Cherry, West Indian Medlar, Bullet Wood	Ayurvedic
Madhuka	*Glycyrrhiza glabra*	Licorice, Liquorice	Ayurvedic
Madhukam	*Scoparia dulcis*	Sweet Broomweed	Folk
Madhukarkatikaa	*Citrus maxima*	Pummelo, Shaddock	Ayurvedic
Madhukparna	*Oroxylum indicum*	Indian Trumpet Flower	Ayurvedic
Madhuli	*Glycyrrhiza glabra*	Licorice, Liquorice	Ayurvedic
Madhulikaa	*Marsdenia tenacissima*	White Turpeth	Ayurvedic
Madhumaalati	*Aganosma dichotoma*	Malati	Ayurvedic
Madhu-maalati	*Dregea volubilis*	Wattakaka	Ayurvedic
Madhuparni	*Spondias pinnata*	Hog-Plum, Wild Mango	Ayurvedic
Madhuparni	*Tinospora cordifolia*	Heart-leaved Tinospora	Ayurvedic

Table Contd.

Indian Name	Botanical Name	English Name	Medicinal System
Madhuparnikaa	*Crinum latifolium*	Wide-leaved Crinum	Ayurvedic
Madhuparnikaa	*Gmelina arborea*	Candahar Tree, White Teak	Ayurvedic
Madhupushpa	*Madhuca indica*	Mahua Tree, Moha	Ayurvedic
Madhupushpa	*Mimusops elengi*	Spanish-Cherry, West Indian Medlar, Bullet Wood	Ayurvedic
Madhura	*Microstylis musifera*	Jivaka	Ayurvedic
Madhuraa	*Foeniculum vulgare*	Fennel	Ayurvedic
Madhuraa	*Lilium polyphyllum*	Kakoli Tuber Lily	Ayurvedic
Madhurasaa	*Glycyrrhiza glabra*	Licorice, Liquorice	Ayurvedic
Madhurasaa	*Marsdenia tenacissima*	White Turpeth	Ayurvedic
Madhurikaa	*Foeniculum vulgare*	Fennel	Ayurvedic
Madhusnuhi	*Smilax china*	China Root	Ayurvedic
Madhusrav	*Madhuca indica*	Mahua Tree, Moha	Ayurvedic
Madhusravaa	*Leptadenia reticulata*	Dodi Vegetable	Ayurvedic
Madhusravaa	*Maerua arenaria*	Desert Maerua, Hemkand	Ayurvedic
Madhutrna	*Saccharum officinarum*	Gannaa, Naishakar	Ayurvedic
Madhuuka (Bheda)	*Bassia longifolia*	Mowra Butter Tree, South Indian Mahua	Ayurvedic
Madhuuka	*Madhuca butyracea*	Phulwara, Indian Butter Tree	Ayurvedic
Madhuuka	*Madhuca indica*	Mahua Tree, Moha	Ayurvedic
Madhuulaka	*Madhuca longifolia*	South Indian Mahua	Folk
Madhuuli	*Eleusine coracana*	Finger Millet, African Millet, Ragi	Ayurvedic
Madhuyashtikaa	*Glycyrrhiza glabra*	Licorice, Liquorice	Ayurvedic
Madhuyash-tyaahvaa	*Glycyrrhiza glabra*	Licorice, Liquorice	Ayurvedic
Madhvaaluka	*Dioscorea esculenta*	Lesser Yam, Karen Potato	Ayurvedic
Madkaarini	*Hyoscyamus niger*	Indian Henbane, Black Henbane	Ayurvedic
Madkarai	*Randia dumetorum*	Common Emetic Nut	Folk/Tamil
Madona Lily	*Lilium candidum*	Madona Lily, Annunciation Lily, White Lily	Folk
Madyantikaa	*Jasminum sambac*	Arabian Jasmine, Tuscan Jasmine, Double Jasmine	Ayurvedic

Table Contd.

Indian Name	Botanical Name	English Name	Medicinal System
Magadhodbhavaa	*Piper longum*	Indian Long Pepper, Joborandi	Ayurvedic
Magarandam	*Jasminum multiflorum*	Downy Jasmine	Siddha/Tamil
Maghaase-Hindi	*Litsea glutinosa*	Common Tallow Lowrel	Unani
Magilam	*Mimusops elengi*	Spanish-Cherry, West Indian Medlar, Bullet Wood	Siddha/Tamil
Mahaabalaa	*Sida rhombifolia*	Red-flowered Mallow	Ayurvedic
Mahaabhadraa	*Gmelina arborea*	Candahar Tree, White Teak	Ayurvedic
Mahaabhari-Vachaa	*Alpinia galanga*	Greater Galangal	Ayurvedic
Mahaabhari-vachaa	*Zingiber zerumbet*	Zerumbet Ginger	Ayurvedic
Mahaagani	*Swietenia mahagoni*	West Indian Mahogany	Folk
Mahaajaalini	*Luffa cylindrica*	Smooth Luffa, Sponge-gourd, Sponge Cucumber	Ayurvedic
Mahaakaala	*Trichosanthes bracteata*	Redball Snakegourd	Ayurvedic
Mahaa-Kaaya	*Zea mays*	Maize, Corn, Indian Corn	Ayurvedic
Mahaakapittha	*Aegle marmelos*	Bael Tree, Bengal Quince	Ayurvedic
Mahaakoshtaki	*Luffa cylindrica*	Smooth Luffa, Sponge-gourd, Sponge Cucumber	Ayurvedic
Mahaalunga	*Citrus medica*	Citron	Ayurvedic
Mahaa-medaa	*Polygonatum cirrhifolium*	Solomon's Seal	Ayurvedic
Mahaa-medaa	*Polygonatum multiflorum*	Solomon's Seal	Ayurvedic
Mahaamuulaa	*Cocculus hirsutus*	Broom-Creeper, Ink-Berry	Ayurvedic
Mahaa-nibu	*Citrus maxima*	Pummelo, Shaddock	Folk
Mahaanimba	*Melia azedarach*	Persian Lilac, Pride of India	Ayurvedic
Mahaaphalaa	*Syzygium cuminii*	Java Plum, Jambolan, Black Plum	Ayurvedic
Mahaapindi	*Gardenia turgida*	Bharangi Bark Tree	Ayurvedic
Mahaapushpa	*Selenicereus grandiflorus*	Night-Blooming Cereus, Sweet-scented Cactus	Ayurvedic
Mahaar Naachni	*Eleusine indica*	Crowfoot Grass, Crab Grass	Folk
Mahaaraashtri	*Spilanthes oleracea*	Brazilian Cress, Para Cress	Ayurvedic

Table Contd.

Indian Name	Botanical Name	English Name	Medicinal System
Mallikaa	*Jasminum sambac*	Arabian Jasmine, Tuscan Jasmine, Double Jasmine	Ayurvedic
Malliveppam	*Olax scandens*	Olax	Folk/Tamil
Malyapushpa	*Crotalaria juncea*	Sun Hemp	Ayurvedic
Mamaram (bark)	*Mangifera indica*	Mango	Siddha/Tamil
Mambulichi	*Spondias pinnata*	Hog-Plum, Wild Mango	Siddha/Tamil
Mamira	*Coptis teeta*	Gold Thread	Ayurvedic
Mamiri	*Caltha palustris*	American Cowslip, Marsh Marigold, Water Buttercup	Folk
Mamiri	*Thalictrum foliolosum*	Meadow Rue	Unani
Manakkarai	*Meyna laxiflora*	Muyna	Siddha/Tamil
Manakkarai	*Vangueria spinosa*	Voa-Vanga	Siddha/Tamil
Manchingi	*Dolichandrone falcate*	Corky-winged-seed Tree	Folk
Manchitti, Sevvallikkodi (Root)	*Rubia cordifolia*	Indian Madder, Bengal Madder	Siddha/Tamil
Mand Dhuup	*Canarium strictum*	Black Dammar	Ayurvedic
Manda	*Ricinus communis*	Castor Seed	Ayurvedic
Mandaar	*Calotropis gigantea*	Swallow Wort	Ayurvedic
Mandaara	*Erythrina indica*	Indian Coral Tree	Ayurvedic
Mandaara	*Nyctanthes arbor-tristis*	Tree of Sorrow, Night Jasmine, Coral Jasmine	Ayurvedic
Mandaka	*Hiptage benghalensis*	Hiptage	Ayurvedic
Mandalpatrikaa	*Dalbergia latifolia*	East Indian Rosewood, Bombay Blackwood	Ayurvedic
Mandapi	*Arachis hypogaea*	Groundnut, Peanut, Monkeynut	Ayurvedic
Mandavalli	*Ipomoea bona-nox*	Moon Flower	Folk
Manduukaparni	*Centella asiatica*	Asiatic Pennywort, Indian Pennywort	Ayurvedic
Manduukaparni	*Hydrocotyle javanica*	Java Pennywort	Folk
Manduuka-parnikaa	*Centella asiatica*	Asiatic Pennywort, Indian Pennywort	Ayurvedic
Manga	*Mangifera indica*	Mango	Folk/Tamil
Mangaiinji	*Curcuma amada*	Mango-ginger, Wild Turmeric	Folk/Tamil

Table Contd.

Indian Name	Botanical Name	English Name	Medicinal System
Mangalyaa	*Lens culinaris*	Lentil	Ayurvedic
Mangalyak	*Lens culinaris*	Lentil	Ayurvedic
Manganari	*Limnophila aromatica*	Turpentine Spinach	Folk
Manganari	*Limnophila indica*	Oil-of-lemons Spinach	Folk
Mangottai Paruppu	*Mangifera indica*	Mango	Siddha/Tamil
Mangusta	*Garcinia mangostana*	Mangosteen, Dodol	Siddha/Tamil
Mangustaan	*Garcinia mangostana*	Mangosteen, Dodol	Folk
Manipungu	*Sapindus laurifolius*	Soapnut Tree of South India	Siddha/Tamil
Manithakkali	*Solanum nigrum*	Black Nightshade	Siddha/Tamil
Manjakadambu	*Adina cordifolia*	Yellow Teak, Saffron Teak	Siddha/Tamil
Manjal	*Curcuma longa*	Turmeric	Siddha/Tamil
Manjal Karisaalai	*Wedelia calendulaceae*	Yellow-flowered Weldia	Siddha/Tamil
Manjalkodi	*Coscinium fenestratum*	False Calumba	Siddha/Tamil
Manjarikaa	*Ocimum sanctum*	Holy Basil, Sacred Basil	Ayurvedic
Manjeeth	*Rubia cordifolia*	Indian Madder, Bengal Madder	Unani
Manji	*Crotalaria juncea*	Sun Hemp	Folk/Tamil
Manjika	*Ipomoea sepiaria*	Big-flowered Morning Glory	Ayurvedic
Manjimedi	*Ficus palmata*	Indian Fig	Folk/Telugu
Manjishthaa	*Rubia cordifolia*	Indian Madder, Bengal Madder	Ayurvedic
Manjitti	*Bixa orellana*	Annatto	Siddha/Tamil
Manjul	*Ficus carica*	Common Fig	Ayurvedic
Manjurukh	*Pluchea indica*	Indian Fleabane	Folk
Manmadabanam	*Jasminum officinale*	Spanish Jasmine	Siddha/Tamil
Manoranjitam	*Artabotrys hexapetalus*	Yling-Yling Vine	Siddha/Tamil
Manupasapu	*Curcuma caesia*	Black Zedorary	Folk/Telugu
Maraad (var.)	*Polygala crotalarioides*	Himalayan Milkwort	Folk
Maraad	*Polygala chinensis*	Senega	Ayurvedic
Maramalli	*Millingtonia hortensis*	Indian Cork Tree	Siddha/Tamil
Maramanjal	*Coscinium fenestratum*	False Calumba	Siddha/Tamil
Marang Chirchiti	*Stachytarpheta jamaicensis*	Brazilian Tea, Bastard Vervain, Aaron's Rod	Folk
Marasaa	*Amaranthus blitum*	Trailing Amaranth, Wild Blite	Folk
Mara-uri	*Antiaris toxicaria*	Sacking Tree, Upas Tree	Folk/Tamil

Table Contd.

Indian Name	Botanical Name	English Name	Medicinal System
Maravalai	*Hedera helix*	Common Ivy, Bentwood	Siddha/Tamil
Maravalli kizhangu	*Manihot esculenta*	Manioc, Tapioca, Cassava	Siddha/Tamil
Maravattai	*Hydnocarpus laurifolia*	Soorty Oil Tree	Siddha/Tamil
Mardu tvak	*Betula utilis*	Himalayan Silver Birch, Indian Paper Tree	Ayurvedic
Marethi	*Spilanthes calva*	Para Cress	Folk
Marethi	*Spilanthes oleracea*	Brazilian Cress, Para Cress	Ayurvedic
Maricha	*Piper nigrum*	Black Pepper	Ayurvedic
Marich-patraka	*Vateria indica*	White Damar, Indian Copal-Tree, Malabar Tallow Tree, Piney Varnish-Tree	Ayurvedic
Marjal	*Iris ensata*	Japanese Iris	Folk
Markataamra	*Spondias pinnata*	Hog-Plum, Wild Mango	Ayurvedic
Markatahastatrna	*Eleusine coracana*	Finger Millet, African Millet, Ragi	Ayurvedic
Markati	*Mucuna prurita*	Cowhage, Horse-eye Bean	Ayurvedic
Marmanjal	*Berberis aristata*	Indian Barberry	Siddha/Tamil
Marorphali	*Helicteres isora*	East Indian Screw Tree	Unani
Maruaa-bel	*Marsdenia roylei*	Marua Vine	Folk
Maruaa-bel	*Marsdenia tenacissima*	White Turpeth	Folk
Maruaa-daanaa	*Strobilanthes callosus*	Carvia Callosa	Folk
Marubaka	*Origanum majorana*	Sweet Marjoram	Ayurvedic
Marubhooruuha	*Capparis aphylla*	Caper Berry	Ayurvedic
Marudam	*Myrica nagi*	Box Myrtle	Siddha/Tamil
Marudam	*Terminalia arjuna*	Arjun Terminalia	Siddha/Tamil
Marudhonri	*Lawsonia inermis*	Henna	Siddha/Tamil
Marudu	*Terminalia paniculata*	Flowering Murdah	Folk/Tamil
Marukkaaraikai	*Randia dumetorum*	Common Emetic Nut	Siddha/Tamil
Marul	*Sansevieria hyacinthoides*	Ceylon Bowstring Hemp	Siddha/Tamil
Marul	*Sansevieria roxburghiana*	Indian Bowstring Hemp	Siddha/Tamil
Maruloomatham	*Xanthium strumarium*	Cocklebur, Burweed	Siddha/Tamil
Marungi	*Syzygium zeylanicum*	Sumaich (Cambodia)	Siddha/Tamil

Table Contd.

Indian Name	Botanical Name	English Name	Medicinal System
Marusambhava	*Raphanus sativus*	Radish	Ayurvedic
Maruva	*Terminalia paniculata*	Flowering Murdah	Folk
Maruvu	*Origanum majorana*	Sweet Marjoram	Siddha/Tamil
Marv	*Salvia spinosa*	Wrinkled-leaf Sage	Unani
Maryaada-valli	*Ipomoea pes-caprae*	Goat's Foot Creeper	Ayurvedic
Marzanjosh	*Origanum majorana*	Sweet Marjoram	Unani
Mashmash	*Prunus armeniaca*	Apricot	Unani
Masi	*Peristrophe bicalyculata*	Panicled Peristrophe	Folk
Masoor	*Lens culinaris*	Lentil	Unani
Masrnaa	*Linum usitatissimum*	Linseed, Flax	Ayurvedic
Mastagi	*Pistacia lentiscus*	Mastic Tree	Unani
Mastaki	*Pistacia lentiscus*	Mastic Tree	Unani
Mastaru	*Grangea maderaspatana*	Madras Carpet	Folk
Mastiyaaraa	*Artemisia absinthium*	Wormwood, Madderwood	Folk
Masura	*Lens culinaris*	Lentil	Ayurvedic
Masurikaa	*Lens culinaris*	Lentil	Ayurvedic
Mate Tea	*Ilex paraguariensis*	Mate Tea, Yerba Mate, Paraguay Tea	Folk
Matsyaadani	*Alternanthera sessilis*	Sessile Joyweed	Ayurvedic
Matsyaadani	*Phyla nodiflora*	Fogfruit, Sawtooth Fogfruit	Ayurvedic
Matsyaakshaka	*Bacopa monnieri*	Thyme-leaved Gratiola	Ayurvedic
Matsyaakshi	*Alternanthera sessilis*	Sessile Joyweed	Ayurvedic
Matsyaakshika	*Alternanthera sessilis*	Sessile Joyweed	Ayurvedic
Matsyagandhaa	*Alternanthera sessilis*	Sessile Joyweed	Ayurvedic
Matsyagandhaa	*Juniperus communis*	Common Juniper	Ayurvedic
Matsyagandhaa	*Lippia nodiflora*	Wild Sage	Ayurvedic
Matsyagandhaa	*Phyla nodiflora*	Fogfruit, Sawtooth Fogfruit	Ayurvedic
Matsya-gandhi	*Alternanthera sessilis*	Sessile Joyweed	Ayurvedic
Matsyashakalaa	*Picrorhiza kurroa*	Picrorhiza	Ayurvedic
Maulsiri	*Mimusops elengi*	Spanish-Cherry, West Indian Medlar, Bullet Wood	Ayurvedic

Table Contd.

Indian Name	Botanical Name	English Name	Medicinal System
Maweez	*Vitis vinifera*	Wine Grape, European Grape	Unani
Mayirkonrai	*Caesalpinia pulcherrima*	Barbados Pride, Peacock Flower	Siddha/Tamil
Mayirmanikkam	*Ipomoea quamoclit*	Cypress Vine, Indian Pink	Siddha/Tamil
Mayura	*Achyranthes aspera*	Prickly Chaff Flower	Ayurvedic
Mayuraka	*Achyranthes aspera*	Prickly Chaff Flower	Ayurvedic
Mayura-shikhaa	*Elephantopus scaber*	Prickly-leaved Elephant's Foot	Ayurvedic
Mayurjuti	*Elephantopus scaber*	Prickly-leaved Elephant's Foot	Folk
Mayurshikhaa	*Actiniopteris dichotoma*	Peacock's Tail	Ayurvedic
Mayurshikhaa	*Adiantum incisum*	Peacock's Tail	Ayurvedic
Medaa (var.)	*Polygonatum multiflorum*	Solomon's Seal	Ayurvedic
Medaa	*Polygonatum cirrhifolium*	Solomon's Seal	Ayurvedic
Medaa	*Polygonatum verticillatum*	Whorl-leaved Solomon's Seal	Ayurvedic
Medaasaka	*Litsea glutinosa*	Common Tallow Lowrel	Ayurvedic
Meethaa Telia	*Aconitum falconeri*	Indian Aconite	Folk
Meethaa Zahar	*Aconitum chasmanthum*	Indian Napellus	Folk
Meghaahvaa	*Cyperus rotundus*	Nut Grass	Ayurvedic
Meghapushpa	*Salix caprea*	Sallow, Goat Willow, Common Willow	Ayurvedic
Megharava	*Amaranthus spinosus*	Spiny Amaranth, Thorny Amaranth, Spiny Pigweed	Ayurvedic
Meghnaad	*Amaranthus spinosus*	Spiny Amaranth, Thorny Amaranth, Spiny Pigweed	Ayurvedic
Mehndi	*Lawsonia inermis*	Henna	Unani
Mela-nelli	*Phyllanthus maderaspatensis*	Kanocha Seed	Siddha/Tamil
Melei veppu	*Chukrasia tabularis*	Bastard Cedar, White Cedar, Indian Red Wood	Siddha/Tamil
Mendika	*Lawsonia inermis*	Henna	Ayurvedic
Meradu (var.)	*Polygala sibirica*	Common Milkwort	Folk
Meradu	*Polygala chinensis*	Senega	Ayurvedic

Table Contd.

Indian Name	Botanical Name	English Name	Medicinal System
Mermahaul	*Euonymus tingens*	Spindle Wood, Wahoo	Folk
Merukan kizhangu	*Alocasia indica*	Giant Taro	Siddha/Tamil
Meshalochana	*Cassia tora*	Sickle Senna, Ringworm Plant	Ayurvedic
Mesha-shringi	*Dolichandrone falcate*	Corky-winged-seed Tree	Ayurvedic
Meshashringi	*Gymnema sylvestre*	Australian Cow Plant, Gymnema	Ayurvedic
Meshavalli	*Gymnema sylvestre*	Australian Cow Plant, Gymnema	Ayurvedic
Meshavi-shaanikaa	*Gymnema sylvestre*	Australian Cow Plant, Gymnema	Ayurvedic
Methi	*Trigonella foenum-graecum*	Fenugreek	Ayurvedic
Methi	*Trigonella foenum-graecum*	Fenugreek	Unani
Methi	*Trigonella incisa*	Winter burr Clover	Folk
Methikaa	*Trigonella foenum-graecum*	Fenugreek	Ayurvedic
Methini	*Trigonella foenum-graecum*	Fenugreek	Ayurvedic
Mezenga	*Zanthoxylum oxyphyllum*	Tumru Tree, Prickly Ash	Folk
Mezereon Hindi	*Clitoria ternatea*	Butterfly Pea, Winged-leaved Clitoria, Mezereon	Unani
Mhaataaraa	*Sonchus asper*	Spinyleaved Sow Thistle	Folk
Michaai	*Ipomoea muricata*	Traveller's Midnight Lilies	Folk
Michren	*Pedicularis pectinata*	Lousewort	Folk
Mi-gang-ew	*Kadsura heteroclita*	Flashy-leaved Kadsura, Fructus kadsurae	Folk/Assam
Mikaaniaa	*Mikania cordata*	Heartleaf Hempvine	Folk
Milagaipoondu	*Vinca pusilla*	Bengal Periwinkle	Folk
Milagay	*Capsicum annuum*	Chilli, Red Pepper	Siddha/Tamil
Milagu	*Piper chaba*	Java Long Pepper	Siddha/Tamil
Milagu	*Piper nigrum*	Black Pepper	Siddha/Tamil
Milagu ver (root)	*Piper nigrum*	Black Pepper	Siddha/Tamil
Milakaranai	*Toddalia asiatica*	Wild Orange Tree, Forest Pepper	Siddha/Tamil

Table Contd.

Indian Name	Botanical Name	English Name	Medicinal System
Milk Thistle	*Silybum marianum*	Holy Thistle, Milk Thistle	Folk
Mimri	*Wendlandia exserta*	Wendlandia	Folk
Minaakshi	*Alternanthera sessilis*	Sessile Joyweed	Ayurvedic
Mindiri	*Anacardium occidentale*	Cashew Nut Tree	Siddha/Tamil
Minnargodi	*Calycopteris floribunda*	White Daisy	Siddha/Tamil
Mirch	*Capsicum annuum*	Chilli, Red Pepper	Unani
Mirchaai	*Vinca pusilla*	Bengal Periwinkle	Folk
Mishi	*Foeniculum vulgare*	Fennel	Ayurvedic
Mishran	*Pedicularis pectinata*	Lousewort	Folk/Punjab
Mishreyaa	*Foeniculum vulgare*	Fennel	Ayurvedic
Misurpurpu	*Lens culinaris*	Lentil	Folk/Tamil
Miswaak	*Salvadora persica*	Mustard Tree, Salt Bush Tree, Tooth Brush Tree	Unani
Mitha Zahar	*Aconitum ferox*	Indian Aconite, Wolfsbane, Monkshood	Folk
Mithaa (sweet) Kiryaat	*Swertia angustifolia*	Hill Chiretta	Folk
Mithaa Neem	*Murraya koenigii*	Curry-Leaf Tree	Folk
Mithaa-dudhiaa	*Polygonatum verticillatum*	Whorl-leaved Solomon's Seal	Folk
Miyilai	*Gordonia obtusa*	Loblolly Bay, Grey Laurel	Folk/South
Mochaa	*Musa paradisiaca*	Banana, Plantain	Ayurvedic
Mochaa	*Salmalia malabarica*	Silk Cotton Tree, Semul Tree	Ayurvedic
Mochaahva	*Salmalia malabarica*	Silk Cotton Tree, Semul Tree	Ayurvedic
Mochaka	*Moringa pterygosperma*	Drumstick, Horse-Radish	Ayurvedic
Mochani	*Lolium temulentum*	Darnel, Bearded Ryegrass	Ayurvedic
Mochras (gum)	*Salmalia malabarica*	Silk Cotton Tree, Semul Tree	Unani
Modhuphal	*Salacia chinensis*	Chinese Salacia	Folk
Mogalingum	*Schrebera swietenioides*	Weaver's Beam Tree	Siddha/Tamil
Mogaraa	*Jasminum malabaricum*	Climbing Mogara	Folk
Mograa	*Jasminum sambac*	Arabian Jasmine, Tuscan Jasmine, Double Jasmine	Unani
Mohri	*Aconitum chasmanthum*	Indian Napellus	Folk

Table Contd.

Indian Name	Botanical Name	English Name	Medicinal System
Mokandar	*Justicia betonica*	Shrimp Plant, Lobster Plant	Folk
Mokhaa	*Momordica balsamina*	Balsam Apple	Folk
Mollukkay	*Tephrosia purpurea*	Purple Tephrosia, Wild Indigo	Folk/Tamil
Molsari	*Mimusops elengi*	Spanish-Cherry, West Indian Medlar, Bullet Wood	Unani
Mom-China	*Sapium sebiferum*	Chinese Tallow Tree	Folk
Monalu	*Terminalia citrina*	Bengal Myrobalan	Folk/Assam
Mongiluppu (Manna)	*Bambusa bambos*	Spiny or Thorny Bamboo	Siddha/Tamil
Mookkirattai	*Boerhavia diffusa*	Red-flowered Hogweed	Siddha/Tamil
Mookkukkadalai	*Cicer arietinum*	Bengal Gram, Chick Pea	Siddha/Tamil
Mookuti	*Vicoa indica*	Banjauri	Folk/Tamil
Moong	*Phaseolus radiatus*	Greengram, Golden Gram	Unani
Moongil	*Bambusa bambos*	Spiny or Thorny Bamboo	Siddha/Tamil
Moongphali	*Arachis hypogaea*	Groundnut, Peanut, Monkeynut	Unani
Moosaambaram (Dried leaf juice)	*Aloe barbadensis*	Curacao Aloe, Barbados Aloe, Indian Aloe, Jaffarabad Aloe	Siddha/Tamil
Moovilai (Root)	*Uraria lagopoides*	Trailing Uraria	Siddha/Tamil
Morang	*Gisekia pharnaceoides*	Jisucao (Chinese)	Folk
Morang-elaichi	*Amomum aromaticum*	Bengal Cardamom, Cardamom	Folk
Morata	*Maerua arenaria*	Desert Maerua, Hemkand	Ayurvedic
Morata	*Saccharum officinarum*	Gannaa, Naishakar	Ayurvedic
Morataa	*Marsdenia tenacissima*	White Turpeth	Ayurvedic
Morepankhi	*Thuja orientalis*	Oriental Arbor-Vitae	Folk
Moriamaram	*Buchanania lanzan*	Almondette Tree, Cheronjee, Buchanan's Mango	Siddha/Tamil
Morinda	*Abies pindrow*	Pindrow-Fir, Silver-Fir, The West-Himalayan Low-Level Fir	Folk
Morinda	*Abies webbiana*	Indian Silver Fir, The West-Himalayan High-Level Fir, The East-Himalayan Fir	Folk
Morindaa	*Picea smithiana*	West Himalayan Spruce	Folk
Mosakathuthalai	*Notonia grandiflora*	Common Fleshy Rag-weed	Siddha/Tamil

Table Contd.

Indian Name	Botanical Name	English Name	Medicinal System
Mostaki	*Lolium temulentum*	Darnel, Bearded Ryegrass	Folk
Motaa-pasuti	*Knema angustifolia*	Pseudo-Redsander Tree	Folk
Moth	*Phaseolus aconitifolius*	Aconite-Bean, Moth	Ayurvedic
Mothibhuiaamvali	*Phyllanthus simplex*	Wild Chanca Piedra	Folk
Motiaabelaa	*Jasminum sambac*	Arabian Jasmine, Tuscan Jasmine, Double Jasmine	Folk
Motirakkanni	*Hugonia mystax*	Climbing Flax	Siddha/Tamil
Motta manji	*Sansevieria hyacinthoides*	Ceylon Bowstring Hemp	Siddha/Tamil
Motta manji	*Sansevieria roxburghiana*	Indian Bowstring Hemp	Siddha/Tamil
Mouz	*Musa paradisiaca*	Banana, Plantain	Unani
Moyna	*Meyna laxiflora*	Muyna	Folk
Mozhuku-peerankai	*Luffa cylindrica*	Smooth Luffa, Sponge-gourd, Sponge Cucumber	Siddha/Tamil
Mrdvikaa	*Vitis vinifera*	Wine Grape, European Grape	Ayurvedic
Mridupushpa	*Albizia lebbeck*	Siris Tree, East Indian Walnut	Ayurvedic
Mrigadaani	*Citrullus colocynthis*	Colocynth Bitter Apple	Ayurvedic
Mrigairvaaru	*Citrullus colocynthis*	Colocynth Bitter Apple	Ayurvedic
Mubaaraka	*Adiantum capillus-veneris*	American Maidenhair Fern, Venus Hair, Rock Fern	Folk
Mubaaraka	*Adiantum lunulatum*	Walking Maidenhair Fern, Black Maidenhair	Folk
Muchakunda (var.)	*Pterospermum canescens*	Hathipaila	Ayurvedic
Muchakunda	*Pterospermum acerifolium*	Hathipaila	Ayurvedic
Muchukunda Champaa	*Pterospermum acerifolium*	Hathipaila	Ayurvedic
Mudaima	*Buchanania axillaris*	Buchanan's Mango, Cuddapah Almond	Siddha/Tamil
Mudaima	*Buchanania lanzan*	Almondette Tree, Cheronjee, Buchanan's Mango	Siddha/Tamil
Mudak-karuththaan	*Cardiospermum halicacabum*	Balloon Vine, Winter Pea, Heartseed	Siddha/Tamil
Mudchembai	*Sesbania bispinosa*	Prickly Sesban, Dhaincha	Siddha/Tamil

Table Contd.

Indian Name	Botanical Name	English Name	Medicinal System
Mudga	*Phaseolus radiatus*	Greengram, Golden Gram	Ayurvedic
Mudgaparni	*Phaseolus adenanthus*	South American Snail Vine	Ayurvedic
Mudgaparni	*Phaseolus trilobus*	Wild Gram	Ayurvedic
Mudgara	*Jasminum malabaricum*	Climbing Mogara	Ayurvedic
Mudiyaakkoon-thal	*Merremia tridentata*	Woodrose, Merremia	Siddha/Tamil
Muduna	*Meyna laxiflora*	Muyna	Folk
Mugavan	*Phaseolus trilobus*	Wild Gram	Folk
Mugdhee	*Jasminum auriculatum*	Cultivated Jasmine	Ayurvedic
Mughilaan	*Acacia arabica*	Babul, Black Babul, Indian Gum Arabic Tree	Unani
Mukhaaluka	*Ipomoea batatas*	Sweet Potato	Ayurvedic
Mukhatari	*Grangea maderaspatana*	Madras Carpet	Folk
Mukhjali	*Drosera peltata*	Sundew	Folk
Mukkampalai	*Alstonia scholaris*	Devil's Tree, Dita Bark Tree	Siddha/Tamil
Mukki	*Garcinia xanthochymus*	Egg Tree	Siddha/Tamil
Muktavarchaa	*Acalypha indica*	Copperleaf Acalypha	Ayurvedic
Mukuulaka	*Pistacia vera*	Pistachio, Green Almond	Ayurvedic
Mulakkeerai	*Amaranthus tricolor*	Chinese Spinach, Garden Amaranth, Fountain Plant	Folk/Tamil
Mulasari	*Lasia spinosa*	Prickly Lasia	Siddha/Tamil
Mulchangan	*Azima tetracantha*	Mistletoe Berrythorn	Siddha/Tamil
Mulethi	*Glycyrrhiza glabra*	Licorice, Liquorice	Unani
Mulkatri	*Solanum indicum*	Poison Berry	Siddha/Tamil
Mull Ilavam	*Salmalia malabarica*	Silk Cotton Tree, Semul Tree	Siddha/Tamil
Mullangi	*Raphanus sativus*	Radish	Siddha/Tamil
Mullarasanam	*Hura crepitans*	Sandbox Tree, Monkey Dinner-bell	Siddha/Tamil
Mulli	*Solanum ferox*	Poison-Berry	Siddha/Tamil
Mullukkeerai	*Amaranthus spinosus*	Spiny Amaranth, Thorny Amaranth, Spiny Pigweed	Siddha/Tamil
Mullu-murukku	*Erythrina stricta*	Scarlet-flowered Coral Tree	Siddha/Tamil

Table Contd.

Indian Name	Botanical Name	English Name	Medicinal System
Mulluvengai	*Bridelia retusa*	Spinous Kino Tree	Siddha/Tamil
Mulvizaj	*Delphinium staphisagria*	Stavesacre	Unani
Mumiri	*Capsella bursa-pastoris*	Shepherd's Purse, St. James's Wort	Folk/Kumaun
Mundi	*Sphaeranthus indicus*	East Indian Globe Thistle	Ayurvedic
Mundi	*Sphaeranthus indicus*	East Indian Globe Thistle	Unani
Mundika	*Sphaeranthus indicus*	East Indian Globe Thistle	Ayurvedic
Munditikaa	*Sphaeranthus indicus*	East Indian Globe Thistle	Ayurvedic
Mungalya	*Phaseolus radiatus*	Greengram, Golden Gram	Ayurvedic
Mungraa	*Raphanus sativus*	Radish	Ayurvedic
Mungus-vel	*Ophiorrhiza mungos*	Mongoose Plant	Folk
Muni	*Sesbania grandiflora*	Agati Sesban, Swamp Pea	Ayurvedic
Munidrum	*Sesbania grandiflora*	Agati Sesban, Swamp Pea	Ayurvedic
Munitaru	*Sesbania grandiflora*	Agati Sesban, Swamp Pea	Ayurvedic
Muniyaaraa	*Polygonum plebeium*	Common Knotweed	Folk/Bihar
Munja	*Saccharum munja*	Munja Culms	Ayurvedic
Munjaataka	*Eulophia campestris*	Salep Orchid	Ayurvedic
Munjaataka	*Eulophia herbacea*	Salep Orchid	Ayurvedic
Munjaataka	*Orchis latifolia*	Orchis, Salep	Ayurvedic
Munjappullu	*Saccharum munja*	Munja Culms	Siddha/Tamil
Munjipul	*Saccharum munja*	Munja Culms	Siddha/Tamil
Munnai	*Premna integrifolia*	Headache Tree	Siddha/Tamil
Munnakaa	*Vitis vinifera*	Wine Grape, European Grape	Ayurvedic
Muql	*Balsamodendron mukul*	Indian Bdellium, Gum Guggul	Unani
Muraa (var.)	*Selinum monnieri*	Snake's Bed	Folk
Muraa	*Erythrina stricta*	Scarlet-flowered Coral Tree	Ayurvedic
Muraa	*Selinum tenuifolium*	Cow Parsley	Ayurvedic
Mural	*Selinum tenuifolium*	Cow Parsley	Siddha/Tamil
Murangi	*Moringa pterygosperma*	Drumstick, Horse-Radish	Ayurvedic
Murasabalam	*Artocarpus integrifolia*	Jackfruit, Jack Tree	Siddha/Tamil
Murgal	*Garcinia indica*	Kokam Butter Tree, Mangosteen Oil Tree	Siddha/Tamil

Table Contd.

Indian Name	Botanical Name	English Name	Medicinal System
Murhari	*Maerua arenaria*	Desert Maerua, Hemkand	Folk
Murmakki	*Balsamodendron myrrha*	Myrrh, Herabol	Unani
Murr	*Selinum tenuifolium*	Cow Parsley	Folk
Murukkan	*Butea monosperma*	Flame of the Forest, Butea Gum, Bengal Kino	Siddha/Tamil
Murungai	*Moringa pterygosperma*	Drumstick, Horse-Radish	Siddha/Tamil
Musabbar (Dried leaf juice)	*Aloe barbadensis*	Curacao Aloe, Barbados Aloe, Indian Aloe, Jaffarabad Aloe	Folk
Musali	*Chlorophytum tuberosum*	White Musali	Unani
Musali Safed	*Chlorophytum arundinaceum*	White Musali	Unani
Musattalai	*Ipomoea pes-caprae*	Goat's Foot Creeper	Folk/Tamil
Mushaippeyetti	*Litsea glutinosa*	Common Tallow Lowrel	Siddha/Tamil
Mushali Shveta	*Chlorophytum arundinaceum*	White Musali	Ayurvedic
Mushali Shveta	*Chlorophytum tuberosum*	White Musali	Ayurvedic
Mushali Sveta	*Asparagus adscendens*	White Musali	Ayurvedic
Mushkbaalaa	*Valeriana wallichii*	Indian Valerian	Folk
Mushkdaanaa	*Hibiscus abelmoschus*	Musk Seed, Ambette Seed, Muskmallow	Unani
Mushkiyaara	*Sambucus ebulus*	Dwarf Elder	Siddha/Tamil
Musht-ul-Ghaul	*Abutilon indicum*	Country Mallow, Flowering Maples, Chinese Bell-flowers	Unani
Musi Milagay	*Capsicum frutescens*	Bird Chilli	Siddha/Tamil
Musilam	*Dioscorea esculenta*	Lesser Yam, Karen Potato	Siddha/Tamil
Muskakaa	*Schrebera swietenioides*	Weaver's Beam Tree	Ayurvedic
Musli Siyaah	*Curculigo orchioides*	Black Musali	Unani
Musna	*Saponaria vaccaria*	Soapwort, Cowcokle	Folk
Musna	*Vaccaria pyramidata*	Soapwort, Cow Herb	Folk
Musta	*Cyperus rotundus*	Nut Grass	Ayurvedic
Mustaa	*Cyperus rotundus*	Nut Grass	Ayurvedic
Mustaka (var.)	*Kyllinga triceps*	Spikesedge, The Sedge of Jamaica	Ayurvedic

Table Contd.

Indian Name	Botanical Name	English Name	Medicinal System
Mustaka	*Cyperus rotundus*	Nut Grass	Ayurvedic
Mustu	*Kyllinga triceps*	Spikesedge, The Sedge of Jamaica	Folk
Musumsukkai	*Melothria maderaspatana*	Rough Bryony	Siddha/Tamil
Musuttai	*Rivea hypocrateriformis*	Midnapore Creeper	Siddha/Tamil
Mutri-Tulasi	*Orthosiphon grandiflorus*	Kidney Tea Plant, Java Tea	Folk
Muttanna	*Cyperus scariosus*	Nut Grass	Folk/South
Muulaipalyirai	*Cassia absus*	Four-leaved Cassia, Pig's Senna	Siddha/Tamil
Muulaka	*Raphanus sativus*	Radish	Ayurvedic
Muulakapotikaa	*Raphanus sativus*	Radish	Ayurvedic
Muuli	*Raphanus sativus*	Radish	Unani
Muulini	*Tylophora indica*	Emetic Swallow Wort, Indian or Country Ipecacuanha	Ayurvedic
Muurad	*Myrtus communis*	Myrtle, Clove Myrtle, Spanish Myrtle	Siddha/Tamil
Muurad-daan	*Myrtus communis*	Myrtle, Clove Myrtle, Spanish Myrtle	Unani
Muurdhaja	*Pavonia odorata*	Fragrant Sticky Mallow	Ayurvedic
Muurvaa (var.)	*Marsdenia roylei*	Marua Vine	Ayurvedic
Muurvaa	*Chonemorpha macrophylla*	Wood Vine	Ayurvedic
Muurvaa	*Dregea volubilis*	Wattakaka	Ayurvedic
Muurvaa	*Marsdenia tenacissima*	White Turpeth	Ayurvedic
Muusaakaani	*Evolvulus nummularius*	Round-leaf Bindweed	Folk
Muusaakarni	*Evolvulus nummularius*	Round-leaf Bindweed	Ayurvedic
Muusaakarni	*Ipomoea reniformis*	Mouse-ear Shrub	Ayurvedic
Muyaa	*Sagittaria trifolia*	Old World Arrowhead	Folk
Muyana	*Vangueria spinosa*	Voa-Vanga	Folk
Muyna	*Meyna laxiflora*	Muyna	Folk
Naadeya	*Salix caprea*	Sallow, Goat Willow, Common Willow	Ayurvedic
Naadeya	*Salix tetrasperma*	Indian Willow	Ayurvedic

Table Contd.

Indian Name	Botanical Name	English Name	Medicinal System
Naadeyi	*Clerodendrum phlomidis*	Glory Bower	Ayurvedic
Naadi Shaaka	*Corchorus capsularis*	White Jute	Folk
Naadihingu	*Gardenia gummifera*	Gummy Cape Jasmine	Ayurvedic
Naadihingu	*Gardenia resinifera*	Brilliant Gardenia, Cambi Resin Tree	Ayurvedic
Naaga	*Mesua ferrea*	Iron-wood, Mesu	Ayurvedic
Naagaa-aiari	*Lippia geminata*	Melissa Lipia	Folk
Naagaarjuni	*Euphorbia hirta*	Euphorbia, Australian Asthma Weed, Pill-bearing Spurge	Ayurvedic
Naagaarjuni	*Euphorbia thymifolia*	Thyme-leaf Spurge	Ayurvedic
Naagabalaa	*Grewia hirsuta*	Veronicalolia, Naagbala	Ayurvedic
Naagabalaa	*Sida spinosa*	Prickly Mallow	Ayurvedic
Naagabalaa	*Urena lobata*	Pink Chinese Burr, Burr Mallow	Ayurvedic
Naagaballi	*Mussaenda frondosa*	White Lady, White Rag Plant	Folk
Naaga-beli	*Lycopodium clavatum*	Common Club Moss	Folk
Naagadaman	*Pedilanthus tithymaloides*	Slipper Plant, Bird-Cactus	Folk
Naagadamani	*Aristolochia indica*	Indian Birthwort	Ayurvedic
Naagadamani	*Crinum asiaticum*	St. John's Lily, Poison Bulb	Ayurvedic
Naagadamani	*Sansevieria hyacinthoides*	Ceylon Bowstring Hemp	Ayurvedic
Naagadamani	*Sansevieria roxburghiana*	Indian Bowstring Hemp	Ayurvedic
Naagadanti	*Croton oblongifolius*	Purging Croton	Ayurvedic
Naagakeshara	*Mesua ferrea*	Iron-wood, Mesu	Ayurvedic
Naagakesharam	*Dillenia pentagyna*	Deer Apple	Siddha/Tamil
Naagakeshram	*Mesua ferrea*	Iron-wood, Mesu	Siddha/Tamil
Naagakinjalika	*Mesua ferrea*	Iron-wood, Mesu	Ayurvedic
Naagapatra	*Crinum asiaticum*	St. John's Lily, Poison Bulb	Ayurvedic
Naagaphani (var.)	*Opuntia vulgaris*	Prickly Pear	Ayurvedic
Naagaphani	*Opuntia dillenii*	Prickly Pear, Slipper Thorn	Ayurvedic
Naagaphani	*Opuntia dillenii*	Prickly Pear, Slipper Thorn	Unani
Naagaphani	*Pedilanthus tithymaloides*	Slipper Plant, Bird-Cactus	Folk

Table Contd.

Indian Name	Botanical Name	English Name	Medicinal System
Nagappu	*Ochrocarpus longifolius*	Red-dye-flowerbud, Pseudo-Mesua ferra	Folk/Tamil
Nagathali	*Opuntia dillenii*	Prickly Pear, Slipper Thorn	Folk/Tamil
Nagavalli	*Piper betle*	Betel Pepper	Folk
Nagesarpu	*Ochrocarpus longifolius*	Red-dye-flowerbud, Pseudo-Mesua ferra	Folk/Tamil
Nagette	*Gordonia obtusa*	Loblolly Bay, Grey Laurel	Folk/Nilgiri
Nagli	*Dendrobium ovatum*	Pigeon Orchid, Cooktown Orchid	Folk
Nahikaa	*Corallocarpus epigaeus*	Indian Bryonia	Ayurvedic
Naichotte Poonde	*Vernonia cinerea*	Ash Coloured Fleabane, Purple Fleabane	Siddha/Tamil
Naioringi	*Stachytarpheta jamaicensis*	Brazilian Tea, Bastard Vervain, Aaron's Rod	Folk/Tamil
Naishakar	*Saccharum officinarum*	Gannaa, Naishakar	Unani
Nak-chhikani	*Centipeda orbicularis*	Sneezewort	Folk
Nak-chhikkini	*Dregea volubilis*	Wattakaka	Ayurvedic
Nakhud	*Cicer arietinum*	Bengal Gram, Chick Pea	Unani
Nakhud	*Primula vulgaris*	Primrose (Evening Primrose is equated with Oenothera biennis), Cowslip	Unani
Nakkukappan	*Melastoma malabathricum*	Indian Rhododendron	Folk
Naktaahvaa	*Curcuma longa*	Turmeric	Ayurvedic
Naktmaal	*Derris indica*	Indian Beech, Pongamia Oil Tree	Ayurvedic
Nala (var.)	*Lobelia leschenaultiana*	Poisonous Pukeweed	Ayurvedic
Nala (var.)	*Lobelia nicotianaefolia*	Wild Tobacco	Ayurvedic
Nala	*Arundo donax*	Great Reed, Spanish-Bamboo-Reed, Giant-Bamboo-Reed	Ayurvedic
Nala	*Phragmites karka*	Common Reed-grass	Ayurvedic
Nalada	*Vetiveria zizanioides*	Vetiver, Khas	Ayurvedic
Naladaa	*Nardostachys jatamansi*	Spikenard, Musk-root	Ayurvedic
Nalal	*Caesalpinia pulcherrima*	Barbados Pride, Peacock Flower	Siddha/Tamil
Nalava	*Leea indica*	Purple-berry Holly	Folk/Tamil

Table Contd.

Indian Name	Botanical Name	English Name	Medicinal System
Nalina	*Nelumbo nucifera*	East Indian Lotus, Sacred Lotus	Ayurvedic
Nalla Karai	*Canthium parviflorum*	Wild Jasmine	Siddha/Tamil
Nalla-Tulasi	*Ocimum sanctum*	Holy Basil, Sacred Basil	Siddha/Tamil
Nallennai (Seed)	*Sesamum indicum*	Sesame, Gingelly	Siddha/Tamil
Nalugu	*Leea crispa*	Grey-berry Holly	Folk
Nalvellai	*Cleome icosandra*	Wild Mustard	Siddha/Tamil
Namaskaari	*Mimosa pudica*	Sensitive-plant, Humble-Plant	Ayurvedic
Namasu	*Pinus roxburghii*	Long-leaved Pine, Three-leaved Pine, Chir Pine	Ayurvedic
Nanaa	*Mentha spicata*	Spearmint, Garden Mint	Unani
Nanal	*Saccharum officinarum*	Gannaa, Naishakar	Siddha/Tamil
Nanda	*Monochoria vaginalis*	Oval-leaved Pondweed, Pickerel Weed	Folk
Nandi Pushpa	*Tabernaemontana coronaria*	East Indian Rosebay	Ayurvedic
Nandi Vriksha	*Ficus arnottiana*	Indian Rock Fig	Ayurvedic
Nandi Vrksha	*Cedrela toona*	Red Cedar, Toon, Indian Mahogany Tree	Ayurvedic
Nandiaa	*Eleusine indica*	Crowfoot Grass, Crab Grass	Folk
Nandimukha (var.)	*Eleusine indica*	Crowfoot Grass, Crab Grass	Ayurvedic
Nandini	*Lepidium sativum*	Gardencress, Tongue Grass	Ayurvedic
Nandivriksha (var.)	*Ficus altissima*	Council Tree, Lofty Fig Tree	Ayurvedic
Nandivriksha	*Ervataemia coronaria*	East Indian Rosebay	Ayurvedic
Nandivriksha	*Tabernaemontana coronaria*	East Indian Rosebay	Ayurvedic
Nandiyaavattam	*Ervataemia coronaria*	East Indian Rosebay	Siddha/Tamil
Nandiyavattam	*Tabernaemontana coronaria*	East Indian Rosebay	Siddha/Tamil
Nandunarai	*Gymnosporia spinosa*	Celastrus Tree	Siddha/Tamil
Nangilaippiratti	*Tylophora indica*	Emetic Swallow Wort, Indian or Country Ipecacuanha	Siddha/Tamil
Nanjundam	*Gardenia turgida*	Bharangi Bark Tree	Siddha/Tamil
Nanjundan	*Balanites aegyptiaca*	Desert Date	Siddha/Tamil

Table Contd.

Indian Name	Botanical Name	English Name	Medicinal System
Nankhwaah	*Trachyspermum ammi*	Ammi, Lovage, Carum, Ajowan	Unani
Nannaari	*Hemidesmus indicus*	Indian Sarsaparilla	Siddha/Tamil
Narakachura	*Curcuma zedoaria*	Zedoary, Zerumbet	Ayurvedic
Narakkarandai	*Blumea lacera*	Nagai Camphor	Siddha/Tamil
Narakul	*Phragmites karka*	Common Reed-grass	Folk
Narakyaa-ood	*Gironniera reticulata*	Diancaoxieshu (Chinese)	Folk
Nargis	*Narcissus tazetta*	Narcissus, Daffodil, Lent Lily	Unani
Narichaa	*Corchorus capsularis*	White Jute	Folk
Naringi	*Limonia crenulata*	Naringi, Beli	Folk
Narivalai	*Clerodendrum indicum*	Turk's Turban, Tube-Flower	Siddha/Tamil
Narivengai	*Ougeinia dalbergioides*	Chariot Tree, Punjab Kino	Folk/Tamil
Narivengayam	*Urginea indica*	Indian Squill, Sea Onion (red and white varieties)	Siddha/Tamil
Narivila	*Feronia limonia*	Wood Apple	Siddha/Tamil
Narkachoor	*Zingiber zerumbet*	Zerumbet Ginger Curcuma caesia is also equated with Narkachoor	Unani
Narkachura	*Curcuma caesia*	Black Zedorary	Ayurvedic
Narkanta	*Solanum albicaule*	Narkanta Prikly Shrub	Folk
Naruvili	*Cordia myxa*	Sabestan Plum	Siddha/Tamil
Naruvili	*Cordia rothii*	Sebestan	Siddha/Tamil
Narvel	*Viburnum foetidum*	Tooth-leaved Guelder Rose	Folk
Nata	*Valeriana officinalis*	Valerian, Garden Heliotrope, Common Valerian	Ayurvedic
Nata	*Valeriana wallichii*	Indian Valerian	Ayurvedic
Nathaichoori	*Borreria articularis*	Shaggy Button Weed	Siddha/Tamil
Natmi	*Amoora cucullata*	Rohitak	Folk (Bengal)
Nattaichuri	*Spermacoce hispida*	Saggy Buttonweed	Siddha/Tamil
Nattirevaichini	*Rheum emodi*	Indian Rhubarb, Himalayan Rhubarb	Siddha/Tamil
Natuvadom	*Terminalia catappa*	Indian Almond, Tropical Almond	Siddha/Tamil
Nauli	*Ipomoea vitifolia*	Funnei-flowered Twiner	Folk
Nava-mallikaa	*Jasminum arborescens*	Tree Jasmine	Ayurvedic

Table Contd.

Indian Name	Botanical Name	English Name	Medicinal System
Nava-Mallikaa	*Jasminum sambac*	Arabian Jasmine, Tuscan Jasmine, Double Jasmine	Ayurvedic
Navananji	*Dicoma tomentosa*	Bitter Dicoma	Folk
Navelangu	*Dalbergia lanceolaria*	Takoliwood	Folk/Tamil
Nawal	*Ipomoea vitifolia*	Funnei-flowered Twiner	Folk
Nay Kumil	*Trewia nudiflora*	False White Teak, Gutel	Folk/Tamil
Nayantaaraa	*Catharanthus roseus*	Madagascar Periwinkle	Folk
Nayikkadugu	*Cleome icosandra*	Wild Mustard	Siddha/Tamil
Nayi-Tulasi	*Ocimum canum*	Hoary Basil	Folk/Tamil
Nayvila	*Limonia crenulata*	Naringi, Beli	Siddha/Tamil
Nedunar	*Kydia calycina*	Pula Tree	Folk
Neelaalu	*Dioscorea prazeri*	Poisonous Black Yam	Ayurvedic
Neelaniryaasa	*Eucalyptus globulus*	Blue-gum Tree, Australian Gum Tree	Ayurvedic
Neelgiri Oil	*Eucalyptus globulus*	Blue-gum Tree, Australian Gum Tree	Unani
Neeli chettu	*Indigofera tinctoria*	Indigo	Folk/Telugu
Neelkanthi	*Ajuga bracteosa*	Bugle	Ayurvedic
Neelkanthi	*Gentiana kurroo*	Himalayan Gentian, Indian Gentian Root	Ayurvedic
Neelothpalam	*Nymphaea stellata*	Indian Blue Water-lily	Siddha/Tamil
Neem-Chameli	*Millingtonia hortensis*	Indian Cork Tree	Folk
Neendavalli	*Naravelia zeylanica*	Naravelia Climber	Folk/Tamil
Neerabraahmi	*Bacopa monnieri*	Thyme-leaved Gratiola	Ayurvedic
Neerada	*Cyperus rotundus*	Nut Grass	Ayurvedic
Neeradimuthu	*Baliospermum montanum*	False Croton	Siddha/Tamil
Neermalli	*Pseudarthria viscida*	Shalparni	Siddha/Tamil
Neermulli	*Asteracantha longifolia*	Hygrophilla	Siddha/Tamil
Neermulli	*Hygrophila auriculata*	Indian Swampweed	Siddha/Tamil
Negali	*Polygala chinensis*	Senega	Ayurvedic
Negali	*Polygala sibirica*	Common Milkwort	Folk
Nelakadalai	*Arachis hypogaea*	Groundnut, Peanut, Monkeynut	Siddha/Tamil
Nell	*Oryza sativa*	Rice	Siddha/Tamil

Table Contd.

Indian Name	Botanical Name	English Name	Medicinal System
Nelli	*Emblica officinalis*	Embic, Indian Gooseberry	Siddha/Tamil
Nellikkaai	*Emblica officinalis*	Embic, Indian Gooseberry	Siddha/Tamil
Nellu	*Leea crispa*	Grey-berry Holly	Folk
Nemi	*Ougeinia dalbergioides*	Chariot Tree, Punjab Kino	Ayurvedic
Nepaali Dhaniyaa	*Zanthoxylum acanthopodium*	Tumru Tree, Prickly Ash	Folk
Nepaali Dhaniyaa	*Zanthoxylum armatum*	Toothache Tree, Indian Prickly Ash	Folk
Nepaal-Nimba	*Schweinfurthia sphaerocarpa*	Nepal Neem	Ayurvedic
Nerani	*Salacia chinensis*	Chinese Salacia	Folk/South
Neri-arishippal	*Liquidambar orientalis*	Storax, Oriental Sweet Gum	Siddha/Tamil
Neriyurishippal	*Altingia excelsa*	Storax, Oriental Sweet Gum	Siddha/Tamil
Neru	*Vinca pusilla*	Bengal Periwinkle	Folk
Nerugobbi	*Asteracantha longifolia*	Hygrophilla	Siddha/Tamil
Nerunjil	*Tribulus terrestris*	Land-Caltrops, Puncture Vine	Folk/Tamil
Nervaalam	*Baliospermum montanum*	False Croton	Siddha/Tamil
Nervaalam	*Croton tiglium*	Purging Croton	Siddha/Tamil
Nettavil	*Antiaris toxicaria*	Sacking Tree, Upas Tree	Folk/Tamil
Nettilingam	*Polyalthia longifolia*	Mast Tree, Fake Asoka Tree, False Devadaru, Cemetry Tree	Siddha/Tamil
Nevali	*Ixora parviflora*	Torchwood Tree	Ayurvedic
Nevari	*Ixora parviflora*	Torchwood Tree	Ayurvedic
Nibam	*Quassia indica*	Niepa Bark Tree	Folk/Tamil
Nichnai	*Rhododendron campanulatum*	Paper-bark Azalea	Folk
Nichula	*Barringtonia acutangula*	Indian Oak	Ayurvedic
Nidigdhaa	*Solanum xanthocarpum*	Wild Eggplant, Yellow-Berried Nightshade	Ayurvedic
Nidigdhikaa	*Solanum xanthocarpum*	Wild Eggplant, Yellow-Berried Nightshade	Ayurvedic
Niepa	*Quassia indica*	Niepa Bark Tree	Folk/Tamil
Nigerian Mahogany	*Khaya senegalensis*	African Mahogany	Folk
Niguudhapatra	*Capparis aphylla*	Caper Berry	Ayurvedic

Table Contd.

Indian Name	Botanical Name	English Name	Medicinal System
Niketan	*Salix tetrasperma*	Indian Willow	Ayurvedic
Nikhari	*Ipomoea eriocarpa*	Tiny Morning Glory, Wooly-Fruited Morning Glory	Folk
Nikochaka	*Pinus gerardiana*	Neosia Pine, Edible Pine, Chilgoza Pine	Ayurvedic
Nikumbha	*Baliospermum montanum*	False Croton	Ayurvedic
Nilaavaarai	*Cassia angustifolia*	Indian senna, Tinnevelly senna	Siddha/Tamil
Nila-chitraka	*Plumbago capensis*	South African Leadwort	Ayurvedic
Nilaisedachi	*Polycarpaea corymbosa*	Old Man's Cap	Siddha/Tamil
Nilakantha-shikhaa	*Adiantum incisum*	Peacock's Tail	Ayurvedic
Nilakanthi	*Chrozophora plicata*	Chrozophora	Folk
Nila-manjari	*Justicia gendarussa*	Blue-flowered Vasaka, Chinese Justicia	Ayurvedic
Nilambari	*Ecbolium linneanum*	Blue Fox Tail Nail Dye	Siddha/Tamil
Nilanaaringa	*Naregamia alata*	Goanese Ipecacuanha	Folk
Nila-nirgundi	*Justicia gendarussa*	Blue-flowered Vasaka, Chinese Justicia	Ayurvedic
Nilanirgundi	*Vitex negundo*	Five-leaved Chaste Tree	Ayurvedic
Nila-paalai	*Wrightia tinctoria*	Pala Indigo Plant	Siddha/Tamil
Nilapoosani	*Ipomoea petaloidea*	False Jalap, Hawaii Morning Glory	Siddha/Tamil
Nilappanan Kizhangu	*Curculigo orchioides*	Black Musali	Siddha/Tamil
Nilappoosani, Palmudukkan kizhangu	*Pueraria tuberosa*	Indian Kudze	Siddha/Tamil
Nilapushpa	*Indigofera tinctoria*	Indigo	Ayurvedic
Nilapushpaka	*Vitex negundo*	Five-leaved Chaste Tree	Ayurvedic
Nilapushpi	*Linum usitatissimum*	Linseed, Flax	Ayurvedic
Nilasaara	*Diospyros embryopteris*	Gaub Persimmon, Riber Ebony	Ayurvedic
Nilasampangi	*Polianthes tuberosa*	Tuberose	Siddha/Tamil
Nila-sindhukaa	*Vitex negundo*	Five-leaved Chaste Tree	Ayurvedic
Nilavalli	*Viscum articulatum*	Napalese Mistletoe	Ayurvedic
Nilavembu	*Andrographis paniculata*	Creat	Siddha/Tamil

Table Contd.

Indian Name	Botanical Name	English Name	Medicinal System
Nilavembu	*Swertia chirayita*	Chiretta	Siddha/Tamil
Nilgiri Pepper	*Piper schmidtii*	Nilgiri Pepper	Folk
Nili	*Barleria strigosa*	Blue-flowered Barleria	Siddha/Tamil
Nili	*Indigofera arrecta*	Natal Indigo, Java Indigo, Bengal Indigo	Ayurvedic
Nili	*Indigofera articulata*	Egyptian Indigo, Arabian Indigo, Wild Indigo, Surat Indigo	Ayurvedic
Nili	*Indigofera aspalathoides*	Wiry Indigo	Ayurvedic
Nili	*Indigofera oblongifolia*	Wild Indigo, Mysore Panicled Indigo	Folk
Nili	*Indigofera pulchella*	Cassia Indigo	Ayurvedic
Nili	*Indigofera tinctoria*	Indigo	Siddha/Tamil
Nili-gulmohar	*Jacaranda acutifolia*	Brazil Rosewood, Green Ebony	Folk
Nilikaa	*Indigofera tinctoria*	Indigo	Ayurvedic
Nilini	*Indigofera tinctoria*	Indigo	Ayurvedic
Nilkanth	*Curcuma caesia*	Black Zedorary	Ayurvedic
Nilofar	*Nelumbo nucifera*	East Indian Lotus, Sacred Lotus	Unani
Nilofar	*Nymphaea alba*	European White Water-lily	Unani
Nilofar	*Nymphaea stellata*	Indian Blue Water-lily	Unani
Nilotpala	*Nymphaea stellata*	Indian Blue Water-lily	Ayurvedic
Nimatotaa	*Picrasma quassioides*	Quassia	Folk
Nimba	*Azadirachta indica*	Neem Tree, Margosa Tree	Ayurvedic
Nimbaka	*Azadirachta indica*	Neem Tree, Margosa Tree	Ayurvedic
Nimbataru	*Erythrina indica*	Indian Coral Tree	Ayurvedic
Nimbi	*Picrasma quassioides*	Quassia	Ayurvedic
Nimbuka	*Citrus aurantifolia*	Acid or Sour Lime, Country Lime	Ayurvedic
Nimbuka	*Citrus limon*	Lemon	Ayurvedic
Nimiri	*Terminalia paniculata*	Flowering Murdah	Folk
Nipa	*Anthocephalus cadamba*	Wild Cinchona	Ayurvedic
Nira	*Pavonia odorata*	Fragrant Sticky Mallow	Ayurvedic
Niradi-muththu	*Hydnocarpus kurzii*	Chalmogra	Siddha/Tamil

Table Contd.

Indian Name	Botanical Name	English Name	Medicinal System
Niradi-muttu	*Hydnocarpus laurifolia*	Soorty Oil Tree	Siddha/Tamil
Nirgundi (white var.)	*Vitex trifolia*	Three-leaved Vitex	Ayurvedic
Nirinji	*Indigofera pulchella*	Cassia Indigo	Siddha/Tamil
Nirkancha	*Monochoria vaginalis*	Oval-leaved Pondweed, Pickerel Weed	Ayurvedic
Nirkkrambu	*Jussiaea suffruticosa*	Swamp Primrose	Siddha/Tamil
Nirkundi	*Vitex negundo*	Five-leaved Chaste Tree	Folk/Tamil
Nirmali	*Strychnos potatorum*	Clearing Nut Tree	Ayurvedic
Nirmudi	*Blumea eriantha*	Nagai Camphor	Folk
Nirpa	*Bauhinia retusa*	Semla Gum Tree	Siddha/Tamil
Nirumari	*Tamarix dioica*	Tamarisk	Siddha/Tamil
Nirvisha	*Delphinium vestitum*	Candle Larkspur, Bee Larkspur	Ayurvedic
Nirvishaa (var.)	*Kyllinga triceps*	Spikesedge, The Sedge of Jamaica	Ayurvedic
Nirvishi	*Delphinium denudatum*	Larkspur	Ayurvedic
Nishaa	*Curcuma caesia*	Black Zedorary	Ayurvedic
Nishaachara	*Angelica glauca*	Angelica	Ayurvedic
Nishi	*Curcuma caesia*	Black Zedorary	Ayurvedic
Nishoth (black var.)	*Ipomoea petaloidea*	False Jalap, Hawaii Morning Glory	Folk
Nishoth	*Operculina turpethum*	Indian Jalap, Turpeth	Unani
Nishotra	*Operculina turpethum*	Indian Jalap, Turpeth	Ayurvedic
Nishotraa	*Eucalyptus globulus*	Blue-gum Tree, Australian Gum Tree	Ayurvedic
Nishpaava	*Dolichos lablab*	Indian Butter Bean, Lablab Bean, Horsebean	Ayurvedic
Nising	*Chlorophytum arundinaceum*	White Musali	Folk
Nithiya Kalyani	*Vinca rosea*	Madagascar Periwinkle	Siddha/Tamil
Nityakalyaani	*Catharanthus roseus*	Madagascar Periwinkle	Folk
Nityakalyaani	*Vinca rosea*	Madagascar Periwinkle	Ayurvedic
Nivadung Paanchkoni	*Cereus grandiflorus*	Cereus, Night Blooming Cereus, Sweet Scented Cactus	Folk

Table Contd.

Indian Name	Botanical Name	English Name	Medicinal System
Nivara	*Oryza sativa*	Rice	Ayurvedic
Nochchi	*Vitex negundo*	Five-leaved Chaste Tree	Siddha/Tamil
Nokkotta	*Eriobotrya japonica*	Loquat, Japanese Medlar	Siddha/Tamil
Nripapaadapa	*Cassia fistula*	Indian Laburnum, Purging Cassia, Golden Shower	Ayurvedic
Nrityakaundaka	*Dactyloctenium aegyptium*	Spider Grass	Ayurvedic
Nukha	*Monochoria vaginalis*	Oval-leaved Pondweed, Pickerel Weed	Folk
Nunaa	*Morinda citrifolia*	Indian Mulberry	Siddha/Tamil
Nunigatcha	*Caesalpinia digyra*	Teri Pods	Siddha/Tamil
Nuql-e-khwazaa (Seeds)	*Buchanania lanzan*	Almondette Tree, Cheronjee, Buchanan's Mango	Unani
Nurakvel	*Kedrostis foetidissima*	Lobed-leaf Foetid Plant	Folk
Nyagrodha	*Ficus beng(h)alensis*	Banyan Tree	Ayurvedic
Nyekki	*Leea indica*	Purple-berry Holly	Folk/Tamil
Oathupul	*Echinochloa crus-galli*	Barnyard Millet	Siddha/Tamil
Odal	*Sarcostigma kleinii*	Ingudi	Folk/Tamil
Odangod	*Reissantia indica*	Atari Vine	Siddha/Tamil
Odiyan	*Lannea coromandelica*	Jhingan	Folk/Tamil
Odrapushpa	*Hibiscus rosa-sinensis*	Rose-of-China, Shoe-flower, Chinese Hibiscus	Ayurvedic
Okkadi-kodi	*Wagatea spicata*	Western Ghat-Wakeri	Folk/Tamil
Ola	*Gordonia obtusa*	Loblolly Bay, Grey Laurel	Folk/South
Ololiuqui	*Rivea corymbosa*	Ololiuqui, Snake Plant	Folk
Omam	*Apium leptophyllum*	Celery	Siddha/Tamil
Omam	*Trachyspermum ammi*	Ammi, Lovage, Carum, Ajowan	Siddha/Tamil
Ood Gharqi	*Aquilaria agallocha*	Aloewood, Eaglewood, Agarwood	Unani
Ood Gharqi	*Paeonia emodi*	Himalayan Paeony	Unani
Ood Gharqi	*Paeonia officinalis*	European Paeony	Unani
Ood Saleeb	*Paeonia emodi*	Himalayan Paeony	Unani
Ood Saleeb	*Paeonia officinalis*	European Paeony	Unani

Table Contd.

Indian Name	Botanical Name	English Name	Medicinal System
Ood-e-Balsaan (Wood)	*Balsamodendron opobalsamum*	Balsam Tree, Balsam of Mecca, Balsam of Gilead	Unani
Ood-ul Hindi	*Aquilaria agallocha*	Aloewood, Eaglewood, Agarwood	Unani
Oomaththai	*Datura metel*	Thornapple, Downy Datura	Siddha/Tamil
Orchaa	*Sonneratia caseolaris*	Berembang, Mangrove Apple	Folk
Origanon	*Zataria multiflora*	Wild Thyme	Unani
Orilaithamarai	*Ionidium suffruticosum*	Charati	Siddha/Tamil
Ottamulli	*Barleria cristata*	Crested Philippine Violet	Siddha/Tamil
Ottanali	*Leea indica*	Purple-berry Holly	Folk/Tamil
Ottatti	*Urena lobata*	Pink Chinese Burr, Burr Mallow	Folk/Tamil
Ottipilu	*Artocarpus lakoocha*	Monkey Jack	Folk/Tamil
Ottupullu	*Triumfetta rhomboidea*	Burbush, Burweed	Siddha/Tamil
Oyster-root	*Tragopogon porrifolius*	Salify, Vegetable-Oyster, Purple Goat's Beard, Oyster Plant	Folk
Paachi	*Pogostemon cablin*	Patchouli	Ayurvedic
Paachi	*Pogostemon patchouli*	Patchouli	Ayurvedic
Paadak kizhangu	*Cissampelos pareira*	Velvet-Leaf Pareira, Pareira Brava	Siddha/Tamil
Paadhal	*Stereospermum personatum*	Trumpet Flower, Yellow Snake Tree	Ayurvedic
Paadiri	*Radermachera xylocarpa*	Padri Tree	Folk
Paadiri	*Stereospermum personatum*	Trumpet Flower, Yellow Snake Tree	Siddha/Tamil
Paahraa	*Stephania glabra*	Indian Tape Vine	Folk
Paakal	*Momordica charantia*	Bitter Gourd, Balsam Pear, Carilla	Siddha/Tamil
Paakar	*Ficus cordifolia*	Rumpf's Fig	Folk
Paakur-muula	*Polygonum hydropiper*	Water Pepper, Pepperwort, Smartweed	Folk
Paalak	*Spinacia oleracea*	Garden Spinach	Unani
Paalaka	*Saussurea lappa*	Kuth, Costus	Ayurvedic
Paalaka-Juuhi	*Rhinacanthus nasuta*	Snake Jasmine	Ayurvedic

Table Contd.

Indian Name	Botanical Name	English Name	Medicinal System
Paalakyaa	*Spinacia oleracea*	Garden Spinach	Ayurvedic
Paalani	*Gentiana kurroo*	Himalayan Gentian, Indian Gentian Root	Ayurvedic
Paalankikaa	*Spinacia oleracea*	Garden Spinach	Ayurvedic
Paalankya	*Spinacia oleracea*	Garden Spinach	Ayurvedic
Paalasha	*Butea monosperma*	Flame of the Forest, Butea Gum, Bengal Kino	Ayurvedic
Paal-Kodi	*Cryptolepis buchanani*	Indian Sarsaparilla	Folk/Tamil
Paalmudukkan kizhangu	*Ipomoea digitata*	Milky Yam	Siddha/Tamil
Paalorey	*Melastoma malabathricum*	Indian Rhododendron	Folk
Paan	*Piper betle*	Betel Pepper	Unani
Paanal	*Glycosmis pentaphylla*	Orangeberry, Ginberry	Folk
Paanari	*Pogostemon cablin*	Patchouli	Folk
Paanch	*Pogostemon patchouli*	Patchouli	Folk
Paani-lajak	*Neptunia oleracea*	Sensitive Plant	Folk
Paani-maricha	*Polygonum hydropiper*	Water Pepper, Pepperwort, Smartweed	Folk
Paani-Sambhaalu	*Vitex trifolia*	Three-leaved Vitex	Folk
Paaniya Valli	*Delima scandens*	Delima	Ayurvedic
Paaniyaamalaka	*Flacourtia jangomas*	Puneala Plum	Ayurvedic
Paaniyaphala	*Euryale ferox*	Gorgan Nut, Fox Nut	Ayurvedic
Paaniyaphala	*Trapa bispinosa*	Water Chestnut	Ayurvedic
Paaniyavalli	*Calycopteris floribunda*	White Daisy	Ayurvedic
Paan-lataa	*Derris uliginosa*	Tuba Root	Folk
Paapadi	*Pavetta indica*	White-Pavetta	Folk
Paaparaa	*Gardenia latifolia*	Boxwood Gardenia	Folk
Paapari	*Buxus wallichiana*	Himalayan Boxwood Tree	Folk
Paapraa (var.)	*Podophyllum sikkimensis*	Sikkim Podophyllum	Folk
Paapraa	*Podophyllum hexandrum*	Indian Podophyllum	Folk
Paapri	*Podophyllum hexandrum*	Indian Podophyllum	Folk
Paaraavata	*Garcinia cowa*	Indo-Malayan Brindleberry	Ayurvedic

Table Contd.

Indian Name	Botanical Name	English Name	Medicinal System
Paaraavatapaadi	*Leea aequata*	Black-berry Holly	Ayurvedic
Paaraavatapadi	*Vitex leucoxylon*	Deccan Vitex	Ayurvedic
Paaraavatpadi	*Celastrus paniculatus*	Staff Tree, Intellect Tree	Ayurvedic
Paaranki	*Garuga pinnata*	Grey Downy Balsam	Ayurvedic
Paaranti	*Ixora coccinea*	Jungleflame Ixora	Ayurvedic
Paarasa Pipala	*Ficus arnottiana*	Indian Rock Fig	Ayurvedic
Paaribhadra	*Azadirachta indica*	Neem Tree, Margosa Tree	Ayurvedic
Paaribhadra	*Erythrina indica*	Indian Coral Tree	Ayurvedic
Paaribhadraka	*Erythrina indica*	Indian Coral Tree	Ayurvedic
Paarijaata	*Nyctanthes arbor-tristis*	Tree of Sorrow, Night Jasmine, Coral Jasmine	Ayurvedic
Paarijaataka	*Erythrina indica*	Indian Coral Tree	Ayurvedic
Paarisha	*Thespesia populnea*	Portia Tree, Tulip Tree, Umbrella Tree, False Rosewood	Ayurvedic
Paarseeka Vachaa	*Iris ensata*	Japanese Iris	Ayurvedic
Paarseeka Vachaa	*Iris germanica*	Orris, Iridis Rhizome, German Iris	Ayurvedic
Paarseeka Vachaa	*Iris nepalensis*	Nepal Iris	Ayurvedic
Paarseeka yavaani	*Hyoscyamus niger*	Indian Henbane, Black Henbane	Siddha/Tamil
Paarshvpippala	*Thespesia populnea*	Portia Tree, Tulip Tree, Umbrella Tree, False Rosewood	Ayurvedic
Paarsika-yavaani	*Hyoscyamus muticus*	Egyptian Henbane	Ayurvedic
Paarsika-yavaani	*Hyoscyamus niger*	Indian Henbane, Black Henbane	Ayurvedic
Paartha	*Terminalia arjuna*	Arjun Terminalia	Ayurvedic
Paashaanabheda	*Aerva javanica*	Javanese Wool Plant	Folk
Paashaanabheda	*Aerva lanata*	Mountain Knot Grass	Ayurvedic
Paashaanabheda	*Bergenia ligulata*	Elephant-Ear, Siberian Saxifrage	Ayurvedic
Paashaana-bheda	*Homonoia riparia*	Willow-leaved Water Croton	Ayurvedic
Paashaanabheda	*Iris pseudacorus*	Yellow Flag	Folk
Paashaanabhedi	*Ammi visnaga*	Khella	Folk
Paashaanbheda	*Rotula aquatica*	Aquatic Rotula	Folk

Table Contd.

Indian Name	Botanical Name	English Name	Medicinal System
Paashikaa	*Myristica malabarica*	Malabar Nutmeg, False Nutmeg, Bombay Nutmeg, Bombay Mace	Ayurvedic
Paataala-garuda	*Cocculus hirsutus*	Broom-Creeper, Ink-Berry	Ayurvedic
Paataalagarudaa	*Corallocarpus epigaeus*	Indian Bryonia	Ayurvedic
Paataalavaasini	*Piper betle*	Betel Pepper	Folk
Paataal-Tumbi	*Ceropegia bulbosa*	Candlestick Ceropegia	Folk
Paatalaa	*Cydonia oblonga*	Quince Fruit	Ayurvedic
Paatalaa	*Stereospermum personatum*	Trumpet Flower, Yellow Snake Tree	Ayurvedic
Paatali	*Stereospermum personatum*	Trumpet Flower, Yellow Snake Tree	Ayurvedic
Paatang	*Heterophragma roxburghii*	Karen Wood	Folk
Paatha	*Chondrodendron tomentosum*	False Pareira Brava	Ayurvedic
Paathaa (Kerala)	*Cyclea arnotii*	Green Jelly Shrub	Folk
Paathaa	*Cissampelos pareira*	Velvet-Leaf Pareira, Pareira Brava	Ayurvedic
Paathaa	*Cissampelos pareira*	Velvet-Leaf Pareira, Pareira Brava	Unani
Paathaa	*Stephania glabra*	Indian Tape Vine	Ayurvedic
Paathri	*Launaea pinnatifida*	Bhonpatri	Folk
Paavali	*Tephrosia purpurea*	Purple Tephrosia, Wild Indigo	Folk/Tamil
Pachabotuka	*Kydia calycina*	Pula Tree	Folk
Pachampachaa	*Berberis aristata*	Indian Barberry	Ayurvedic
Pachiyalari	*Thevetia peruviana*	Yellow Oleander	Siddha/Tamil
Pachumullai	*Premna latifolia*	Dusky Fire Brand Bark	Siddha/Tamil
Padanbethi	*Bergenia ligulata*	Elephant-Ear, Siberian Saxifrage	Siddha/Tamil
Padangam	*Caesalpinia pulcherrima*	Barbados Pride, Peacock Flower	Ayurvedic
Padar-malligai	*Jasminum officinale*	Spanish Jasmine	Siddha/Tamil
Padauk	*Pterocarpus dalbergioides*	Andaman Paduak, Andaman Redwood	Folk/Trade

Table Contd.

Indian Name	Botanical Name	English Name	Medicinal System
Padimukam	*Prunus cerasoides*	Wild Himalayan Cherry, Bird Cherry	Siddha/Tamil
Padma	*Clerodendrum serratum*	Blue-flowered Glory Tree, Beetle Killer	Ayurvedic
Padma	*Nelumbo nucifera*	East Indian Lotus, Sacred Lotus	Ayurvedic
Padmaadyaa	*Prunus cerasoides*	Wild Himalayan Cherry, Bird Cherry	Ayurvedic
Padmaakha	*Prunus cerasoides*	Wild Himalayan Cherry, Bird Cherry	Ayurvedic
Padmaata	*Cassia tora*	Sickle Senna, Ringworm Plant	Ayurvedic
Padma-bijaabha	*Euryale ferox*	Gorgan Nut, Fox Nut	Ayurvedic
Padmachaarini	*Nervilia aragoana*	Tall Shield Orchid	Ayurvedic
Padmagandhi	*Prunus cerasoides*	Wild Himalayan Cherry, Bird Cherry	Ayurvedic
Padma-Guduuchi	*Tinospora malabarica*	Tinospora	Ayurvedic
Padmaka	*Prunus cerasoides*	Wild Himalayan Cherry, Bird Cherry	Ayurvedic
Padmapatra	*Inula racemosa*	Elecampane	Ayurvedic
Paduthalai	*Lippia nodiflora*	Wild Sage	Siddha/Tamil
Paeyaavarai	*Cassia occidentalis*	Coffee Senna, Foetid Cassia, Negro Coffee	Siddha/Tamil
Pagoda Tree	*Sophora japonica*	Japanese Pagoda Tree, Chinese Scholar Tree, Umbrella Tree	Folk
Pagumbar	*Elaeocarpus tuberculatus*	Western Ghat Olive-Nut Tree	Siddha/Tamil
Pahaari Gaajar	*Eryngium caeruleum*	Turnip-shaped Himalayan Carrot	Folk
Pahaari Kiretta	*Swertia angustifolia*	Hill Chiretta	Folk
Pahaari Peepal	*Piper sylvaticum*	Mountain Long Pepper	Folk
Pahargungri	*Sophora mollis*	Himalayan Laburnum, Low Mountain Laurel	Folk/Kumaun
Pai Karumbu	*Saccharum spontaneum*	Thatch Grass, Wild Sugarcane	Siddha/Tamil
Pala	*Ehretia buxifolia*	Carmonia Shrub	Folk
Pala	*Wrightia tomentosa*	Red-flowered Wrightia	Siddha/Tamil
Palaandu	*Allium cepa*	Onion	Ayurvedic

Table Contd.

Indian Name	Botanical Name	English Name	Medicinal System
Palaashi	*Curcuma zedoaria*	Zedoary, Zerumbet	Ayurvedic
Palai	*Manilkara kauki*	Kauki	Siddha/Tamil
Palampasi	*Sida veronicaefolia*	Prostrate Mallow	Siddha/Tamil
Palamunpala	*Alstonia venenata*	Devil's Tree, Dita Bark Tree	Folk/Malayalam
Palankash	*Balsamodendron mukul*	Indian Bdellium, Gum Guggul	Ayurvedic
Palasam	*Butea monosperma*	Flame of the Forest, Butea Gum, Bengal Kino	Siddha/Tamil
Palay-keerai	*Holostemma annularis*	Holostemma Creeper	Folk/Tamil
Palisa	*Grewia asiatica*	Indian Phalsa	Siddha/Tamil
Palit	*Erigeron canadensis*	Canadian Fleabane	Ayurvedic
Pallipundu	*Striga asiatica*	Witchweed	Siddha/Tamil
Paluppakai	*Momordica dioica*	Small Bitter Gourd, burr Cucumber	Siddha/Tamil
Pambahdaanaa	*Gossypium herbaceum*	Asiatic Cotton, Levant Cotton, Uppam Cotton	Unani
Pambalimasu	*Citrus maxima*	Pummelo, Shaddock	Siddha/Tamil
Panai	*Borassus flabellifer*	Palmyra Palm, Brab Tree	Siddha/Tamil
Panaimaram	*Borassus flabellifer*	Palmyra Palm, Brab Tree	Siddha/Tamil
Panapuuduu	*Viscum articulatum*	Napalese Mistletoe	Folk
Panasa	*Artocarpus integrifolia*	Jackfruit, Jack Tree	Ayurvedic
Panasagandhi	*Artabotrys hexapetalus*	Yling-Yling Vine	Ayurvedic
Panchaangula	*Ricinus communis*	Castor Seed	Ayurvedic
Panchaanguli	*Dactyloctenium aegyptium*	Spider Grass	Ayurvedic
Panch-mukhi	*Elaeocarpus ganitrus*	Utrasum Bead Tree	Ayurvedic
Pancholi	*Pogostemon patchouli*	Patchouli	Ayurvedic
Panchparni	*Adansonia digitata*	Baobab, Monkey Bread Tree, African Calabash	Ayurvedic
Panchuli	*Limnanthemum cristatum*	Aquatic Pseudo-Chiretta Plant	Folk
Pandadi	*Perilepta auriculata*	Pandai	Folk
Pandharphali	*Securinega suffruticosa*	Securinega	Folk
Pandiki	*Kydia calycina*	Pula Tree	Folk
Pandikutti	*Ceriops candolleana*	Compound Cymed Mangrove	Siddha/Tamil
Pandre	*Turraea villosa*	Wild Honeysuckle	Folk

Table Contd.

Indian Name	Botanical Name	English Name	Medicinal System
Paneer	*Withania coagulans*	Vegetable Rennet, Indian Cheese-maker	Unani
Paneer-band	*Withania coagulans*	Vegetable Rennet, Indian Cheese-maker	Unani
Paneraa	*Sorghum vulgare*	Sorghum, Broomcorn	Folk
Panibira	*Luffa echinata*	Bristly Luffa	Siddha/Tamil
Paniru	*Lepidagathis cristata*	Spotted White-flowered Pluchea	Folk
Panivaragu	*Panicum miliaceum*	Common Millet, Proso Millet, Hog Millet	Folk/Tamil
Paniyaalaa	*Flacourtia jangomas*	Puneala Plum	Folk
Panjuli	*Kirganelia reticulata*	Black-berried Featherfoil	Folk
Pankaja	*Nelumbo nucifera*	East Indian Lotus, Sacred Lotus	Ayurvedic
Pannaikeerai	*Celosia argentea*	Wild Cook's Comb	Siddha/Tamil
Pannu-kilangu	*Dioscorea bulbifera*	Patoto Yam, Bulb-bearing Yam, Air Potato, Dog Yam	Siddha/Tamil
Panturasi	*Oenanthe javanica*	Water Dropwort	Folk
Panuitteku	*Kleinhovia hospita*	Crowned Bol Tree	Folk
Panwaar	*Cleome brachycarpa*	Bastard Mustard	Unani
Panwaar	*Cleome icosandra*	Wild Mustard	Unani
Papata	*Pavetta indica*	White-Pavetta	Ayurvedic
Papitaa	*Carica papaya*	Papaya, Papaw	Ayurvedic
Papitaa Desi	*Carica papaya*	Papaya, Papaw	Unani
Papitaa Vilaayati	*Strychnos ignatii*	Ignatus Beans	Unani
Pappaali	*Carica papaya*	Papaya, Papaw	Siddha/Tamil
Pappara-mulli	*Solanum ferox*	Poison-Berry	Siddha/Tamil
Papparapuli	*Adansonia digitata*	Baobab, Monkey Bread Tree, African Calabash	Siddha/Tamil
Pappayi	*Carica papaya*	Papaya, Papaw	Siddha/Tamil
Pappili	*Ventilago denticulata*	Ventilago Black Vine	Folk
Pappili-chaka	*Ventilago madraspatana*	Ventilago Vermilion Vine	Siddha/Tamil
Paral	*Osyris wightiana*	African Sandalwood, Zanzibar Lawa Wood	Folk
Parangi chchakkai	*Smilax china*	China Root	Siddha/Tamil
Parangikayi	*Cucurbita maxima*	Red Gourd, Red Pumpkin	Siddha/Tamil

Table Contd.

Indian Name	Botanical Name	English Name	Medicinal System
Parangisaam-birani	*Boswellia serrata*	Indian Frankincense, Indian Olibanum	Siddha/Tamil
Parapalanamu	*Glossocardia bosvallia*	Pathari, Seri	Siddha/Tamil
Paratathali	*Actinodaphne hookeri*	Pisa	Siddha/Tamil
Parjani	*Berberis aristata*	Indian Barberry	Ayurvedic
Parjanyaa	*Berberis aristata*	Indian Barberry	Ayurvedic
Parkati	*Ficus lacor*	White Fig	Ayurvedic
Parnabija (var.)	*Kalanchoe integra*	Never Die	Ayurvedic
Parnabija (var.)	*Kalanchoe laciniata*	Plakkie (South India)	Ayurvedic
Parnabija	*Bryophyllum pinnatum*	Air Plant, Mexican Love Plant	Ayurvedic
Parnabija	*Kalanchoe pinnata*	Christmastree Plant	Ayurvedic
Parnaka	*Marsilea minuta*	Dwarf Waterclover, Pepperwort	Ayurvedic
Parna-yavaani	*Coleus amboinicus*	Indian Borage	Ayurvedic
Parpaatakam	*Mollugo cerviana*	Carpetweed	Siddha/Tamil
Parpata	*Fumaria officinalis*	Fumitory	Ayurvedic
Parpata	*Fumaria parviflora*	Fumitory	Ayurvedic
Parpata	*Fumaria vaillantii*	Yellow Fumitory	Ayurvedic
Parpata	*Glossocardia bosvallia*	Pathari, Seri	Ayurvedic
Parpata	*Mollugo cerviana*	Carpetweed	Ayurvedic
Parpata	*Mollugo spergula*	Falsely-whorled Carpetweed	Ayurvedic
Parpata	*Polycarpaea corymbosa*	Old Man's Cap	Ayurvedic
Parpata	*Rungia pectinata*	Matheran Wild Flower	Ayurvedic
Parpata	*Rungia repens*	Creeping Rungia	Ayurvedic
Parpataka	*Fumaria parviflora*	Fumitory	Ayurvedic
Parpataki	*Gardenia latifolia*	Boxwood Gardenia	Ayurvedic
Parpoti (var.)	*Physalis peruviana*	Cape Gooseberry	Ayurvedic
Parpoti	*Zanonia indica*	Zanonia	Folk
Parpotikaa	*Physalis minima*	Sun-berry	Ayurvedic
Parsiaavashaan	*Adiantum capillus-veneris*	American Maidenhair Fern, Venus Hair, Rock Fern	Unani
Parsnip	*Pastinaca sativa*	Parsnip	Folk
Paruppukeerai	*Chenopodium album*	Fat Hen, Lamb's Quarters, White Goosefoot, Wild Spinach, Pigweed	Siddha/Tamil

Table Contd.

Indian Name	Botanical Name	English Name	Medicinal System
Paruppukirai	*Portulaca oleracea*	Common Purslane	Siddha/Tamil
Parusha	*Grewia asiatica*	Indian Phalsa	Ayurvedic
Parushaka	*Grewia asiatica*	Indian Phalsa	Ayurvedic
Parushaka	*Grewia sclerophylla*	Bhokota	Ayurvedic
Parushaka	*Phoenix pusilla*	Wild Coromandel Palm	Ayurvedic
Paruttikkootam	*Gossypium herbaceum*	Asiatic Cotton, Levant Cotton, Uppam Cotton	Siddha/Tamil
Parwal	*Trichosanthes dioica*	Patol, Pointed Gourd	Unani
Pasali	*Talinum triangulare*	Ceylon Spinach, Surinam Purslane, Flame Flower, Sweet Heart, Water Leaf, Ceylon Spinach	Folk/Tamil
Pashm vazg	*Ceratophyllum demersum*	Coontail, Hornwort	Unani
Pashugandhaa	*Gynandropsis gynandra*	African Spider Plant	Ayurvedic
Pashumehan-kaarika	*Lepidium sativum*	Gardencress, Tongue Grass	Ayurvedic
Pashumo-hanikaa	*Viscum monoicum*	Himalayan Mistletoe	Ayurvedic
Pashupaashi	*Myristica malabarica*	Malabar Nutmeg, False Nutmeg, Bombay Nutmeg, Bombay Mace	Ayurvedic
Passaam	*Gymnema sylvestre*	Australian Cow Plant, Gymnema	Siddha/Tamil
Patadi	*Spathodea campanulata*	Syringe Tree, Fountain Tree, African Tulip Tree	Siddha/Tamil
Patalai Kaiantakerai	*Wedelia calendulaceae*	Yellow-flowered Weldia	Siddha/Tamil
Patanga	*Caesalpinia sappan*	Sappan	Ayurvedic
Pataranjaka	*Caesalpinia sappan*	Sappan	Ayurvedic
Patavaa	*Hibiscus sabdariffa*	Roselle, Jamaican Sorrel, Natal Sorrel, Red Sorrel	Folk
Pater	*Typha australis*	Lesser Indian Reed-Mace	Folk
Patharchattaa	*Elytraria crenata*	Dasmori	Folk
Pathiri	*Myristica malabarica*	Malabar Nutmeg, False Nutmeg, Bombay Nutmeg, Bombay Mace	Siddha/Tamil

Table Contd.

Indian Name	Botanical Name	English Name	Medicinal System
Pekadukkai	*Terminalia paniculata*	Flowering Murdah	Folk/Tamil
Penarisangai	*Paederia foetida*	Skunk Vine	Siddha/Tamil
Penar-valli	*Zanonia indica*	Zanonia	Folk/Tamil
Pencolum	*Sapium indicum*	Tallow Tree	Siddha/Tamil
Pendhar	*Randia uliginosa*	Himalayan Randia	Folk
Pendraa	*Randia uliginosa*	Himalayan Randia	Folk
Pentagul	*Dalbergia sympathetica*	Pentagul Tree	Folk
Penwaad Taarutaa	*Cassia tora*	Sickle Senna, Ringworm Plant	Unani
Peraamutti	*Pavonia odorata*	Fragrant Sticky Mallow	Siddha/Tamil
Peraamutti	*Pavonia zeylanica*	Fragrant Swamp Mallow	Folk/Telugu
Perandai	*Cissus quadrangula*	Square Stalked Vine, Adamant Creeper	Siddha/Tamil
Peranjoli	*Hymenodictyon excelsum*	Bridal Couch Tree	Siddha/Tamil
Perarattai	*Alpinia galanga*	Greater Galangal	Siddha/Tamil
Pereecham/ pazham (Fruit)	*Phoenix dactylifera*	Date Palm	Siddha/Tamil
Perelam	*Amomum aromaticum*	Bengal Cardamom, Cardamom	Folk/Tamil
Perettaikkirai	*Ipomoea reniformis*	Mouse-ear Shrub	Siddha/Tamil
Peria elam	*Amomum subulatum*	Greater or Nepal Cardamom	Folk/Tamil
Peria-Tulasi	*Ocimum gratissimum*	Shrubby Basil	Folk/Tamil
Periya Elumuchhai	*Citrus limon*	Lemon	Siddha/Tamil
Periyaitcham	*Phoenix sylvestris*	Wild Date Palm	Folk/Tamil
Periyattalargai	*Mucuna monosperma*	Negro Bean	Siddha/Tamil
Perru	*Ailanthus excelsa*	Tree of Heaven, Maharukh	Siddha/Tamil
Peru Navel	*Syzygium jambos*	Rose Apple	Siddha/Tamil
Perugilai	*Clerodendrum infortunatum*	Glory Bower	Siddha/Tamil
Peruka	*Psidium guajava*	Guava	Ayurvedic
Perumal Arali	*Plumeria alba*	White Champaka	Siddha/Tamil
Perumaram	*Ailanthus excelsa*	Tree of Heaven, Maharukh	Siddha/Tamil
Perumaram	*Ailanthus malabarica*	Ailanto	Siddha/Tamil
Perumbukalli	*Euphorbia neriifolia*	Holy Milk Hedge, Dog's Tongue	Siddha/Tamil

Table Contd.

Indian Name	Botanical Name	English Name	Medicinal System
Perumkaayam	*Ferula foetida*	Asafoetida	Siddha/Tamil
Perumpoolai	*Aerva javanica*	Javanese Wool Plant	Siddha/Tamil
Perumvalli kizhangu	*Dioscorea alata*	Wild Yam, Greater Yam, Asiatic Yam	Siddha/Tamil
Perunanal	*Phragmites karka*	Common Reed-grass	Siddha/Tamil
Perunaruvili	*Cordia wallichii*	Sebestan	Siddha/Tamil
Perungambil	*Gardenia latifolia*	Boxwood Gardenia	Siddha/Tamil
Perungayam	*Ferula narthex*	Narthex Asafoetida	Siddha/Tamil
Perungoli	*Salvadora persica*	Mustard Tree, Salt Bush Tree, Tooth Brush Tree	Siddha/Tamil
Perungondrai	*Delonix regia*	Flamboyant Flame Tree, Gold Mohur	Siddha/Tamil
Perungondrai	*Peltophorum pterocarpum*	Copper Pod, Rusty Shield-Bearer	Siddha/Tamil
Perungunni	*Physalis peruviana*	Cape Gooseberry	Siddha/Tamil
Perunkanchori	*Laportea crenulata*	Devil Nettle, Fever Nettle	Siddha/Tamil
Perunkarai	*Randia uliginosa*	Himalayan Randia	Siddha/Tamil
Perunkurinjan	*Marsdenia tenacissima*	White Turpeth	Siddha/Tamil
Peruppi	*Ailanthus excelsa*	Tree of Heaven, Maharukh	Siddha/Tamil
Peruvaagai	*Oroxylum indicum*	Indian Trumpet Flower	Siddha/Tamil
Peruvidukol	*Atylosia goensis*	Maashparni	Siddha/Tamil
Peshaavari-Bhuutakeshi	*Selinum vaginatum*	Tang-kuen	Folk
Pethaa	*Benincasa hispida*	Ash Gourd, White Gourd, Wax Gourd, White Pumpkin	Unani
Pey Ellu	*Guizotia abyssinica*	Nigerseed	Folk/Tamil
Peyatti	*Ficus hispida*	Devil's Fig, Rough-leaved Fig	Siddha/Tamil
Peykkandal	*Rhizophora mucronata*	True Mangrove	Siddha/Tamil
Peyppudal	*Trichosanthes dioica*	Patol, Pointed Gourd	Siddha/Tamil
Peyu	*Zingiber cassumunar*	Cassumunar Ginger	Ayurvedic
Phaalsaa	*Grewia asiatica*	Indian Phalsa	Unani
Phaang	*Rivea hypocrateriformis*	Midnapore Creeper	Folk
Phaang	*Rivea ornate*	Oliliuqui	Folk
Phaangalaa	*Pogostemon benghalensis*	Bengal Pogostemon	Folk

Table Contd.

Indian Name	Botanical Name	English Name	Medicinal System
Phaangalaa	*Pogostemon parviflorus*	Orissa Pogostemon	Folk
Phaapar	*Fagopyrum esculentum*	Buckwheat	Folk
Phaavaaniaa	*Paeonia emodi*	Himalayan Paeony	Unani
Phaggarmuul	*Arctium lappa*	Common/Great Burdock	Folk (Kashmir)
Phalakantaka	*Pergularia extensa*	Hairknot Plant, Whitlow Plant	Ayurvedic
Phalendraa	*Syzygium cuminii*	Java Plum, Jambolan, Black Plum	Ayurvedic
Phalepushpaa	*Leucas aspera*	White Dead Nettle	Ayurvedic
Phalgu	*Ficus carica*	Common Fig	Ayurvedic
Phalgu	*Ficus hispida*	Devil's Fig, Rough-leaved Fig	Ayurvedic
Phalgu	*Ficus palmata*	Indian Fig	Ayurvedic
Phalini	*Callicarpa macrophylla*	Perfumed Cherry	Ayurvedic
Phanasa	*Artocarpus integrifolia*	Jackfruit, Jack Tree	Folk
Phanat	*Quercus incana*	Grey Oak	Folk
Phanijjaka	*Origanum majorana*	Sweet Marjoram	Ayurvedic
Phanji (var.)	*Rivea ornate*	Ololiuqui	Ayurvedic
Phanji	*Clerodendrum serratum*	Blue-flowered Glory Tree, Beetle Killer	Ayurvedic
Phanji	*Rivea hypocrateriformis*	Midnapore Creeper	Ayurvedic
Phenila	*Sapindus laurifolius*	Soapnut Tree of South India	Ayurvedic
Phenila	*Sapindus mukorossi*	Chinese Soap Berry, Soap Nut Tree of North India	Ayurvedic
Phen-kamal	*Saussurea gossypiphora*	Himalayan Saw-wort	Folk
Philunaa	*Parthenocissus himalayana*	Kandur Tree	Folk
Phindak	*Crataegeus oxyacantha*	English Hawthorn	Folk
Phoot-Kanda	*Elsholtzia cristata*	Himalayan Pseudo-Basil	Folk
Phullaa	*Verbascum thapsus*	Cow's Lungwort, Common Mullein	Ayurvedic
Phulwaaraa	*Madhuca butyracea*	Phulwara, Indian Butter Tree	Folk
Phutium	*Bidens pilosa*	Beggar's Tick, Devil's Needle	Folk
Phutuka	*Melastoma malabathricum*	Indian Rhododendron	Folk
Picchila	*Cordia myxa*	Sabestan Plum	Ayurvedic
Picchilaa	*Dalbergia sissoo*	Sissoo, South Indian Redwood	Ayurvedic

Table Contd.

Indian Name	Botanical Name	English Name	Medicinal System
Picchita-taru	*Persea macrantha*	Machilus	Folk
Pichhi	*Parthenium hysterophorus*	Congress Grass	Folk
Pichhila	*Salmalia malabarica*	Silk Cotton Tree, Semul Tree	Ayurvedic
Pichi	*Jasminum officinale*	Spanish Jasmine	Siddha/Tamil
Pichu	*Gossypium herbaceum*	Asiatic Cotton, Levant Cotton, Uppam Cotton	Ayurvedic
Pichuka	*Prunus persica*	Peach	Ayurvedic
Pichumanda	*Azadirachta indica*	Neem Tree, Margosa Tree	Ayurvedic
Pichumandaka	*Azadirachta indica*	Neem Tree, Margosa Tree	Ayurvedic
Pichumarda	*Azadirachta indica*	Neem Tree, Margosa Tree	Ayurvedic
Picinpattai	*Litsea monopetala*	Yati	Siddha/Tamil
Pidikarunai	*Typhonium trilobatum*	Bengal Arum	Siddha/Tamil
Pikavallabha	*Mangifera indica*	Mango	Ayurvedic
Pikku	*Luffa cylindrica*	Smooth Luffa, Sponge-gourd, Sponge Cucumber	Siddha/Tamil
Pilappu-shiragam	*Carum bulbocastanum*	Black Caraway	Siddha/Tamil
Pili-badkadi	*Siegesbeckia orientalis*	The Holy Herb, Sieges-beckia	Folk
Pilimbi	*Averrhoa bilimbi*	Bilimbi, Tree Sorrel	Folk/Tamil
Pilu	*Careya arborea*	Kumbi, Slow-Match Tree	Folk
Pilu	*Juglans regia*	Walnut Tree	Ayurvedic
Pilu	*Salvadora oleoides*	Mustard Tree, Salt Bush Tree, Tooth Brush Tree	Ayurvedic
Pilu	*Salvadora persica*	Mustard Tree, Salt Bush Tree, Tooth Brush Tree	Ayurvedic
Pilukaa	*Salvadora persica*	Mustard Tree, Salt Bush Tree, Tooth Brush Tree	Ayurvedic
Piluparni	*Coccinia indica*	Ivy-Gourd	Ayurvedic
Piluparni	*Maerua arenaria*	Desert Maerua, Hemkand	Ayurvedic
Piluphalaa	*Cissampelos pareira*	Velvet-Leaf Pareira, Pareira Brava	Ayurvedic
Pimento	*Pimenta dioica*	Allspice Tree, Jamaica Pepper Tree, Pimento Tree	Folk
Pimpri	*Ficus benjamina*	Java Fig	Folk
Pinari	*Sterculia foetida*	Kola Seeds, Gurru Nuts	Siddha/Tamil

Table Contd.

Indian Name	Botanical Name	English Name	Medicinal System
Pindaalu	*Randia uliginosa*	Himalayan Randia	Ayurvedic
Pindaaluka	*Colocasia esculenta*	Taro, Edible Yam	Ayurvedic
Pindaar	*Randia uliginosa*	Himalayan Randia	Folk
Pindaara	*Trewia nudiflora*	False White Teak, Gutel	Ayurvedic
Pindakhar-juurikaa	*Phoenix dactylifera*	Date Palm	Ayurvedic
Pindaphalaa	*Lagenaria siceraria*	Bitter Bottle-Gourd	Ayurvedic
Pindapushpa	*Saraca asoca*	Ashoka Tree	Ayurvedic
Pindi	*Randia dumetorum*	Common Emetic Nut	Ayurvedic
Pinditaka	*Meyna laxiflora*	Muyna	Ayurvedic
Pinditaka	*Randia uliginosa*	Himalayan Randia	Ayurvedic
Pinditaka	*Vangueria spinosa*	Voa-Vanga	Ayurvedic
Pingyat	*Crataegeus oxyacantha*	English Hawthorn	Folk
Pinnakkuppundu	*Melochia corchorifolia*	Chocolate-Weed	Siddha/Tamil
Pippali	*Piper longum*	Indian Long Pepper, Joborandi	Ayurvedic
Pippalikam	*Piper longum*	Indian Long Pepper, Joborandi	Ayurvedic
Piraayan	*Streblus asper*	Siamese Rough Brush	Siddha/Tamil
Piramathandu	*Argemone mexicana*	Prickly Poppy, Mexican Poppy	Siddha/Tamil
Pirambu	*Calamus rotang*	Rotang, Rattan, Chair Bottom Cane	Siddha/Tamil
Pirambu	*Calamus travancoricus*	Travancore Cane	Siddha/Tamil
Piramivazhukkai	*Bacopa monnieri*	Thyme-leaved Gratiola	Siddha/Tamil
Pirang	*Trigonella corniculata*	Kasuri Fenugreek	Unani
Pirattai-keerai	*Corchorus capsularis*	White Jute	Folk/Tamil
Piriyaa-Haalim	*Nasturtium officinale*	Watercress	Folk
Pirlu	*Thysanolaena agrostis*	Bouquet-Grass, Broom-Grass, Tiger-Grass, Amliso	Folk
Pisaa	*Actinodaphne hookeri*	Pisa	Folk
Pishaacha Kaarpaasa	*Abroma augusta*	Perennial Indian Hemp, Devil's Cotton	Ayurvedic
Pisi	*Litsea stocksii*	Yati	Folk
Pistaa (Kernel)	*Pistacia vera*	Pistachio, Green Almond	Unani
Pita Kanchana	*Bauhinia tomentosa*	Yellow Bauhinia, St. Thomas Tree, Bell Bauhinia	Ayurvedic

Table Contd.

Indian Name	Botanical Name	English Name	Medicinal System
Pita Kovidaara	*Bauhinia tomentosa*	Yellow Bauhinia, St. Thomas Tree, Bell Bauhinia	Ayurvedic
Pitaanga	*Eugenia uniflora*	Surinam Cherry	Ayurvedic
Pitabhringaraaja	*Wedelia calendulaceae*	Yellow-flowered Weldia	Ayurvedic
Pitabhringi	*Wedelia calendulaceae*	Yellow-flowered Weldia	Ayurvedic
Pitachandana	*Coscinium fenestratum*	False Calumba	Ayurvedic
Pitadaaru	*Adina cordifolia*	Yellow Teak, Saffron Teak	Ayurvedic
Pitadugdhaa	*Argemone mexicana*	Prickly Poppy, Mexican Poppy	Ayurvedic
Pitadugdhaa	*Euphorbia thomsoniana*	Hirvi Spurge	Ayurvedic
Pita-Karavira	*Thevetia peruviana*	Yellow Oleander	Ayurvedic
Pitamuuli	*Rheum emodi*	Indian Rhubarb, Himalayan Rhubarb	Ayurvedic
Pitamuulikaa	*Thalictrum foliolosum*	Meadow Rue	Ayurvedic
Pitana	*Ficus lacor*	White Fig	Ayurvedic
Pitanaasha	*Artocarpus lakoocha*	Monkey Jack	Ayurvedic
Pitaphalaka	*Streblus asper*	Siamese Rough Brush	Ayurvedic
Pitapushpaka	*Acacia arabica*	Babul, Black Babul, Indian Gum Arabic Tree	Ayurvedic
Pitarangaa	*Thalictrum foliolosum*	Meadow Rue	Ayurvedic
Pita-Ranjak Padapa	*Reseda luteola*	Dyer's Rocket, Weld	Folk
Pitarohini	*Gmelina arborea*	Candahar Tree, White Teak	Ayurvedic
Pitasaara	*Coscinium fenestratum*	False Calumba	Ayurvedic
Pitashaala	*Pterocarpus marsupium*	Indian Kino Tree, Malabar Kino Tree	Ayurvedic
Pita-vriksha	*Pinus roxburghii*	Long-leaved Pine, Three-leaved Pine, Chir Pine	Ayurvedic
Pittapaaparaa	*Fumaria parviflora*	Fumitory	Folk
Pittapaaparaa	*Fumaria vaillantii*	Yellow Fumitory	Folk
Pittapaaparaa	*Polycarpaea corymbosa*	Old Man's Cap	Folk
Pitta-vela	*Naregamia alata*	Goanese Ipecacuanha	Folk
Pitti	*Ventilago denticulata*	Ventilago Black Vine	Folk
Pivari	*Abroma augusta*	Perennial Indian Hemp, Devil's Cotton	Ayurvedic

Table Contd.

Indian Name	Botanical Name	English Name	Medicinal System
Piyaabaansaa	*Barleria prionitis*	Common Yellow Nail Dye Plant	Unani
Piyaar	*Buchanania lanzan*	Almondette Tree, Cheronjee, Buchanan's Mango	Ayurvedic
Piyaaraangaa	*Thalictrum foliolosum*	Meadow Rue	Ayurvedic
Piyaaz	*Allium cepa*	Onion	Unani
Piyaaz-Dasti	*Urginea indica*	Indian Squill, Sea Onion (red and white varieties)	Unani
Piyaazi	*Asphodelus fistulosus*	Asphodel	Unani
Piyaaz-Sahraayi	*Urginea indica*	Indian Squill, Sea Onion (red and white varieties)	Unani
Pizh	*Typha laxmannii*	Scented Flag	Folk/Kashmir
Plaksha	*Ficus lacor*	White Fig	Ayurvedic
Plaksha	*Ficus microcarpa*	Indian Laurel Fig	Ayurvedic
Plaksha	*Ficus talboti*	Pakar Tree	Ayurvedic
Plavithil	*Dendrophthoe falcata*	Mango and Citrus Parasite	Siddha/Tamil
Plihaghna	*Aphanamixis polystachya*	Amoora	Ayurvedic
Plihaghna	*Tecomella undulata*	Rohida Tree	Ayurvedic
Podinaka	*Mentha spicata*	Spearmint, Garden Mint	Ayurvedic
Pods-Sungraa	*Raphanus sativus*	Radish	Ayurvedic
Poduthalai	*Phyla nodiflora*	Fogfruit, Sawtooth Fogfruit	Siddha/Tamil
Poi	*Basella alba*	Indian Spinach	Folk
Poiychaviral	*Citrullus vulgaris*	Watermelon	Siddha/Tamil
Pola	*Kydia calycina*	Pula Tree	Folk
Polao	*Kydia calycina*	Pula Tree	Folk
Pon Ichi	*Ficus benjamina*	Java Fig	Siddha/Tamil
Pondanganari	*Premna tomentosa*	Bastard Teak	Siddha/Tamil
Poniol	*Flacourtia indica*	Ramontchi, Madagascar Plum, Mauritius Plum, Governor's Plum	Folk
Ponkoranti	*Salacia oblonga*	Saptrangi	Folk
Ponnaavaarai	*Cassia occidentalis*	Coffee Senna, Foetid Cassia, Negro Coffee	Siddha/Tamil
Ponnaavaarai	*Cassia sophera*	Sophera Senna	Folk

Table Contd.

Indian Name	Botanical Name	English Name	Medicinal System
Ponnam-pomaraiva	*Vanda spathulata*	Plantain Tree, Tree-top Plantain	Folk/South
Ponnankanni Keerai	*Alternanthera sessilis*	Sessile Joyweed	Siddha/Tamil
Ponnuikan kungiliyam	*Pistacia lentiscus*	Mastic Tree	Siddha/Tamil
Poolankizangu	*Hedychium spicatum*	Spiked Ginger Ivy	Siddha/Tamil
Poonai kaanchori	*Tragia involucrata*	Indian Stinging-Nettle	Siddha/Tamil
Poonaik-kanchori	*Alhagi pseudalhagi*	Camel Thorn, Persian Manna Plant	Siddha/Tamil
Poonaikkaali	*Mucuna prurita*	Cowhage, Horse-eye Bean	Siddha/Tamil
Poondu	*Vicoa indica*	Banjauri	Folk/Tamil
Poovarsu	*Thespesia populnea*	Portia Tree, Tulip Tree, Umbrella Tree, False Rosewood	Siddha/Tamil
Popli	*Osyris wightiana*	African Sandalwood, Zanzibar Lawa Wood	Folk
Porashu	*Chloroxylon swietenia*	Indian Satinwood Tree	Siddha/Tamil
Posha	*Litsea stocksii*	Yati	Folk
Poshkar	*Senecio jacquemontianus*	Jacquemont's Senecio	Folk
Post-daanaa (seed)	*Papaver somniferum*	Opium Poppy	Ayurvedic
Potagala	*Typha elephantina*	Elephant Grass, Indian Reed-Mace, Bulrush	Ayurvedic
Potaki	*Basella alba*	Indian Spinach	Ayurvedic
Potgala	*Arundo donax*	Great Reed, Spanish-Bamboo-Reed, Giant-Bamboo-Reed	Ayurvedic
Potralai Kaiyan Tagarai	*Wedelia calendulaceae*	Yellow-flowered Weldia	Siddha/Tamil
Potri	*Kydia calycina*	Pula Tree	Folk
Pottipallam	*Physalis peruviana*	Cape Gooseberry	Siddha/Tamil
Praachibalaa	*Peristrophe bicalyculata*	Panicled Peristrophe	Ayurvedic
Praachinaamalaka	*Flacourtia jangomas*	Puneala Plum	Ayurvedic
Praagraha	*Cassia fistula*	Indian Laburnum, Purging Cassia, Golden Shower	Ayurvedic
Praan	*Allium porrum*	Leek	Folk/Kashmir

Table Contd.

Indian Name	Botanical Name	English Name	Medicinal System
Prabhaakara	*Calotropis gigantea*	Swallow Wort	Ayurvedic
Prahaarvalli	*Soymida febrifuga*	Indian Red-Wood, Bastard Cedar	Ayurvedic
Prakirya	*Holoptelea integrifolia*	Indian Elm, Kanju Wood	Ayurvedic
Prameha-harati	*Justicia betonica*	Shrimp Plant, Lobster Plant	Folk
Prapunnaada	*Cassia obtusifolia*	Arsenic Weed, Sicklepod	Ayurvedic
Prapunnaada	*Cassia tora*	Sickle Senna, Ringworm Plant	Ayurvedic
Prarohi	*Ficus arnottiana*	Indian Rock Fig	Ayurvedic
Prasaarini	*Merremia quinquefolia*	Five-fingered Morning Glory, Rock Rosemary	Ayurvedic
Prasaarini	*Paederia foetida*	Skunk Vine	Ayurvedic
Prasaarini	*Sida veronicaefolia*	Prostrate Mallow	Ayurvedic
Prasaha	*Solanum ferox*	Poison-Berry	Ayurvedic
Prataanikaa	*Orthosiphon tomentosus*	Cat's Whiskers	Ayurvedic
Prativishaa	*Aconitum palmatum*	Himalayan Aconite	Ayurvedic
Prativishnuka	*Pterospermum acerifolium*	Hathipaila	Ayurvedic
Pratyakpushpaa	*Achyranthes aspera*	Prickly Chaff Flower	Ayurvedic
Pratyak-shreni	*Baliospermum montanum*	False Croton	Ayurvedic
Pravaaljaati	*Jasminum officinale*	Spanish Jasmine	Ayurvedic
Prishniparni	*Uraria alopecuroides*	Jackal's Tail	Ayurvedic
Prishniparni	*Uraria crinita*	Ekor Kuching, Cat's Tail	Ayurvedic
Prishniparni	*Uraria lagopoides*	Trailing Uraria	Ayurvedic
Prishniparni	*Uraria picta*	Trailing Uraria	Ayurvedic
Prithakparni	*Uraria picta*	Trailing Uraria	Ayurvedic
Prithivikaa	*Amomum subulatum*	Greater or Nepal Cardamom	Ayurvedic
Prithvikaa	*Carum carvi*	Caraway	Ayurvedic
Prithvikaa	*Elettaria cardamomum*	Lesser Cardamom	Ayurvedic
Priyaal	*Buchanania axillaris*	Buchanan's Mango, Cuddapah Almond	Ayurvedic
Priyaala	*Buchanania lanzan*	Almondette Tree, Cheronjee, Buchanan's Mango	Ayurvedic
Priyaka	*Anthocephalus cadamba*	Wild Cinchona	Ayurvedic
Priyaka	*Callicarpa macrophylla*	Perfumed Cherry	Ayurvedic

Table Contd.

Indian Name	Botanical Name	English Name	Medicinal System
Priyaka	*Curcuma longa*	Turmeric	Ayurvedic
Priyaka	*Pterocarpus marsupium*	Indian Kino Tree, Malabar Kino Tree	Ayurvedic
Priyangu	*Aglaia roxburghiana*	Priyangu Mahogany	Ayurvedic
Priyangu	*Callicarpa macrophylla*	Perfumed Cherry	Ayurvedic
Priyangu Dhaanya (Millet)	*Setaria italica*	Italian Millet, Fox-tail Millet	Ayurvedic
Priyangukaa	*Callicarpa macrophylla*	Perfumed Cherry	Ayurvedic
Prshniparni	*Desmodium gangeticum*	Shaalparni, Beggarweed (Uraria Picta: also used as Shaalparni)	Ayurvedic
Prthushimba	*Oroxylum indicum*	Indian Trumpet Flower	Ayurvedic
Prthvikaa	*Nigella sativa*	Black Cumin, Small Fennel	Ayurvedic
Prukkaa	*Delphinium brunonianum*	Musk Larkspur	Ayurvedic
Pu	*Aesculus hippocastanum*	Horse Chestnut Tree	Folk
Puchikalli	*Opuntia cochinellifera*	Cochineal Cactus	Siddha/Tamil
Pudal	*Trichosanthes anguina*	Snake-Gourd	Siddha/Tamil
Pudinaa (var.)	*Micromeria capitellata*	Pseudo-Mint	Folk
Pudinaa	*Mentha spicata*	Spearmint, Garden Mint	Ayurvedic
Pudinaa Kohi	*Mentha spicata*	Spearmint, Garden Mint	Unani
Pudinaa Nahari	*Mentha aquatica*	Water Mint, Wild Mint	Unani
Pudinaa-Barri	*Mentha longifolia*	English Horsemint	Unani
Pudvali	*Trichosanthes anguina*	Snake-Gourd	Folk
Pula	*Kydia calycina*	Pula Tree	Folk
Pulaachi	*Schleichera oleosa*	Lac Tree, Macassar Oil Tree, Honey Tree, Ceylon Oak	Siddha/Tamil
Puli	*Tamarindus indica*	Tamarind Tree	Siddha/Tamil
Pulichai-keerai	*Hibiscus sabdariffa*	Roselle, Jamaican Sorrel, Natal Sorrel, Red Sorrel	Siddha/Tamil
Pulichakkai	*Averrhoa bilimbi*	Bilimbi, Tree Sorrel	Siddha/Tamil
Pulichan	*Uvaria narum*	Cinnamon-leaved Uvaria	Siddha/Tamil
Pulichhai	*Hibiscus cannabinus*	Bimlipatam Jute, Kenaf, Mesta, Deccan Hemp	Folk/Tamil
Pulinak-kagondai	*Wagatea spicata*	Western Ghat-Wakeri	Siddha/Tamil
Pulivanji	*Zehneria umbellata*	Zehneria	Siddha/Tamil

Table Contd.

Indian Name	Botanical Name	English Name	Medicinal System
Qinn	*Pinus roxburghii*	Long-leaved Pine, Three-leaved Pine, Chir Pine	Unani
Qinnab	*Cannabis sativa*	Hemp, Indian Hemp	Unani
Quillaia	*Quillaja saponaria*	Chilean Soap Bark	Folk
Quinine	*Cinchona officinalis*	Crown or Loxa Bark	Ayurvedic
Qurtum (Seed)	*Carthamus tinctorius*	Safflower	Unani
Qust	*Saussurea lappa*	Kuth, Costus	Unani
Raai	*Brassica juncea*	Chinese Mustard, Brown Mustard	Folk
Raai	*Brassica nigra*	Black Mustard	Folk
Raaj Kasheruka	*Scirpus tuberosus*	Sea Clubrush	Ayurvedic
Raajaarka	*Calotropis gigantea*	Swallow Wort	Ayurvedic
Raajabalaa	*Sida veronicaefolia*	Prostrate Mallow	Ayurvedic
Raajadruma	*Cassia fistula*	Indian Laburnum, Purging Cassia, Golden Shower	Ayurvedic
Raajakoshataki	*Luffa cylindrica*	Smooth Luffa, Sponge-gourd, Sponge Cucumber	Ayurvedic
Raajakshavaka	*Brassica napus*	Mustard, Indian Rape	Ayurvedic
Raajaputrikaa	*Physalis alkekengi*	Strawberry Tomato, Winter Cherry	Ayurvedic
Raajchampaa	*Calophyllum inophyllum*	Indian Laurel, Alexandrian Laurel	Ayurvedic
Raajeeva	*Nelumbo nucifera*	East Indian Lotus, Sacred Lotus	Ayurvedic
Raajhans	*Adiantum lunulatum*	Walking Maidenhair Fern, Black Maidenhair	Folk
Raajika	*Brassica nigra*	Black Mustard	Ayurvedic
Raajikaa	*Brassica juncea*	Chinese Mustard, Brown Mustard	Ayurvedic
Raajiphala	*Trichosanthes dioica*	Patol, Pointed Gourd	Ayurvedic
Raaj-Jambu	*Syzygium jambos*	Rose Apple	Ayurvedic
Raajmah (seed)	*Phaseolus vulgaris*	Kidney Bean, French Bean, Haricot Bean	Unani
Raajodumbara	*Ficus carica*	Common Fig	Ayurvedic

Table Contd.

Indian Name	Botanical Name	English Name	Medicinal System
Raaj-Paathaa (South)	*Stephania hernandiifolia*	Japanese Tape Vine	Ayurvedic
Raaj-Paathaa	*Cyclea arnotii*	Green Jelly Shrub	Folk
Raajvrksha	*Cassia fistula*	Indian Laburnum, Purging Cassia, Golden Shower	Ayurvedic
Raal	*Vateria indica*	White Damar, Indian Copal-Tree, Malabar Tallow Tree, Piney Varnish-Tree	Unani
Raal Dhuup	*Canarium strictum*	Black Dammar	Ayurvedic
Raam Kurthi	*Glycine max*	Soybean, Soya	Folk
Raam Tulasi	*Dracocephalum moldavica*	Dragon's Head	Ayurvedic
Raamabaanam	*Hemionitis arifolia*	Male Fern	Folk
Raamadhaani	*Ventilago denticulata*	Ventilago Black Vine	Folk
Raamaka	*Acacia leucophloea*	White Babul	Ayurvedic
Raamapatri	*Myristica malabarica*	Malabar Nutmeg, False Nutmeg, Bombay Nutmeg, Bombay Mace	Ayurvedic
Raamaphala	*Annona reticulata*	Bull's Heart, Common Custard Apple	Ayurvedic
Raamasenaka	*Swertia chirayita*	Chiretta	Ayurvedic
Raamattha	*Ferula foetida*	Asafoetida	Ayurvedic
Raam-begun	*Solanum ferox*	Poison-Berry	Folk
Raam-daanaa (Grain)	*Amaranthus caudatus*	Love-Lies-Bleeding, Tassel Flower	Ayurvedic
Raamethaa	*Lasiosiphon eriocephalus*	Wooly-headed Gnidia	Folk
Raampat	*Strobilanthes flaccidifolius*	Assam Indigo	Folk
Raamshara	*Saccharum munja*	Munja Culms	Ayurvedic
Raam-til	*Guizotia abyssinica*	Nigerseed	Folk
Raam-Tulasi	*Ocimum gratissimum*	Shrubby Basil	Ayurvedic
Raamturai	*Abelmoschus esculentus*	Gumbo, Lady Finger, Okra	Folk
Raan-bhendi	*Thespesia lampas*	Indian Hemp	Folk
Raan-ghevaraa	*Rhynchosia minima*	Rhynchosia	Folk

Table Contd.

Indian Name	Botanical Name	English Name	Medicinal System
Raani-phool	*Polygonum plebeium*	Common Knotweed	Folk
Raan-Tulasi	*Ocimum gratissimum*	Shrubby Basil	Ayurvedic
Raasana (Andhra Pradesh)	*Dodonaea viscosa*	Jamacia Switch Sorrel	Ayurvedic
Raasanaa	*Saccolabium papillosum*	Small Warty Acampe	Folk
Raasnaa	*Pluchea lanceolata*	Rasana Shrub	Ayurvedic
Raasnaa	*Vanda roxburghii*	Tassellata	Ayurvedic
Raasnikaa	*Pluchea lanceolata*	Rasana Shrub	Ayurvedic
Raatri	*Curcuma caesia*	Black Zedorary	Ayurvedic
Raatripraphulla	*Selenicereus grandiflorus*	Night-Blooming Cereus, Sweet-scented Cactus	Ayurvedic
Raayasan	*Pluchea lanceolata*	Rasana Shrub	Folk
Ragat-Rohido	*Maba nigrescens*	Karuti Ebony	Folk
Raghaa	*Picea smithiana*	West Himalayan Spruce	Folk
Ragi	*Eleusine coracana*	Finger Millet, African Millet, Ragi	Siddha/Tamil
Rai Jaamun	*Syzygium cerasoideum*	Piaman Tree	Folk
Raihan	*Ocimum basilicum*	Sweet Basil, Basil Herb	Unani
Raisalla	*Abies pindrow*	Pindrow-Fir, Silver-Fir, The West-Himalayan Low-Level Fir	Folk
Raisalla	*Abies webbiana*	Indian Silver Fir, The West-Himalayan High-Level Fir, The East-Himalayan Fir	Folk
Raitung	*Rhus parviflora*	Sumach	Folk
Rajani	*Curcuma caesia*	Black Zedorary	Ayurvedic
Rajanigandhaa	*Polianthes tuberosa*	Tuberose	Ayurvedic
Rajapoo	*Rosa centifolia*	Cabbage Rose, Provence Rose, Hundred-leaved Rose	Folk/Tamil
Rakshogna	*Brassica napus*	Mustard, Indian Rape	Ayurvedic
Rakta Kambal	*Adenanthera pavonina*	Coral Wood, Red Wood	Ayurvedic
Rakta Kanchan	*Bauhinia purpurea*	Camel's Foot Tree, Pink Bauhinia, Butterfly Tree, Geramium Tree, Orchid Tree	Folk
Rakta Kanchana	*Adenanthera pavonina*	Coral Wood, Red Wood	Ayurvedic
Rakta Posta	*Papaver rhoeas*	Corn Poppy, Red Poppy	Ayurvedic

Table Contd.

Indian Name	Botanical Name	English Name	Medicinal System
Raktaalu	*Dioscorea bulbifera*	Patoto Yam, Bulb-bearing Yam, Air Potato, Dog Yam	Ayurvedic
Raktaalu	*Ipomoea batatas*	Sweet Potato	Ayurvedic
Raktaanga	*Mallotus philippensis*	Kamala Tree, Monkey Face Tree	Ayurvedic
Raktaangi	*Rubia cordifolia*	Indian Madder, Bengal Madder	Ayurvedic
Raktabeeja	*Sapindus laurifolius*	Soapnut Tree of South India	Ayurvedic
Rakta-chandana (var.)	*Pterocarpus dalbergioides*	Andaman Paduak, Andaman Redwood	Ayurvedic
Raktachandana	*Pterocarpus santalinus*	Red Sandalwood, Red Sanders	Ayurvedic
Rakta-chitraka	*Plumbago indica*	Rose-coloured Leadwort	Ayurvedic
Rakta-Granjana	*Beta vulgaris*	Beet Root, Garden Beet, Chard	Ayurvedic
Raktajhinti	*Barleria cristata*	Crested Philippine Violet	Folk
Raktaka	*Moringa pterygosperma*	Drumstick, Horse-Radish	Ayurvedic
Rakta-Kaarpaasa	*Gossypium herbaceum*	Asiatic Cotton, Levant Cotton, Uppam Cotton	Ayurvedic
Raktakanda	*Ipomoea batatas*	Sweet Potato	Ayurvedic
Raktakusumaa	*Punica granatum*	Pomegranate	Ayurvedic
Raktamaricha	*Capsicum annuum*	Chilli, Red Pepper	Ayurvedic
Raktaniryaas	*Daemonorops draco*	East Indian Dragon's Blood	Ayurvedic
Raktapaadi	*Adiantum lunulatum*	Walking Maidenhair Fern, Black Maidenhair	Ayurvedic
Raktapaadi	*Mimosa pudica*	Sensitive-plant, Humble-Plant	Ayurvedic
Raktaphala	*Coccinia indica*	Ivy-Gourd	Ayurvedic
Raktapindaka	*Ipomoea batatas*	Sweet Potato	Ayurvedic
Raktaprasava	*Nerium oleander*	Indian Oleander, White Oleander	Ayurvedic
Rakta-punarnavaa	*Boerhavia diffusa*	Red- flowered Hogweed	Ayurvedic
Raktapushpa	*Erythrina indica*	Indian Coral Tree	Ayurvedic
Raktapushpa	*Nerium oleander*	Indian Oleander, White Oleander	Ayurvedic
Raktapushpa	*Punica granatum*	Pomegranate	Ayurvedic
Raktapushpa	*Salmalia malabarica*	Silk Cotton Tree, Semul Tree	Ayurvedic
Raktapushpaka	*Butea monosperma*	Flame of the Forest, Butea Gum, Bengal Kino	Ayurvedic
Rakta-Rohidaa	*Rhamnus wightii*	Bitter Ragtrora	Ayurvedic

Table Contd.

Indian Name	Botanical Name	English Name	Medicinal System
Raktarohidi	*Chloroxylon swietenia*	Indian Satinwood Tree	Folk
Rakta-Rohido	*Maba nigrescens*	Karuti Ebony	Folk
Rakta-rohitaka	*Polygonum glabrum*	Denseflower Knotweed	Ayurvedic
Raktasaara (Heartwood extract)	*Acacia catechu*	Cutch tree, Catechu	Ayurvedic
Raktasaara	*Caesalpinia sappan*	Sappan	Ayurvedic
Raktasaara	*Pterocarpus santalinus*	Red Sandalwood, Red Sanders	Ayurvedic
Raktaskandana	*Anaphalis neelgerriana*	Katplaster	Ayurvedic
Rakta-Taruni	*Rosa multiflora*	Japanese Rose, Seven Sister's Rose, Baby Rose	Ayurvedic
Rakta-Taruni	*Rosa rubra*	French Rose	Ayurvedic
Raktavalli	*Ventilago denticulata*	Ventilago Black Vine	Ayurvedic
Rakta-Vyaaghrairanda	*Jatropha gossypifolia*	Physic Nut, Purging Nut	Ayurvedic
Raktayashtikaa	*Rubia cordifolia*	Indian Madder, Bengal Madder	Ayurvedic
Raktikaa	*Abrus precatorius*	Indian Wild Liquorice, Jequirity, Crab's Eye, Precatory Bean	Ayurvedic
Ramabanam mullai	*Jasminum flexile*	Jasmine, Juhi	Siddha/Tamil
Rambhaa	*Musa paradisiaca*	Banana, Plantain	Ayurvedic
Ramguwaa	*Knema angustifolia*	Pseudo-Redsander Tree	Folk
Ramyaka	*Melia azedarach*	Persian Lilac, Pride of India	Ayurvedic
Ran Bhindi	*Hibiscus surattensis*	Wild Sour, Bush Sorrel	Ayurvedic
Ran-Baingan	*Solanum torvum*	West Indian Turkey Berry	Folk
Ranchimani	*Andrographis echioides*	Creat	Folk
Randhuni	*Apium graveolens*	Celery	Folk
Rangan	*Ixora coccinea*	Jungleflame Ixora	Folk
Rangan	*Ixora parviflora*	Torchwood Tree	Ayurvedic
Rangoon-ki-Bel	*Quisqualis indica*	Rangoon Creeper	Ayurvedic
Ranjaka	*Lawsonia inermis*	Henna	Ayurvedic
Ranjana	*Caesalpinia sappan*	Sappan	Ayurvedic
Ranjani	*Indigofera tinctoria*	Indigo	Ayurvedic
Ran-limbu	*Limonia crenulata*	Naringi, Beli	Folk

Table Contd.

Indian Name	Botanical Name	English Name	Medicinal System
Ran-methi	*Desmodium triflorum*	Matty Trefoil	Folk
Ran-mogaraa	*Jasminum malabaricum*	Climbing Mogara	Folk
Ransla	*Abies pindrow*	Pindrow-Fir, Silver-Fir, The West-Himalayan Low-Level Fir	Folk
Rasaa	*Pluchea lanceolata*	Rasana Shrub	Ayurvedic
Rasaal	*Mangifera indica*	Mango	Ayurvedic
Rasagadimaanu	*Solanum erianthum*	Mullen Nightshade	Folk
Rasanaa	*Pluchea lanceolata*	Rasana Shrub	Ayurvedic
Rasaut (Extract)	*Berberis aristata*	Indian Barberry	Unani
Rasbhari	*Physalis peruviana*	Cape Gooseberry	Folk
Rasona	*Allium sativum*	Garlic	Ayurvedic
Rasonaka	*Allium sativum*	Garlic	Ayurvedic
Rasunia	*Kandelia rheedii*	Backwater Kandal Tree	Folk
Rataalu	*Ipomoea batatas*	Sweet Potato	Ayurvedic
Rataalu	*Ipomoea batatas*	Sweet Potato	Unani
Ratangaruur	*Elaeodendron glaucum*	Jamrasi Gum Tree	Folk
Ratanjot (var.)	*Geranium nepalense*	Nepal Geranium, Nepalese Crane's Bill	Folk
Ratanjot	*Alkanna tinctoria*	Alkanet, Dyers' or Spanish Bugloss	Unani
Ratanjot	*Clausena pentaphylla*	Clausena	Folk
Ratanjot	*Geranium wallichianum*	Wallich Crane's Bill	Ayurvedic
Ratanjot	*Mycrotomia benthami*	Pseudo-Ratanjot	Folk
Ratanjot	*Onosma echioides*	Goldendrop, Red-dye Onosma	Unani
Ratanjot	*Potentilla nepalensis*	Nepal Cinquefoil	Folk
Ratapaati	*Ajuga bracteosa*	Bugle	Folk
Ratnagandhi	*Caesalpinia pulcherrima*	Barbados Pride, Peacock Flower	Ayurvedic
Ratna-purush	*Ionidium suffruticosum*	Charati	Folk
Ratthapaalai	*Alkanna tinctoria*	Alkanet, Dyers' or Spanish Bugloss	Siddha/Tamil
Ratti	*Abrus precatorius*	Indian Wild Liquorice, Jequirity, Crab's Eye, Precatory Bean	Folk

Table Contd.

Indian Name	Botanical Name	English Name	Medicinal System
Sevaar	*Vallisneria spiralis*	Eel-Grass, Tape Grass, Wild Celery	Folk
Sevai	*Sandoricum indicum*	European Elder	Siddha/Tamil
Sevati	*Rosa alba*	Common English Dog Rose, White Cottage Rose	Ayurvedic
Sevati	*Rosa alba*	Common English Dog Rose, White Cottage Rose	Unani
Sevya	*Vetiveria zizanioides*	Vetiver, Khas	Ayurvedic
Shaabara Lodhra	*Symplocos racemosa*	Lodh Tree, Sapphire Berry	Ayurvedic
Shaabiraj	*Atropa acuminata*	Indian Belladonna, Indian Atropa	Unani
Shaahtaraa	*Fumaria officinalis*	Fumitory	Unani
Shaahtaraa	*Fumaria parviflora*	Fumitory	Unani
Shaahtaraa	*Fumaria vaillantii*	Yellow Fumitory	Unani
Shaaka	*Tectona grandis*	Teak Tree	Ayurvedic
Shaaka-shreshtha	*Leptadenia reticulata*	Dodi Vegetable	Ayurvedic
Shaaka-turshak	*Rumex acetosella*	Sheep Sorrel	Unani
Shaakhota	*Streblus asper*	Siamese Rough Brush	Ayurvedic
Shaakhotaka	*Streblus asper*	Siamese Rough Brush	Ayurvedic
Shaala	*Shorea robusta*	Sal Tree	Ayurvedic
Shaalaparni	*Desmodium gangeticum*	Shaalparni, Beggarweed	Ayurvedic
Shaalaparni	*Pseudarthria viscida*	Shalparni	Ayurvedic
Shaaleya	*Raphanus sativus*	Radish	Ayurvedic
Shaali	*Oryza sativa*	Rice	Ayurvedic
Shaaliparni	*Desmodium gangeticum*	Shaalparni, Beggarweed	Ayurvedic
Shaalmali	*Salmalia malabarica*	Silk Cotton Tree, Semul Tree	Ayurvedic
Shaalmali-veshtaka	*Salmalia malabarica*	Silk Cotton Tree, Semul Tree	Ayurvedic
Shaaluraparni	*Bacopa monnieri*	Thyme-leaved Gratiola	Ayurvedic
Shaandilya	*Aegle marmelos*	Bael Tree, Bengal Quince	Ayurvedic
Shaarada	*Alstonia scholaris*	Devil's Tree, Dita Bark Tree	Ayurvedic
Shaaradi	*Indigofera tinctoria*	Indigo	Ayurvedic
Shaaradi	*Lippia nodiflora*	Wild Sage	Ayurvedic
Shaaradi	*Phyla nodiflora*	Fogfruit, Sawtooth Fogfruit	Ayurvedic

Table Contd.

Indian Name	Botanical Name	English Name	Medicinal System
Shaaraf	*Ipomoea petaloidea*	False Jalap, Hawaii Morning Glory	Unani
Shaavaka	*Tamarix indica*	Takut Galls	Ayurvedic
Shaavara	*Symplocos racemosa*	Lodh Tree, Sapphire Berry	Ayurvedic
Shaay	*Camellia sinensis*	Tea Plant	Unani
Shadgranthaa	*Acorus calamus*	Sweet Flag, Calamus	Ayurvedic
Shaeppam-kizhangu	*Colocasia esculenta*	Taro, Edible Yam	Siddha/Tamil
Shahtuut	*Morus alba*	Chinese White-Mulberry	Unani
Shaikharika	*Achyranthes aspera*	Prickly Chaff Flower	Ayurvedic
Shaila	*Parmelia perlata*	Parmelia Lichen	Ayurvedic
Shailaja	*Swertia ciliata*	Black Chiretta	Ayurvedic
Shailaja	*Swertia densifolia*	Dense-leaved Chiretta	Ayurvedic
Shailaka	*Parmelia perlata*	Parmelia Lichen	Ayurvedic
Shailbhava	*Juglans regia*	Walnut Tree	Ayurvedic
Shaileya	*Cetraria islandica*	Cetraria, Iceland Lichen, Liceland Moss	Ayurvedic
Shaileya	*Parmelia perlata*	Parmelia Lichen	Ayurvedic
Shaileyaka	*Parmelia perlata*	Parmelia Lichen	Ayurvedic
Shailuusha	*Aegle marmelos*	Bael Tree, Bengal Quince	Ayurvedic
Shaivaala	*Ceratophyllum demersum*	Coontail, Hornwort	Ayurvedic
Shaivaala	*Vallisneria spiralis*	Eel-Grass, Tape Grass, Wild Celery	Ayurvedic
Shakarkand	*Ipomoea batatas*	Sweet Potato	Unani
Shakataahya	*Anogeissus latifolia*	Axle-wood, Button Tree, Ghatti Tree	Ayurvedic
Shakkankeerai	*Rumex vesicarius*	Bladder-Dock, Country Sorrel	Siddha/Tamil
Shakra	*Holarrhena antidysenterica*	Easter Tree, Ivory Tree, Tellicherry	Ayurvedic
Shakraahvya	*Holarrhena antidysenterica*	Easter Tree, Ivory Tree, Tellicherry	Ayurvedic
Shakulaadani	*Lippia nodiflora*	Wild Sage	Ayurvedic
Shakulaadani	*Phyla nodiflora*	Fogfruit, Sawtooth Fogfruit	Ayurvedic
Shakuldaani	*Picrorhiza kurroa*	Picrorhiza	Ayurvedic
Shalayaka	*Randia dumetorum*	Common Emetic Nut	Ayurvedic

Table Contd.

Indian Name	Botanical Name	English Name	Medicinal System
Shallaki	*Boswellia serrata*	Indian Frankincense, Indian Olibanum	Ayurvedic
Shalya	*Aegle marmelos*	Bael Tree, Bengal Quince	Ayurvedic
Shamaa	*Echinochloa colonum*	Shama Millet	Folk
Shamaa	*Echinochloa frumentacea*	Japanese Barnyard Millet	Folk
Shami (var.)	*Prosopis stephaniana*	Syrian Mestique Gum Tree	Ayurvedic
Shami	*Prosopis spicigera*	Mestique Gum Tree	Ayurvedic
Shamipatraa	*Mimosa pudica*	Sensitive-plant, Humble-Plant	Ayurvedic
Shampaaka	*Cassia fistula*	Indian Laburnum, Purging Cassia, Golden Shower	Ayurvedic
Shamshaad	*Buxus wallichiana*	Himalayan Boxwood Tree	Folk
Shamshaad	*Myrsine africana*	Pseudo-Embelia	Folk
Shana	*Crotalaria juncea*	Sun Hemp	Ayurvedic
Shana	*Crotalaria verrucosa*	Sun Hemp	Ayurvedic
Shanapushpi	*Crotalaria juncea*	Sun Hemp	Ayurvedic
Shanapushpi	*Crotalaria verrucosa*	Sun Hemp	Ayurvedic
Shana-pushpikaa	*Cajanus cajan*	Pigeon Pea, Red Gram	Ayurvedic
Shankaahuli	*Evolvulus alsinoides*	Blue-flowered Shankhpushpi	Unani
Shankapushpi	*Evolvulus alsinoides*	Blue-flowered Shankhpushpi	Ayurvedic
Shankhaahvaa	*Convolvulus pluricaulis*	Conch-flowered Bindweed	Ayurvedic
Shankhaaluka	*Dioscorea glabra*	Gluey Yam	Ayurvedic
Shankhaaluka	*Nervilia aragoana*	Tall Shield Orchid	Ayurvedic
Shankhani	*Ipomoea nil*	Pharbitis Seeds	Ayurvedic
Shankhapushpi	*Convolvulus pluricaulis*	Conch-flowered Bindweed	Ayurvedic
Shankhapushpi	*Lavandula bipinnata*	Wild Lavender	Ayurvedic
Shankheshwara	*Xanthium strumarium*	Cocklebur, Burweed	Ayurvedic
Shankhini	*Ctenolepis cerasiformis*	Ctenolepis	Ayurvedic
Shankh-phuli	*Canscora decussata*	Conch-flowered Bindweed	Folk
Shankuphalaa	*Prosopis spicigera*	Mestique Gum Tree	Ayurvedic
Shaqaaqul	*Polygonatum verticillatum*	Whorl-leaved Solomon's Seal	Unani
Shaqaaqul-e-Hindi	*Asparagus adscendens*	White Musali	Unani

Table Contd.

Indian Name	Botanical Name	English Name	Medicinal System
Shaqaaq-ul-Misri	*Pastinaca secacul*	Wild Parsnip	Unani
Shaqaaq-un-Nomaan	*Anemone obtusiloba*	Wind-Flower, Wood Anemone, Pasque Flower, Pulsatilla	Unani
Shara	*Saccharum munja*	Munja Culms	Ayurvedic
Sharapunkhaa	*Tephrosia purpurea*	Purple Tephrosia, Wild Indigo	Ayurvedic
Sharifaa	*Annona squamosa*	Custard Apple, Sugar Apple, Sweet-sop	Unani
Sharmili	*Mimosa pudica*	Sensitive-plant, Humble-Plant	Unani
Sharunai	*Trianthema portulacastrum*	Horse Purslane	Siddha/Tamil
Sharvari	*Curcuma longa*	Turmeric	Ayurvedic
Shashi	*Cinnamomum camphora*	Camphor Tree	Ayurvedic
Shash-shruti	*Emilia sonchifolia*	Emilia Salad	Ayurvedic
Shataahvaa	*Anethum sowa*	Indian Dill, Sowa	Ayurvedic
Shataahvaa	*Foeniculum vulgare*	Fennel	Ayurvedic
Shataakratilataa	*Cardiospermum halicacabum*	Balloon Vine, Winter Pea, Heartseed	Ayurvedic
Shataavari	*Asparagus racemosus*	Indian Asparagus, Wild Asparagus	Ayurvedic
Shataavari Vilaayati	*Asparagus officinalis*	Asparagus, Sparrow Grass	Ayurvedic
Shatakumbhak	*Nerium indicum*	Indian Oleander, White Oleander	Ayurvedic
Shataparvaa	*Acorus calamus*	Sweet Flag, Calamus	Ayurvedic
Shatapatri	*Chrysanthemum indicum*	Chrysanthemum	Ayurvedic
Shatapatri	*Rosa centifolia*	Cabbage Rose, Provence Rose, Hundred-leaved Rose	Ayurvedic
Shatapushpaa	*Anethum sowa*	Indian Dill, Sowa	Ayurvedic
Shatapushpaa	*Foeniculum vulgare*	Fennel	Ayurvedic
Shathi	*Hedychium spicatum*	Spiked Ginger Ivy	Ayurvedic
Shati (South)	*Kaempferia galanga*	Marba	Folk
Shati	*Curcuma zedoaria*	Zedoary, Zerumbet	Ayurvedic
Shati	*Hedychium coronarium*	Ginger Ivy	Ayurvedic
Shati	*Hedychium spicatum*	Spiked Ginger Ivy	Ayurvedic

Table Contd.

Indian Name	Botanical Name	English Name	Medicinal System
Shatkabhedi	*Aerva lanata*	Mountain Knot Grass	Ayurvedic
Shatmuuli	*Asparagus racemosus*	Indian Asparagus, Wild Asparagus	Ayurvedic
Shatpadi	*Asparagus racemosus*	Indian Asparagus, Wild Asparagus	Ayurvedic
Shatparvaa	*Bambusa bambos*	Spiny or Thorny Bamboo	Ayurvedic
Shatparvaa	*Cynodon dactylon*	Bermuda Grass, Bahama Grass, Couch Grass	Ayurvedic
Shatparvaa	*Picrorhiza kurroa*	Picrorhiza	Ayurvedic
Shatpatrikaa	*Rosa centifolia*	Cabbage Rose, Provence Rose, Hundred-leaved Rose	Ayurvedic
Shatvalli	*Cynodon dactylon*	Bermuda Grass, Bahama Grass, Couch Grass	Ayurvedic
Shatvedhani	*Rumex crispus*	Yellow Dock, Curled Dock	Ayurvedic
Shatviryaa	*Asparagus racemosus*	Indian Asparagus, Wild Asparagus	Ayurvedic
Shatviryaa	*Cynodon dactylon*	Bermuda Grass, Bahama Grass, Couch Grass	Ayurvedic
Shaukaraan	*Conium maculatum*	Spotted Hemlock, Poison Hemlock	Unani
Shaundi	*Piper longum*	Indian Long Pepper, Joborandi	Ayurvedic
Sheeta-bhiru	*Vitex negundo*	Five-leaved Chaste Tree	Ayurvedic
Sheetalchini	*Piper cubeba*	Cubeb, Tailed Pepper	Ayurvedic
Sheetavalli	*Ipomoea eriocarpa*	Tiny Morning Glory, Wooly-Fruited Morning Glory	Ayurvedic
Sheet-phala	*Adansonia digitata*	Baobab, Monkey Bread Tree, African Calabash	Ayurvedic
Sheetraj Hindi	*Plumbago zeylanica*	Ceylon Leadwort	Unani
Shelu	*Cordia myxa*	Sabestan Plum	Ayurvedic
Shemai-seeragam	*Carum bulbocastanum*	Black Caraway	Siddha/Tamil
Shemai-tutti	*Althaea officinalis*	Marshmallow, Hollyhock	Siddha/Tamil
Shembudu	*Waltheria indica*	Boater Bush, Buff Coat' Leather Coat, Sleepy Morning	Siddha/Tamil
Shempuvan	*Euphoria longan*	Longan	Siddha/Tamil
Shephaali	*Nyctanthes arbor-tristis*	Tree of Sorrow, Night Jasmine, Coral Jasmine	Ayurvedic

Table Contd.

Indian Name	Botanical Name	English Name	Medicinal System
Shephaalikaa	*Nyctanthes arbor-tristis*	Tree of Sorrow, Night Jasmine, Coral Jasmine	Ayurvedic
Shephaalikaa	*Vitex negundo*	Five-leaved Chaste Tree	Ayurvedic
Sherundi	*Ochna jabotapita*	Bird's Eye Bush	Folk/Tamil
Shibt	*Anethum sowa*	Indian Dill, Sowa	Unani
Shiddar	*Quercus incana*	Grey Oak	Folk
Shighraa	*Baliospermum montanum*	False Croton	Ayurvedic
Shigru (Red var.)	*Moringa concanensis*	Drumstick, Horse-Radish	Ayurvedic
Shigru (white var.)	*Moringa pterygosperma*	Drumstick, Horse-Radish	Ayurvedic
Shikaakaai	*Acacia concinna*	Soap-nut Acacia	Unani
Shikhari	*Achyranthes aspera*	Prickly Chaff Flower	Ayurvedic
Shikhi	*Blepharis edulis*	Acanthus	Ayurvedic
Shilaa Supaari	*Quercus incana*	Grey Oak	Folk
Shilaabheda	*Bergenia ligulata*	Elephant-Ear, Siberian Saxifrage	Ayurvedic
Shilaabhit	*Bergenia ligulata*	Elephant-Ear, Siberian Saxifrage	Ayurvedic
Shilaadaaru	*Parmelia perlata*	Parmelia Lichen	Ayurvedic
Shilaa-pushpa	*Didymocarpus pedicellata*	Rock Flower, Stone-Breaker	Ayurvedic
Shilaapushpa	*Parmelia perlata*	Parmelia Lichen	Ayurvedic
Shilaarasa	*Altingia excelsa*	Storax, Oriental Sweet Gum	Ayurvedic
Shilaatikaa	*Trianthema portulacastrum*	Horse Purslane	Ayurvedic
Shilaa-valkaa	*Didymocarpus pedicellata*	Rock Flower, Stone-Breaker	Ayurvedic
Shilodbhava	*Parmelia perlata*	Parmelia Lichen	Ayurvedic
Shimai chamantipu	*Anthemis nobilis*	Roman Chamomile, Double Chamomile	Folk/Tamil
Shimai eluppai	*Achras zapota*	Sapota, Sapodilla Plum, Chicle	Siddha/Tamil
Shimaimathala	*Cydonia oblonga*	Quince Fruit	Siddha/Tamil
Shimaishembu	*Carum carvi*	Caraway	Siddha/Tamil
Shimbi	*Phaseolus lunatus*	Double Bean, Lima Bean, Burma Bean	Ayurvedic

Table Contd.

Indian Name	Botanical Name	English Name	Medicinal System
Shriparni	*Premna integrifolia*	Headache Tree	Ayurvedic
Shriparnikaa	*Myrica nagi*	Box Myrtle	Ayurvedic
Shriphala	*Aegle marmelos*	Bael Tree, Bengal Quince	Ayurvedic
Shriphalaa	*Indigofera tinctoria*	Indigo	Ayurvedic
Shriprasuunaka	*Syzygium aromaticum*	Clove	Ayurvedic
Shrisangya	*Syzygium aromaticum*	Clove	Ayurvedic
Shrivalli	*Acacia concinna*	Soap-nut Acacia	Ayurvedic
Shrivara	*Mussaenda frondosa*	White Lady, White Rag Plant	Folk
Shrivati	*Mussaenda frondosa*	White Lady, White Rag Plant	Ayurvedic
Shriveshtaka (Oleo-resin)	*Pinus roxburghii*	Long-leaved Pine, Three-leaved Pine, Chir Pine	Ayurvedic
Shrngaata	*Trapa bispinosa*	Water Chestnut	Ayurvedic
Shrngaataka	*Trapa bispinosa*	Water Chestnut	Ayurvedic
Shrngamuula	*Trapa bispinosa*	Water Chestnut	Ayurvedic
Shrngavera	*Zingiber officinale*	Ginger	Ayurvedic
Shrngibera	*Zingiber officinale*	Ginger	Ayurvedic
Shubhaa	*Bambusa bambos*	Spiny or Thorny Bamboo	Ayurvedic
Shukaayi	*Volutarella ramosa*	Volutarella	Unani
Shuka-dhaanya	*Hordeum vulgare*	Barley	Ayurvedic
Shukanaasaa	*Corallocarpus epigaeus*	Indian Bryonia	Ayurvedic
Shukapushpa	*Taxus baccata*	European Yew	Ayurvedic
Shukchin	*Smilax lanceifolia*	Himalayan China Root	Folk
Shukla-ajaaji	*Cuminum cyminum*	Cumin	Ayurvedic
Shuklakandaa	*Aconitum heterophyllum*	Atis Root, Aconite	Ayurvedic
Shukranaashana	*Cannabis sativa*	Hemp, Indian Hemp	Ayurvedic
Shukrapushpikaa	*Gloriosa superba*	Glory Lily, Super Lily, Tiger's Claws	Ayurvedic
Shulundu-kora	*Ixora parviflora*	Torchwood Tree	Siddha/Tamil
Shunthi (Dried rhizome)	*Zingiber officinale*	Ginger	Ayurvedic
Shutthi	*Vernonia javanica*	Java Fleabane	Siddha/Tamil
Shuukashimbi	*Mucuna prurita*	Cowhage, Horse-eye Bean	Ayurvedic
Shuukraan	*Hyoscyamus muticus*	Egyptian Henbane	Unani

Table Contd.

Indian Name	Botanical Name	English Name	Medicinal System
Shuulaghni	*Ocimum sanctum*	Holy Basil, Sacred Basil	Ayurvedic
Shuulikaa	*Acacia arabica*	Babul, Black Babul, Indian Gum Arabic Tree	Ayurvedic
Shuunyamadhya	*Arundo donax*	Great Reed, Spanish-Bamboo-Reed, Giant-Bamboo-Reed	Ayurvedic
Shvadamshtraa	*Tribulus terrestris*	Land-Caltrops, Puncture Vine	Ayurvedic
Shveta Apaamaarga	*Achyranthes bidentata*	White Chaff Flower	Ayurvedic
Shveta Babbuula	*Acacia senegal*	Gum Arabic Tree	Ayurvedic
Shveta Khadira	*Acacia suma*	White Babul	Ayurvedic
Shveta Kutaja	*Wrightia tinctoria*	Pala Indigo Plant	Ayurvedic
Shveta Punarnavaa	*Boerhavia verticillata*	White-flowered Hogweed	Ayurvedic
Shveta Saarivaa	*Hemidesmus indicus*	Indian Sarsaparilla	Ayurvedic
Shveta Sarshapa	*Brassica alba*	White Mustard	Ayurvedic
Shveta Taruni	*Rosa alba*	Common English Dog Rose, White Cottage Rose	Ayurvedic
Shveta Vachaa	*Iris ensata*	Japanese Iris	Ayurvedic
Shveta Vachaa	*Iris germanica*	Orris, Iridis Rhizome, German Iris	Ayurvedic
Shvetaarka	*Calotropis gigantea*	Swallow Wort	Ayurvedic
Shveta-chaamara	*Saccharum spontaneum*	Thatch Grass, Wild Sugarcane	Ayurvedic
Shvetachandana	*Santalum album*	White Sandalwood	Ayurvedic
Shveta-Garjan	*Dipterocarpus alatus*	Gurjun	Ayurvedic
Shveta-jiraka	*Cuminum cyminum*	Cumin	Ayurvedic
Shveta-murga	*Celosia argentea*	Wild Cook's Comb	Folk
Shveta-punarnavaa	*Trianthema portulacastrum*	Horse Purslane	Ayurvedic
Shvetaraaji	*Trichosanthes anguina*	Snake-Gourd	Ayurvedic
Shveta-Shaalmali	*Ceiba pentandra*	White Silk Cotton Tree	Ayurvedic
Shveta-sursaa	*Eruca sativa*	Rocket-Salad	Ayurvedic
Shveta-vachaa	*Paris polyphylla*	Herb Paris, Tingling Rootstock Plant	Ayurvedic
Shyaama	*Cryptolepis buchanani*	Indian Sarsaparilla	Ayurvedic

Table Contd.

Indian Name	Botanical Name	English Name	Medicinal System
Shyaamaa	*Ipomoea petaloidea*	False Jalap, Hawaii Morning Glory	Ayurvedic
Shyaamaa	*Operculina turpethum*	Indian Jalap, Turpeth	Ayurvedic
Shyaamaaka	*Echinochloa frumentacea*	Japanese Barnyard Millet	Ayurvedic
Shyaamabija	*Ipomoea nil*	Pharbitis Seeds	Ayurvedic
Shyaamalataa	*Ichnocarpus frutescens*	Black Creeper	Ayurvedic
Shyaamguptaa	*Mucuna prurita*	Cowhage, Horse-eye Bean	Ayurvedic
Shyaamkandaa	*Aconitum palmatum*	Himalayan Aconite	Ayurvedic
Shyamaa	*Callicarpa macrophylla*	Perfumed Cherry	Ayurvedic
Shyamalataa	*Cryptolepis buchanani*	Indian Sarsaparilla	Ayurvedic
Shyonaaka	*Oroxylum indicum*	Indian Trumpet Flower	Ayurvedic
Sibr (Dried leaf juice)	*Aloe barbadensis*	Curacao Aloe, Barbados Aloe, Indian Aloe, Jaffarabad Aloe	Unani
Siddaartha	*Eruca sativa*	Rocket-Salad	Ayurvedic
Siddha	*Lagerstroemia parviflora*	Lendi, Benteak	Ayurvedic
Siddhaartha	*Brassica alba*	White Mustard	Ayurvedic
Siddhaartha	*Brassica campestris*	Field Mustard, Turnip Rape	Ayurvedic
Siddhaartha	*Brassica napus*	Mustard, Indian Rape	Ayurvedic
Siddhaarthaka	*Brassica napus*	Mustard, Indian Rape	Ayurvedic
Siddhaarthasita	*Brassica napus*	Mustard, Indian Rape	Ayurvedic
Siddhaka	*Lagerstroemia parviflora*	Lendi, Benteak	Ayurvedic
Siddhapushpa	*Nerium indicum*	Indian Oleander, White Oleander	Ayurvedic
Sigakai	*Acacia concinna*	Soap-nut Acacia	Siddha/Tamil
Sigra	*Moringa pterygosperma*	Drumstick, Horse-Radish	Ayurvedic
Sihoraa	*Streblus asper*	Siamese Rough Brush	Folk
Sikhi	*Plumbago zeylanica*	Ceylon Leadwort	Ayurvedic
Sikkaa	*Hovenia dulcis*	Japanese Raisin Tree, Coral Tree	Folk
Silaajit	*Styrax officinale*	The True Storax Tree	Folk
Silaaras (var.)	*Liquidambar formosana*	Fragrant Maple	Unani

Table Contd.

Indian Name	Botanical Name	English Name	Medicinal System
Silaaras	*Liquidambar orientalis*	Storax, Oriental Sweet Gum	Unani
Silaarasa	*Styrax officinale*	The True Storax Tree	Ayurvedic
Silamishri	*Orchis latifolia*	Orchis, Salep	Siddha/Tamil
Silhak (var.)	*Liquidambar formosana*	Fragrant Maple	Ayurvedic
Silhaka	*Altingia excelsa*	Storax, Oriental Sweet Gum	Ayurvedic
Silhaka	*Liquidambar orientalis*	Storax, Oriental Sweet Gum	Ayurvedic
Silhaka	*Styrax officinale*	The True Storax Tree	Ayurvedic
Silingi	*Osmanthus fragrans*	Sweet Olive Tree	Folk
Siltimur	*Lindera neesiana*	Spicebush, Benjamin Bush	Folk
Simaidevadaru	*Pinus roxburghii*	Long-leaved Pine, Three-leaved Pine, Chir Pine	Siddha/Tamil
Simainayuruvi	*Stachytarpheta jamaicensis*	Brazilian Tea, Bastard Vervain, Aaron's Rod	Siddha/Tamil
Simaiyalavinai	*Peganum harmala*	Wild Rue, Foreign Henna, Syrian Rue	Siddha/Tamil
Simbitikaa	*Cydonia oblonga*	Quince Fruit	Ayurvedic
Simeyaranelli	*Malpighia punicifolia*	West Indian Cherry	Folk
Simhaasya	*Adhatoda vasica*	Malabar Nut, Vasaca	Ayurvedic
Simhakeshara	*Mimusops elengi*	Spanish-Cherry, West Indian Medlar, Bullet Wood	Ayurvedic
Simhaparni	*Adhatoda vasica*	Malabar Nut, Vasaca	Ayurvedic
Simhapushpi	*Uraria picta*	Trailing Uraria	Ayurvedic
Simhavadanaa	*Adhatoda vasica*	Malabar Nut, Vasaca	Ayurvedic
Simhi	*Solanum ferox*	Poison-Berry	Ayurvedic
Simsipaa	*Dalbergia latifolia*	East Indian Rosewood, Bombay Blackwood	Ayurvedic
Sinappu	*Lagerstroemia indica*	Common Crape Myrtle	Folk/Tamil
Sinchitikaa	*Malus pumila*	Cultivated Apple	Ayurvedic
Sindhuka	*Vitex negundo*	Five-leaved Chaste Tree	Ayurvedic
Sindhuvaarak	*Vitex negundo*	Five-leaved Chaste Tree	Ayurvedic
Sinduri	*Bixa orellana*	Annatto	Ayurvedic
Sinduriyaa	*Bixa orellana*	Annatto	Ayurvedic
Sinduvaarak	*Vitex trifolia*	Three-leaved Vitex	Ayurvedic
Singara	*Trapa bispinosa*	Water Chestnut	Siddha/Tamil

Table Contd.

Indian Name	Botanical Name	English Name	Medicinal System
Singarauti	*Pentatropis microphylla*	Ambervel, Beak-shaped Elliptic Flower	Folk
Singhaaraa	*Castanea sativa*	Spanish Chestnut, Sweet Chestnut	Folk
Singhaaraa	*Trapa bispinosa*	Water Chestnut	Unani
Singhtunda	*Euphorbia neriifolia*	Holy Milk Hedge, Dog's Tongue	Ayurvedic
Singri	*Raphanus sativus*	Radish	Ayurvedic
Sinna Kambil	*Gardenia gummifera*	Gummy Cape Jasmine	Siddha/Tamil
Sinnangurinji	*Nilgirianthus ciliatus*	Kurunji	Siddha/Tamil
Sinnun	*Fraxinus hookery*	European Ash, Weeping Ash	Folk
Sipandaan	*Lepidium sativum*	Gardencress, Tongue Grass	Unani
Sipil	*Bupleurum flacutum*	Hare's Ear	Folk
Siras	*Albizia lebbeck*	Siris Tree, East Indian Walnut	Unani
Sirikramaa	*Gloriosa superba*	Glory Lily, Super Lily, Tiger's Claws	Ayurvedic
Sirmaa	*Hippophae rhamnoides*	Seabuckthorn, Sand Thorn	Folk
Sirrali (Seed)	*Linum usitatissimum*	Linseed, Flax	Siddha/Tamil
Sirrukaanchori	*Tragia involucrata*	Indian Stinging-Nettle	Siddha/Tamil
Siru Pasalai-keerai	*Portulaca quadrifida*	Chicken Weed	Siddha/Tamil
Siru seruppadai	*Glinus lotoides*	Lotus Sweetjuice, Damascisa	Siddha/Tamil
Siru thekku	*Pygmaeopremna herbacea*	Bharangi Tree, Qian jie cao (Chinese)	Siddha/Tamil
Sirukeerai	*Amaranthus caudatus*	Love-Lies-Bleeding, Tassel Flower	Siddha/Tamil
Siru-keerai	*Amaranthus tricolor*	Chinese Spinach, Garden Amaranth, Fountain Plant	Folk/Tamil
Sirunagappo	*Mesua ferrea*	Iron-wood, Mesu	Siddha/Tamil
Sirunerunchil	*Tribulus terrestris*	Land-Caltrops, Puncture Vine	Siddha/Tamil
Sirunochi	*Vitex trifolia*	Three-leaved Vitex	Siddha/Tamil
Sirupoolai	*Aerva lanata*	Mountain Knot Grass	Siddha/Tamil
Siruppunaikkali	*Passiflora foetida*	Stinking Passion Flower	Folk/Tamil
Sirupulladi Moovilai (root)	*Desmodium gangeticum*	Shaalparni, Beggarweed	Siddha/Tamil

Table Contd.

Indian Name	Botanical Name	English Name	Medicinal System
Sirusavakku	*Tamarix indica*	Takut Galls	Siddha/Tamil
Siruvalli Kilangu	*Dioscorea esculenta*	Lesser Yam, Karen Potato	Siddha/Tamil
Siruyilandai	*Ximenia americana*	Tallow-Wood, False Sandal-Wood	Folk/Tamil
Sisau	*Dalbergia sissoides*	Malabar Blackwood	Folk
Sismulia	*Murdannia scapiflora*	Few-flowered Dewflower	Folk
Sitaabhra	*Cinnamomum camphora*	Camphor Tree	Ayurvedic
Sitaakesh	*Ipomoea quamoclit*	Cypress Vine, Indian Pink	Folk
Sitaaphala	*Annona squamosa*	Custard Apple, Sugar Apple, Sweet-sop	Ayurvedic
Sitaaphalam	*Annona squamosa*	Custard Apple, Sugar Apple, Sweet-sop	Siddha/Tamil
Sitammapogunalu	*Cuscuta epithymum*	Lesser Doddar, Hellweed, Devil's Guts	Folk/Telugu
Sithamutti	*Pavonia zeylanica*	Fragrant Swamp Mallow	Siddha/Tamil
Sittirappaladai	*Uraria picta*	Trailing Uraria	Siddha/Tamil
Sittrapaladi	*Euphorbia thymifolia*	Thyme-leaf Spurge	Siddha/Tamil
Sivaar	*Ceratophyllum demersum*	Coontail, Hornwort	Folk
Sivadari	*Erythroxylum coca*	Coca, Cocaine Plant	Siddha/Tamil
Sivakraandi	*Convolvulus pluricaulis*	Conch-flowered Bindweed, White-flowered Shankhpushpi	Siddha/Tamil
Sivanaarvembu	*Indigofera aspalathoides*	Wiry Indigo	Siddha/Tamil
Sivanarvembu	*Justica tranquebariensis*	Pindi	Folk
Sivappattusha-vukku	*Tamarix aphylla*	Athel, Tamarisk	Siddha/Tamil
Sivappu	*Papaver rhoeas*	Corn Poppy, Red Poppy	Siddha/Tamil
Sivappu kashmakki	*Hibiscus sabdariffa*	Roselle, Jamaican Sorrel, Natal Sorrel, Red Sorrel	Siddha/Tamil
Sivappu Mandaarai	*Bauhinia purpurea*	Camel's Foot Tree, Pink Bauhinia, Butterfly Tree, Geramium Tree, Orchid Tree	Siddha/Tamil
Sivappumanchori	*Bauhinia variegata*	Mountain Ebony, Buddhist Bauhinia	Siddha/Tamil
Sivappuparutthi	*Gossypium arboreum*	Tree Cotton, Desi Cotton	Siddha/Tamil

Table Contd.

Indian Name	Botanical Name	English Name	Medicinal System
Sivapputtutti	*Abroma augusta*	Perennial Indian Hemp, Devil's Cotton	Siddha/Tamil
Siyaah Musli	*Murdannia scapiflora*	Few-flowered Dewflower	Siddha/Tamil
Skandhaphala	*Cocos nucifera*	Coconut Palm	Ayurvedic
Skullcap	*Scutellaria galericulata*	Scurvey Grass, Marsh Skullcap	Folk
Smar-e-Gul	*Rosa damascena*	Damask Rose	Unani
Snehphala	*Sesamum indicum*	Sesame, Gingelly	Ayurvedic
Snigdh-pinditaka	*Vangueria spinosa*	Voa-Vanga	Ayurvedic
Snuhi	*Euphorbia antiquorum*	Triangular Spurge	Ayurvedic
Snuhi	*Euphorbia neriifolia*	Holy Milk Hedge, Dog's Tongue	Ayurvedic
Snuhi	*Euphorbia nivulia*	Corky-barked Spurge	Ayurvedic
Snuhi	*Euphorbia royleana*	Thor Spurge	Ayurvedic
Snuk	*Euphorbia neriifolia*	Holy Milk Hedge, Dog's Tongue	Ayurvedic
Snuk	*Euphorbia royleana*	Thor Spurge	Ayurvedic
Sodakku Thakkali	*Physalis minima*	Sun-berry	Siddha/Tamil
Soma	*Psoralea corylifolia*	Purple Fleabane	Ayurvedic
Somakaa	*Berberis aristata*	Indian Barberry	Ayurvedic
Soma-kalp	*Ephedra gerardiana*	Ephedra	Folk
Somakshiri	*Sarcostemma brevistigma*	Moon Plant, Soma Plant	Ayurvedic
Somalataa	*Sarcostemma brevistigma*	Moon Plant, Soma Plant	Ayurvedic
Somamum	*Sarcostemma brevistigma*	Moon Plant, Soma Plant	Siddha/Tamil
Somanthiri	*Xylocarpus granatum*	The Puzzle Fruit Tree	Folk/Tamil
Somaraaji	*Centratherum anthelminticum*	Purple Flea-bane, Achenes	Ayurvedic
Somaraaji	*Psoralea corylifolia*	Purple Fleabane	Ayurvedic
Somavalka	*Acacia catechu*	Cutch tree, Catechu	Ayurvedic
Soma-valka	*Ficus dalhousiae*	Carica Fig	Ayurvedic
Somavalkala	*Acacia suma*	White Babul	Ayurvedic
Soma-valli	*Ephedra gerardiana*	Ephedra	Ayurvedic
Somavalli	*Psoralea corylifolia*	Purple Fleabane	Ayurvedic

Table Contd.

Indian Name	Botanical Name	English Name	Medicinal System
Somavalli	*Sarcostemma brevistigma*	Moon Plant, Soma Plant	Ayurvedic
Somavalli	*Sarcostemma brevistigma*	Moon Plant, Soma Plant	Siddha/Tamil
Somavallik	*Psoralea corylifolia*	Purple Fleabane	Ayurvedic
Sombu	*Foeniculum vulgare*	Fennel	Siddha/Tamil
Somi-maram	*Soymida febrifuga*	Indian Red-Wood, Bastard Cedar	Siddha/Tamil
Somvalli	*Crinum latifolium*	Wide-leaved Crinum	Ayurvedic
Somyaa	*Desmodium gangeticum*	Shaalparni, Beggarweed	Ayurvedic
Sonaamukhi	*Cassia angustifolia*	Indian senna, Tinnevelly senna	Unani
Sonaamukhi	*Cassia obovata*	Spanish, Sudan Senna	Folk
Sonaa-paathaa	*Oroxylum indicum*	Indian Trumpet Flower	Folk
Sonapaati	*Tecoma stans*	Yellow Elder, Yellow Bells	Siddha/Tamil
Sonapushpaka	*Bauhinia variegata*	Mountain Ebony, Buddhist Bauhinia	Ayurvedic
Soorai	*Ziziphus oenoplia*	Jackal Jujube	Siddha/Tamil
Sophkrit	*Semecarpus anacardium*	Marking-Nut	Ayurvedic
Sorapinnai	*Rhizophora mucronata*	True Mangrove	Siddha/Tamil
Sosan	*Iris ensata*	Japanese Iris	Unani
Sosan	*Iris nepalensis*	Nepal Iris	Folk
Sottai-kala	*Flacourtia indica*	Ramontchi, Madagascar Plum, Mauritius Plum, Governor's Plum	Siddha/Tamil
Sowdangigida	*Solanum erianthum*	Mullen Nightshade	Folk
Soyaa	*Anethum sowa*	Indian Dill, Sowa	Unani
Soyabean	*Glycine max*	Soybean, Soya	Folk
Spergularia	*Spergularia rubra*	Red Sand-Spurry, Sandwort, Arenaria Rubra	Folk
Sphotaa	*Hemidesmus indicus*	Indian Sarsaparilla	Ayurvedic
Sphuurjaka	*Diospyros embryopteris*	Gaub Persimmon, Riber Ebony	Ayurvedic
Sprikkaa	*Anisomeles malabarica*	Malabar Catmint	Ayurvedic
Sprikkaa	*Delphinium brunonianum*	Musk Larkspur	Ayurvedic
Sprikkaa	*Delphinium zalil*	Zalil Larkspur	Ayurvedic

Table Contd.

Indian Name	Botanical Name	English Name	Medicinal System
Sprk	*Schizachyrium exile*	Fakara Beardgrass	Ayurvedic
Sprkaa	*Schizachyrium exile*	Fakara Beardgrass	Ayurvedic
Spruce (trade)	*Picea smithiana*	West Himalayan Spruce	Folk
Sraavikaa	*Claviceps purpurea*	Ergot of Rye, Fungus of Rye	Ayurvedic
Sransi	*Salvadora persica*	Mustard Tree, Salt Bush Tree, Tooth Brush Tree	Ayurvedic
Sriparni	*Gmelina arborea*	Candahar Tree, White Teak	Ayurvedic
Sruva-vriksha	*Flacourtia indica*	Ramontchi, Madagascar Plum, Mauritius Plum, Governor's Plum	Ayurvedic
Sruva-Vriksha	*Gymnosporia spinosa*	Celastrus Tree	Ayurvedic
Stalai	*Jatropha gossypifolia*	Physic Nut, Purging Nut	Siddha/Tamil
Sthaavaravisha	*Aconitum ferox*	Indian Aconite, Wolfsbane, Monkshood	Ayurvedic
Sthala-Padam	*Hibiscus mutabilis*	Cotton-Rose, Chinese-Rose, Confederate Rose	Ayurvedic
Sthal-Kamal	*Hibiscus mutabilis*	Cotton-Rose, Chinese-Rose, Confederate Rose	Ayurvedic
Sthauneya	*Taxus baccata*	European Yew	Ayurvedic
Sthauneyaka	*Taxus baccata*	European Yew	Ayurvedic
Sthavira	*Argyreia speciosa*	Elephant Creeper	Ayurvedic
Sthavira	*Parmelia perlata*	Parmelia Lichen	Ayurvedic
Sthaviradaaru	*Argyreia speciosa*	Elephant Creeper	Ayurvedic
Sthiraa	*Desmodium gangeticum*	Shaalparni, Beggarweed	Ayurvedic
Sthiraa	*Mimusops elengi*	Spanish-Cherry, West Indian Medlar, Bullet Wood	Ayurvedic
Sthiraayu	*Salmalia malabarica*	Silk Cotton Tree, Semul Tree	Ayurvedic
Sthirapushpa	*Mimusops elengi*	Spanish-Cherry, West Indian Medlar, Bullet Wood	Ayurvedic
Sthirphala	*Berberis aristata*	Indian Barberry	Ayurvedic
Sthula-elaa	*Amomum aromaticum*	Bengal Cardamom, Cardamom	Ayurvedic
Sthula-elaa	*Amomum subulatum*	Greater or Nepal Cardamom	Ayurvedic
Sthula-eranda	*Jatropha curcas*	Physic Nut, Purging Nut	Ayurvedic

Table Contd.

Indian Name	Botanical Name	English Name	Medicinal System
Sthula-granthi	*Zingiber zerumbet*	Zerumbet Ginger	Ayurvedic
Sthulajiraka	*Nigella sativa*	Black Cumin, Small Fennel	Ayurvedic
Sthulavalkal	*Symplocos racemosa*	Lodh Tree, Sapphire Berry	Ayurvedic
Sthuulagranthi	*Alpinia galanga*	Greater Galangal	Ayurvedic
Subul-e-Barri	*Asarum europaeum*	Asarbacca, Hazelwort, Wild Nard	Unani
Sudaab	*Ruta graveolens*	Garden Rue	Unani
Sudarshana	*Crinum asiaticum*	St. John's Lily, Poison Bulb	Ayurvedic
Sudarshana	*Crinum latifolium*	Wide-leaved Crinum	Ayurvedic
Suddaab	*Ruta graveolens*	Garden Rue	Unani
Sudhaa	*Euphorbia neriifolia*	Holy Milk Hedge, Dog's Tongue	Ayurvedic
Sudhaa-muuli	*Eulophia campestris*	Salep Orchid	Ayurvedic
Sudukadu Mallikai	*Vinca rosea*	Madagascar Periwinkle	Siddha/Tamil
Sugandha udgaar	*Carum carvi*	Caraway	Ayurvedic
Sugandhaa	*Alpinia galanga*	Greater Galangal	Ayurvedic
Sugandha-baalaa	*Valeriana hardwickii*	Himalayan Valerian	Folk
Sugandhabaalaa	*Valeriana leschenaultii*	Nilgiri Valerian	Folk
Sugandha-baalaa	*Valeriana officinalis*	Valerian, Garden Heliotrope, Common Valerian	Folk
Sugandhabaalaa	*Valeriana pyrolaefolia*	Smaller-rhizome Jatamansi	Folk
Sugandhabaalaa	*Valeriana wallichii*	Indian Valerian	Ayurvedic
Sugandha-Kuutth	*Saussurea lappa*	Kuth, Costus	Folk
Sugandhapatra	*Eucalyptus globulus*	Blue-gum Tree, Australian Gum Tree	Ayurvedic
Sugandha-vachaa	*Kaempferia galanga*	Maraba	Ayurvedic
Sugandhbaalaa	*Pavonia odorata*	Fragrant Sticky Mallow	Ayurvedic
Sugandhi Paanadi	*Pogostemon patchouli*	Patchouli	Folk
Sugandhikaa	*Vitex negundo*	Five-leaved Chaste Tree	Ayurvedic
Sugandhimuula	*Vetiveria zizanioides*	Vetiver, Khas	Ayurvedic
Sugandh-kokilaa	*Luvunga scandens*	Woody Clove Vine	Folk
Sugandh-vaastuuka	*Chenopodium ambrosioides*	Indian Wormseed, Sweet Pigweed, Mexican Tea	Ayurvedic

Table Contd.

Indian Name	Botanical Name	English Name	Medicinal System
Suganthipala	*Hemidesmus indicus*	Indian Sarsaparilla	Siddha/Tamil
Sukaandaka	*Ranunculus sceleratus*	Blister Buttercup, Celery-leaved Crowfoot	Ayurvedic
Sukaayi	*Volutarella ramosa*	Volutarella	Folk
Sukatsing	*Sarcococca saligna*	Christmas Box	Folk
Sukhaatmaka	*Origanum majorana*	Sweet Marjoram	Ayurvedic
Sukhadarshana	*Crinum latifolium*	Wide-leaved Crinum	Ayurvedic
Sukshm patraka	*Betula utilis*	Himalayan Silver Birch, Indian Paper Tree	Ayurvedic
Sukshmailaa	*Elettaria cardamomum*	Lesser Cardamom	Ayurvedic
Sukshmapatra	*Acacia arabica*	Babul, Black Babul, Indian Gum Arabic Tree	Ayurvedic
Sukshmapatra	*Fumaria parviflora*	Fumitory	Ayurvedic
Suktaa	*Tamarindus indica*	Tamarind Tree	Ayurvedic
Sulabhaa	*Ocimum sanctum*	Holy Basil, Sacred Basil	Ayurvedic
Sulambuli	*Garcinia mangostana*	Mangosteen, Dodol	Siddha/Tamil
Sulemaani Khajuur	*Phoenix sylvestris*	Wild Date Palm	Folk
Sulomaasha	*Leea aequata*	Black-berry Holly	Ayurvedic
Sulomashaa	*Nardostachys jatamansi*	Spikenard, Musk-root	Ayurvedic
Sulomshaa	*Peristrophe bicalyculata*	Panicled Peristrophe	Ayurvedic
Sult	*Avena sativa*	Oat, Common Oat	Unani
Sultaan Champaa	*Calophyllum inophyllum*	Indian Laurel, Alexandrian Laurel	Ayurvedic
Sum	*Fraxinus hookery*	European Ash, Weeping Ash	Folk
Sumaaq	*Rhus coriaria*	European or Sicilian Sumach	Unani
Sumaaq	*Rhus parviflora*	Sumach	Unani
Sumanaa	*Jasminum officinale*	Spanish Jasmine	Ayurvedic
Sumanganaa	*Sida cordifolia*	Country Mallow	Ayurvedic
Sumbul	*Ferula sumbul*	Musk Root	Folk
Sumbul-e-Hindi	*Nardostachys jatamansi*	Spikenard, Musk-root	Unani
Sundaikkirai	*Neptunia oleracea*	Sensitive Plant	Siddha/Tamil
Sunishannaka	*Marsilea minuta*	Dwarf Waterclover, Pepperwort	Ayurvedic
Sunn	*Crotalaria juncea*	Sun Hemp	Unani

Table Contd.

Indian Name	Botanical Name	English Name	Medicinal System
Sunthi (Dried rhizome)	*Zingiber officinale*	Ginger	Siddha/Tamil
Supaari	*Areca catechu*	Areca Nut, Betel Nut	Unani
Suprasaraa	*Sida veronicaefolia*	Prostrate Mallow	Ayurvedic
Suraahva	*Cupressus sempervirens*	Mediterranean Cypress	Ayurvedic
Suraal	*Pueraria tuberosa*	Indian Kudze	Folk
Suraalu	*Dioscorea bulbifera*	Patoto Yam, Bulb-bearing Yam, Air Potato, Dog Yam	Ayurvedic
Surabhi	*Selinum tenuifolium*	Cow Parsley	Ayurvedic
Surabhichhada	*Feronia limonia*	Wood Apple	Ayurvedic
Surabhidaaru	*Curcuma amada*	Mango-ginger, Wild Turmeric	Ayurvedic
Surabhidaaruka	*Pinus roxburghii*	Long-leaved Pine, Three-leaved Pine, Chir Pine	Ayurvedic
Surabhini-nimba	*Murraya koenigii*	Curry-Leaf Tree	Ayurvedic
Surabhipatra	*Syzygium cuminii*	Java Plum, Jambolan, Black Plum	Ayurvedic
Surabhuruha	*Cedrus deodara*	Himalayan Cedar, Deodar	Ayurvedic
Suradaaru	*Cedrus deodara*	Himalayan Cedar, Deodar	Ayurvedic
Suradruma	*Cedrus deodara*	Himalayan Cedar, Deodar	Ayurvedic
Surai	*Euphorbia royleana*	Thor Spurge	Folk
Suraikai	*Lagenaria siceraria*	Bitter Bottle-Gourd	Siddha/Tamil
Suraikayi	*Cucurbita pepo*	Pumpin, Marrow	Siddha/Tamil
Surajaan Talkh	*Colchicum luteum*	Hermodactyls, Colchicum, Meadow Saffron, Golden Collyrium	Unani
Surajkaanti	*Belamcanda chinensis*	Leopard Lily	Folk/Assam
Surali	*Celosia argentea*	Wild Cook's Comb	Folk
Suram	*Cupressus sempervirens*	Mediterranean Cypress	Folk/Tamil
Suram	*Cupressus sempervirens*	Mediterranean Cypress	Siddha/Tamil
Suranga	*Caesalpinia sappan*	Sappan	Ayurvedic
Surangi	*Ochrocarpus longifolius*	Red-dye-flowerbud, Pseudo-Mesua ferra	Folk
Surapadi	*Leea aequata*	Black-berry Holly	Folk
Surapunnaaga	*Ochrocarpus longifolius*	Red-dye-flowerbud, Pseudo-Mesua ferra	Ayurvedic

Table Contd.

Indian Name	Botanical Name	English Name	Medicinal System
Surasa	*Balsamodendron myrrha*	Myrrh, Herabol	Ayurvedic
Surasa	*Ocimum sanctum*	Holy Basil, Sacred Basil	Ayurvedic
Surasaa	*Ocimum sanctum*	Holy Basil, Sacred Basil	Ayurvedic
Surataru	*Cedrus deodara*	Himalayan Cedar, Deodar	Ayurvedic
Suravaari Harad	*Terminalia citrina*	Bengal Myrobalan	Folk
Suravalli	*Ocimum sanctum*	Holy Basil, Sacred Basil	Ayurvedic
Suretaa	*Polycarpon prostratum*	Four-leaved Allseed	Folk
Suriaa	*Xylia xylocarpa*	Irul Tree	Folk
Surkh Kaner	*Nerium oleander*	Red Oleander, Rose Bay	Unani
Surkh Mirch	*Capsicum annuum*	Chilli, Red Pepper	Unani
Surkh Mirch	*Capsicum frutescens*	Bird Chilli	Unani
Surmai Nila	*Indigofera articulata*	Egyptian Indigo, Arabian Indigo, Wild Indigo, Surat Indigo	Folk
Surudu	*Symphorema involucratum*	Bhingri	Folk
Surulpattai	*Alkanna tinctoria*	Alkanet, Dyers' or Spanish Bugloss	Siddha/Tamil
Surya	*Calotropis procera*	Swallow-wort, Milk Weed, King's Crown	Ayurvedic
Suryakanti	*Helianthus annuus*	Sunflower	Siddha/Tamil
Sushaavi	*Momordica charantia*	Bitter Gourd, Balsam Pear, Carilla	Ayurvedic
Sushavi	*Calycopteris floribunda*	White Daisy	Ayurvedic
Sushavi	*Carum carvi*	Caraway	Ayurvedic
Sushavi	*Nigella sativa*	Black Cumin, Small Fennel	Ayurvedic
Sushena	*Carissa carandas*	Christ's Thorn, Bengal Currant	Ayurvedic
Sushenaa	*Operculina turpethum*	Indian Jalap, Turpeth	Ayurvedic
Susravaa	*Boswellia serrata*	Indian Frankincense, Indian Olibanum	Ayurvedic
Susunishaak	*Marsilea minuta*	Dwarf Waterclover, Pepperwort	Ayurvedic
Sutajva	*Drypetes roxburghii*	Putrajiva	Ayurvedic
Suthani	*Dioscorea esculenta*	Lesser Yam, Karen Potato	Folk

Table Contd.

Indian Name	Botanical Name	English Name	Medicinal System
Sutherlandia	*Sutherlandia frutescens*	Bladdersenna, Cancerwort, Cape Baloon Pea	Folk
Sutiktak	*Azadirachta indica*	Neem Tree, Margosa Tree	Ayurvedic
Sutrasowa	*Myrtus communis*	Myrtle, Clove Myrtle, Spanish Myrtle	Folk
Suuchi	*Atropa acuminata*	Indian Belladonna, Indian Atropa	Ayurvedic
Suuchikaa pushpaa	*Pandanus fascicularis*	Screw Pine	Ayurvedic
Suuchyagra	*Desmostachya bipinnata*	Sacrificial Grass	Ayurvedic
Suuchyagra	*Imperata cylindrica*	Thatch Grass	Ayurvedic
Suukshmamuulaa	*Sesbania sesban*	Common Sesban	Ayurvedic
Suukshma-patraa	*Sesbania sesban*	Common Sesban	Ayurvedic
Suurajmukhi	*Helianthus annuus*	Sunflower	Ayurvedic
Suurana	*Amorphophallus campanulatus*	Elephant's Foot Yam	Ayurvedic
Suurana	*Tacca pinnatifida*	Fiji Arrowroot, Tahiti Arrowroot	Ayurvedic
Suuryaahvya	*Calotropis procera*	Swallow-wort, Milk Weed, King's Crown	Ayurvedic
Suuryaasani	*Teramnus labialis*	Blue Wiss	Ayurvedic
Suuryaavart	*Chrozophora plicata*	Chrozophora	Ayurvedic
Suuryaavarta	*Helianthus annuus*	Sunflower	Ayurvedic
Suuryaparni	*Phaseolus trilobus*	Wild Gram	Ayurvedic
Suurya-vallabha	*Eclipta alba*	Trailing Eclipta Plant	Unani
Suvaa	*Marsdenia tenacissima*	White Turpeth	Ayurvedic
Suvaasaraa	*Lepidium sativum*	Gardencress, Tongue Grass	Ayurvedic
Suvahaa	*Eucalyptus globulus*	Blue-gum Tree, Australian Gum Tree	Ayurvedic
Suvahaa	*Operculina turpethum*	Indian Jalap, Turpeth	Ayurvedic
Suvahaa	*Pluchea lanceolata*	Rasana Shrub	Ayurvedic
Suvahaa	*Vitex negundo*	Five-leaved Chaste Tree	Ayurvedic
Suvarchalaa (var.)	*Malva sylvestris*	Common Mallow, Blue Mallow, High Mallow	Ayurvedic

Table Contd.

Indian Name	Botanical Name	English Name	Medicinal System
Tengari	*Tabernaemontana coronaria*	East Indian Rosebay	Folk
Tenkai	*Cocos nucifera*	Coconut Palm	Siddha/Tamil
Tennacham	*Sida rhombifolia*	Red-flowered Mallow	Siddha/Tamil
Tenti	*Capparis aphylla*	Caper Berry	Unani
Tesu	*Butea monosperma*	Flame of the Forest, Butea Gum, Bengal Kino	Folk
Tezhak	*Veronica beccabunga*	Brooklime	Folk
Tezma	*Iris kumaonensis*	Kumaon Iris	Folk
Thaalikeerai	*Ipomoea sepiaria*	Big-flowered Morning Glory	Siddha/Tamil
Thaamarai	*Nelumbo nucifera*	East Indian Lotus, Sacred Lotus	Siddha/Tamil
Thaanrikkaai	*Terminalia bellirica*	Belleric Myrobalan, Bastard Myrobalan	Siddha/Tamil
Thaanyo	*Bupleurum flacutum*	Hare's Ear	Folk
Thadachi	*Grewia asiatica*	Indian Phalsa	Siddha/Tamil
Thaelkodukkup-pondu	*Heliotropium indicum*	Scorpion Tail	Siddha/Tamil
Thaeyilai	*Camellia sinensis*	Tea Plant	Siddha/Tamil
Thaikala	*Garcinia pedunculata*	Bengal Brindleberry	Folk
Thaivelai	*Gynandropsis gynandra*	African Spider Plant	Siddha/Tamil
Thalay	*Pandanus fascicularis*	Screw Pine	Folk/Tamil
Thali	*Actinodaphne hookeri*	Pisa	Siddha/Tamil
Thandri	*Terminalia bellirica*	Belleric Myrobalan, Bastard Myrobalan	Siddha/Tamil
Thandu-keerai	*Amaranthus tricolor*	Chinese Spinach, Garden Amaranth, Fountain Plant	Folk/Tamil
Thaneervittan Kizhangu	*Asparagus racemosus*	Indian Asparagus, Wild Asparagus	Siddha/Tamil
Thanella	*Gardenia turgida*	Bharangi Bark Tree	Ayurvedic
Thanga arali	*Tecoma stans*	Yellow Elder, Yellow Bells	Siddha/Tamil
Thangi	*Corylus avellana*	Turkish Hazel	Folk
Tharbuzapalam	*Citrullus vulgaris*	Watermelon	Siddha/Tamil
Tharubai	*Desmostachya bipinnata*	Sacrificial Grass	Siddha/Tamil

Table Contd.

Indian Name	Botanical Name	English Name	Medicinal System
Thavasai murungai	*Sauropus androgynus*	Star Goose Berry	Siddha/Tamil
Thazhai	*Pandanus fascicularis*	Screw Pine	Folk/Tamil
Thazhuthaazhai	*Clerodendrum phlomidis*	Glory Bower	Siddha/Tamil
Theiarbawm	*Kadsura heteroclita*	Flashy-leaved Kadsura, Fructus kadsurae	Folk/Assam
Thekku	*Tectona grandis*	Teak Tree	Siddha/Tamil
Thelkaa	*Viburnum nervosum*	Rosy-flowered Guelder Rose	Folk
Thelkodukkukai	*Martynia annua*	Devil's Claw, Tiger Claw	Siddha/Tamil
Thengpren-keorong	*Microcos paniculata*	Kadamb	Folk/Assam
Thetrankottai	*Strychnos potatorum*	Clearing Nut Tree	Siddha/Tamil
Thettran	*Strychnos potatorum*	Clearing Nut Tree	Siddha/Tamil
Thevathaaram	*Cedrus deodara*	Himalayan Cedar, Deodar	Siddha/Tamil
Thippa Ragi	*Eleusine indica*	Crowfoot Grass, Crab Grass	Folk
Thippili	*Piper longum*	Indian Long Pepper, Joborandi	Siddha/Tamil
Thippili ver (root)	*Piper longum*	Indian Long Pepper, Joborandi	Siddha/Tamil
Thiratchai, Draksha	*Vitis vinifera*	Wine Grape, European Grape	Siddha/Tamil
Tholoo-pavai	*Momordica dioica*	Small Bitter Gourd, burr Cucumber	Siddha/Tamil
Thorilla	*Gordonia obtusa*	Loblolly Bay, Grey Laurel	Folk/South
Thottalsurungi	*Mimosa pudica*	Sensitive-plant, Humble-Plant	Siddha/Tamil
Thoyya-keerai	*Digera muricata*	Gitana Weed	Siddha/Tamil
Thuhar	*Euphorbia dracunculoides*	Dragon Spurge	Unani
Thulvkka Saamanthi	*Calendula officinalis*	Pot-Marigold, Marigold, Calendula	Siddha/Tamil
Thumbai	*Leucas aspera*	White Dead Nettle	Siddha/Tamil
Thumbi	*Diospyros melanoxylon*	Coromandel Ebony, Persimmon	Siddha/Tamil
Thunera	*Taxus baccata*	European Yew	Ayurvedic
Thungtu	*Viola pilosa*	Banafshah-oil Violet	Folk
Thuno	*Taxus baccata*	European Yew	Folk

Table Contd.

Indian Name	Botanical Name	English Name	Medicinal System
Thura	*Fumaria parviflora*	Fumitory	Siddha/Tamil
Thurinjippazham	*Citrus aurantifolia*	Acid or Sour Lime, Country Lime	Siddha/Tamil
Thurinjippazham	*Citrus medica*	Citron	Siddha/Tamil
Thuruksaamanthi	*Tagetes erecta*	Big Marigold, Aztec or African Marigold	Siddha/Tamil
Thusimullai	*Euphorbia dracunculoides*	Dragon Spurge	Siddha/Tamil
Thutthi	*Abutilon indicum*	Country Mallow, Flowering Maples, Chinese Bell-flowers	Siddha/Tamil
Thuuhar	*Euphorbia neriifolia*	Holy Milk Hedge, Dog's Tongue	Ayurvedic
Thuuhar	*Euphorbia royleana*	Thor Spurge	Unani
Thuvar kandan	*Kandelia rheedii*	Backwater Kandal Tree	Siddha/Tamil
Thuvarai	*Cajanus cajan*	Pigeon Pea, Red Gram	Siddha/Tamil
Tibali	*Dalbergia sympathetica*	Pentagul Tree	Folk
Tibbati Ginseng	*Chlorophytum arundinaceum*	White Musali	Folk
Tidhaaraa Sehunda	*Euphorbia antiquorum*	Triangular Spurge	Folk
Tiger Lily	*Hemerocallis fulva*	Common Yellow Day-lily, Tawny Day-lily, Orange Day-lily	Folk
Tiger Lily	*Lilium tigrinum*	Tiger Lily, Crumple Lily	Folk
Tikhur	*Curcuma angustifolia*	East Indian Arrowroot, Travancore Starch	Unani
Tikshnagandhaa	*Acorus calamus*	Sweet Flag, Calamus	Ayurvedic
Tikshnagandhaa	*Brassica juncea*	Chinese Mustard, Brown Mustard	Ayurvedic
Tikshnagandhaa	*Moringa pterygosperma*	Drumstick, Horse-Radish	Ayurvedic
Tikshnapatra	*Enicostemma littorale*	Indian Gentian	Ayurvedic
Tikshnashuka	*Hordeum vulgare*	Barley	Ayurvedic
Tikshnatandulaa	*Piper longum*	Indian Long Pepper, Joborandi	Ayurvedic
Tikshnavriksha	*Salvadora persica*	Mustard Tree, Salt Bush Tree, Tooth Brush Tree	Ayurvedic
Tiktaalaavu	*Lagenaria siceraria*	Bitter Bottle-Gourd	Ayurvedic

Table Contd.

Indian Name	Botanical Name	English Name	Medicinal System
Tiktaka	*Azadirachta indica*	Neem Tree, Margosa Tree	Ayurvedic
Tiktaka	*Zanonia indica*	Zanonia	Ayurvedic
Tiktakarkatikaa	*Cucumis sativus*	Cucumber	Ayurvedic
Tiktakoshtaki	*Luffa acutangula*	Ribbed or Ridged Gourd (bitter var.)	Ayurvedic
Tiktamuulaa	*Coptis teeta*	Gold Thread	Ayurvedic
Tiktaparvaa	*Cynodon dactylon*	Bermuda Grass, Bahama Grass, Couch Grass	Ayurvedic
Tikta-Patoli	*Trichosanthes cucumerina*	Coiled Snakegourd	Ayurvedic
Tiktashaaka	*Crataeva nurvala*	Steaved Tree, Sacred Barna	Ayurvedic
Tiktavalli	*Marsdenia tenacissima*	White Turpeth	Ayurvedic
Tiktikaa	*Abrus precatorius*	Indian Wild Liquorice, Jequirity, Crab's Eye, Precatory Bean	Ayurvedic
Til	*Sesamum indicum*	Sesame, Gingelly	Unani
Tila	*Sesamum indicum*	Sesame, Gingelly	Ayurvedic
Tilachaang	*Salix fragilis*	Crack Willow, Kashmir Willow	Folk/ (Himachal)
Tilak	*Wendlandia tinctoria*	Wendlandia	Ayurvedic
Tilaka	*Wendlandia exserta*	Wendlandia	Ayurvedic
Tilaparna	*Eucalyptus globulus*	Blue-gum Tree, Australian Gum Tree	Ayurvedic
Tilaparni	*Cleome icosandra*	Wild Mustard	Ayurvedic
Tilaparni	*Gynandropsis gynandra*	African Spider Plant	Ayurvedic
Tilapushpi (Non-classical)	*Digitalis lanata*	Grecian Foxglove	Ayurvedic
Tilapushpi (Non-classical) Purple var.	*Digitalis purpurea*	Digitalis, Foxglove	Ayurvedic
Tilen	*Viburnum nervosum*	Rosy-flowered Guelder Rose	Folk
Tilia	*Tilia cordata*	Small-leaved Lime, Linden, Basswood	Folk
Tilia Kachnaag	*Aconitum violaceum*	Himalayan Aconite	Folk
Tiliari	*Sarcococca saligna*	Christmas Box	Folk
Tiliyaa	*Wendlandia exserta*	Wendlandia	Folk

Table Contd.

Indian Name	Botanical Name	English Name	Medicinal System
Tiliyaa-koraa	*Tiliacora acuminata*	Bega Climber	Folk/Bengal
Tilki	*Wendlandia exserta*	Wendlandia	Folk
Tillai	*Excoecaria agallocha*	Blinding Tree	Siddha/Tamil
Tillakada	*Euphorbia dracunculoides*	Dragon Spurge	Siddha/Tamil
Tilvaka	*Viburnum coriaceum*	Guelder Rose, Snowball Tree	Ayurvedic
Tilvaka	*Viburnum nervosum*	Rosy-flowered Guelder Rose	Ayurvedic
Tilvaka	*Viburnum prunifolium*	Black Haw	Ayurvedic
Timidaa	*Dactyloctenium aegyptium*	Spider Grass	Folk
Timoi	*Viburnum nervosum*	Rosy-flowered Guelder Rose	Folk
Timru	*Diospyros montana*	Mountain Persimmon	Folk
Timur	*Zanthoxylum acanthopodium*	Tumru Tree, Prickly Ash	Folk
Timur	*Zanthoxylum oxyphyllum*	Tumru Tree, Prickly Ash	Folk
Tinduka (var.)	*Diospyros kaki*	Japanese Persimmon	Ayurvedic
Tinduka (var.)	*Diospyros melanoxylon*	Coromandel Ebony, Persimmon	Ayurvedic
Tinduka (var.)	*Diospyros tomentosa*	Nepal Ebony Persimmon	Ayurvedic
Tinduka	*Diospyros ebenum*	Ebony Persimmon, Malabar Ebony, Ceylon Ebony	Ayurvedic
Tinduka	*Diospyros embryopteris*	Gaub Persimmon, Riber Ebony	Ayurvedic
Tinduki	*Diospyros embryopteris*	Gaub Persimmon, Riber Ebony	Ayurvedic
Tinisha	*Ougeinia dalbergioides*	Chariot Tree, Punjab Kino	Ayurvedic
Tinishaa	*Ougeinia dalbergioides*	Chariot Tree, Punjab Kino	Ayurvedic
Tinpaani	*Naregamia alata*	Goanese Ipecacuanha	Folk
Tinpatiyaa	*Oxalis acetosella*	Common Wood-Sorrel	Folk
Tinpatiyaa	*Oxalis corniculata*	Indian Sorrel	Folk
Tintidi	*Rhus parviflora*	Sumach	Ayurvedic
Tintidika	*Garcinia indica*	Kokam Butter Tree, Mangosteen Oil Tree	Ayurvedic
Tintidika	*Tamarindus indica*	Tamarind Tree	Ayurvedic
Tintidiphala	*Croton tiglium*	Purging Croton	Ayurvedic
Tintindeeka	*Rhus parviflora*	Sumach	Ayurvedic

Table Contd.

Indian Name	Botanical Name	English Name	Medicinal System
Tirruli	*Reissantia indica*	Atari Vine	Folk
Tirukalli	*Euphorbia tirucalli*	Milk-Bush, Milk Hedge, Indian Tree Spurge, Aveloz, Petroleum Plant	Siddha/Tamil
Tiruneetrup-pachhilai	*Ocimum basilicum*	Sweet Basil, Basil Herb	Siddha/Tamil
Tirutaalli	*Ipomoea marginata*	Purple Heart Morning Glory	Folk
Tiruvaatti	*Bauhinia tomentosa*	Yellow Bauhinia, St. Thomas Tree, Bell Bauhinia	Siddha/Tamil
Tita	*Viburnum coriaceum*	Guelder Rose, Snowball Tree	Folk
Titaa	*Coptis teeta*	Gold Thread	Folk
Titaaphul	*Phlogacanthus thyrsiflorus*	Nongmangkha, Banheka	Folk
Titakhana	*Exacum bicolor*	Pseudo-Chiretta	Folk
Titali	*Euphorbia dracunculoides*	Dragon Spurge	Folk
Titalokiyaa	*Veronica beccabunga*	Brooklime	Folk
Titapat	*Corchorus aestuans*	White Jute	Folk
Titapat	*Corchorus capsularis*	White Jute	Folk
Titari	*Euphorbia thomsoniana*	Hirvi Spurge	Folk
Titpaati	*Laminum amplexicaule*	Henbit Dead Nettle	Folk
Titpaati	*Roylea cinerea*	Roylea Mint	Folk
Titween	*Artemisia absinthium*	Wormwood, Madderwood	Folk
Tivar	*Sonneratia caseolaris*	Berembang, Mangrove Apple	Folk
Tivaria	*Avicennia officinalis*	White Mangrove	Folk
Todari	*Lepidium iberis*	Peppercress	Unani
Todari	*Ziziphus rugosa*	White Jujube	Siddha/Tamil
Toddalia	*Paullinia asiatica*	Lopez Root Tree, Wild Orange Tree, Forest Pepper	Folk
Togaru	*Morinda citrifolia*	Indian Mulberry	Siddha/Tamil
Tohlab	*Ranunculus trichophyllus*	Water Crowfoot, Water Fennel	Folk
Tolu	*Rubus ellipticus*	Gach Strawberry	Folk
Tondsha	*Limonia crenulata*	Naringi, Beli	Folk

Table Contd.

Indian Name	Botanical Name	English Name	Medicinal System
Tongollati	*Eupatorium cannabinum*	Hemp Agrimony, Water Hemp, Hemp Eupatorium	Folk
Tooduvalai	*Solanum trilobatum*	Climbing Brinjal	Siddha/Tamil
Toon	*Garuga pinnata*	Grey Downy Balsam	Folk
Toona	*Cedrela toona*	Red Cedar, Toon, Indian Mahogany Tree	Folk
Topaakudaa	*Syzygium cerasoideum*	Piaman Tree	Folk
Torana	*Ziziphus rugosa*	White Jujube	Folk
Tosad kesari	*Wahlenbergia marginata*	Tenane (South Africa)	Folk
Totaro	*Berberis chitria*	Barberry	Folk
Toya	*Coleus vettiveroides*	Coleus	Ayurvedic
Toya	*Pavonia odorata*	Fragrant Sticky Mallow	Ayurvedic
Toya-pippali	*Alternanthera sessilis*	Sessile Joyweed	Ayurvedic
Toyavalli	*Ranunculus sceleratus*	Blister Buttercup, Celery-leaved Crowfoot	Ayurvedic
Traani	*Ephedra gerardiana*	Ephedra	Folk
Traapusha	*Cucumis sativus*	Cucumber	Ayurvedic
Traayamaana	*Gentiana kurroo*	Himalayan Gentian, Indian Gentian Root	Ayurvedic
Traayamaanaa	*Ficus heterophylla*	Oak-Leaf Fig	Ayurvedic
Traayanta	*Gentiana kurroo*	Himalayan Gentian, Indian Gentian Root	Ayurvedic
Traayanti	*Ficus heterophylla*	Oak-Leaf Fig	Ayurvedic
Traayanti	*Gentiana kurroo*	Himalayan Gentian, Indian Gentian Root	Ayurvedic
Traayantikaa	*Gentiana kurroo*	Himalayan Gentian, Indian Gentian Root	Ayurvedic
Trailokyavijayaa	*Cannabis sativa*	Hemp, Indian Hemp	Ayurvedic
Trapusha	*Cucumis sativus*	Cucumber	Ayurvedic
Trapushi	*Cucumis sativus*	Cucumber	Ayurvedic
Trepatra	*Trifolium pratense*	Red Clover	Folk/Punjab
Tribhandi	*Eucalyptus globulus*	Blue-gum Tree, Australian Gum Tree	Ayurvedic
Tribhandi	*Operculina turpethum*	Indian Jalap, Turpeth	Ayurvedic

Table Contd.

Indian Name	Botanical Name	English Name	Medicinal System
Tribhuvanavijayaa	*Cannabis sativa*	Hemp, Indian Hemp	Ayurvedic
Tridhaari	*Euphorbia antiquorum*	Triangular Spurge	Folk
Trika	*Trapa bispinosa*	Water Chestnut	Ayurvedic
Trikanta	*Tribulus terrestris*	Land-Caltrops, Puncture Vine	Ayurvedic
Trikantaka	*Acanthospermum hispidum*	Bristly Starbur	Ayurvedic
Trikantaka	*Pedalium murex*	Caltrops (bigger var.)	Ayurvedic
Trikantaka	*Tribulus terrestris*	Land-Caltrops, Puncture Vine	Ayurvedic
Trikona	*Trapa bispinosa*	Water Chestnut	Ayurvedic
Trikonaphala	*Trapa bispinosa*	Water Chestnut	Ayurvedic
Trikoshaki	*Melothria maderaspatana*	Rough Bryony	Ayurvedic
Trikota	*Trapa bispinosa*	Water Chestnut	Ayurvedic
Trinadhwaj	*Bambusa bambos*	Spiny or Thorny Bamboo	Ayurvedic
Trinnimba	*Swertia chirayita*	Chiretta	Ayurvedic
Trinraj	*Borassus flabellifer*	Palmyra Palm, Brab Tree	Ayurvedic
Trinshunya	*Pandanus fascicularis*	Screw Pine	Ayurvedic
Tripaadi	*Desmodium triflorum*	Matty Trefoil	Ayurvedic
Tripaadikaa	*Adiantum lunulatum*	Walking Maidenhair Fern, Black Maidenhair	Ayurvedic
Triparni	*Desmodium gangeticum*	Shaalparni, Beggarweed	Ayurvedic
Triputaa	*Amomum subulatum*	Greater or Nepal Cardamom	Ayurvedic
Triputaa	*Elettaria cardamomum*	Lesser Cardamom	Ayurvedic
Triputaa	*Eucalyptus globulus*	Blue-gum Tree, Australian Gum Tree	Ayurvedic
Triputaa	*Operculina turpethum*	Indian Jalap, Turpeth	Ayurvedic
Triputi	*Ricinus communis*	Castor Seed	Ayurvedic
Trisandhi	*Mirabilis jalapa*	Four-O'Clock Plant, Marvel of Peru	Ayurvedic
Trishati	*Gmelina arborea*	Candahar Tree, White Teak	Ayurvedic
Trita	*Symplocos racemosa*	Lodh Tree, Sapphire Berry	Ayurvedic
Trivrta	*Operculina turpethum*	Indian Jalap, Turpeth	Ayurvedic
Trnaraaja	*Cocos nucifera*	Coconut Palm	Ayurvedic
Trnarasa	*Saccharum officinarum*	Gannaa, Naishakar	Ayurvedic
Truti	*Amomum subulatum*	Greater or Nepal Cardamom	Ayurvedic

Table Contd.

Indian Name	Botanical Name	English Name	Medicinal System
Turagaahvaa	*Withania ashwagandha*	Winter Cherry	Ayurvedic
Turaga-gandhaa	*Withania ashwagandha*	Winter Cherry	Ayurvedic
Turanj	*Citrus medica*	Citron	Unani
Turanjabeen (Manna)	*Alhagi pseudalhagi*	Camel Thorn, Persian Manna Plant	Unani
Turanjeen	*Fraxinus ornus*	Flake Manna	Unani
Turapoondu	*Mollugo spergula*	Falsely-whorled Carpetweed	Siddha/Tamil
Turb Fajal	*Raphanus sativus*	Radish	Unani
Turbud	*Operculina turpethum*	Indian Jalap, Turpeth	Unani
Turmus	*Lupinus albus*	While Lupine, Wolfsbohne	Unani
Tursh	*Rumex acetosella*	Sheep Sorrel	Unani
Turushka	*Altingia excelsa*	Storax, Oriental Sweet Gum	Ayurvedic
Turushka	*Liquidambar orientalis*	Storax, Oriental Sweet Gum	Ayurvedic
Turushka	*Styrax officinale*	The True Storax Tree	Ayurvedic
Turushkaa	*Hyoscyamus muticus*	Egyptian Henbane	Ayurvedic
Turushkaa	*Hyoscyamus niger*	Indian Henbane, Black Henbane	Ayurvedic
Tushaara	*Cinnamomum camphora*	Camphor Tree	Ayurvedic
Tut-gandhaa	*Ephedra gerardiana*	Ephedra	Folk
Tutthaa	*Elettaria cardamomum*	Lesser Cardamom	Ayurvedic
Tutthaa	*Indigofera tinctoria*	Indigo	Ayurvedic
Tuula	*Gossypium herbaceum*	Asiatic Cotton, Levant Cotton, Uppam Cotton	Ayurvedic
Tuulaphala	*Calotropis procera*	Swallow-wort, Milk Weed, King's Crown	Ayurvedic
Tuulini	*Salmalia malabarica*	Silk Cotton Tree, Semul Tree	Ayurvedic
Tuunikaa	*Cedrela toona*	Red Cedar, Toon, Indian Mahogany Tree	Ayurvedic
Tuuri	*Datura stramonium*	Thornapple, Jimsonweed, Stramonium	Ayurvedic
Tuut	*Morus alba*	Chinese White-Mulberry	Unani
Tuut Siyaah	*Morus nigra*	Black Mulberry	Unani
Tuut-malangaa	*Lallemantia royleana*	Balanga Seed	Folk
Tuvadi	*Scutia myrtina*	Chimat Fruit	Folk

Table Contd.

Indian Name	Botanical Name	English Name	Medicinal System
Tuvara	*Avicennia officinalis*	White Mangrove	Ayurvedic
Tuvara	*Cajanus cajan*	Pigeon Pea, Red Gram	Ayurvedic
Tuvaraka (var.)	*Gynocardia odorata*	Oleum Gynocardiae	Ayurvedic
Tuvaraka	*Hydnocarpus kurzii*	Chalmogra	Ayurvedic
Tuvaraka	*Hydnocarpus laurifolia*	Soorty Oil Tree	Ayurvedic
Tuvari	*Cajanus cajan*	Pigeon Pea, Red Gram	Ayurvedic
Tuvari	*Eruca sativa*	Rocket-Salad	Ayurvedic
Tuvari	*Ocimum basilicum*	Sweet Basil, Basil Herb	Ayurvedic
Tuvarikaa	*Eruca sativa*	Rocket-Salad	Ayurvedic
Tvak	*Cinnamomum cassia*	Chinese Cinnamon, Cassia bark	Ayurvedic
Tvak	*Cinnamomum zeylanicum*	Cinnamon, Ceylon Cinnamon	Ayurvedic
Tvakkshiri (Manna)	*Bambusa bambos*	Spiny or Thorny Bamboo	Ayurvedic
Tvakshira	*Curcuma angustifolia*	East Indian Arrowroot, Travancore Starch	Ayurvedic
Tvakshiri	*Curcuma angustifolia*	East Indian Arrowroot, Travancore Starch	Ayurvedic
Uch Ellu	*Guizotia abyssinica*	Nigerseed	Folk/Tamil
Uchchattaa	*Blepharis edulis*	Acanthus	Folk
Uchunti	*Ageratum conyzoides*	Goat Weed, White Weed	Ayurvedic
Udaka	*Coleus vettiveroides*	Coleus	Ayurvedic
Uddaalaka	*Cordia wallichii*	Sebestan	Ayurvedic
Uddaalaka Shita	*Cordia myxa*	Sabestan Plum	Ayurvedic
Udichya	*Coleus vettiveroides*	Coleus	Ayurvedic
Udichya	*Pavonia odorata*	Fragrant Sticky Mallow	Ayurvedic
Udkirya	*Derris indica*	Indian Beech, Pongamia Oil Tree	Ayurvedic
Udumbara	*Ficus racemosa*	Cluster Fig, Country Fig	Ayurvedic
Udumbarparni	*Baliospermum montanum*	False Croton	Ayurvedic
Ugraa	*Acorus calamus*	Sweet Flag, Calamus	Ayurvedic
Ugragandha	*Allium sativum*	Garlic	Ayurvedic
Ugragandhaa	*Acorus calamus*	Sweet Flag, Calamus	Ayurvedic

Table Contd.

Indian Name	Botanical Name	English Name	Medicinal System
Ugragandhaa	*Alpinia galanga*	Greater Galangal	Ayurvedic
Ugragandhaa	*Gynandropsis gynandra*	African Spider Plant	Ayurvedic
Ugragandhaa	*Hymenodictyon excelsum*	Bridal Couch Tree	Ayurvedic
Ukhal	*Fagopyrum tataricum*	Tatary Duckwheat	Ayurvedic
Ulankarei	*Elaeocarpus serratus*	Wild Olive Tree, Ceylon Olive	Siddha/Tamil
Ulat-kambal	*Abroma augusta*	Perennial Indian Hemp, Devil's Cotton	Unani
Ulli	*Xylopia parviflora*	Netawu, Atuketiya	Folk/Karnataka
Ullippoondu	*Allium sativum*	Garlic	Siddha/Tamil
Ulunthu	*Phaseolus mungo*	Kidney Bean, Black Gram	Siddha/Tamil
Uluukhala	*Balsamodendron mukul*	Indian Bdellium, Gum Guggul	Ayurvedic
Umaa	*Linum usitatissimum*	Linseed, Flax	Ayurvedic
Unamkodi	*Erycibe paniculata*	Kari Climber (Assam)	Siddha/Tamil
Unarjal	*Iris ensata*	Japanese Iris	Folk
Undir-chaa-kaan	*Lactuca runcinata*	Wild Lettuce	Folk
Undurukarnikaa	*Ipomoea reniformis*	Mouse-ear Shrub	Ayurvedic
Unmatta	*Datura metel*	Thornapple, Downy Datura	Ayurvedic
Unmatta	*Datura stramonium*	Thornapple, Jimsonweed, Stramonium	Ayurvedic
Unnaab	*Ziziphus jujuba* Mill.	Chinese Tsao	Unani
Unnayangodi	*Lettsomia elliptica*	Silverweed	Folk/Tamil
Unnichedi	*Lantana camara*	Lantana, Wild Sage, Surinam Tea Plant	Siddha/Tamil
Unnu	*Grewia tiliaefolia*	Dhaman	Siddha/Tamil
Unsul-e-Hindi	*Urginea indica*	Indian Squill, Sea Onion (red and white varieties)	Unani
Ununjil	*Onosma bracteatum*	Borage	Siddha/Tamil
Upakunchikaa (var.)	*Nigella damascena*	Love-in-a-mist	Ayurvedic
Upakunchikaa	*Carum carvi*	Caraway	Ayurvedic
Upattam	*Avicennia officinalis*	White Mangrove	Folk
Upkulyaa	*Piper longum*	Indian Long Pepper, Joborandi	Ayurvedic
Upkunchikaa	*Elettaria cardamomum*	Lesser Cardamom	Ayurvedic

Table Contd.

Indian Name	Botanical Name	English Name	Medicinal System
Upkunchikaa	*Nigella sativa*	Black Cumin, Small Fennel	Ayurvedic
Uplet	*Saussurea hypoleuca*	Himalayan Saw-wort	Folk
Upodika	*Portulaca oleracea*	Common Purslane	Ayurvedic
Upodikaa	*Basella alba*	Indian Spinach	Ayurvedic
Upothaki	*Trianthema portulacastrum*	Horse Purslane	Ayurvedic
Upperichedi	*Lobelia nicotianaefolia*	Wild Tobacco	Siddha/Tamil
Uppilankodi	*Pentatropis microphylla*	Ambervel, Beak-shaped Elliptic Flower	Siddha/Tamil
Uppu Sananga	*Cressa cretica*	Mediterranean Bindweed	Siddha/Tamil
Uralli	*Litsea glutinosa*	Common Tallow Lowrel	Siddha/Tamil
Urd-Siyaah	*Phaseolus mungo*	Kidney Bean, Black Gram	Unani
Urni	*Corylus colurna*	Turkish Hazel	Folk
Urumaana	*Prunus armeniaca*	Apricot	Ayurvedic
Uruvaka	*Ricinus communis*	Castor Seed	Ayurvedic
Urvaaru	*Cucumis melo*	Musk Melon, Sweet Melon	Ayurvedic
Usaare Rewand	*Rheum officinale*	Rhubarb	Unani
Usaar-e-revand	*Garcinia hanburyi*	Siam Gamboge	Unani
Ushaare-revand	*Garcinia morella*	Indian Gamboge	Ayurvedic
Ushah	*Dorema ammoniacum*	Ammoniacum, Gum Ammoniac	Unani
Ushaka	*Dorema ammoniacum*	Ammoniacum, Gum Ammoniac	Ayurvedic
Ushaq	*Dorema ammoniacum*	Ammoniacum, Gum Ammoniac	Unani
Ushbaa	*Smilax ornata*	Jamaica Sarsaparilla	Unani
Ushbaa	*Smilax ovalifolia*	Wild China Root	Unani
Ushbaa Hindi	*Hemidesmus indicus*	Indian Sarsaparilla	Unani
Ushbaa Maghrabi	*Smilax aristolochiaefolia*	Mexican Sarsaparilla	Unani
Ushira	*Andropogon muricatus*	Vetiver, Cuscus	Ayurvedic
Ushira	*Vetiveria zizanioides*	Vetiver, Khas	Ayurvedic
Ushittgarai	*Cassia tora*	Sickle Senna, Ringworm Plant	Siddha/Tamil
Ushnaa	*Usnea longissima*	Lichen	Unani

Table Contd.

Indian Name	Botanical Name	English Name	Medicinal System
Ushnaan	*Salsola kali*	Glass-Wort, Russian Thistle, Prickly-Saltwort	Unani
Ushtrakaandi	*Blepharis linariaefolia*	Acanthus	Ayurvedic
Usimalligai	*Jasminum auriculatum*	Cultivated Jasmine	Siddha/Tamil
Usipallai	*Oxystelma secamone*	Dudhni, Chamuuk plaa lot (Thai)	Folk
Usippalai	*Oxystelma secamone*	Dudhni, Chamuuk plaa lot (Thai)	Folk/Tamil
Usqurdiyun	*Teucrium chamaedrys*	Germander, Wall Germander	Unani
Ustukhuddus	*Lavandula stoechas*	Arabian or French Lavender	Unani
Ustukhudduus	*Brunella vulgaris*	Self-heal	Unani
Usturak	*Styrax officinale*	The True Storax Tree	Folk
Utangan (Sindh)	*Blepharis linariaefolia*	Acanthus	Ayurvedic
Utangana	*Blepharis edulis*	Acanthus	Ayurvedic
Utaran	*Pergularia extensa*	Hairknot Plant, Whitlow Plant	Folk
Uththaamani	*Pergularia extensa*	Hairknot Plant, Whitlow Plant	Siddha/Tamil
Utigun	*Laportea crenulata*	Devil Nettle, Fever Nettle	Folk
Utkantaka	*Echinops echinatus*	Globe-Thistle, Camel's Thistle	Ayurvedic
Utkat	*Cinnamomum tamala*	Indian Cassia Lignea	Ayurvedic
Utkata	*Cinnamomum zeylanicum*	Cinnamon, Ceylon Cinnamon	Ayurvedic
Utpala	*Nymphaea alba*	European White Water-lily	Ayurvedic
Utpala	*Nymphaea rubra*	Indian Red Water-lily	Ayurvedic
Utpalsaarivaa	*Hemidesmus indicus*	Indian Sarsaparilla	Ayurvedic
Utraj	*Citrus limon*	Lemon	Unani
Uttaanpatraka	*Ricinus communis*	Castor Seed	Ayurvedic
Uttamaarani	*Pergularia extensa*	Hairknot Plant, Whitlow Plant	Ayurvedic
Uttamkanyaka	*Vernonia cinerea*	Ash Coloured Fleabane, Purple Fleabane	Ayurvedic
Uttraccham	*Elaeocarpus serratus*	Wild Olive Tree, Ceylon Olive	Siddha/Tamil
Uttundaka	*Echinops echinatus*	Globe-Thistle, Camel's Thistle	Ayurvedic
Uudakiraayita	*Exacum bicolor*	Pseudo-Chiretta	Folk
Uuntakataaraa	*Tricholepis angustifolia*	Camel's Thistle	Folk

Table Contd.

Indian Name	Botanical Name	English Name	Medicinal System
Uunta-Kateraa	*Echinops echinatus*	Globe-Thistle, Camel's Thistle	Folk
Uushaka	*Dorema ammoniacum*	Ammoniacum, Gum Ammoniac	Ayurvedic
Uushna	*Piper nigrum*	Black Pepper	Ayurvedic
Uushnaa	*Piper longum*	Indian Long Pepper, Joborandi	Ayurvedic
Uva	*Dillenia indica*	Elephant Apple	Folk
Uyyakondan	*Jasminum rottlerianum*	Wild jasmine (Western Ghats)	Siddha/Tamil
Vaadumai	*Amygdalus communis*	Almond	Siddha/Tamil
Vaadumai	*Prunus amygdalus*	Almond	Siddha/Tamil
Vaagei	*Albizia amara*	Siris Tree, East Indian Walnut	Siddha/Tamil
Vaagei	*Albizia lebbeck*	Siris Tree, East Indian Walnut	Siddha/Tamil
Vaajidanta	*Adhatoda vasica*	Malabar Nut, Vasaca	Ayurvedic
Vaajigandhaa	*Withania ashwagandha*	Winter Cherry	Ayurvedic
Vaajikari	*Withania ashwagandha*	Winter Cherry	Ayurvedic
Vaakeri	*Caesalpinia digyra*	Teri Pods	Ayurvedic
Vaakeri	*Rourea minor*	Leenhaits, Hong ye teng (Chinese)	Folk
Vaakeri	*Wagatea spicata*	Western Ghat-Wakeri	Folk
Vaakuchi	*Psoralea corylifolia*	Purple Fleabane	Ayurvedic
Vaalaka	*Coleus vettiveroides*	Coleus	Ayurvedic
Vaalaka	*Pavonia odorata*	Fragrant Sticky Mallow	Ayurvedic
Vaalmilagu	*Piper cubeba*	Cubeb, Tailed Pepper	Siddha/Tamil
Vaaluluvai	*Celastrus paniculatus*	Staff Tree, Intellect Tree	Siddha/Tamil
Vaalunja	*Salix tetrasperma*	Indian Willow	Folk
Vaamana-haati	*Clerodendrum indicum*	Turk's Turban, Tube-Flower	Ayurvedic
Vaamanahaati	*Clerodendrum serratum*	Blue-flowered Glory Tree, Beetle Killer	Ayurvedic
Vaamataruni	*Ventilago madraspatana*	Ventilago Vermilion Vine	Ayurvedic
Vaana	*Saccharum munja*	Munja Culms	Ayurvedic
Vaanira	*Salix caprea*	Sallow, Goat Willow, Common Willow	Ayurvedic
Vaanira	*Salix tetrasperma*	Indian Willow	Folk
Vaapya	*Saussurea lappa*	Kuth, Costus	Ayurvedic

Table Contd.

Indian Name	Botanical Name	English Name	Medicinal System
Vajjradram	*Euphorbia neriifolia*	Holy Milk Hedge, Dog's Tongue	Ayurvedic
Vajjri	*Euphorbia neriifolia*	Holy Milk Hedge, Dog's Tongue	Ayurvedic
Vajra	*Euphorbia neriifolia*	Holy Milk Hedge, Dog's Tongue	Ayurvedic
Vajraanga	*Aconitum ferox*	Indian Aconite, Wolfsbane, Monkshood	Ayurvedic
Vajra-bhang	*Hyoscyamus muticus*	Egyptian Henbane	Folk
Vajradanti	*Dicoma tomentosa*	Bitter Dicoma	Folk
Vajra-kanda	*Amorphophallus campanulatus*	Elephant's Foot Yam	Ayurvedic
Vajrakanda	*Plesmonium margaritiferum*	Kharhar Tuber	Ayurvedic
Vajrakanda	*Urginea indica*	Indian Squill, Sea Onion (red and white varieties)	Ayurvedic
Vajra-kantaka	*Euphorbia antiquorum*	Triangular Spurge	Ayurvedic
Vajratundi	*Euphorbia antiquorum*	Triangular Spurge	Ayurvedic
Vakkanai	*Diospyros montana*	Mountain Persimmon	Siddha/Tamil
Vakkanatan	*Diospyros montana*	Mountain Persimmon	Siddha/Tamil
Vakraa	*Pistacia integerrima*	Horn-shaped Gall Tree, Kakra Gall Tree	Ayurvedic
Vakrapushpa	*Sesbania grandiflora*	Agati Sesban, Swamp Pea	Ayurvedic
Valampiri	*Helicteres isora*	East Indian Screw Tree	Siddha/Tamil
Valkala vrksha	*Antiaris toxicaria*	Sacking Tree, Upas Tree	Ayurvedic
Vallaarai	*Centella asiatica*	Asiatic Pennywort, Indian Pennywort	Siddha/Tamil
Vallaimusali	*Chlorophytum arundinaceum*	White Musali	Siddha/Tamil
Vallaimusali	*Chlorophytum tuberosum*	White Musali	Siddha/Tamil
Vallari	*Malpighia punicifolia*	West Indian Cherry	Folk
Valli Kanjiram	*Strychnos rheedei*	Snakewood	Siddha/Tamil
Valli kilangu	*Dioscorea esculenta*	Lesser Yam, Karen Potato	Siddha/Tamil
Valli-kantakaarikaa	*Solanum dulcamara*	Woody Night Shade, Bittersweet, Bitter Nightshade, Felonwort	Ayurvedic

Table Contd.

Indian Name	Botanical Name	English Name	Medicinal System
Valli-kantakaarikaa	*Solanum trilobatum*	Climbing Brinjal	Ayurvedic
Vallipana	*Lygodium flexuosum*	Wolfberry, Scrambling Fern	Folk
Valliphala	*Berberis aristata*	Indian Barberry	Ayurvedic
Valuluvai	*Gymnosporia spinosa*	Celastrus Tree	Siddha/Tamil
Valval	*Acacia leucophloea*	White Babul	Siddha/Tamil
Van Haridraa	*Curcuma aromatica*	Wild Turmeric, Yellow Zedoary	Ayurvedic
Vanachchhedi	*Lantana camara*	Lantana, Wild Sage, Surinam Tea Plant	Ayurvedic
Vana-gobhi	*Launaea pinnatifida*	Bhonpatri	Folk
Vanajai	*Clerodendrum inerme*	Smooth Volkameria	Ayurvedic
Vana-kulattha	*Atylosia scarabaeoides*	Peanut Grass	Ayurvedic
Vana-malli	*Jasminum angustifolium*	Wild Jasmine	Ayurvedic
Vana-mallikaa	*Jasminum rottlerianum*	Wild jasmine (Western Ghats)	Ayurvedic
Vana-methi	*Indigofera trifoliata*	Three-Leaved Indigo	Folk
Vana-methikaa	*Melilotus indica*	Sweet Clover, Annual Yellow Sweet Clover, Small-flowered Melilot	Ayurvedic
Vana-nimbuukaa	*Glycosmis pentaphylla*	Orangeberry, Ginberry	Ayurvedic
Vana-Palaandu	*Scilla indica*	South Indian Squill	Ayurvedic
Vana-palaandu	*Urginea indica*	Indian Squill, Sea Onion (red and white varieties)	Ayurvedic
Vana-Patola	*Trichosanthes cucumerina*	Coiled Snakegourd	Ayurvedic
Vana-Pippali	*Piper sylvaticum*	Mountain Long Pepper	Ayurvedic
Vanardraka	*Zingiber cassumunar*	Cassumunar Ginger	Ayurvedic
Vana-Tulasi	*Ocimum canum*	Hoary Basil	Ayurvedic
Vanaveri	*Pentatropis spiralis*	Ambervel	Folk
Vana-Yavaani	*Thymus serphyllum*	Mother-of-thyme, Wild Thyme	Ayurvedic
Van-bhendi	*Urena lobata*	Pink Chinese Burr, Burr Mallow	Folk
Vandaka Raasnaa	*Vanda roxburghii*	Tassellata	Folk
Vandhyaavari	*Vicoa indica*	Banjauri	Ayurvedic

Table Contd.

Indian Name	Botanical Name	English Name	Medicinal System
Vangasena	*Sesbania grandiflora*	Agati Sesban, Swamp Pea	Ayurvedic
Vanitaa	*Callicarpa macrophylla*	Perfumed Cherry	Ayurvedic
Vanjula	*Salix caprea*	Sallow, Goat Willow, Common Willow	Ayurvedic
Vansha	*Bambusa bambos*	Spiny or Thorny Bamboo	Ayurvedic
Vanshalochana (Manna)	*Bambusa bambos*	Spiny or Thorny Bamboo	Ayurvedic
Vansharochanaa (Manna)	*Bambusa bambos*	Spiny or Thorny Bamboo	Ayurvedic
Vanya Taruni	*Rosa macrophylla*	Himalayan Rose	Ayurvedic
Vanya-jiraka	*Centratherum anthelminticum*	Purple Flea-bane, Achenes	Ayurvedic
Vanya-Kaahuu	*Lactuca serriola*	Wild Lettuce, Prickly Lettuce	Ayurvedic
Vanya-Mansala	*Careya arborea*	Kumbi, Slow-Match Tree	Ayurvedic
Vanya-yamaani	*Seseli indicum*	Wild Seseli	Ayurvedic
Vara	*Crocus sativus*	Saffron, Crocus	Ayurvedic
Varaahakarni	*Withania ashwagandha*	Winter Cherry	Ayurvedic
Varaanga	*Cinnamomum zeylanicum*	Cinnamon, Ceylon Cinnamon	Ayurvedic
Varadaa	*Withania ashwagandha*	Winter Cherry	Ayurvedic
Varadaaru	*Tectona grandis*	Teak Tree	Ayurvedic
Varagu	*Paspalum scrobiculatum*	Kodo Millet	Siddha/Tamil
Varaka	*Echinochloa colonum*	Shama Millet	Ayurvedic
Varana	*Crataeva nurvala*	Steaved Tree, Sacred Barna	Ayurvedic
Varanga	*Carallia brachiata*	Freshwater Mangrove	Folk
Varatikta	*Fumaria parviflora*	Fumitory	Ayurvedic
Varatiktaaa	*Cissampelos pareira*	Velvet-Leaf Pareira, Pareira Brava	Ayurvedic
Varatuli	*Dichrostachys cinerea*	Chinese Lantern, Kalihari Christmastree	Folk
Varavarnini	*Curcuma longa*	Turmeric	Ayurvedic
Vard	*Rosa damascena*	Damask Rose	Unani
Vard Abyaz	*Rosa alba*	Common English Dog Rose, White Cottage Rose	Unani
Vard Abyaz Barri	*Rosa alba*	Common English Dog Rose, White Cottage Rose	Unani

Table Contd.

Indian Name	Botanical Name	English Name	Medicinal System
Vardaar	*Rourea minor*	Leenhaits, Hong ye teng (Chinese)	Folk
Vard-e-Ahmar	*Rosa damascena*	Damask Rose	Unani
Vardhamaana	*Ricinus communis*	Castor Seed	Ayurvedic
Vardhipatraka	*Dolichos biflorus*	Horsegram	Ayurvedic
Vari	*Asparagus racemosus*	Indian Asparagus, Wild Asparagus	Ayurvedic
Varnya	*Crocus sativus*	Saffron, Crocus	Ayurvedic
Varsanam-pillu	*Echinochloa colonum*	Shama Millet	Siddha/Tamil
Varshaabhu	*Boerhavia diffusa*	Red-flowered Hogweed	Ayurvedic
Varshaabhu	*Trianthema decandra*	Horse Purslane	Ayurvedic
Varshaabhu	*Trianthema govindia*	Horse Purslane	Ayurvedic
Varshaabhu	*Trianthema portulacastrum*	Horse Purslane	Ayurvedic
Vartaki	*Solanum ferox*	Poison-Berry	Ayurvedic
Varuna	*Crataeva nurvala*	Steaved Tree, Sacred Barna	Ayurvedic
Vasaakaa	*Adhatoda vasica*	Malabar Nut, Vasaca	Folk
Vasaiyila-keerai	*Spinacia oleracea*	Garden Spinach	Siddha/Tamil
Vasambu	*Acorus calamus*	Sweet Flag, Calamus	Siddha/Tamil
Vasanaavi	*Aconitum ferox*	Indian Aconite, Wolfsbane, Monkshood	Siddha/Tamil
Vasandagala-malligai	*Hiptage benghalensis*	Hiptage	Siddha/Tamil
Vashira	*Achyranthes aspera*	Prickly Chaff Flower	Ayurvedic
Vashiraa	*Phyla nodiflora*	Fogfruit, Sawtooth Fogfruit	Ayurvedic
Vaslakkirai	*Basella alba*	Indian Spinach	Siddha/Tamil
Vasmaa	*Indigofera oblongifolia*	Wild Indigo, Mysore Panicled Indigo	Unani
Vastikaa	*Trigonella foenum-graecum*	Fenugreek	Ayurvedic
Vastika-parnika	*Marsilea minuta*	Dwarf Waterclover, Pepperwort	Ayurvedic
Vastraranjaka	*Carthamus tinctorius*	Safflower	Ayurvedic
Vasuka	*Calotropis gigantea*	Swallow Wort	Ayurvedic
Vasuka	*Calotropis procera*	Swallow-wort, Milk Weed, King's Crown	Ayurvedic

Table Contd.

Indian Name	Botanical Name	English Name	Medicinal System
Vasuka	*Osmanthus fragrans*	Sweet Olive Tree	Ayurvedic
Vata	*Ficus beng(h)alensis*	Banyan Tree	Ayurvedic
Vatanarayanan	*Delonix regia*	Flamboyant Flame Tree, Gold Mohur	Folk/Telugu
Vatapatri	*Kalanchoe laciniata*	Christmastree Plant	Ayurvedic
Vathomkolli	*Naravelia zeylanica*	Naravelia Climber	Folk/Tamil
Vatsa	*Holarrhena antidysenterica*	Easter Tree, Ivory Tree, Tellicherry	Ayurvedic
Vatsaadani	*Tinospora cordifolia*	Heart-leaved Tinospora	Ayurvedic
Vatsaadani	*Tinospora malabarica*	Tinospora	Ayurvedic
Vatsabija (Seed)	*Holarrhena antidysenterica*	Easter Tree, Ivory Tree, Tellicherry	Ayurvedic
Vatsaka	*Holarrhena antidysenterica*	Easter Tree, Ivory Tree, Tellicherry	Ayurvedic
Vatsanaabha	*Aconitum atrox*	Himalayan Napellus	Ayurvedic
Vatsanaabha	*Aconitum chasmanthum*	Indian Napellus	Ayurvedic
Vatsanaabha	*Aconitum deinorrhizum*	Indian Aconite	Ayurvedic
Vatsanaabha	*Aconitum falconeri*	Indian Aconite	Ayurvedic
Vatsanaabha	*Aconitum ferox*	Indian Aconite, Wolfsbane, Monkshood	Ayurvedic
Vatsanaabha	*Aconitum laciniatum*	Himalayan Aconite	Ayurvedic
Vatsanaabha	*Aconitum luridum*	Himalayan Aconite	Ayurvedic
Vatsanaabha	*Aconitum spicatum*	Nepal Aconite	Ayurvedic
Vatsanaabha	*Aconitum violaceum*	Himalayan Aconite	Ayurvedic
Vatsanaagaka	*Aconitum ferox*	Indian Aconite, Wolfsbane, Monkshood	Ayurvedic
Vattavalli	*Entada scandens*	Garbee Bean, Mackay Bean, Elephant Creeper	Siddha/Tamil
Vayangarai	*Flacourtia jangomas*	Puneala Plum	Siddha/Tamil
Vayasyaa	*Emblica officinalis*	Embic, Indian Gooseberry	Ayurvedic
Vayhasthaa	*Lilium polyphyllum*	Kakoli Tuber Lily	Ayurvedic
Vazhuthunai (root)	*Solanum indicum*	Poison Berry	Siddha/Tamil
Vedanguruni	*Radermachera xylocarpa*	Padri Tree	Folk/Tamil
Veddayala	*Acacia farnesiana*	Cassie Flower, Sweet Acacia	Siddha/Tamil

Table Contd.

Indian Name	Botanical Name	English Name	Medicinal System
Vedhi	*Ferula foetida*	Asafoetida	Ayurvedic
Vegaa	*Celastrus paniculatus*	Staff Tree, Intellect Tree	Ayurvedic
Vekhali	*Pittosporum floribundum*	Ginger-bark Pittosporum	Folk
Velampasi	*Ceratophyllum demersum*	Coontail, Hornwort	Siddha/Tamil
Velampisin (gum)	*Acacis arabica*	Babul, Black Babul, Indian Gum Arabic Tree	Siddha/Tamil
Velari	*Dodonaea viscosa*	Jamacia Switch Sorrel	Siddha/Tamil
Velimungil	*Justicia betonica*	Shrimp Plant, Lobster Plant	Siddha/Tamil
Veli-paruthi	*Pergularia extensa*	Hairknot Plant, Whitlow Plant	Folk/Tamil
Vel-itti	*Dalbergia sissoides*	Malabar Blackwood	Siddha/Tamil
Vel-khantudi	*Ceropegia juncea*	Leafless Godlet Flower	Folk/Marathi
Vella	*Embelia ribes*	Embelia	Ayurvedic
Vella Champakam	*Plumeria alba*	White Champaka	Folk/ Malayalam
Vellai Kadambam	*Anthocephalus cadamba*	Wild Cinchona	Siddha/Tamil
Vellai Kundarakam	*Vateria indica*	White Damar, Indian Copal-Tree, Malabar Tallow Tree, Piney Varnish-Tree	Siddha/Tamil
Vellai kunthirikam	*Vateria indica*	White Damar, Indian Copal-Tree, Malabar Tallow Tree, Piney Varnish-Tree	Siddha/Tamil
Vellai Naval	*Syzygium hemisphericum*	Jambosa	Siddha/Tamil
Vellai saaranai	*Trianthema decandra*	Horse Purslane	Siddha/Tamil
Vellaibolam	*Balsamodendron myrrha*	Myrrh, Herabol	Siddha/Tamil
Vellaikeerai	*Ipomoea aquatica*	Swamp Cabbage	Siddha/Tamil
Vellaimandarai	*Bauhinia acuminata*	Dwarf White Bauhinia	Siddha/Tamil
Vellaippula	*Securinega suffruticosa*	Securinega	Siddha/Tamil
Vellai-yilai	*Mussaenda frondosa*	White Lady, White Rag Plant	Siddha/Tamil
Vellaja	*Piper nigrum*	Black Pepper	Ayurvedic
Vellambal	*Nymphaea rubra*	Indian Red Water-lily	Folk/Tamil

Table Contd.

Indian Name	Botanical Name	English Name	Medicinal System
Vella-muttangam	*Scaevola frutescens*	Fan Flower, Malay Rice Paper Plant	Siddha/Tamil
Vellantaru	*Dichrostachys cinerea*	Chinese Lantern, Kalihari Christmastree	Ayurvedic
Vellargu	*Enicostemma littorale*	Indian Gentian	Siddha/Tamil
Vellari	*Cucumis sativus*	Cucumber	Siddha/Tamil
Vellarikkai	*Cucumis melo*	Musk Melon, Sweet Melon	Folk/Tamil
Vellaynaga	*Anogeissus latifolia*	Axle-wood, Button Tree, Ghatti Tree	Siddha/Tamil
Vellei Kadambu	*Hymenodictyon excelsum*	Bridal Couch Tree	Siddha/Tamil
Vellerukku	*Calotropis procera*	Swallow-wort, Milk Weed, King's Crown	Siddha/Tamil
Velliloththiram	*Symplocos racemosa*	Lodh Tree, Sapphire Berry	Siddha/Tamil
Velliloththiram pattai (Bark)	*Symplocos racemosa*	Lodh Tree, Sapphire Berry	Siddha/Tamil
Velli-madandai	*Mussaenda frondosa*	White Lady, White Rag Plant	Siddha/Tamil
Velukku	*Kydia calycina*	Pula Tree	Folk
Velvayalam	*Acacia leucophloea*	White Babul	Siddha/Tamil
Vembu	*Azadirachta indica*	Neem Tree, Margosa Tree	Siddha/Tamil
Ven Kottam	*Costus speciosus*	Canereed, Wild Ginger	Siddha/Tamil
Vendai	*Abelmoschus esculentus*	Gumbo, Lady Finger, Okra	Siddha/Tamil
Vendayam	*Trigonella foenum-graecum*	Fenugreek	Siddha/Tamil
Vendi	*Kydia calycina*	Pula Tree	Folk
Vengai	*Pterocarpus dalbergioides*	Andaman Paduak, Andaman Redwood	Siddha/Tamil
Vengai	*Pterocarpus marsupium*	Indian Kino Tree, Malabar Kino Tree	Siddha/Tamil
Venge-maram	*Bridelia montana*	Spinous Kino Tree	Siddha/Tamil
Venilai Valli	*Dioscorea oppositifolia*	Cylindrical Red Yam	Siddha/Tamil
Venivel	*Podophyllum hexandrum*	Indian Podophyllum	Folk
Venkaayam	*Allium cepa*	Onion	Siddha/Tamil
Venkadugu	*Brassica alba*	White Mustard	Siddha/Tamil
Venkodiveli	*Agaricus campestris*	Field Mushroom, Edible Mushroom	Siddha/Tamil

Table Contd.

Indian Name	Botanical Name	English Name	Medicinal System
Venkungiliyam (resin)	*Shorea robusta*	Sal Tree	Siddha/Tamil
Vennangu	*Pterospermum acerifolium*	Hathipaila	Siddha/Tamil
Ven-poosani	*Benincasa hispida*	Ash Gourd, White Gourd, Wax Gourd, White Pumpkin	Siddha/Tamil
Venta	*Kydia calycina*	Pula Tree	Folk
Venu	*Bambusa bambos*	Spiny or Thorny Bamboo	Ayurvedic
Venupatrikaa	*Gardenia gummifera*	Gummy Cape Jasmine	Ayurvedic
Veppan	*Azadirachta indica*	Neem Tree, Margosa Tree	Siddha/Tamil
Veppu	*Azadirachta indica*	Neem Tree, Margosa Tree	Siddha/Tamil
Verikkumatti	*Citrullus colocynthis*	Colocynth Bitter Apple	Siddha/Tamil
Verkadalai	*Arachis hypogaea*	Groundnut, Peanut, Monkeynut	Siddha/Tamil
Vetasa	*Salix caprea*	Sallow, Goat Willow, Common Willow	Ayurvedic
Vetasaamla	*Garcinia pedunculata*	Bengal Brindleberry	Ayurvedic
Vetchi	*Ixora coccinea*	Jungleflame Ixora	Siddha/Tamil
Vetra	*Calamus rotang*	Rotang, Rattan, Chair Bottom Cane	Ayurvedic
Vetra	*Calamus tenuis*	Barcilly Canc	Ayurvedic
Vetra	*Calamus travancoricus*	Travancore Cane	Ayurvedic
Vetra	*Daemonorops jenkinsianus*	Calamus	Ayurvedic
Vetrilai	*Piper betle*	Betel Pepper	Siddha/Tamil
Vettangi	*Caesalpinia sappan*	Sappan	Siddha/Tamil
Vettiver	*Vetiveria zizanioides*	Vetiver, Khas	Siddha/Tamil
Vettiveru	*Andropogon muricatus*	Vetiver, Cuscus	Siddha/Tamil
Vettukkaaya-thalai	*Tridax procumbens*	Mexican Daisy	Siddha/Tamil
Vibhitaka	*Terminalia bellirica*	Belleric Myrobalan, Bastard Myrobalan	Ayurvedic
Vidaari (var.)	*Pueraria lobata*	Tropical Kudze	Ayurvedic
Vidaari (var.)	*Trichosanthes cordata*	Snake-Gourd	Ayurvedic/ Bengal
Vidaari	*Pueraria tuberosa*	Indian Kudze	Ayurvedic

Table Contd.

Indian Name	Botanical Name	English Name	Medicinal System
Visha	*Aconitum ferox*	Indian Aconite, Wolfsbane, Monkshood	Ayurvedic
Vishaa	*Aconitum heterophyllum*	Atis Root, Aconite	Ayurvedic
Vishaalaa	*Citrullus colocynthis*	Colocynth Bitter Apple	Ayurvedic
Vishaalaa	*Trichosanthes bracteata*	Redball Snakegourd	Ayurvedic
Vishaaltvak	*Alstonia scholaris*	Devil's Tree, Dita Bark Tree	Ayurvedic
Vishaalya	*Baliospermum montanum*	False Croton	Ayurvedic
Vishaalyaa	*Gloriosa superba*	Glory Lily, Super Lily, Tiger's Claws	Ayurvedic
Vishaani	*Pistacia integerrima*	Horn-shaped Gall Tree, Kakra Gall Tree	Ayurvedic
Vishaanikaa	*Dolichandrone falcate*	Corky-winged-seed Tree	Ayurvedic
Vishaanikaa	*Pergularia extensa*	Hairknot Plant, Whitlow Plant	Ayurvedic
Vishaarada	*Mimusops elengi*	Spanish-Cherry, West Indian Medlar, Bullet Wood	Ayurvedic
Visha-chhatraka	*Amanita muscaria*	Fly Agaric, Aga, Soma (Constituent)	Ayurvedic
Vishadhvansi	*Cyperus rotundus*	Nut Grass	Ayurvedic
Visha-ghaasa	*Lolium temulentum*	Darnel, Bearded Ryegrass	Folk
Vishaghn	*Amaranthus spinosus*	Spiny Amaranth, Thorny Amaranth, Spiny Pigweed	Ayurvedic
Vishakanegale	*Vinca pusilla*	Bengal Periwinkle	Folk
Vishakhar-parikaa	*Trianthema portulacastrum*	Horse Purslane	Ayurvedic
Vishalyakarani	*Eupatorium triplinerve*	Ayapana Tea	Ayurvedic
Vishamchhada	*Alstonia scholaris*	Devil's Tree, Dita Bark Tree	Ayurvedic
Vishamoongil	*Crinum asiaticum*	St. John's Lily, Poison Bulb	Siddha/Tamil
Vishamoongil	*Crinum latifolium*	Wide-leaved Crinum	Siddha/Tamil
Vishamushti	*Strychnos nux-vomica*	Nux Vomica	Ayurvedic
Vishamushtikaa	*Strychnos nux-vomica*	Nux Vomica	Ayurvedic
Vishani	*Microstylis wallichii*	Rshabhaka	Ayurvedic
Visha-phala	*Actaea spicata*	Baneberry Grapewort	Folk
Vishapushpaka	*Randia dumetorum*	Common Emetic Nut	Ayurvedic

Table Contd.

Indian Name	Botanical Name	English Name	Medicinal System
Visha-tinduka	*Diospyros montana*	Mountain Persimmon	Ayurvedic
Vishatinduka	*Strychnos nux-vomica*	Nux Vomica	Ayurvedic
Vishikha-punkhaa	*Tephrosia purpurea*	Purple Tephrosia, Wild Indigo	Ayurvedic
Vishlumbha	*Cucumis trigonus*	Wild Cucumber	Folk
Vishnukraandi	*Convolvulus pluricaulis*	Conch-flowered Bindweed, White-flowered Shankhpushpi	Siddha/Tamil
Vishnukraantaa	*Clitoria ternatea*	Butterfly Pea, Winged-leaved Clitoria, Mezereon	Ayurvedic
Vishnukraantaa	*Convolvulus pluricaulis*	Conch-flowered Bindweed, White-flowered Shankhpushpi	Ayurvedic
Vishnukraanti	*Convolvulus pluricaulis*	Conch-flowered Bindweed, White-flowered Shankhpushpi	Ayurvedic
Vishnukrandi	*Evolvulus alsinoides*	Blue-flowered Shankhpushpi	Siddha/Tamil
Vishvaa	*Zingiber officinale*	Ginger	Ayurvedic
Vishvaaushadha	*Zingiber officinale*	Ginger	Ayurvedic
Vishvabheshaja	*Zingiber officinale*	Ginger	Ayurvedic
Vishwaa	*Aconitum heterophyllum*	Atis Root, Aconite	Ayurvedic
Vishwambharaa	*Andrographis paniculata*	Creat	Ayurvedic
Visra	*Raphanus sativus*	Radish	Ayurvedic
Vitakhadir	*Acacia leucophloea*	White Babul	Ayurvedic
Vitakhadira	*Acacia farnesiana*	Cassie Flower, Sweet Acacia	Ayurvedic
Vittunu-kiraanthi	*Evolvulus alsinoides*	Blue-flowered Shankhpushpi	Siddha/Tamil
Vitunna	*Celosia argentea*	Wild Cook's Comb	Ayurvedic
Vitunnaka	*Coriandrum sativum*	Coriander	Ayurvedic
Vivir	*Salix alba*	White Willow, European Willow	Folk
Vrahitaphala	*Berberis aristata*	Indian Barberry	Ayurvedic
Vrantphala	*Juglans regia*	Walnut Tree	Ayurvedic
Vrddha	*Parmelia perlata*	Parmelia Lichen	Ayurvedic
Vriddha Tulasi	*Ocimum gratissimum*	Shrubby Basil	Ayurvedic
Vriddhadaaraka	*Argyreia speciosa*	Elephant Creeper	Ayurvedic
Vriddhadaaraka	*Ipomoea petaloidea*	False Jalap, Hawaii Morning Glory	Ayurvedic
Vriddhadaaru	*Argyreia speciosa*	Elephant Creeper	Ayurvedic

Table Contd.

Indian Name	Botanical Name	English Name	Medicinal System
Woundwort	*Stachys palustris*	Marsh Hedge-Nettle, Woundwort (purple-flowered), Allheal	Folk
Woundwort	*Stachys sylvatica*	Hedge Woundwort	Folk
Yaalki	*Memecylon edule*	Iron Wood	Folk
Yaanaichhuvadi	*Elephantopus scaber*	Prickly-leaved Elephant's Foot	Siddha/Tamil
Yaasa	*Alhagi pseudalhagi*	Camel Thorn, Persian Manna Plant	Ayurvedic
Yaasa-sharkaraa (Manna)	*Alhagi pseudalhagi*	Camel Thorn, Persian Manna Plant	Ayurvedic
Yaasmin	*Jasminum officinale*	Spanish Jasmine	Unani
Yaava-naala	*Sorghum vulgare*	Sorghum, Broomcorn	Ayurvedic
Yabaruj	*Atropa acuminata*	Indian Belladonna, Indian Atropa	Unani
Yagnika	*Imperata cylindrica*	Thatch Grass	Ayurvedic
Yagyaanga	*Ficus racemosa*	Cluster Fig, Country Fig	Ayurvedic
Yagyabhuushana	*Desmostachya bipinnata*	Sacrificial Grass	Ayurvedic
Yagyabhuushana	*Imperata cylindrica*	Thatch Grass	Ayurvedic
Yajnyavrksha	*Flacourtia indica*	Ramontchi, Madagascar Plum, Mauritius Plum, Governor's Plum	Ayurvedic
Yamaani	*Trachyspermum ammi*	Ammi, Lovage, Carum, Ajowan	Ayurvedic
Yamaanikaa	*Trachyspermum ammi*	Ammi, Lovage, Carum, Ajowan	Ayurvedic
Yashti	*Glycyrrhiza glabra*	Licorice, Liquorice	Ayurvedic
Yashtika	*Glycyrrhiza glabra*	Licorice, Liquorice	Ayurvedic
Yashtimadhu	*Glycyrrhiza glabra*	Licorice, Liquorice	Ayurvedic
Yashtimadhuka	*Glycyrrhiza glabra*	Licorice, Liquorice	Ayurvedic
Yashtipushpa	*Putranjiva roxburghii*	Child-life Tree, Indian Amulet Plant, Spurious Wild Olive	Ayurvedic
Yashtyaahva	*Glycyrrhiza glabra*	Licorice, Liquorice	Ayurvedic
Yastikaahva	*Glycyrrhiza glabra*	Licorice, Liquorice	Ayurvedic
Yathu	*Fritillaria cirrhosa*	Himalayan Fritillaria Bulb	Folk
Yava	*Hordeum vulgare*	Barley	Ayurvedic

Table Contd.

Indian Name	Botanical Name	English Name	Medicinal System
Yavaani	*Hyoscyamus niger*	Indian Henbane, Black Henbane	Ayurvedic
Yavaani	*Trachyspermum ammi*	Ammi, Lovage, Carum, Ajowan	Ayurvedic
Yavaanikaa	*Trachyspermum ammi*	Ammi, Lovage, Carum, Ajowan	Ayurvedic
Yavaasa	*Alhagi pseudalhagi*	Camel Thorn, Persian Manna Plant	Ayurvedic
Yavaasaka	*Alhagi pseudalhagi*	Camel Thorn, Persian Manna Plant	Ayurvedic
Yavam	*Hordeum vulgare*	Barley	Folk/Tamil
Yavandeshaja	*Styrax officinale*	The True Storax Tree	Ayurvedic
Yavaneshta	*Allium sativum*	Garlic	Ayurvedic
Yavatiktaa	*Erythraea roxburghii*	Pseudo-Chiretta	Ayurvedic
Yavikaa	*Avena sativa*	Oat, Common Oat	Ayurvedic
Yavphala	*Bambusa bambos*	Spiny or Thorny Bamboo	Ayurvedic
Yavtikta	*Andrographis paniculata*	Creat	Ayurvedic
Yelandai	*Ziziphus jujuba*	Indian Jujube, Common Jujube	Siddha/Tamil
Yelikkaad-hukeerai	*Ipomoea reniformis*	Mouse-ear Shrub	Siddha/Tamil
Yesti	*Reissantia grahamii*	Pristimera Root	Folk
Yettikkottai	*Strychnos nux-vomica*	Nux Vomica	Siddha/Tamil
Yojanavalli	*Rubia cordifolia*	Indian Madder, Bengal Madder	Ayurvedic
Yonipushpaa	*Clitoria ternatea*	Butterfly Pea, Winged-leaved Clitoria, Mezereon	Ayurvedic
Yoshitapriyaa	*Curcuma longa*	Turmeric	Ayurvedic
Ysjudemaram	*Graptophyllum picum*	Caricature Plant, Jamaican Cotton	Folk/Tamil
Yucca	*Yucca filamentosa*	Adam's Needle, Golden Sword	Folk
Yugmakantaka	*Acacia arabica*	Babul, Black Babul, Indian Gum Arabic Tree	Ayurvedic
Yuktaa	*Pluchea lanceolata*	Rasana Shrub	Ayurvedic
Yuktrasaa	*Pluchea lanceolata*	Rasana Shrub	Ayurvedic

Table Contd.

Indian Name	Botanical Name	English Name	Medicinal System
Yuuthi	*Jasminum auriculatum*	Cultivated Jasmine	Ayurvedic
Yuuthikaa	*Jasminum auriculatum*	Cultivated Jasmine	Ayurvedic
Yuuthikaparni	*Rhinacanthus nasuta*	Snake Jasmine	Ayurvedic
Yuuthiparni	*Rhinacanthus nasuta*	Snake Jasmine	Ayurvedic
Zaafraan	*Crocus sativus*	Saffron. Crocus	Unani
Zabeeb	*Vitis vinifera*	Wine Grape, European Grape	Unani
Zahari Sontakkaa	*Allemanda cathartica*	Golden Trumpet	Folk
Zaitoon	*Olea europaea*	Olive	Unani
Zakhm-e-Hayaat	*Bryophyllum pinnatum*	Air Plant, Mexican Love Plant	Unani
Zakhm-e-Hayaat	*Kalanchoe integra*	Never Die	Unani
Zakhm-e-Hayaat	*Kalanchoe laciniata*	Christmastree Plant	Unani
Zakhm-e-Hayaat	*Kalanchoe pinnata*	Christmastree Plant	Unani
Zalil	*Delphinium zalil*	Zalil Larkspur	Unani
Zamikand	*Amorphophallus campanulatus*	Elephant's Foot Yam	Unani
Zanjabeel (Dried rhizome)	*Zingiber officinale*	Ginger	Unani
Zanjabeel-e-Ratab (Fresh rhizome)	*Zingiber officinale*	Ginger	Unani
Zanjabeel-e-yaabis	*Zingiber officinale*	Ginger	Unani
Zaraavand-Hindi	*Aristolochia indica*	Indian Birthwort	Unani
Zaraawand Taweel	*Aristolochia longa*	European Birthwort	Unani
Zarambaad	*Curcuma caesia*	Black Zedorary	Unani
Zarambaad	*Curcuma zedoaria*	Zedoary, Zerumbet	Unani
Zarambaad	*Zingiber zerumbet*	Zerumbet Ginger	Unani
Zard Chob	*Curcuma longa*	Turmeric	Unani
Zard-e-Vard (Stamens)	*Rosa damascena*	Damask Rose	Unani
Zarir	*Delphinium zalil*	Zalil Larkspur	Unani
Zarishk (Fruit)	*Berberis aristata*	Indian Barberry	Unani
Zarnab	*Flacourtia jangomas*	Puneala Plum	Unani
Zarnab	*Taxus baccata*	European Yew	Unani
Zeeraa Siyaah	*Carum carvi*	Caraway	Unani

Table Contd.

Indian Name	Botanical Name	English Name	Medicinal System
Zergul	*Calendula officinalis*	Pot-Marigold, Marigold, Calendula	Unani
Zerwati	*Reissantia grahamii*	Pristimera Root	Folk
Zirgulaki	*Hypecoum leptocarpum*	Waziri Opium Herb	Folk
Zurraa Makkaa	*Zea mays*	Maize, Corn, Indian Corn	Unani
Zuufaa	*Hyssopus officinalis*	Hyssop	Unani
Zuufaa Yaabis	*Hyssopus officinalis*	Hyssop	Unani

Part Three

APPENDICES

Facsimile of the Preface of "A Catalogue of Indian Synonyms of the medicinal plants, products, inorganic substances, & c., proposed to be included in the Pharmacopoeia of India".

PREFACE.

A few years since, I had an occasion to pay attention to the vernacular synonymes in some works on Materia Medica and Botany. While I was much impressed with the importance and usefulness of the subject, I found it blended with a great inaccuracy and confusion. I was about rectifying these defects in a work, when it was my privilege to be called upon officially to contribute to the Pharmacopœia of India, *vide* Circular Memorandum No. 2824, dated 7th August 1865, from the Secretary to the Principal Inspector General of the Medical Department, which was accompanied with the 'Proceedings of the Madras Government, Financial Department, 28th July 1865,' and Dr. E. J. Waring's lists of medicinal plants, &c.

On the receipt of these documents, I immediately thought of the subject I was previously meditating upon, and with a wish to see the Pharmacopœia as free as possible from the defects just alluded to, I prepared a Table of Vernacular Synonymes of the medicinal plants, drugs, &c., proposed to be included in that work. The Table was composed of 12 languages, besides the Latin and English; viz., Arabic, Persian, Hindustani, Dukhni, Tamil, Telugu, Malyalim, Canarese, Bengali, Mahratti, Guzratti, and Burmese, and the synonymes in all these languages were expressed in their native characters as well as in English.

In preparing this Table, although I consulted a few works, yet, for the reason already mentioned, I thought it advisable to depend chiefly upon the names found out by myself. With this view, I had personally examined with several native practitioners, druggists, &c., all the plants known as medicinal in many localities of Madras, eluding the Agri-horticultural Society's and other gardens, and ascertained their names without any reference to books. The drugs in the bazaar, together with several other plants which were sent for from distant places, were next examined, and their names found out in the same manner.

The Table was then forwarded, as a part of my contribution, to the Committee of the Pharmacopœia of India, on the 7th February 1866, and returned to me on the 9th July of the same year, with a copy of the following Despatches and Orders :—

'*Proceedings of the Madras Government, Financial Department, 6th July* 1866.

No. 7. Read the following Despatch from the Right Honorable the Secretary of State for India, to His Excellency the Right Honorable the Governor in Council, Fort Saint George ; dated India Office, London, 31st May 1866, No. 43.

Letters from Dr. Waring, dated the 26th April and 15th May 1866, with enclosures in originals.
Letter to Dr. Waring, dated the 4th May 1866.

I forward herewith copies of correspondence with Surgeon E. J. Waring, M.D., with enclosures in original, and I have to request that the necessary measures may be taken by you for meeting, if practicable, the wishes of the Pharmacopœia of India Committee, in regard to the printing at Madras of Mr. Moodeen Sheriff's Table of Medicinal Plants, under that Officer's supervision.

From Surgeon E. J. Waring, M.D., Editor of the Pharmacopœia of India, to the Under Secretary of State for India, &c., &c., &c. ; dated 3A, Talbot Road, Bayswater, 26th April 1866.

By desire of the "Pharmacopœia of India" Committee, I have the honor herewith to transmit a Table compiled by Native Surgeon Moodeen Sheriff of Triplicane Dispensary, Madras, containing the names of upwards of four hundred Medicinal plants of India, in twelve Eastern languages, in Vernacular and English characters

Excerpt from Foreword:Pharmacopoeia of India (1868).djvu/14 from Wikisource (digitalized by Microsoft).

value of knowledge thus gained, it is impossible to place too high an estimate, familiarizing, as it will, the embryo practitioner with remedies which are at hand in the remotest corners of our Indian empire, rendering him in a great measure independent of costly imported articles, and effecting a considerable annual saving to the State.

Amongst the returns received from India was one from Native Surgeon Moodeen Sheriff, of Madras, containing the vernacular names of indigenous plants and drugs, in twelve of the native languages of India, a work of immense labour, reflecting the greatest credit on the intelligence and industry of the compiler. This Catalogue, having been submitted to eminent Oriental scholars at home, and pronounced generally correct, it was resolved to append to the Pharmacopœia. It was accordingly forwarded to Madras, for the purpose of being printed under Mr. Moodeen Sheriff's superintendence. Unexpected circumstances, however, having arisen there to delay its publication, it has been deemed advisable, rather than to defer the publication of this work, to issue the Catalogue in a separate or supplementary volume.

In connexion with this branch of the subject, much valuable assistance has been rendered by Col. W. H. Sykes, M.P., Sir Walter Elliot, K.S.I., Dr. Fitzedward Hall, Mr. C. P. Brown, and Mr. G. H. K. Thwaites, of Ceylon.

The processes employed in the manufacture of chemical preparations have generally been omitted. To have inserted them would have tended materially to increase the size of the volume without any corresponding advantage, seeing that such articles could only be prepared at the Government Medical Stores, and perhaps in the laboratories of a few of the larger private firms in the Presidency towns, the needful appliances not existing elsewhere; and at these establishments the British Pharmacopœia will of course be available, and the directions contained in that work should always be followed, excepting in those cases

- Central Council for Research in Unani Medicine (CCRUM), published literature.
- *Unani Dravyagunaadarsh* (Hindi) by Daljit Singh, Ayurvedic and Tibbi Academy, Uttar Pradesh, Lucknow, 1974.

Siddha/Tamil synonyms have been selected from the following sources:

- *A Catalogue of Indian Synonyms of the Medicinal Plants of India* by Moodeen Sheriff, 1869 (synonyms in Latin, English and 12 reginal languages).
- *Formulary of Siddha Medicine*, Indian Medical Practitioners' Cooperative Pharmacy and Store Ltd. (IMPCOPS), Chennai.
- *The Wealth of India* (Vol. II-XI), Revised Edns (1-3), CSIR (NISCAIR).
- *Glossary of Indian Medicinal Plants* by R.N. Chopra et al., CSIR (NISCAIR).
- *Ayurvedic Drugs and their Plant Sources,* V.V. Sivarajan, Indira Balachandran, Oxford and IBH, New Delhi, 1994.
- *Dictionary of Indian Medicinal Plants,* by Akhtar Husain et al., Central Institute of Medicinal and Aromatic Plants, Lucknow, 1992.

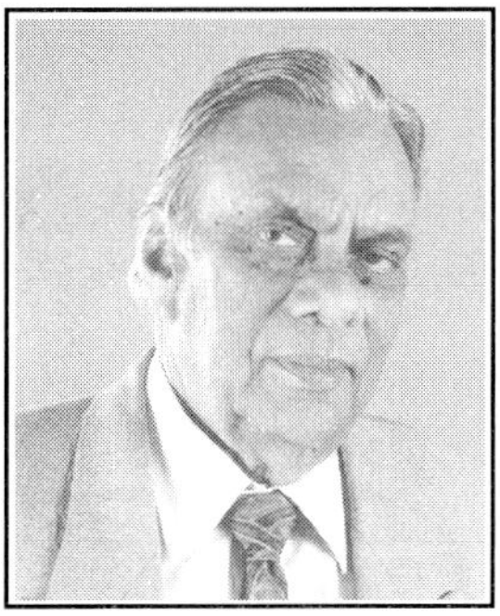

About the Author

C.P. KHARE

C.P. Khare was born on December 18, 1932, and has been a herbalist for more than sixty years.

He was born into a family of herbal physicians, studied the original Ayurvedic texts in Sanskrit and Unani in Urdu and acquired first-hand knowledge of the cultivation, processing and usage of herbs.

In 1952, he took up journalism. Since then he has edited and contributed many features based on his clinical experience to various journals. He has been a Director and Chairman of India's largest magazine publishing group for the last forty years and herbal drug research consultant to a major herbal pharmaceutical company for the last twenty-two years.

As founder President and Director of the Society for New Age Herbals, which started functioning as a centre in 1990 in Delhi, he sought the cooperation and participation of physicians of modern as well as traditional medicines, pharmacologists and scientists to modify, restructure and reassess the age-old herbal formulations in the context of ongoing experimental and clinical research, and to promote evidence-based herbal medicine in India.

His reference works are the outcome of in-depth study and analysis of classical as well as modern herbal treatises. They have secured a prominent place in more than 500 prestigious universities, teaching institutions and libraries in the USA, Canada, Holland, Spain, Australia, New Zealand, Hong Kong, China and Singapore.

Dictionary of Synonyms: Indian Medicinal Plants is his latest reference work.

OTHER WORKS BY C.P. KHARE

- *Indian Herbal Medicine: Application of Research Findings* (Third edition, Vishv Books, New Delhi, 2010)
- *Indian Herbal Remedies/Encyclopedia of Indian Medicinal Plants* (Two edns., Springer, Germany, 2004)
- *Indian Medicinal Plants: An Illustrated Dictionary* (Springer, USA, 2007)
- *The Modern Ayurveda: Milestones Beyond the Classical Age* (Editor-in-Chief) (CRC, Boca Raton, USA, 2012)

Index

Botanical Synonyms

Index

Part One
Botanical Names